X-Linked Mental Retardation

OXFORD MONOGRAPHS ON MEDICAL GENETICS

1. R. B. McConnell: *The genetics of gastrointestinal disorders*
2. A. C. Kopé: *The distribution of the blood groups in the United Kingdom*
3. E. Slater and V. A. Cowie: *The genetics of locomotor disorders*
4. C. O. Carter and T. J. Fairbank: *The genetics of locomotor disorders*
5. A. E. Mourant, A. C. Kopé, and K. Domaniewska-Sobezak: *The distribution of the human blood groups and other polymorphisms*
6. A. E. Mourant, A. C. Kopé and K. Domaniewska-Sobezak: *Blood groups and diseases*
7. A. G. Steinbert and C. E. Cook: *The distribution of the human immunoglobulin allotypes*
8. D. Tills, A. C. Kopé and R. E. Tills: *The distribution of the human blood groups and other polymorphisms: Supplement I*
10. D. Z. Loesch: *Quantitative dermatoglyphics: classification, genetics, and pathology*
11. D. J. Bond and A. C. Chandley: *Aneuploidy*
12. P. F. Benson and A. H. Fensom: *Genetic biochemical disorders*
13. G. R. Sutherland and F. Hecht: *Fragile sites on human chromosomes*
14. M. d'A Crawfurd: *The genetics of renal tract disorders*
16. C. R. Scriver and B. Childs: *Garrod's inborn factors in disease*
18. M. Baraitser: *The genetics of neurological disorders*
19. R. J. Gorlin, M. M. Cohen, Jr., and L. S. Levin: *Syndromes of the head and neck, third edition*
20. R. A. King, J. I. Rotter, and A. G. Motulsky: *The genetics basis of common diseases*
21. D. Warburton, J. Byrne, and N. Canki: *Chromosome anomalies and prenatal development: an atlas*
22. J. J. Nora, K. Berg, and A. H. Nora: *Cardiovascular diseases: gneetics, epidemiology, and prevention*
24. A. E. H. Emery: *Duchenne muscular dystrophy, second edition*
25. E. G. D. Tuddenham and D. N. Cooper: *The molecular genetics of haemostasis and its inherited disorders*
26. A. Boué: *Fetal medicine*
27. R. E. Stevenson, J. G. Hall, and R. M. Goodman: *Human malformations*
28. R. J. Gorlin, H. V. Toriello, and M. M. Cohen, Jr.: *Hereditary hearing loss and its syndromes*
29. R. J. M. Gardner and G. R. Sutherland: *Chromosome abnormalities and genetic counseling, second edition*
30. A. S. Teebi and T. I. Farag: *Genetic disorders among Arab populations*
31. M. M. Cohen, Jr.: *The child with multiple birth defects*
32. W. W. Weber: *Pharmacogenetics*
33. V. P. Sybert: *Genetic skin disorders*
34. M. Baraitser: *Genetics of neurological disorders, third edition*
35. H. Ostrer: *Non-mendelian genetics in humans*
36. E. Traboulsi: *Genetic diseases of the eye*
37. G. L. Semenza: *Transcription factors and human disease*
38. L. Pinsky, R. P. Erickson, and R. N. Schimke: *Genetic disorders of human sexual development*
39. R. E. Stevenson, C. E. Schwartz, and R. J. Schroer: *X-linked mental retardation*

OXFORD MONOGRAPHS ON MEDICAL GENETICS NO. 39

X-Linked Mental Retardation

Roger E. Stevenson
Charles E. Schwartz
Richard J. Schroer

New York Oxford
OXFORD UNIVERSITY PRESS
2000

Oxford University Press

Oxford New York
Athens Auckland Bangkok Bogotá Buenos Aires Calcutta
Cape Town Chennai Dar es Salaam Delhi Florence Hong Kong Istanbul
Karachi Kuala Lumpur Madrid Melbourne Mexico City Mumbai
Nairobi Paris São Paulo Singapore Taipei Tokyo Toronto Warsaw
and associated companies in
Berlin Ibadan

Published by Oxford University Press, Inc.,
198 Madison Avenue, New York, New York, 10016
http://www.oup-usa.org

Library of Congress Cataloging-in-Publication Data
Stevenson, Roger E., 1940–
X-linked mental retardation /
Roger E. Stevenson, Charles E. Schwartz, Richard J. Schroer.
p. cm. Includes bibliographical references and index.
ISBN 0-19-512981-4
1. X-linked mental retardation.
I. Schwartz, Charles E.
II. Schroer, Richard J.
III. Title.
RC574.S77 2000 616.85'88042—dc21 99-14645

9 8 7 6 5 4 3 2 1

Printed in the United States of America
on acid-free paper

X-Linked Mental Retardation is
dedicated to all persons with
this disability, to their families,
to the physicians who
provide medical care, and
to the scientists who
seek to understand the
underlying biology.

Preface

In the earliest days of human development, the brain dominates the embryological landscape. As other organ systems develop and the fetus grows, the brain becomes less imposing anatomically, but progressively more formidable functionally. Soon after postnatal life begins, it engages the environment and issues responses that bind the child to parents and to others. It permits the acquisition of skills that serve as benchmarks of developmental progress. Ultimately, the brain defines the essence of human existence through the control of thought processes and neurological function.

A certain fragility of the developing brain is suggested by the high prevalence in the population of significant impairments of cognitive and adaptive performance. Such impairments may be associated with faulty formation or function of the brain; these occur in one to three percent of the population and are grouped under the general term mental retardation. The high frequency with which developmental failure of the brain occurs is found in no other organ system, which indicates that the developing brain may be easily damaged or that even minor damage may be readily expressed. Alternatively, other organ systems may have structural or functional redundancy that gives them greater capacity in reserve.

Mental retardation, a significant impairment of cognitive and adaptive functions, is a human condition with numerous dimensions. For the affected individual, it represents a cloak that limits capacity to learn, ability for self-expression, freedom of movement, and achievement of goals. For society, it represents a disability characterized by reduced productivity, some measure of dependency, and vulnerability to discrimination and exploitation. For public health, it is a common abnormality, one that is distributed throughout all strata of the population and that imposes a costly and lifelong burden. For medicine, mental retardation represents an aberration in the formation and/or function of the central nervous system that demands evaluation and explanation.

The partition of mental retardation by cause is informative on several counts. Scientifically, it confirms that the developing brain is susceptible to a wide variety of faulty genetic instructions, environmental influences, or combinations of these two forces. Only with recognition of the causes can specific strategies for prevention be devised. From a practical clinical standpoint, knowledge of causes gives the clinician a basis from which to judiciously select diagnostic tests, predict natural history, calculate recurrence risks, direct counseling, and make reasonable medical and educational plans.

A pervasive finding among persons with mental retardation has been the excess of males. In most populations, this excess is about 20%–40%. While greater mortality among females with mental retardation or hormonal contributions to the causation of mental retardation may be possible explanations for the sexual dichotomy, neither has been substantiated. Rather, the biological inequity between males and females conferred by the different number of sex chromosomes has been regarded as primarily responsible for the excess. Accepting a male excess of 30%, one would estimate that X-linked mental retardation (XLMR) is one of the most common causal categories of mental retardation, equaling that of chromosome aberrations. With our current ability to identify mental retardation due to X-linked genes in clinical populations, however, we can account for only a fraction of this number.

X-linked mental retardation has been divided into two broad categories, syndromic and nonsyndromic (or nonspecific). In syndromic XLMR, somatic, neurologic, behavioral, or metabolic abnormalities accompany the mental retardation and often constitute a recognizable pattern. In nonsyndromic XLMR, males have no somatic, neurologic, behavioral, or metabolic findings that distinguish them from nonaffected brothers or from other males with mental retardation.

A large number of families with syndromic and nonsyndromic forms of XLMR have been reported, mainly during the past 50 years. Although there have been recent advances in confirming diagnoses by biochemical or molecular testing, the identification of most XLMR conditions is based on family history and phenotype. This book is intended to provide the clinician, scientist, and student with a background in biology of the X chromosome (Chapter 1), a summary of the emergence of the concept of XLMR (Chapter 2), and a resource to differentiate the various types of XLMR on the basis of craniofacial or other somatic findings, neurologic signs or symptoms, and behavioral manifestations (Chapters 3–5). A minimum of ten X-linked genes is required to account for the numerous families that have been identified with nonsyndromic XLMR. This important category of XLMR is the subject of Chapter 3. There are separate genes for most if not all of the 130 syndromic forms of XLMR. Somatic manifestations, growth and development, cognitive and adaptive function, neurological and neuroanatomical findings, and, if present, metabolic aberrations for each of these entities are described in atlas form in Chapter 5.

Delineation of the various forms of XLMR has been possible only through the contributions of affected families and their physicians. To them, we are indebted and to them we dedicate this monograph. Researchers worldwide have followed up the clinical observations with systematic biological investigations, including a wide variety of imaging, histologic, molecular, and cytogenetic studies, which have permitted description of the phenotype and chromosomal localization of most X-linked mental retardation syndromes. Isolation of the responsible genes has been possible in a lesser percentage of cases.

We thank our clinical and research colleagues who have taught us about X-linked mental retardation, in particular, Herbert Lubs (University of Miami),

Fernando Arena (University of Miami), Hunt Willard (Case Western Reserve University), Jean-Louis Mandel (Institut de Chimie Biologique, Strasbourg), Grant Sutherland (Women's and Children's Hospital, Adelaide), and Michel Fontés (INSERM, Marseille). Our clinical colleagues at the Greenwood Genetic Center, Robert Saul, Curtis Rogers, Laurie Seaver, Katie Clarkson, Richard Simensen, William Allen, Steven Skinner, and Joseph Geer, and our laboratory team, Harold Taylor, Katy Phelan, Bernhard Häne, Jack Tarleton, Anand Srivastava, Ron Michaelis, John Longshore, Fatima Abidi, Michael Friez, Khalid Alaoui, Melanie May, Andy Hartung, Retecher Nelson, Lisbeth Ouzts, Darci Horne, and Mike Chandler, have made important contributions to *X-Linked Mental Retardation*. They have made suggestions on content, reviewed drafts of the manuscript, and taken on additional responsibilities to give us time to devote to this effort.

Numerous authors and publishers have provided figures to illustrate XLMR syndromes. Individual credits are given in the figure legends. Literature searches, citation verification, and other library resources have been provided by Ellen Dewkett. Karen Buchanan has organized the materials used to produce this monograph and has provided invaluable assistance and advice.

The production of *X-Linked Mental Retardation* gave us the opportunity to work again with Jeffrey House, Nancy Wolitzer, and Susan Hannan at Oxford University Press. Their valuable suggestions from concept through production have enabled us to work with some degree of efficiency and equanimity.

Greenwood, S.C. R.E.S.
May 1999 C.E.S.
R.J.S.

Contents

X-Linked Mental Retardation

1

The X Chromosome

The sex chromosomes in humans stand alone in having letter designations rather than Arabic numerals. The tradition arose from the study of male reproductive cells in insects and was later adapted for humans. Henking (1891) assigned the letter X to a "chromatin-element" of unknown significance which he observed to be passed undivided to one or the other pole during the anaphase of spermatocytes from *Pyrrhocoris apterus*.[1] Subsequent studies, also on insects, established that the chromatin-element was a chromosome.[2,3] McClung (1902) first suggested that the X chromosome was important in sex determination.[4] Although other terms (monosome, accessory chromosome, heterosome, chromatin nucleolus, idiochromosome) were utilized by various investigators, the term *X chromosome* gained favored status early in this century.[5]

Historical Notes

Throughout the first half of this century, the number of chromosomes in humans was uncertain. The exact nature of sex chromosome constitution was equally clouded. Determination of the number of human chromosomes was based initially on naturally occurring mitosis in tissue sections. Hansemann analyzed three such cells in 1891, finding in them 18, 24, and "more than 40" chromosomes.[6] Other cytologists reported a variety of numbers: Bardeleben (1898) counted 16 chromosomes; Guyer (1910) counted 22; Flemming (1897), Duesberg (1906), and Branca (1910) counted 24; Moore and Arnold (1906) counted 32; and Wilcox (1900) counted 36.[7–13] These inconsistencies were due in greatest measure to inadequate chromosome separation and variable quality of tissue sections in terms of preservation, thickness, and staining. These impediments notwithstanding, Winiwarter (1912) concluded that the chromosome number differed in the two sexes, females having a 48 count with two X chromosomes and males having a 47 count with one X chromosome.[14] Painter (1921) assigned the term *Y chromosome* to the small chromosome which was paired with the X chromosome in human spermatocytes and which segregated from the X chromosome in meiosis I.[15] Although he found "in the clearest equatorial plates so far studied only 46 chromosomes," he eventually concurred with Winiwarter that 48 was the correct chromosome number in humans.

For the ensuing three decades, 48 was generally accepted as the correct chromosome number in humans.[16–19] The sex chromosome constitution remained unsettled, however, primarily due to the insistence by Winiwarter and others that the Y chromosome did not exist in humans.[20,21] Others accepted the existence of the Y chromosome but questioned its function. Roberts (1940) stated that the Y chromosome had nothing to do directly with sex determination.[22] That task was assigned in females to sex-containing genes on the autosomes and the two X chromosomes, and in males to sex-controlling genes on the autosomes balanced against the sex-controlling genes on a single X chromosome.

Barr and Bertram (1949) demonstrated sexual dimorphism in interphase nuclei of mammals, females having a dense staining body adjacent to the nuclear membrane and males lacking this nuclear characteristic.[23] A second sexual dimorphism—a drumstick-like appendage of the nucleus in polymorphonuclear leucocytes of females—was shown by Davidson and Robertson Smith in 1954.[24] Although the correct interpretation of Barr bodies and Davidson drumsticks would not be made until later (see below), the phenomena were considered related to the sex chromosomes and, for a time, were utilized as an indirect method with which to predict the sex chromosome constitution, particularly in humans with abnormalities of sexual development.[25–27]

It was thus of some surprise to the scientific community in 1956 when Tjio and Levan reported finding 46 chromosomes in fibroblasts cultured from fetal lung (Fig. 1–1).[28] No attempt was made in this initial report to distinguish the sex chromosomes. The chromosome number was quickly confirmed in human testicular tissue by Ford and Hamerton and establishment of the sex chromosome constitution as XX in females and XY in males followed.[29–31] Within a few years, refinements in tissue culture and metaphase preparations permitted chromosome analysis to become commonplace in laboratories throughout the world. Numerical chromosome aberrations were first reported in 1959, opening an era when an answer to nearly all human maladies was sought in the chromosomes (Table 1–1).[32,33] Cancer, malformations, mental retardation, abortion, sexual aberrations, and other disorders were investigated.

A rich yield rewarded investigators who sought the explanation of spontaneous abortion in chromosome analysis. In 1961, Penrose and Delhanty demonstrated triploidy in a macerated fetus. In the reports that followed, chromosome aberrations were found in approximately one-half of early spontaneous abortions.[34] The 45,X karyotype was found most frequently, but tetraploidy, triploidy, and numerous trisomies not seen in liveborn infants constituted a major portion of chromosomally abnormal abortuses (Table 1–2).[35–38]

Aneuploidies involving the X chromosome were prominent among the aberrations found in abortion material and in children with growth disorders and disabilities (Table 1–2). The vast majority, perhaps 95%, of conceptions with monosomy X resulted in abortions. With this exception, the X chromosome

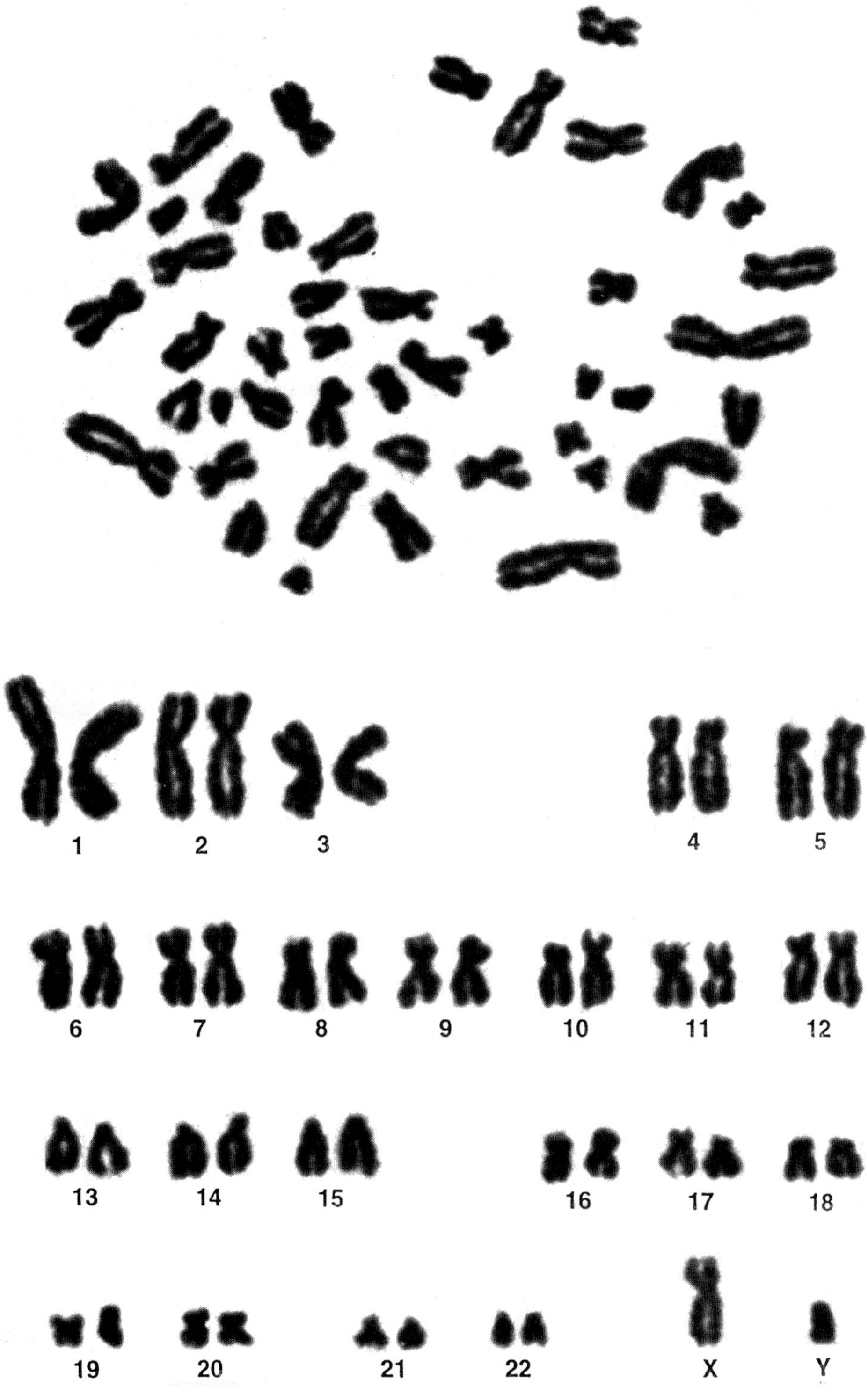

Figure 1–1. Metaphase spread (left) from fibroblasts cultured from fetal lung which established 46 as the chromosome number in humans.[28] The sex chromosome constitution was not reported. A karyotype (right) prepared from this metaphase spread indicates that the sex chromosome constitution was likely 46,XY (courtesy of Dr. M.C. Phelan and Beth Christianson).

TABLE 1–1. Sequence of Discovery of Chromosome Aberrations

1959	Trisomy 21; 45,X; 47,XXY; 47,XXX
1960	Trisomy 18; trisomy 13; 48,XXXY; 48,XXYY; 49,XXXXY
1961	47,XYY; 48,XXXX
1963	del 5p; del 18p; 49,XXXXX
1964	del 18q
1965	del 4p
1969	Fragile X
1971	Mosaic trisomy 8
1973	Partial trisomy 9

aneuploidies were quite compatible with life, in general causing less severe somatic manifestations and intellectual impairments than the autosomal aneuploidies.

Prenatal diagnosis of chromosome aberrations became possible in 1966, when Steele and Breg combined the technique of amniocentesis with culture of amniotic fluid cells.[39] The reliability and safety of the combined procedures contributed to rapid acceptance of the techniques for testing pregnancies determined to be at increased risk of chromosome aberrations because of advanced maternal age,

TABLE 1–2. Prevalence of Chromosomal Aberrations Among Spontaneous Abortions[34–38]

Type Aberration	*Percent*
All Chromosome Aberrations	40
Trisomies	20
T-16	8
T-13, 15, 21, 22	2*
T-2, 7, 8, 14, 18	1*
T-4, 9, 10, 20	0.5*
T-3, 5, 6, 12, 17	0.1*
T-1, 11, 19	<0.1*
Sex chromosome	<0.5*
Monosomy X	8
Autosomal Monosomy	<0.1
Polyploidies	9
Triploidy	7
Tetraploidy	2
Other Rearrangements	3
Mosaicism	2
Unbalanced rearrangement	1
Balanced rearrangement	<0.5

*Approximate rate for each of the trisomies named.

a prior pregnancy with a chromosome aberration, or a balanced chromosome rearrangement in a parent.

Soon after technical improvements for making metaphase chromosome preparations were widely adopted, a group of pioneer cytogeneticists convened a meeting to head off a potential quagmire of confusing chromosome nomenclature. At the first conference in 1960 (Denver), the 14 cytogeneticists and three consultants proposed a standard system of nomenclature for human mitotic chromosomes.[40] They agreed to serially number the autosomes 1–22 in descending order of length and maintain the X and Y designations for the sex chromosomes. Autosomes were placed in seven groups: 1–3, 4–5, 6–12, 13–15, 16–18, 19–20, and 21–22. At the second conference (London) held 3 years later, the participants accepted an alternative designation for the chromosome groups by letters: A for chromosomes 1–3, B for 4–5, C for 6–12 plus X, D for 13–15, E for 16–18, F for 19–20, and G for 21–22 plus Y.[41] This convention acknowledged that most of the individual chromosomes could not be identified and was utilized for nearly a decade. Subsequent conferences have continued to deal with nomenclature, chromosome structure and identification, culture conditions, and staining.[42–46]

The first phase of exploiting cytogenetics to explain human disorders reached a plateau by the late 1960s. The introduction of banding techniques by Caspersson et al. in 1971, demonstration of fragile sites by Sutherland in 1977, and adoption of methods to analyze prophase and prometaphase chromosomes in the 1980s brought new life to cytogenetics.[48–50] A greater understanding of the chromosomal basis for malformations, mental retardation, cancer, and other human disorders accompanied these advances. Progress has continued through the merging of cytogenetic and molecular techniques by which fluorescent molecular probes are hybridized to metaphase or prometaphase chromosome preparations.[51–54] This fluorescent *in situ* hybridization (FISH) technique permits detection of deletions, duplications, and rearrangements which are beyond the resolution of light microscopy.

Anatomy of the X Chromosome

With the utilization of new staining methods of the early 1970s, it became possible to identify each chromosome on the basis of distinctive banding patterns and to separate the sex chromosomes from the autosomes.[43–48] The X chromosome is a medium-sized chromosome characterized by a submetacentric centromere. It can be distinctly banded using Giemsa, quinacrine, and 5-bromodeoxyuridine (BrdU)-acridine orange, and thereby easily distinguished from chromosomes 6 and 7, those of nearest size and centromere locations. Likewise the Y can be consistently distinguished from chromosomes 21 and 22.

The X chromosome accounts for 5.1%–5.8% of the combined length of the autosomes or 4.9%–5.5% of the total haploid length (chromosomes 1–22 plus X). Assuming a total of 80,000 human genes, even distribution of genes on the autosomes and the X chromosome, and a negligible number of genes on the Y chromosome, the X chromosome may contain 3900–4400 genes.

While a full isochore map of the X chromosome has not been constructed, several generalizations may be made. Giemsa light bands, composed predominantly of guanine-rich and cytosine-rich H1, H2 and H3 isochores, make up 51% of the X chromosome.[55] The H1, H2, and H3 isochores constitute about 35% of the human genome. Genes in these isochores are relatively small and densely packed, have short introns, and tend to code for proteins having less than 500 amino acids. In contrast, Geimsa dark bands are composed of adenine-rich and thymidine-rich isochores (L1 and L3 classes), make up 49% of the X chromosome and about 65% of the genome, and have a low density of genes. Genes in the AT-rich regions tend to be large with long introns.

With clarification of the sex chromosome constitution in 1956, it became possible to assign a number of genes to the X chromosome.[56] These early assignments were based on pedigree characteristics which permitted phenotypes caused by genes on the X chromosome to be distinguished from those caused by autosomal genes. The differences are determined primarily by the presence of a single X chromosome in males and two X chromosomes in females and by the obligatory transfer of the male's single X chromosome to all daughters but not to sons. Characteristics of X-linked recessive phenotypes include the following:

1. Only males are affected.
2. Sons of carrier females have a 50% risk of being affected.
3. Daughters of carrier females have a 50% risk of being carriers.
4. Male to male transmission does not occur.
5. All daughters of affected males will be carriers.
6. Unaffected males cannot transmit the phenotype.

Characteristics common in X-linked dominant phenotypes include the following:

1. Males and females are affected in a 1:2 ratio.
2. Male to male transmission does not occur.
3. Affected males transmit the phenotype to all of their daughters.
4. Offspring of affected females have a 50% risk of being affected whether male or female.
5. Only one parent is usually affected.
6. Heterozygous females are affected less severely than are hemizygous males.

Regional Mapping of X-Linked Genes

A number of genes were known to be located on the X chromosome prior to the first autosomal gene assignment, that of the Duffy blood group to chromosome 1, in 1968. The early X chromosome linkages were based on the pedigree considerations noted above, which precluded the likelihood that the genes could be autosomal. Among these were the genes for color blindness, hemophilia, and Duchenne muscular dystrophy, conditions known for the prior century to be expressed exclusively or nearly so in males. In his first catalogue of gene loci on the X chromosome, published in 1964, McKusick accepted 59 entities with strong pedigree evidence for X-linkage and 21 entities with less evidence for X-linkage (Table 1–3).[56] He excluded eight entities which had previously been considered to show X-linkage.

Regional mapping of several genes known to be X-linked became possible in the 1960s and 1970s utilizing balanced X:autosome translocations and other X chromosome rearrangements. Lubs's identification of a family in which a constriction in the distal q arm of the X chromosome segregated with mental retardation in males constituted, in fact, the first more or less precise mapping of an X-linked gene.[57] He stated in his 1969 report that "either the secondary constriction itself or a closely linked recessive gene may account for the pattern of X-linked inheritance." As a generalization, the X chromosome involved in an X:autosome translocation remains active; hence if an X-linked gene is disrupted by the rearrangement, a phenotype may result. Further, since these translocations have been found primarily in females, the appearance of an X-linked phenotype not usually expressed in a female provides a clue to the existence of an X chromosome rearrangement. The initial localizations provided a skeleton upon which other entities could be mapped through linkage analysis (Table 1–4).[58–71]

Development of restriction fragment length polymorphisms (RFLPs) and microsatellite polymorphisms provided the tools necessary to escalate the pace of mapping genes on the X chromosome.[72–75] The first gene localization on the X chromosome accomplished through these molecular means was hypoxanthine guanine phosphoribosyl transferase in 1983.[76] A remarkable array of X-linked genes, small and large, of great and negligible clinical importance, has been added to the chromosome's regional anatomy in the years since.[77] Of the 59 entities accepted as X-linked in McKusick's initial catalogue (1964), 41 have been mapped and 29 have been cloned.[56,77]

The rapid assignment of X-linked genes has been accompanied by a less spectacular pace of gene isolation and mutation analysis.[77] Notable in the chronology of isolation of X-linked genes are those encoding clotting factor IX (1982), hypoxanthine guanine phosphoribosyl transferase (1983), clotting factor VIII (1985), glucose-6-phosphate dehydrogenase (1986), dystrophin (1987), fragile site mental retardation 1 protein (1991), L1 cell adhesion molecule (1992), and the SHOX homeobox protein (1998).[78–85] Mutational analyses are in common clinical usage for the confirmation of Duchenne/Becker muscular dystrophy, fragile X syndrome, and hemophilia A and B due to factor VIII and factor IX deficiency, respectively.

Inactivation

In at least four circumstances, regions of chromosomes can become altered, rendering the involved region functionally inert. The phenomenon is called *inacti-*

vation, involves no change in the DNA code, and is reversed in oogonia prior to meiosis. Inactivation involving most of the X chromosome was first proposed in 1961 by Lyon and is now a well-accepted phenomenon.[86] One X chromosome in normal females and all but one X chromosome in individuals with multiple X chromosomes become inactivated during the 1000–2000 cell stage of embryogenesis. Inactivation appears random; that is, either the maternal or the paternal chromosome can be inactivated, but once this is established it remains fixed for all descendants of the initially inactivated cell. With the exception of the pseudoautosomal regions at Xpter and Xqter and a segment of the proximal long arm (Xq) which contains the inactivation gene (XIST), most of the X chromosome participates in the inactivation (Fig. 1–2).[87–91] Because of this phenome-

Table 1–3. X-Linked Phenotypes Listed by McKusick in 1961[56]

A. Conditions for which X-Linkage Is Considered Proved or Very Likely	
1. Partial color blindness, deutan series	29. Congenital deafness
2. Partial color blindness, protan series	30. Progressive deafness
3. Total color blindness	31. Mental deficiency
4. Glucose-6-phosphate dehydrogenase	32. Börjeson syndrome
deficiency	33. Spinal ataxia
5. Xg blood group system	34. Cerebellar ataxia with extrapyramidal
6. Muscular dystrophy, Duchenne type	involvement
7. Muscular dystrophy, Becker type	35. Spastic paraplegia
8. Hemophilia A	36. Progressive bulbar paralysis
9. Hemophilia B	37. Charcot-Marie-Tooth peroneal muscular
10. Agammaglobulinemia	atrophy
11. Hunter syndrome	38. Diffuse cerebral sclerosis (Pelizaeus-
12. Late spondylo-epiphyseal dysplasia	Merzbacher)
13. Aldrich syndrome	39. Diffuse cerebral sclerosis (Scholz)
14. Hypophosphatemia	40. Hydrocephalus
15. Hypoparathyroidism	41. Parkinsonism
16. Nephrogenic diabetes insipidus	42. Ocular albinism
17. Neurohypophyseal diabetes insipidus	43. External ophthalmoplegia and myopia
18. Lowe oculo-cerebro-renal syndrome	44. Microphthalmia
19. Hypochromic anemia	45. Microphthalmia, with digital anomalies
(Cooley-Rundles-Falls type)	46. Nystagmus
20. Angiokeratoma diffusum	47. Megalocornea
corporis universale	53. Retinitis pigmentosa
21. Dyskeratosis congenita	48. Hypoplasia of iris with glaucoma
22. Dystrophia bullosa hereditaria, typus	54. Macular dystrophy
maculatus	49. Congenital total cataract
23. Keratosis follicularis spinulosa	55. Retinoschisis
cum ophiasi	50. Congenital cataract with microcornea
24. Ichthyosis vulgaris	56. Pseudoglioma
25. Anhidrotic ectodermal dysplasia	51. Stationary night blindness with
26. Amelogenesis imperfecta,	57. Van den Bosch syndrome
hypomaturation type	myopia
27. Amelogenesis imperfecta,	58. Menkes syndrome
hypoplastic type	52. Choroideremia
28. Absence of central incisors	59. Albinism-deafness syndrome

(continued)

TABLE 1–3. Continued

B. Conditions for which the Evidence of X-Linkage is Considered Inconclusive

1. Inability to smell cyanide
2. Incontinentia pigmenti
3. Wildervanck syndrome
4. Male hypogonadism
5. Male hypogonadism and ichthyosis
6. Testicular feminization syndrome
7. Male pseudohermaphroditism
8. Kallmann syndrome
9. Anosmia
10. Zonular cataract and nystagmus
11. Myoclonic nystagmus
12. Combined Charcot-Marie-Tooth disease and Friedreich ataxia
13. Choroidal sclerosis
14. White occipital lock of hair
15. Diffuse corticomeningeal angiomatosis
16. Albright hereditary osteodystrophy
17. Aptitude for spatial visualization
18. Microcephaly with spastic diplegia
19. Familial obstructive jaundice
20. Paget disease of bone
21. Phosphorylase-deficient glycogen storage disease of liver

C. Conditions Probably not X-Linked Although this Genetic Mechanism Has Been Suggested

1. Leber optic atrophy
2. Gynecomastia
3. Acrokeratosis verruciformis
4. The OFD syndrome
5. Plain radial loop, right index finger
6. Spiegler-Brooke tumors
7. Familial periodic paralysis
8. Mohr syndrome

non, normal females are genetically mosaic, a portion of their cells having one active X chromosome and the remaining cells having the alternative X chromosome active. The inactive X chromosome can be identified in interphase nuclei as a dense staining body (the so-called Barr body) adjacent to the nuclear membrane; in polymorphonuclear leucocytes it manifests as drumstick-shaped extensions from the nucleus and in dividing cells as the late-replicating X chro-

TABLE 1–4. Gene Localizations Based on X Chromosome Deletions or X:Autosome Translocations

Year	*Clinical Disorder*	*Chromosomal Localization*
1972	Ectodermal dysplasia, anhidrotic or hypohidrotic[58]	Xq12.2-q13.1
1977	Duchenne pseudohypertrophic muscular dystrophy[59]	Xp21.3-p21.1
1978	Becker pseudohypertrophic muscular dystrophy[60]	Xp21.3-p21.1
1980	Aarskog syndrome[61]	Xp11.2
1982	Aicardi syndrome[62]	Xp22
1982	Goeminne syndrome[63]	Xq28-qter
1983	Hunter syndrome (IDS* deficiency)[64]	Xq27.3-q28
1985	Incontinentia pigmenti–1[65]	Xp11.21-cen
1986	Hemophilia B (factor IX deficiency)[66]	Xq26.3-q27.1
1986	Lowe syndrome[67]	Xq25-q26.1
1987	Menkes syndrome[68]	Xq13.2-q13.3
1987	Tapetochoroidal dystrophy[69]	Xq21.1-q21.3
1990	Rett syndrome[70]	Xp22.11 or p 11.22
1992	Norrie disease[71]	Xp11.4-p11.3

*IDS, iduronate-2-sulfatase.

mosome.[23, 24] At the molecular level, X chromosome inactivation is thought to be achieved by methylation of DNA.[91]

Two segments located adjacent to the telomeres of the X chromosome which are exempt from inactivation have been termed *pseudoautosomal regions* (PARs).[88,89] Sequences in these regions are found on both the X and the Y chromosomes. The major pseudoautosomal region (XpPAR, PAR1) spans the distal 2.6 Mb of Xp and is the primary site of meiotic pairing and recombination between Xp and Yp.[92–98] While the gene content of the pseudoautosomal region is incompletely understood, seven genes have been identified (Fig. 1–2). Mutations and deletions in one of the seven, SHOX, have been demonstrated in Leri-Weill dyschondrosteosis.[99,100] As predicted from clinical experience, homozygous mutations of this gene have been found in Langer mesomelic chondrodysplasia.

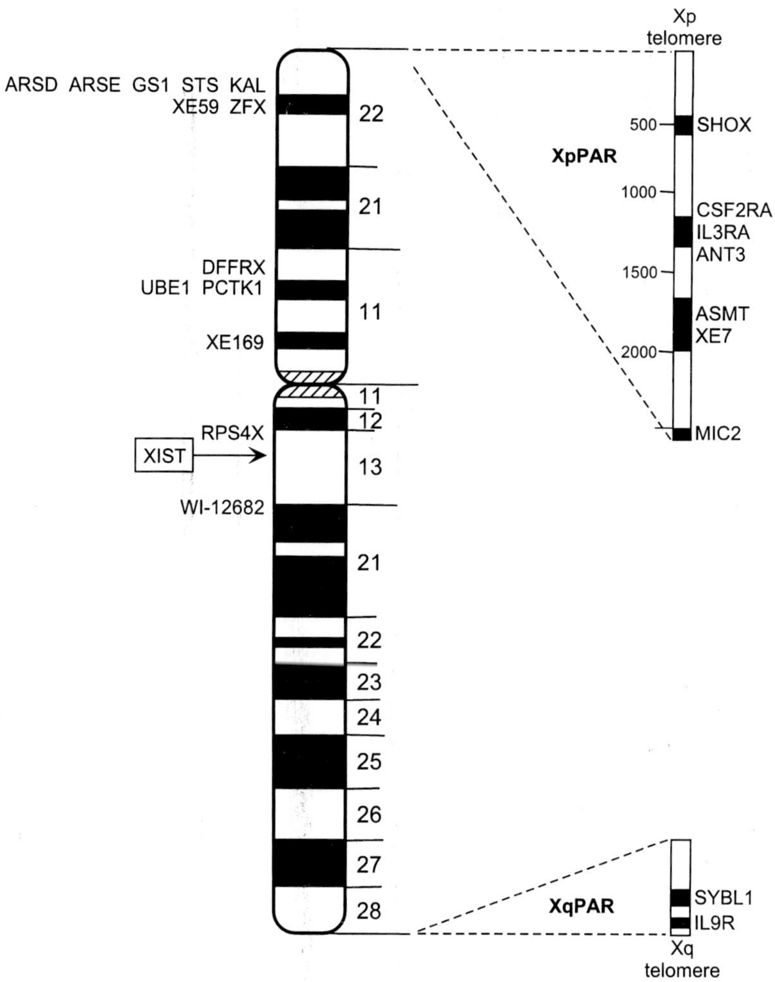

FIGURE 1–2. The two major pseudoautosomal regions (PAR) located at the X chromosome telomeres. Seven genes have been identified on the XpPAR and two on the XqPAR. Other genes on the X chromosome that escape inactivation are shown on the left.[88,89,98,101,105]

A smaller pseudoautosomal region (XqPAR, PAR2), 320 kb in size, is located at the Xq and Yq termini.[88,89,101] At least two genes, IL9R and SYBL1, are located in this PAR. It is of interest that IL9R is expressed from the X and Y chromosomes but that SYBL1, the more centromeric of the two genes, is expressed from the active X but not from the inactive X chromosome or the Y chromosome. Xq-Yq interchanges within this region of homology have been demonstrated.

In addition to genes in the Xp/Yp and Xq/Yq pseudoautosomal regions, a number of other genes on the X chromosome escape inactivation.[90,91,102–105] Some of these interspersed genes have Y homologues; others do not.

Inactivation of segments of other chromosomes is presumed to be responsible for partitioning of gene activity temporally (e.g., genes that are active during embryogenesis may become inactive thereafter) and by cell type (e.g., genes that are transcribed in hepatic cells may not be transcribed in muscle cells and vice versa).

Considerable attention has recently been given to the potential of certain genes to be expressed differently depending on whether they were inherited from the mother or the father.[106,107] This special type of altered gene activity has been called *imprinting*. As with other types of nonpermanent DNA modification, imprinting may involve methylation of DNA, generally persists for life, and may be reversible during gametogenesis.

One of the most conspicuous of the imprinting phenomena has been documented during the past decade. Termed *uniparental disomy*, the phenomenon occurs when both contributions of a particular chromosome (or portion of a particular chromosome) are derived from the same parent.[106] Maternal disomy for chromosome 15 accounts for about 25% of cases of Prader-Willi syndrome and paternal disomy for chromosome 15 accounts for about 2%–5% of cases of Angelman syndrome.[107,108] Uniparental disomy has also been implicated in some cases of Beckwith-Wiedemann syndrome (paternal 11p), a Russell-Silver–like syndrome (maternal 7), neonatal diabetes mellitus (paternal 6), and a variety of disorders with growth disturbances and learning disabilities.[109–115]

Several instances of complete or segmental uniparental disomy for the X chromosome have been described.[116–118] Maternal whole X chromosome disomy has been demonstrated in two normal females as has maternal isodisomy for the terminal q arm. A 6-year-old girl with maternal whole X chromosome isodisomy was found to have Duchenne muscular dystrophy caused by homozygosity for a deletion of the dystrophin gene.[117] Paternal uniparental disomy for the X chromosome has been described in a girl with short stature, short neck, broad chest, cubitus valgus, and partial ovarian insufficiency.[118] The relationship of the paternal uniparental disomy and the patient's Turner syndrome features was not clear because of a low-grade 45,X/46,XX mosaicism demonstrated in lymphocyte cultures. No instance of paternal derivation of both X and Y chromosomes has been recognized.

Segmental X disomy has been demonstrated in several XY males with Xq sequences translocated onto Yq.[119] The males had severe mental retardation, hypotonia, and seizures. Genes involved in the translocation were hyperexpressed.

Table 1–5. Chromosome Number and Sex Chromosome Constitution in Selected Organisms*

	Chromosome Number	*Sex Chromosome*	
		Female	*Male*
Mammals			
Primates			
Human	46	XX	XY
Gorilla	48	XX	XY
Chimpanzee	48	XX	XY
Ringtailed lemur	56	XX	XY
Spider monkey	34	XX	XY
Cetacea			
Killer whale	44	XX	XY
Carnivora			
Black bear	74	XX	XY
Cat	38	XX	XY
Chiroptera			
Mexican free-tailed bat	48	XX	XY
Insectivora			
Shrew	50	XX	XY
Lagomorpha			
Jackrabbit	48	XX	XY
Proboscidea			
Elephant	56	XX	XY
Xenarthra			
Nine-banded armadillo	64	XX	XY
Artiodactyla			
White-tailed deer	74	XX	XY
Giraffe	30	XX	XY
Indian muntjac deer	6,7	XX	XY,YZ
Perissodactyla			
Horse	64	XX	XY
Donkey	62	XX	XY
Cape zebra	32	XX	XY
Rodentia			
Mouse	40	XX	XY
Marsupialia			
Wallaby	10,11	XX	XY_1Y_2
Gray kangaroo	16	XX	XY
Opossum	22	XX	XY
Birds			
California condor	14	ZW	ZZ
Turkey	16	ZW	ZZ
Chicken	12	ZW	ZZ

(continued)

TABLE 1–5. Continued

	Chromosome Number	Sex Chromosome Female	Sex Chromosome Male
Amphibians			
Frog (Xenopus)	36	XY (?)	XX (?)
Reptiles†			
Lizard	33,34	X	XX
Sea Turtle	57,58	X	XX
Fish†	48–104	—	—
Insects			
Drosophila	8	XX	XY

Data courtesy of Kurt Benirschke, M.D., University of California, San Diego.

†Fish and many reptiles have no recognized sex chromosomes.

Evolutionary Conservation

The sex chromosome constitution in humans is the same as all other mammals and many other lower forms (Table 1–5).[120] However, in some cases males are the homogametic sex and females the heterogametic sex.

Ohno has reviewed evidence that the "original X chromosome of a common ancestor has been preserved in its entirety by diverse species of placental mammals of today. Despite the enormous array of karyotypes displayed by various species of mammals, in the great majority, including man and the mouse (*Mus musculus*), the X is nearly identical in size, comprising a little more than 5% of the genome."[121] The X chromosome has been more or less extensively rearranged in the various species and individual genes altered by mutations, duplications, and deletions.[122–128] However, the relationship among large blocks of the X chromosome has remained in tact. Blair et al., for example, finds that the human–mouse comparative map is composed of a minimum of eight blocks of homologous loci, a situation which could be produced by the occurrence of three inversions of these subchromosomal blocks during evolution from a single ancestral X chromosome (Fig. 1–3).[125]

With few exceptions, X-linked genes in humans are X-linked in all placental mammals. In a sense, genes that were present on the original ancestral X chromosome have been fixed in that location. It is plausible that X-linked genes are kept from translocating to the autosomes because such a move would result in loss of inactivation and a concurrent change in gene dosage, which would be a disadvantage to the organism.

The Other Sex Chromosome

Ohno has traced the evolution of the Y chromosome in heterogametic organisms from a second X chromosome in homogametic organisms.[121, 129] Degeneration

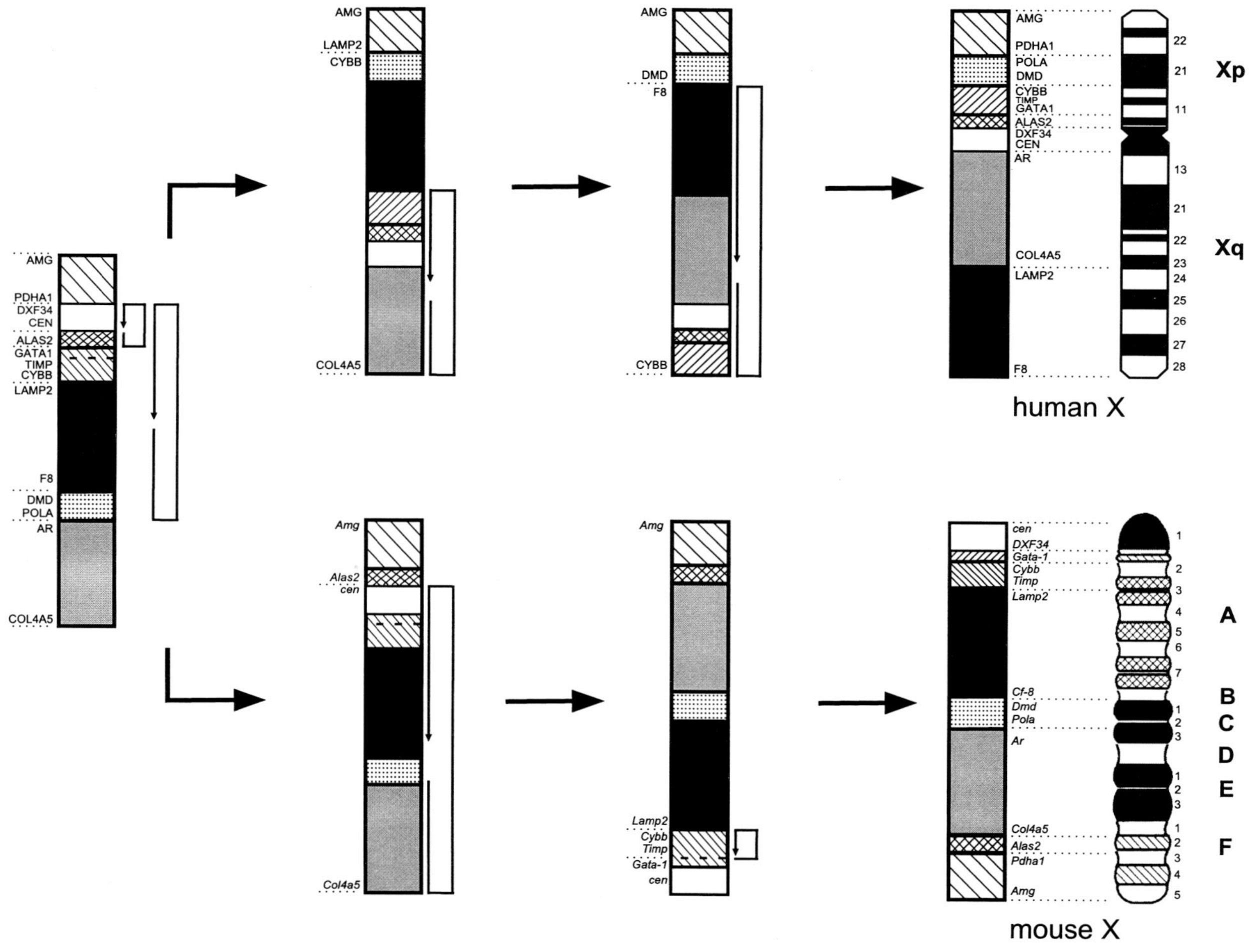

AMG
PDHA1
DXF34
CEN
ALAS2
GATA1
TIMP
CYBB
LAMP2
F8
DMD
POLA
AR
COL4A5
AMG
LAMP2
CYBB
COL4A5
AMG
DMD
F8
CYBB
AMG
PDHA1
POLA
DMD
CYBB
TIMP
GATA1
ALAS2
DXF34
CEN
AR
COL4A5
LAMP2
F8
22
21
11
13
21
22
23
24
25
26
27
28
Xp
Xq
human X
Amg
Alas2
cen
Col4a5
Amg
Lamp2
Cybb
Timp
Gata-1
cen
cen
DXF34
Gata-1
Cybb
Timp
Lamp2
Cf-8
Dmd
Pola
Ar
Col4a5
Alas2
Pdha1
Amg
1
2
3
4
5
6
7
1
2
3
1
2
3
1
2
3
4
5
A
B
C
D
E
F
mouse X

of the residual genetic content followed a series of structural rearrangements and deletions. In the process, the Y chromosome has become the smallest in the human genome, measuring 38% of the X chromosome and only 2% of the haploid autosomal length. Were it not for retention of the sex-determining property resident in the SRY gene, the Y chromosome would be a relatively unimportant chromosome since it has few genes which are expressed.[88–105]

X-Linked Genes and Intelligence

That there may be a concentration of genes on the X chromosome concerned with intelligence via their impact on the structure and function of the brain is an idea that has been posed by a number of observers.[130–136] Turner suggests that such genes for intelligence could have been rapidly spread by dominant males, escalating the evolutionary pace of ascendance of humans above other creatures.[136]

Certainly at this phase of resolution of the human genome, there are relatively more genes on the X chromosome which might influence intelligence than on an equal span of the autosomal genome or on any other individual chromosome, and perhaps even more than on the entire autosomal genome.[137] This may merely reflect the greater ease in identifying genes on the X chromosome because hemizygosity is so good at bringing genes to light. No other natural genetic phenomenon so clearly exposes genes to observation. Trisomy and chromosome rearrangements, consanguinity, uniparental disomy, and other phenomena either do so less clearly or less commonly. Hence, there exists a strong bias toward identifying genes on the X chromosome which would not be present if the same gene were located on an autosome.

That there exists greater variability of intelligence among males as measured by available cognitive instruments has provided further evidence for the importance of X-linked genes that influence intelligence.[138–140] This greater variability essentially changes the conformation of the bell-shaped curve of male cognition when compared to that of the female. Males have fewer performers in the middle (mean) range than females and more in the extremes beyond 2 standard deviations (SD). The argument goes that one predicts greater variability because of hemizygosity for genes on the X chromosome, the males feeling the full influence of these intelligence genes, whether positive or negative,

←

FIGURE 1–3. Blair et al. have postulated the model on p. 14 for the evolution of the current arrangement of conserved segments on the human and mouse X chromosomes from an ancestral chromosome.[125] A minimum of eight blocks of homologous loci are rearranged through a series of three inversions to form the current arrangement of the human X or the mouse X. Each homologous block is shaded in the same manner throughout and the proximal and distal loci that define the blocks are indicated on the postulated ancestral chromosome and the human and mouse X chromosomes. Dotted lines between the loci indicate the positions of the evolutionary breakpoints. The comparative maps of the human and mouse X chromosomes are shown alongside their G-banded cytogenetic maps.

whereas in females a second X chromosome serves to modify the influence, lessening the impact of positive or negative influences of specific genes for intelligence.[130]

These arguments assume that the test instruments themselves do not permit this performance variability based on some influence other than X-linked genes. They further assume that the variability is real and that it is not due to an epigenetic phenomenon such as hormonal influence or sexual dimorphism from social enhancement/impediments.

This book is devoted to the concept that the detrimental effect of genes on the X chromosome contributes substantially to the excess of males with intelligence beyond 2 SD below the mean. Males with low cognitive function are likely to come to attention since services must be provided by families and by society. An equal excess of males in the IQ range beyond 2 SD above the mean would have a greater chance of going unnoticed. In fact, in no case has a gene for superior intelligence been mapped or cloned. Lubs has called for the identification of pedigrees which might demonstrate such a phenomenon.[133] Even if such pedigrees exist, they may be difficult to find since they do not require ascertainment for services, nor do they necessarily achieve distinction that segregates them from society.

Opposing the idea of disproportionate influence of the X chromosome in determining intelligence is the observation that microdeletions almost anywhere in the autosomal genome produce mental retardation. While not quantitative in any sense, this gives a clue that genes that influence intelligence via brain structure or function are widely distributed through the human genome. Further, evidence that a broad spectrum of genes are expressed in the brain during and/or following the developmental period has been an important contribution of molecular studies.[141–146] Only the accumulation of information on genes from all parts of the genome and delineation of the function of these genes will resolve the issue of distribution of genes for intelligence. Until such time, Turner's gentle reminder to the male that the intelligence of his sons "is solely dependent on his partner" should be considered with some reservation.[132]

REFERENCES

1. Henking H: Untersuchungen über die ersten Entwicklungsvorgänge in den elern von Insekten. II. Ueber spermatogenese un deren Beziehung zur Eientwicklung bei *Pyrrhocoris apterus*. Z wiss Zool 51:685, 1891.
2. Montgomery TH Jr: The spermatogenesis in *Pentatoma* up to the formation of the spermatid. Zool Jahrb 12:1, 1899.
3. McClung CE: A peculiar nuclear element in the male reproductive cells of insects. Zool Bull 2:187, 1899.
4. McClung CE: The accessory-chromosome—sex determinant? Biol Bull 3:43, 1902.
5. Wilson EB: The Cell in Development and Heredity. MacMillan, New York, 1925, pp. 748–749.
6. Hansemann D von: Ueber pathologische mitosen. Arch Pathol Anat Physiol 123:356, 1891.
7. Bardeleben K von: Weitere Beiträge zur Spermatogenese beim Menschen. (Further observations on spermatogenesis in man.) Jen Z Nat 31:475, 1898.

8. Guyer MF: Accessory chromosomes in man. Bull Biol 19:219, 1910.
9. Flemming W von: Über die chromosomenzahl beim menschen. (Number of chromosomes in man.) Anat Anz 14:178, 1897.
10. Duesberg J: Sur le nombre des chromosomes chez l'homme. (On the number of chromosomes in men.) Anat Anz 28:415, 1906.
11. Branca A: Précis d'histologie (Outline of Histology), 1 vol. Baillière, Paris, 1910.
12. Moore JES, Arnold G: On the constancy of form among the synaptic gemini (heterotype chromosomes) in certain animals. Proc R Soc Lond [Biol] 77:563, 1905–1906.
13. Wilcox EV: Human spermatogenesis. Anat Anz 17:316, 1900.
14. Winiwarter H de: Etudes sur la spermatogenése humaine. I. Cellule de Sertoli. II. Hétérochromosome et mitoses de l'épithelium séminal. Arch Biol 27:91, 1912.
15. Painter TS: The Y-chromosome in mammals. Science 53:503, 1921.
16. Painter T: The sex chromosomes of man. Am Nat 58:506, 1924.
17. King RL, Beams HW: The sex chromosomes in man, with reference to the first spermatocyte. Anat Rec 65:165, 1936.
18. Koller PC: The genetical and mechanical properties of sex chromosomes. III. Man. Proc R Soc Edinb (Pt 2, Sec B) 57:194, 1937.
19. Sachs L: The chromosome constancy of the normal mammalian uterus. Heredity 8:117, 1954.
20. Winiwarter H de, Oguma K: La formule chromosiale humaine. Arch Biol 40:541, 1930.
21. Oguma K: The segmentary structure of the human X-chromosome compared with that of rodents. J Morphol 61:59, 1937.
22. Roberts JAF: An Introduction to Medical Genetics. Oxford University Press, London, 1940, p. 89.
23. Barr ML, Bertram EG: A morphological distinction between neurones of the male and female, and the behaviour of the nucleolar satellite during accelerated nucleoprotein synthesis. Nature 163:676, 1949.
24. Davidson WM, Robertson Smith D: A morphological sex difference in polymorphonuclear neutrophil leucocytes. Br Med J 2:6, 1954.
25. Sachs L, Danon M: The diagnosis of the sex chromosomes in human tissues. Genetica 28:201, 1956.
26. Moore KL, Graham MA, Barr ML: The detection of chromosomal sex in hermaphrodites from a skin biopsy. Surg Gynecol Obstet 96:641, 1953.
27. Polaris PE, Hunter WF, Lennox B: Chromosomal sex in Turner's syndrome with coarctation of the aorta. Lancet 267:120, 1954.
28. Tjio JH, Levan A: The chromosome number of man. Hereditas 42:1, 1956.
29. Ford CE, Hamerton JL: The chromosomes of man. Nature 178:1020, 1956.
30. Ford CE, Jacobs PA, Lajtha LG: Human somatic chromosomes. Nature 181:1565, 1958.
31. Tjio JH, Puck TT: The somatic chromosomes of man. PNAS 441:1229, 1958.
32. Lejeune J: Le mongolisme. Premier example d'aberration autosomique humaine. Ann Genet Semaine Hop 1:41, 1959.
33. Jacobs PA, Strong JA: A case of human intersexuality having a possible XXY sex determining mechanism. Nature 183:302, 1959.
34. Penrose LS, Delhanty JDA: Triploid cell cultures from a macerated fetus. Lancet 1:1261, 1961.
35. Carr DH: Chromosome studies in abortuses and stillborn infants. Lancet 2:603, 1963.
36. Hall B, Kallen B: Chromosome studies in abortuses and stillborn infants. Lancet 1:110, 1964.
37. Boue J, Boue A, Lazar P: The epidemiology of human spontaneous abortions with chromosomal anomalies. In: Aging Gametes. RJ Blandau, ed. Karger, Basel, 1975, p. 330.
38. Warburton D, Stein Z, Kline J, et al.: Chromosome abnormalities in spontaneous

abortion: data from the New York City study. In: Human Embryonic and Fetal Death. IH Porter, EB Hook, eds. Academic Press, New York, 1980, p. 261.
39. Steele MW, Breg WR: Chromosome analysis of human amniotic fluid cells. Lancet 1:383, 1966.
40. The Denver Conference: A proposed standard system of nomenclature of human mitotic chromosomes. Lancet 1:1063, 1960.
41. The London Conference on the Normal Human Karyotype. Cytogenet 2:264, 1963.
42. Chicago Conference: Standardization in Human Cytogenetics. Birth Defects: Orig Art Series II(2), 1966.
43. Paris Conference (1971): Standardization in Human Cytogenetics. Birth Defects Orig Art Series VIII(7), 1972.
44. Paris Conference (1971), Supplement (1975): Standardization in Human Cytogenetics. Birth Defects Orig Art Series XI(9), 1975.
45. An International System for Human Cytogenetic Nomenclature (1978). Report of the Standing Committee on Human Cytogenetic Nomenclature (Stockholm Conference). S. Karger, Basel, Switzerland, 1978.
46. An International System for Human Cytogenetic Nomenclature (1985). Report of the Standing Committee on Human Cytogenetic Nomenclature. S. Karger, Basel, Switzerland, 1985.
47. An International System for Human Cytogenetic Nomenclature (1995). Recommendation of the International Standing Committee on Human Cytogenetic Nomenclature (Memphis Conference). S. Karger, Basel, Switzerland, 1995.
48. Caspersson T, Lomakka G, Zech L: The 24 fluorescence patterns of human metaphase chromosomes—distinguishing characters and variability. Hereditas 67:89, 1971.
49. Sutherland GR: Heritable fragile sites on human chromosomes. I. Factors affecting expression in lymphocyte culture. Am J Hum Genet 31:125, 1979.
50. Yunis J: High resolution of human chromosomes. Science 191:1268, 1976.
51. Harper ME, Ullrich A, Saunders GF: Localization of the human insulin gene to the distal end of the short arm of chromosome 11. Proc Natl Acad Sci USA 78:4458, 1981.
52. Langer PR, Waldrop AA, Ward DC: Enzymatic synthesis of biotin-labeled polynucleotides: novel nucleic acid affinity probes. Proc Natl Acad Sci USA 78:6633, 1981.
53. Speicher MR, Ballard SG, Ward DC: Karyotyping human chromosomes by combinatorial multi-fluor FISH. Nat Genet 12:368, 1996.
54. Schröck E, duManoir S, Veldman T, et al.: Multicolor spectral karyotyping of human chromosomes. Science 273:494, 1996.
55. Gardiner K: Base composition and gene distribution critical patterns in mammalian genome organization. Trends Genet 12:519, 1996.
56. McKusick VA: On the X Chromosome of Man. Waverly Press, Baltimore, 1964.
57. Lubs HA: A marker X chromosome. Am J Hum Genet 21:231, 1969.
58. Cohen MM, Lin CC, Sybert V, et al.: Two human X-autosome translocations identified by autoradiography and fluorescence. Am J Hum Genet 24:583, 1972.
59. Greenstein RM, Reardon MP, Chan TS: An X-autosome translocation in a girl with Duchenne muscular dystrophy (DMD): evidence for DMD gene localization. (Abstract) Pediatr Res 11:457, 1977.
60. Verellen C, Markovic V, DeMeyer R, et al.: Expression of an X-linked recessive disease in a female due to nonrandom inactivation of the X chromosome. (Abstract) Am J Hum Genet 30:97A, 1978.
61. Tyrkus M, Bawle E, Lipman S, et al.: Aarskog-Scott syndrome inherited as an X-linked dominant with full male–female expression. (Abstract) Am J Hum Genet 32: 134A, 1980.
62. Ropers HH, Zuffardi O, Bianchi E, et al.: Agenesis of corpus callosum, ocular, and skeletal anomalies (X-linked dominant Aicardi's syndrome) in a girl with balanced X/3 translocation. Hum Genet 61:364, 1982.

63. Zuffardi O, Fraccaro M: Gene mapping and serendipity: the locus for torticollis, keloids, cryptorchidism, adrenal dysplasia (31430, McKusick) is at Xq28, distal to the G6PD locus. Hum Genet 62:280, 1982.
64. Mossman J, Blunt S, Stephens R, et al.: Hunter's disease in a girl: association with X:5 chromosomal translocation disrupting the Hunter gene. Arch Dis Child 58:911, 1983.
65. Hodgson SV, Neville B, Jones RWA, et al.: Two cases of X/autosome translocation in females with incontinentia pigmenti. Hum Genet 71:231, 1985.
66. Vianna-Morgante AM, Batista DAS, Levisky RB, et al.: X;autosome translocations in females with X-linked recessive diseases. (Abstract) 7th Int Congr Hum Genet, Berlin, p. 97, 1986.
67. Hodgson SV, Heckmatt JZ, Hughes E, et al.: A balanced de novo X/autosome translocation in a girl with manifestations of Lowe syndrome. Am J Med Genet 23:837, 1986.
68. Kapur S, Higgins JV, Delp K, et al.: Menkes syndrome in a girl with X-autosome translocation. Am J Med Genet 26:503, 1987.
69. Nussbaum RL, Lesko JG, Lewis RA: Isolation of anonymous DNA sequences from within a submicroscopic X chromosomal deletion in a patient with choroideremia, deafness, and mental retardation. Proc Natl Acad Sci USA 84:6521, 1987.
70. Journel H, Melki J, Turleau C, et al.: Rett phenotype with X/autosome translocation: possible mapping to the short arm of chromosome X. Am J Med Genet 35:142, 1990.
71. Berger W, Meindl A, van de Pol TJR, et al.: Isolation of a candidate gene for Norrie disease by positional cloning. Nat Genet 1:199, 1992.
72. Botstein D, White RL, Skolnick M, et al.: Construction of a genetic linkage map in man using restriction fragment length polymorphisms. Am J Hum Genet 32:314, 1980.
73. Cooper DN, Smith BA, Cooke HJ, et al.: An estimate of unique DNA sequence heterozygosity in the human genome. Hum Genet 69:201, 1985.
74. Vogt P: Potential genetic functions of tandem repeated DNA sequence blocks in the human genome are based on a highly conserved 'chromatin folding code.' Hum Genet 84:301, 1990.
75. Williamson R, Bowcock A, Kidd K, et al.: Report of the DNA Committee and catalogues of cloned and mapped genes, markers formatted for PCR and DNA polymorphisms. Cytogenet Cell Genet 58:1190, 1991.
76. Nussbaum RL, Crowder WE, Nyhan WL, et al.: A three allele restriction-fragment-length polymorphism at the hypoxanthine phosphoribosyltransferase locus in man. Proc Natl Acad Sci USA 80:4035, 1983.
77. Lubs H, Chiurazzi P, Arena J, et al.: XLMR genes: Update 1998. Am J Med Genet, 83:237, 1999.
78. Kurachi K, Davie EW: Isolation and characterization of a cDNA coding for human factor IX. Proc Natl Acad Sci USA 79:6461–6464, 1982.
79. Jolly DJ, Okayama H, Berg P, et al.: Isolation and characterization of a full-length expressible cDNA for human hypoxanthine phosphoribosyltransferase. Proc Natl Acad Sci USA 80:477, 1983.
80. Antonarakis SE, Waber PG, Kittur SD, et al.: Hemophilia A: detection of molecular defects and of carriers by DNA analysis. N Engl J Med 313:842, 1985.
81. Martini G, Toniolo D, Vulliamy T, et al.: Structural analysis of the X-linked gene encoding human glucose 6-phosphate dehydrogenase. EMBO J 5:1849, 1986.
82. Koenig M, Hoffman EP, Bertelson CJ, et al.: Complete cloning of the Duchenne muscular dystrophy (DMD) cDNA and preliminary genomic organization of the DMD gene in normal and affected individuals. Cell 50:509, 1987.
83. Verkerk AJMH, Pieretti M, Sutcliffe JS, et al.: Identification of a gene (FMR-1) containing a CGG repeat coincident with a breakpoint cluster region exhibiting length variation in fragile X syndrome. Cell 65:905, 1991.

84. Rosenthal A, Joulet M, Kenwrick S: Aberrant splicing of neural cell adhesion molecule L1 mRNA in a family with X-linked hydrocephalus. Nat Genet 2:107, 1992.
85. Rao E, Weiss B, Fukami M, et al.: Pseuduautosomal deletions encompassing a novel homeobox gene cause growth failure in idiopathic short stature and Turner syndrome. Nat Genet 16:54, 1997.
86. Lyon MF: Gene action in the X-chromosome of the mouse (*Mus musculus* L.). Nature 190:372, 1961.
87. Disteche CM: Escape from X inactivation in human and mouse. Trends Genet 11:17, 1995.
88. Rappold GA: The pseudoautosomal regions of the human sex chromosomes. Hum Genet 92:315, 1993.
89. Freije D, Helms C, Watson MS, et al.: Identification of a second pseudoautosomal region near the Xq and Yq telomeres. Science 258:1784, 1992.
90. Ellison J, Passage M, Yu LC, et al.: Directed isolation of human genes that escape X inactivation. Somat Cell Mol Genet 18:259, 1992.
91. Miller AP, Gustashaw K, Wolff DJ, et al.: Three genes that escape X chromosome inactivation are clustered within a 6 Mb YAC contig and STS map in Xp11.21-11.22. Hum Mol Genet 4:731, 1995.
92. Burgoyne PS: Genetic homology and crossing over in the X and Y chromosomes of the mammals. Hum Genet 6185, 1982.
93. Chandley AC, Goetz P, Hargreave JB, et al.: On the nature and extent of the XY pairing at meiotic prophase in man. Cytogenet Cell Genet 28:241, 1984.
94. Lin L, Hamer DH: Recombination and allelic association in the Xq/Yq homology region. Hum Mol Genet 4:2013, 1995.
95. Yen PH, Ellison J, Salido EC, et al.: Isolation of a new gene from the distal short arm of the human X chromosome that escapes X-inactivation. Hum Mol Genet 1:47, 1992.
96. des Portes V, Bachner L, Brüls T, et al.: X-linked neurodegenerative syndrome with congenital ataxia, late-onset progressive myoclonic encephalopathy and selective macular degeneration, linked to Xp22.33-pter. Am J Med Genet 64:69, 1996.
97. Schiebel K, Winkelmann M, Mertz A, et al.: Abnormal XY interchange between a novel isolated protein kinase gene, *PRKY,* and its homologue, *PRKX,* accounts for one third of all (Y+)XX males and (Y−)XY females. Hum Mol Genet 6:1985, 1997.
98. Gianfrancesco F, Esposito T, Montanini L, et al.: A novel pseudoautosomal gene encoding a putative GTP-binding protein resides in the vicinity of the Xp/Yp telomere. Hum Mol Genet 7:407, 1998.
99. Belin V, Cusin V, Viot G, et al.: *SHOX* mutations in dyschondrosteosis (Leri-Weill syndrome). Nat Genet 19:67, 1998.
100. Shears DJ, Vassal HJ, Goodman FR, et al.: Mutation and deletion of the pseudoautosomal gene *SHOX* cause Leri-Weill dyschondrosteosis. Nat Genet 19:70, 1998.
101. D'Esposito M, Matarazzo MR, Ciccodicola A: Differential expression pattern of Xq-PAR-linked genes SYBL1 and IL9R correlates with the structure and evolution of the region. Hum Mol Genet 6:1917, 1997.
102. Schneider-Gadicke A, Beer-Romero P, Brown LG, et al.: ZFX has a gene structure similar to ZFY, the putative sex determinant, and escapes X inactivation. Cell 57:1247, 1989.
103. Jones MH, Furlong RA, Burkin H, et al: The *Drosophila* developmental gene fat facets has a human homologue in Xp11.4 which escapes X-inactivation and has related sequences on Yq11.2. Hum Mol Genet 5:1695, 1996.
104. Esposito T, Gianfrancesco F, Ciccodicola A, et al.: Escape from X-inactivation of two new genes associated with DXS6974E and DXS7020E. Genomics 43:183, 1997.
105. Brown CJ, Carrel L, Willard HF: Expression of genes from the human active and inactive X chromosomes. Am J Hum Genet 60:1333, 1997.

106. Hall JG: Genomic imprinting: review and relevance to human diseases. Am J Hum Genet 46:857, 1990
107. Nicholls RD, Knoll JHM, Butler MG, et al.: Genetic imprinting suggested by maternal heterodisomy in non-deletion Prader-Willi syndrome. Nature 342:281, 1989.
108. Malcolm S, Nichols M, Clayton-Smith J, et al.: Angelman syndrome can result from uniparental paternal isodisomy. Am J Hum Genet 47(Suppl):A227, 1990.
109. Engel E, DeLozier-Blanchet CD: Uniparental disomy, isodisomy, and imprinting: probable effects in man and strategies for their detection. Am J Med Genet 40:432, 1991.
110. Nicholls RD: Letter to the Editor. Uniparental disomy as the basis for an association of rare disorders. Am J Med Genet 41:273, 1991.
111. Henry I, Bonaiti-Pellié C, Chehensse V, et al.: Uniparental paternal disomy in a genetic cancer-predisposing syndrome. Nature 351:665, 1991.
112. Spence JE, Perciaccante RG, Greig GM, et al.: Uniparental disomy as a mechanism for human genetic disease. Am J Hum Genet 42:217, 1988.
113. Henry I, Puech A, Riesewijk A, et al.: Somatic mosaicism for partial paternal isodisomy in Wiedemann-Beckwith syndrome: a post-fertilization event. Eur J Hum Genet 1:19-29, 1993.
114. Kotzot D, Schmitt S, Bernasconi F, et al.: Uniparental disomy 7 in Silver-Russell syndrome and primordial growth retardation. Hum Mol Genet 4:583, 1995.
115. Abramowicz MJ, Andrien M, Dupont E, et al.: Isodisomy of chromosome 6 in a newborn with methylmalonic acidemia and agenesis of pancreatic beta cells causing diabetes mellitus. J Clin Invest 94:418, 1994.
116. Avivi L, Korenstein A, Braier-Goldstein O, et al.: Uniparental disomy of sex chromosomes in man. Am J Hum Genet 51:A11, 1992.
117. Quan F, Janas J, Toth-Fejel S, et al.: Uniparental disomy of the entire X chromosome in a female with Duchenne muscular dystrophy. Am J Hum Genet 60:160, 1997.
118. Schinzel AA, Robinson WP, Binkert F, et al.: Exclusively paternal X chromosomes in a girl with short stature. Hum Genet 92:175, 1993.
119. Lahn BT, Ma N, Breg WR: Xq-Yq interchange resulting in supernormal X-linked gene expression in severely retarded males with 46,Xyq-karyotype. Nat Genet 8:243, 1994.
120. Makino S: Genetics and Cytology. I. Chromosome Numbers: Annuals, in Biology Data Book, Ed. 2. Altman PL, Dittmer DS, eds. FASEB, Bethesda, 1972.
121. Ohno S: Sex Chromosomes and Sex-Linked Genes. Springer-Verlag, New York, 1967, pp. 5–46, 85.
122. Ohno S: Ancient linkage groups and frozen accidents. Nature 244:259, 1973.
123. Mandel J-L, Monaco AP, Nelson DL, et al.: Genome analysis and the human X chromosome. Science 258:103, 1992.
124. Brown SDM, Avner P, Boyd Y, et al.: Mouse X chromosome. Mamm Genome 4:S269, 1993.
125. Blair HJ, Reed V, Steven H, et al.: New insights into the man–mouse comparative map of the X chromosome. Genomics 19:215, 1994.
126. Rivella S, Tamanini F, Bione S, et al.: A comparative transcriptional map of a region of 250 kb on the human and mouse X chromosome between the G6PD and the FLN1 genes. Genomics 28:377, 1995.
127. Palmer S, Perry J, Ashworth A: A contravention of Ohno's law in mice. Nat Genet 10:472, 1995.
128. Dinulos MB, Bassi MT, Rugarli EI, et al.: A new region of conservation is defined between human and mouse X chromosomes. Genomics 35:244, 1996.
129. Graves JAM: The origin and function of the mammalian Y chromosome and Y-borne genes—an evolving understanding. Bio Essays 178:311, 1995.
130. Lehrke RG: X-linked mental retardation and verbal disability. Birth Defects Orig Art Series X(1):1, 1974.

131. Turner G, Partington MW: Genes for intelligence on the X chromosome. J Med Genet 28:429, 1991.
132. Turner G: Intelligence and the X chromosome. Lancet 347:1814, 1996.
133. Lubs H: The other side of the coin—an hypothesis concerning the importance of genes for high intelligence and evolution of the X chromosome. Am J Med Genet 85:206, 1999.
134. Morton NE (and reply by Turner G, Partington MW): Genes for intelligence on the X chromosome. J Med Genet 29:71, 1992.
135. Hook EB (and author's reply by Turner G): Intelligence and the X chromosome. Lancet 348:826, 1996.
136. Turner G: Finding genes on the X chromosome by which *Homo* may have become *sapiens*. Am J Hum Genet 58:1109, 1996.
137. McKusick VA: Mendelian Inheritance in Man, Ed. 12. Johns Hopkins University Press, Baltimore, 1998.
138. Roberts JAF: On the difference between the sexes in dispersion of intelligence. Br Med J I:727, 1945.
139. Wechsler D: The Measurement and Appraisal of Adult Intelligence, Ed 4. Williams & Wilkins, Baltimore, 1958, pp. 144–149.
140. Hedges LV, Nowell A: Sex differences in mental test scores, variability, and numbers of high-scoring individuals. Science 269:41, 1995.
141. Wilkinson DG, Krumlauf R: Molecular approaches to the segmentation of the hindbrain. Trends Neurosci 13:335, 1990.
142. Wilkinson DG: In Situ Hybridization: A Practical Approach. Alan R Liss, New York, 1992.
143. Moorman AFM, DeBoer PAJ, Vermeulen JLM, et al.: Practical aspects of radioisotopic *in situ* hybridization on RNA. Histochem J 25:251, 1993.
144. Lopes da Silva S, Horssen AM, Chang C van, et al.: Expression of nuclear hormone receptors in the rat supraoptic nucleus. Endocrinology 136:2276, 1995.
145. Schaick HAS van, Smidt MP, Rovescalli AC: Homeobox gene *Prx3* expression in rodent brain and extraneural tissues. Proc Natl Acad Sci USA 94:12993, 1997.
146. Lako M, Lindsay S, Bullen P, et al.: A novel mammalian *Wnt* gene, *WNT8B*, shows brain-restricted expression in early development, with sharply delimited expression boundaries in the developing forebrain. Hum Mol Genet 7:813, 1998.

2

Emergence of the Concept of X-Linked Mental Retardation

Until the 20th century, mental retardation was an informal designation, based primarily on how well an individual adapted in society. In 1905, Binet and Simon published the first test of mental function.[1] This crude test was the foundation upon which subsequent Binet and other tests to predict school achievement were developed. Goddard[2] and Terman[3] translated the Binet test into English (Stanford-Binet), standardized it for use in the United States, quantitated performance in terms of an intelligence quotient (IQ), and concluded that a low IQ (below 70) could be equated with mental retardation. Although others insisted that inability to adapt in society was a mandatory component of mental retardation, the IQ score alone was widely used as the basis for the designation for many years.[3–5] Since the 1950s, both intellectual function and adaptive behavior have been considered equally in determining mental retardation.[6–8]

The most recent definition issued by the American Association on Mental Retardation (1992)[8] states:

> Mental retardation refers to substantial limitations in present functioning. It is characterized by significantly subaverage intellectual functioning, existing concurrently with related limitations in two or more of the following applicable adaptive skill areas: communication, self-care, home living, social skills, community use, self-direction, health and safety, functional academics, leisure and work.

The definition is further qualified by the requirement that mental manifestations be present prior to age 18 years. Subcategories are based upon levels of support needed for adaptation rather than cognitive testing.

Various classifications have been used to partition persons with mental retardation in order to study the underlying biology and to plan for educational, medical, recreational, and other support needs.[7,9–12] The most widely used stratification is based on severity as determined by performance on standardized cognitive tests. Considerable variations in severity stratification and terminology have been used over the years, but they may be generalized under the following correlates:

Mild mental retardation	IQ 50–70
Moderate mental retardation	IQ 35–49
Severe mental retardation	IQ 20–34
Profound mental retardation	IQ <20

Mental retardation occurs as an isolated phenomenon and in the company of other maladies, especially malformations, neurological dysfunction, impairments of the special senses, cerebral palsy, seizures, and behavioral disturbances.[7,11] When mental retardation is consistently associated with somatic, neurological, or behavioral manifestations, it may be termed *syndromal mental retardation.* Such cases generally have a single, specific, and identifiable heritable or environmental cause. In the absence of consistent somatic, neurological, or behavioral manifestations, mental retardation is termed *nonsyndromic* or *nonspecific.*

Mental retardation interferes with performance of essential tasks at each age. In infancy it subdues responsiveness to the environment and delays acquisition of basic motor skills such as sitting up, crawling, or pulling to a standing position. During the preschool years, it impedes development of self-care skills, language utilization, and behavioral conformation. During the school years, academic performance lags because of impairments in problem solving and abstract reasoning. Adult life is characterized by limitations in achieving economic independence and integration into society.

Determination of the prevalence of mental retardation is complicated by difficulties in ascertainment.[12–20] A birth prevalence (incidence) can only be estimated retrospectively, totaling all cases that manifest mental retardation by age 18 years.[18] Such a determination will necessarily fall short of the true figure because of failure to include cases that die early in life prior to the time they would have manifested signs and symptoms and incomplete ascertainment of mild mental retardation. The designation of mental retardation in infancy and early childhood is fraught with uncertainties since delay of motor milestones, behavioral disturbances, or speech impairments may occur due to neuromuscular or other disorders in individuals who are not and will not become mentally retarded.

Prevalence figures determined during the school years are perhaps most meaningful. With few exceptions, individuals with mental retardation will show manifestations during school age. The demands of the academic environment serve to expose limitations in cognitive and adaptive functions. Prevalence figures for adults are considerably lower than during childhood, again reflecting an ascertainment bias. Adults who fail to gain economic independence and satisfactory integration into society may receive societal support through mechanisms other than identification as having mental retardation.

Studies from the first half of the 20th century found prevalence rates approaching 3% of the population in many different locations.[9,13,20] This figure should be revised downward in light of more contemporary studies.[12,14–19,21] Among 10-year-old schoolchildren in the United States, the prevalence of mental retardation averages 1.17%, with a range of 0.2% to 3.9% in different states.[21]

Numerous observers have pointed out that the distribution of intelligence, in general, conforms to the normal distribution curve of continuous traits, but with a conspicuous deviation of the curve beyond 2 standard deviations below the mean.[7,11,22–24] This has been interpreted to indicate that the curve is in fact a composite of two curves.[24] The first and major curve is indeed the bell-shaped curve of normal distribution, with the apex, representing the largest number of individuals, arbitrarily assigned a value of one or 100 and with the numbers of individuals in each category above and below the mean decreasing in a predictable manner (Fig. 2–1). The portion of the curve between 2 SD above and 2 SD below the mean encompasses 95% of the population (percentile 2.5 to percentile 97.5). The IQ score at percentile 2.5 approximates 70, i.e., 2.5% of individuals in a population will be expected to score 70 or less on a properly standardized intelligence test. Most members of this group will score between 50 and 70, the testing range consistent with mild mental retardation, have no other features to distinguish them from the general population and often have a first-degree relative similarly affected. This nonsyndromic subtype is often termed *culturofamilial mental retardation.*

Superimposed on this intelligence curve is a smaller curve comprised of the numbers of individuals who fall substantially below −2 SD. These numbers cause the shoulder at the lower end of the intelligence curve. This group is comprised mainly of individuals with an IQ below 50. As a generalization, these individu-

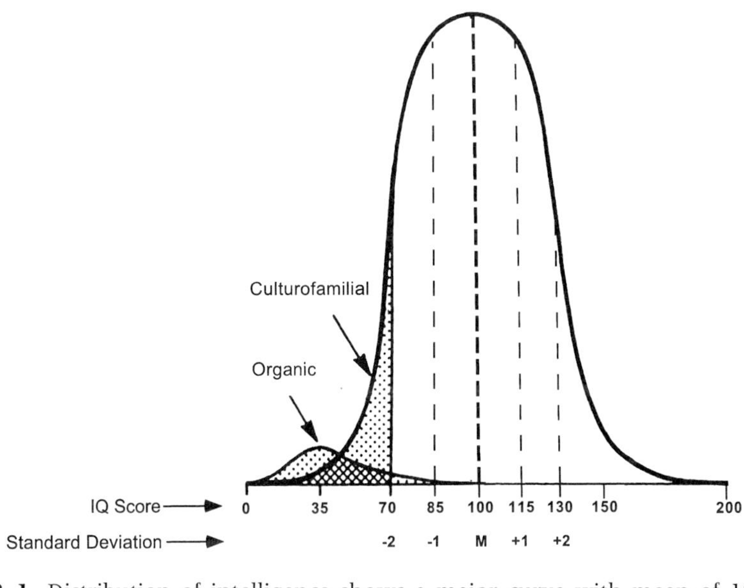

FIGURE 2–1. Distribution of intelligence shows a major curve with mean of 100 representing the general population and a minor curve with a mean of 35 primarily representing persons with specific organic injury from genetic or environmental insults (adapted from Dingman and Tarjan[24]).

als have sustained a single and major insult of genetic or environmental nature to their central nervous system.[11,12,25] They often have other somatic manifestations such as short stature and congenital malformations.[12,25]

The observation in contemporary studies that only about 1% of the population has IQ scores below 70 and that half of those have severe mental retardation suggests an upward migration of IQ performance and the need for restandardization of intelligence measures.[12,14–19,21]

As with other disorders of human formation and function, mental retardation may result from genetic influences, environmental insults, or some combination of the two.[11,12,25,26] Assignment of causation has been possible in only about half of the cases. Heritable and environmental influences claim nearly equal shares of the cases for whom causation can be determined, although the specific percentages vary considerably among the available studies.[11,12,15,16,26–48]

It was from among individuals with severe mental retardation, i.e., those who clearly segregate themselves from those who function near the lower range of normal intelligence, that specific heritable and environmental causes first became delineated. Notable among the first heritable causes to be identified were amaurotic familial idiocy,[49,50] Laurence-Moon-Biedl syndrome (now divided into Laurence-Moon and Bardet-Biedl syndromes[51,52]), phenylketonuria,[53] and X-linked mental retardation with retinitis pigmentosa.[54] It was further noted that certain heritable conditions—neurofibromatosis, tuberous sclerosis, and craniofacial dysostosis—were sometimes complicated by mental retardation.[9] The ranks of single-gene (Mendelian) disorders recognized to cause mental retardation have grown steadily over the past half century. Mental retardation may be associated with as many as 130 (23%) of the 558 X-linked and 661 (7.2%) of the 9265 autosomal genes and genetic disorders listed in McKusick's *Mendelian Inheritance in Man*.[55] There can be little doubt that many of the 60,000–100,000 gene loci yet to be delineated will also influence central nervous system function.

The role of chromosome aberrations as a cause of mental retardation became apparent after Tjio and Levan's 1956 report establishing 46 as the normal number of chromosomes in human cells.[56] A sequence of discoveries followed documenting trisomy, monosomy, segmental duplication (partial trisomy), and segmental deletion (partial monosomy) in individuals with mental retardation, particularly those with associated malformations (Table 2–1).[57,58] Collectively, chromosome aberrations constitute the single most frequent identifiable cause of mental retardation. In recent years, the coupling of cytogenetic and molecular techniques has permitted the demonstration of submicroscopic deletions and duplications and uniparental disomy as additional chromosomal causes of mental retardation.[59–61]

Damage to central nervous system function from prenatal, perinatal, and postnatal environmental insults has been recognized or suspected as a cause of mental retardation for centuries. A wide range of environmental insults of mechanical, immunological, radiological, thermal, chemical, nutritional, and infectious nature have been incriminated.[62] Key observations relating iodine deficiency (Marine and Kimball 1917),[63] X-rays (Goldstein and Murphy 1929),[64] rhesus blood group incompatibility (Levine et al. 1941),[65] rubella infection (Gregg

TABLE 2–1. Sequence of Discovery of Selected Chromosome Aberrations Associated with Mental Retardation

1959	Trisomy 21, Klinefelter syndrome (47,XXY); triple X syndrome (47,XXX)
1960	Trisomy 18, trisomy 13
1963	Deletion 5p (cri du chat syndrome); deletion 18p
1964	Deletion 18q
1965	Deletion 4p (Wolf-Hirschhorn syndrome)
1969	Fragile X syndrome
1973	Partial 9p trisomy
1983	Deletion 17p (Miller-Dieker syndrome)
1986	Deletion 17p (Smith-Magenis syndrome)
1986, 1989	Paternal deletion 15q and maternal disomy 15 (Prader-Willi syndrome)
1987, 1991	Maternal deletion 15q and paternal disomy 15 (Angelman syndrome)
1992	Deletion 22q (velocardiofacial syndrome)
1993	Deletion 7q (Williams syndrome)
1993	Deletion 16p (Rubinstein-Taybi syndrome)

1941),[66] and alcohol (Jones et al. 1973)[67] to brain injury have focused attention on the hazards of environmental agents, especially during the prenatal period. The nervous system becomes progressively more resistant to injury as it matures through fetal development, infancy, and early childhood. Nonetheless, some agents such as viruses and bacteria can damage the brain even after this period. Although widely debated, there can be little doubt that prolonged hypoxia can cause irreparable injury to the immature and mature nervous system as well.[68,69]

Multifactorial causation is perhaps the most common but least understood etiology of mental retardation. Implicit in the concept of multifactorial causation is the notion that individual genetic and environmental factors which alone may lack the power to cause mental retardation can do so through their additive influence. In an individual case, multiple genetic and environmental influences may contribute. Although multifactorial causation is assumed to be responsible for most cases of mild mental retardation, it should be recognized that in no case have the specific genetic and environmental components been identified.

Some perspective regarding causation may be gained from studies of unselected populations of individuals with mental retardation (Tables 2–2 and 2–3).[11,12,15,19,26–41,46–48,70–72] When all ages are considered together, the cause can be determined in about half of cases. When only those under age 20 are included, a cause can be found in 55% of those with mild mental retardation and 65% of those with severe mental retardation. Genetic causes account for 25%–35% of mild mental retardation and 25%–35% of severe mental retardation. Among those with severe mental retardation, chromosome aberrations make up the most common genetic subcategory, and among those with mild mental retardation culturofamilial makes up the most common subcategory. Environmental causes account for 15%–25% of mild mental retardation and 20%–30% of severe mental retardation.

Table 2–2. Causation of Severe Mental Retardation: Comparison of Selected Studies from the Literature

Causation	*Anderson et al.*[72] *1996* *USA, South Carolina* *Institutions,* *Community* *Age < 20 Years* *IQ < 50*	*Anderson et al.*[72] *1996* *USA, South Carolina* *Institutions,* *Community* *Age > 19 Years* *IQ < 50*	*Yeargin-Allsopp et al.*[19] *1997* *USA, Georgia* *Full Population* *10-Year-Olds* *IQ < 50*	*Wellesley et al.*[47] *1991* *Australia* *Handicap* *Registry* *Age 6–16 Years* *IQ < 55*	*Molteno et al.*[27] *1990* *South Africa* *Institutions,* *Special Schools* *Age 1–12 Years* *IQ < 60*	*McQueen et al.*[29] *1986* *Canada* *Full* *Population* *Age 7–10 Years* *IQ < 55*	*Fryns et al.*[28] *1986* *Belgium* *Institutions* *Age 1–25* *Years* *IQ < 45*
1 Chromosomal	123 (10.5)*	568 (15.1)	26 (12.6)	157 (19.3)	198 (17.5)	58 (26.2)	26 (15.0)
2 Single gene	113 (9.6)	238 (6.3)	8 (3.9)	52 (6.4)	6 (0.5)	17 (7.7)	34 (19.7)
3 Multifactorial	35 (3.0)	34 (0.9)	3 (1.5)	36 (4.4)	25 (2.2)	5 (2.3)	2 (1.2)
4 Culturofamilial	63 (5.4)	108 (2.9)	0 (0)	67 (8.2)	0 (0)	1 (0.5)	0 (0)
5 Known syndrome	30 (2.6)	55 (1.5)	2 (1.0)	59 (7.2)	32 (2.8)	2 (0.9)	7 (4.0)
6 Other genetic	10 (0.9)	45 (1.2)	1 (0.5)	0 (0)	17 (1.5)	0 (0)	3 (1.7)
7 Injury, prenatal	3 (0.3)	17 (0.5)	0 (0)	19 (2.3)	0 (0)	0 (0)	0 (0)
8 Injury, perinatal	69 (5.9)	153 (4.1)	22 (10.7)	54 (6.6)	105 (9.3)	17 (7.7)	14 (8.1)
9 Injury, postnatal	30 (2.6)	76 (2.0)	5 (2.4)	20 (2.5)	27 (2.4)	0 (0)	2 (1.2)
10 Infection, prenatal	17 (1.4)	44 (1.2)	4 (1.9)	19 (2.3)	9 (0.8)	2 (0.9)	5 (2.9)
11 Infection, perinatal	15 (1.3)	12 (0.3)	0 (0)	0 (0)	0 (0)	0 (0)	0 (0)
12 Infection, postnatal	53 (4.5)	230 (6.1)	9 (4.4)	47 (5.8)	122 (10.8)	7 (3.2)	8 (4.6)
13 Chemical, prenatal	24 (2.0)	12 (0.3)	6 (2.9)	11 (13.5)	20 (1.8)	15 (6.8)	6 (3.5)
14 Chemical, perinatal	3 (0.3)	17 (0.5)	0 (0)	0 (0)	7 (0.6)	3 (1.4)	2 (1.2)
15 Chemical, postnatal	1 (0.1)	15 (0.4)	0 (0)	0 (0)	0 (0)	0 (0)	1 (0.6)
16 Prematurity	111 (9.4)	91 (2.4)	0 (0)	28 (3.4)	61 (5.4)	10 (4.5)	23 (13.3)
17 Other environmental	9 (0.8)	12 (0.3)	3 (1.5)	0 (0)	57 (5.0)	0 (0)	3 (1.7)
18 Unknown	467 (39.7)	2046 (54.2)	117 (56.7)	246 (30.2)	448 (39.5)	84 (38.0)	37 (21.4)
Total	1176†	3773	206	815	1134	221	173

(continued)

Table 2–2. Causation of Severe Mental Retardation: Comparison of Selected Studies from the Literature—*Continued*

Causation	*Czeizel et al.*[31] *1980* *Hungary* *Institutions, Special Schools* *Age 7–14 Years* *mod-severe MR*	*Hunter et al.*[32] *1980* *Canada* *Institutions* *Age < 20 Years* *IQ ≤ 50*	*Morrison*[33] *1977* *New Zealand* *All Sources* *Age < 65 Years* *IQ < 52*	*Laxova et al.*[35] *1977* *England* *Home, Institutions* *Age 0–10 Years* *IQ < 50*	*Kushlick and Cox*[15] *1973* *England* *Home, Institutions* *Age 15–19 Years* *IQ ≤ 54*	*Moser and Wolf*[11] *1971* *USA, Massachusetts* *Institution* *Age 0–89 years* *IQ ≤ 50*	*IQ 50–70*
1 Chromosomal	38 (12.8)	55 (13.5)	450 (20.0)	48 (32.9)	167 (27.5)	247 (22.9)	10 (3.4)
2 Single gene	41 (13.9)	47 (11.6)	24 (1.1)	21 (14.4)	4 (0.7)	56 (4.1)‡	
3 Multifactorial	0 (0)	15 (3.7)	47 (2.1)	7 (4.8)	5 (0.8)	0 (0)	0 (0)
4 Culturofamilial	17 (5.7)	1 (0.2)	0 (0)	0 (0)	25 (4.1)	44 (3.2)‡	
5 Known syndrome	0 (0)	5 (1.2)	1 (0)	2 (1.4)	0 (0)	10 (0.7)‡	
6 Other genetic	0 (0)	4 (1.0)	19 (0.8)	0 (0)	2 (0.3)	11 (0.8)‡	
7 Injury, prenatal	0 (0)	4 (1.0)	12 (0.5)	0 (0)	0 (0)	0 (0)	0 (0)
8 Injury, perinatal	98 (33.1)	26 (6.4)	146 (6.5)	7 (4.8)	84 (13.8)	71 (6.6)	17 (5.8)
9 Injury, postnatal	0 (0)	19 (4.7)	74 (3.3)	1 (0.7)	0 (0)	16 (1.5)	2 (0.7)
10 Infection, prenatal	14 (4.7)	10 (2.5)	43 (1.9)	1 (0.7)	2 (0.3)	34 (3.2)	4 (1.4)
11 Infection, perinatal	0 (0)	1 (0.2)	0 (0)	0 (0)	0 (0)	0 (0)	0 (0)
12 Infection, postnatal	29 (9.8)	28 (6.9)	158 (7.0)	3 (2.1)	21 (3.5)	41 (3.8)	13 (4.4)
13 Chemical, prenatal	0 (0)	8 (2.0)	37 (1.7)	0 (0)	0 (0)	0 (0)	0 (0)
14 Chemical, perinatal	4 (1.4)	11 (2.7)	0 (0)	0 (0)	27 (4.4)	4 (0.4)	3 (1.0)
15 Chemical, postnatal	0 (0)	0 (0)	8 (0.4)	0 (0)	0 (0)	2 (0.2)	0 (0)
16 Prematurity	0 (0)	13 (3.2)	54 (2.4)	0 (0)	1 (0.2)	97 (9.0)	36 (12.2)
17 Other environmental	6 (2.0)	7 (1.7)	0 (0)	0 (0)	1 (0.2)	1 (0.07)‡	
18 Unknown	49 (16.6)	152 (37.4)	1172 (52.2)	56 (38.4)	269 (44.2)	398(37.0)–95(6.9)‡–160(54.2)	
Total	296	406	2245	146	608	1077	295

MR, mental retardation.

*Number and percentage (in parentheses) of persons with mental retardation assigned to the causation category given in the first column.

†Total number of individuals with mental retardation in the study indicated in the column heading.

‡Severity of MR for these cases not provided.

TABLE 2–3. Causation of Mild Mental Retardation: Comparison of Selected Studies from the Literature

Causation	*Anderson et al.*[72] *1996 USA, South Carolina Institutions, Community Age < 20 Years IQ 50–70*	*Anderson et al.*[72] *1996 USA, South Carolina Institutions, Community Age > 19 Years IQ 50–70*	*Yeargin-Allsopp et al.*[19] *1997 USA, Georgia Full Population 10 Year Olds IQ 50–70*	*Wellesley et al.*[47] *1991 Australia Handicap Registry Age 6–16 Years IQ 55–70*	*Blomquist et al.*[30] *1981 Sweden MR Registry Age < 20 Years IQ 50–69*	*Czeizel et al.*[31] *1980 Hungary Institutions, Special Schools Age 7–14 Years Mild MR*	*Kushlick and Cox*[15] *1973 England Home, Institution Age 15–19 Years IQ 55–70*	*Moser and Wolf*[11] *1971 USA, Massachusetts Institution Age 0–89 Years*	
								IQ ≤ 50	*IQ 50–70*
1 Chromosomal	72 (9.8)*	47 (3.9)	9 (1.7)	49 (8.0)	13 (7.6)	34 (3.5)	18 (3.3)	247 (22.9)	10 (3.4)
2 Single gene	44 (6.0)	56 (4.6)	8 (1.6)	22 (3.6)	15 (8.8)	55 (5.6)	4 (0.7)	56 (4.1)‡	
3 Multifactorial	16 (2.2)	20 (1.7)	4 (0.8)	11 (1.8)	28 (16.4)	0 (0)	1 (0.2)	0 (0)	0 (0)
4 Culturofamilial	130 (17.8)	113 (9.4)	0 (0)	111 (18.1)	0 (0)	523 (53.4)	52 (9.7)	44 (3.2)‡	
5 Known syndrome	16 (2.2)	13 (1.1)	1 (0.2)	23 (3.7)	1 (0.6)	0 (0)	0 (0)	10 (0.7)‡	
6 Other genetic	6 (0.8)	12 (1.0)	1 (0.2)	0 (0)	0 (0)	0 (0)	0 (0)	11 (0.8)‡	
7 Injury, prenatal	2 (0.3)	0 (0)	0 (0)	10 (1.6)	0 (0)	0 (0)	0 (0)	0 (0)	0 (0)
8 Injury, perinatal	24 (3.3)	20 (1.7)	17 (3.3)	36 (5.9)	9 (5.3)	169 (17.2)	56 (10.4)	71 (6.6)	17 (5.8)
9 Injury, postnatal	4 (0.5)	47 (3.9)	6 (1.2)	20 (3.3)	4 (2.3)	0 (0)	0 (0)	16 (1.5)	2 (0.7)
10 Infection, prenatal	2 (0.3)	8 (0.7)	2 (0.4)	6 (1.0)	2 (1.2)	8 (0.8)	2 (0.4)	34 (3.2)	4 (1.4)
11 Infection, perinatal	12 (1.6)	2 (0.2)	3 (0.6)	0 (0)	1 (0.6)	0 (0)	0 (0)	0 (0)	0 (0)
12 Infection, postnatal	7 (1.0)	38 (3.1)	4 (0.8)	18 (2.9)	0 (0)	48 (4.9)	29 (5.4)	41 (3.8)	13 (4.4)
13 Chemical, prenatal	24 (3.3)	6 (0.5)	9 (1.8)	9 (1.5)	2 (1.2)	0 (0)	0 (0)	0 (0)	0 (0)
14 Chemical, perinatal	1 (0.1)	4 (0.3)	0 (0)	0 (0)	1 (0.6)	7 (0.7)	16 (3.0)	4 (0.4)	3 (1.0)
15 Chemical, postnatal	0 (0)	1 (0.1)	0 (0)	0 (0)	0 (0)	0 (0)	0 (0)	2 (0.2)	0 (0)
16 Prematurity	76 (10.4)	27 (2.2)	0 (0)	23 (3.7)	1 (0.6)	0 (0)	0 (0)	97 (9.0)	36 (12.2)
17 Other environmental	2 (0.3)	1 (0.1)	1 (0.2)	0 (0)	11 (6.4)	13 (1.3)	0 (0)	1 (0.7)‡	
18 Unknown	293 (40.1)	792 (65.6)	444 (87.2)	277 (45.0)	83 (48.5)	123 (12.6)	361 (67.0)	398(37.0)—95(6.9)‡	—160(54.2)
Total	731†	1207	509	615	171	980	539	1077	295

MR, mental retardation.

*Number and percentage (in parentheses) of persons with mental retardation assigned to the causation category given in the first column.

†Total number of persons with mental retardation in the study indicated in the column heading.

‡Severity of MR for these cases not provided.

Excess of Males with Mental Retardation

More than any other single factor, the excess of males among persons with mental retardation has forced consideration of the concept of X-linked mental retardation.[73–77] The male excess was noted from the earliest time that mental retardation was distinguished from other human maladies, was found among all grades of severity of mental deficiency, and was documented among persons with mental retardation in diverse populations worldwide.

Among early studies in which total and near total ascertainment was not possible, alternative explanations were sought for the male excess. In particular, social and bureaucratic factors were seen to influence the sex ratio of persons admitted to service programs and institutions.[74–76] Perceived or actual tendencies toward truancy, delinquency, aggressiveness, violence, and other behavioral aberrations among males with mental retardation favored more male admissions. Concerns regarding sexual exploitation of young women with mental retardation favored female admissions, particularly during the teen and early adult years. Allocation of beds by sex artificially fixed the male:female ratio according to administrative decisions. The degree to which each of these factors influenced the sex ratios reported in many early citations cannot be determined with any certainty.

From 1850 until the end of the 19th century, the U.S. Census recorded the number of mentally deficient persons by sex and race. While it is almost certain that the total numbers were underreported, the sex ratio always favored males.[78–80] Figures from the Eleventh Census of 1890 are typical.[80] Of the total 95,571 persons recorded as mentally retarded ("feeble-minded and idiotic"), 52,940 were males and 42,631 were females. Whites and blacks were alike in this regard. Among whites, the excess of males was 25%; among blacks, the excess was 21%.

A significant benchmark in the study of causation of mental deficiency resulted from investigations conducted in the 1930s under the auspices of Great Britain's Medical Research Council, the Darwin Trust, and the Royal Eastern Counties' Institution.[9,81] Referred to as the Colchester Survey, the study included 1280 institutionalized individuals with a wide range of mental retardation. Males outnumbered females among all severities of mental retardation except those with IQs above 70 who were deemed mentally retarded because of antisocial behavior (Table 2–4). The male excess was correlated directly with the severity of

TABLE 2–4. Male Excess Noted in Colchester Survey, 1938, by IQ Level[9]

IQ	*Males*	*Females*	*M:F*
0–19	139	81	1.72
20–49	248	185	1.34
50–70	235	213	1.10
>70 (with antisocial behavior)	88	91	0.96
All	710	570	1.25

TABLE 2–5. Male Excess Noted Among 7285 Individuals with Mental Retardation in South Carolina, by IQ Level[82]

Severity	*IQ*	*Males*	*Females*	*M:F*
Profound	<20	1166	964	1.21
Severe	20–34	835	610	1.37
Moderate	35–49	833	619	1.35
Mild	50–70	1130	841	1.34
Borderline/low normal	>70	180	107	1.68

mental retardation. An explanation for the male excess was not offered. Penrose acknowledged that there might be a "constitutional difference between the sexes which causes males to be more variable than females in respect of intelligence" but that there was "insufficient evidence here to support the view that sex-linked genes play a significant part in the aetiology of mental defect."[9]

Contemporary figures show equal or greater male excess among persons with mental retardation who are institutionalized as well as those who are enrolled in community service programs and public schools (Tables 2–5 through 2–7).[82,83] Surveys from many locations around the world confirm the universal recognition of the male excess among persons with mental retardation (Table 2–7).[14–48]

Confirmation of the male excess in studies with more complete ascertainment required an explanation other than selection factors that favored identification of males. The major biological inequity between males and females stems from the sex chromosome constitution. Whereas a deleterious gene on a male's single X chromosome may cause mental retardation, the same deleterious gene in a female may be silenced by the presence of a normal allele on her second X chromosome.

X-Linked Mental Retardation

Tables 2–8 through 2–12 chronicle the major observations fundamental to emergence of the concept of X-linked mental retardation. This chronicle has been partitioned into five eras on the basis of certain key clinical observations, benchmarks in the understanding of the genetics of mental retardation, and advances in genetic technology.

Era I: 1868–1942

In era I, the period prior to 1943, a number of distinctive syndromes in which mental retardation was one component were described.[84–94] As a group, these entities are notable in having somatic or neurologic manifestations which contribute in major measure to the conditions' importance apart from the impact of impaired cognitive function. Further, mental retardation associated with these conditions occurs inconsistently, inexplicably affecting some individuals and exempting others.

Table 2–6. Mental Retardation (MR) in U.S. Public School System, By Sex[83]

MR Severity	*# of States Reporting*	*Males*	*Females*	*M:F*
Mild	17	107,922	78,234	1.38
Moderate	5	6,624	4,086	1.62
Severe/profound	5	1,421	1,151	1.23

Table 2–7. Sex Ratio Among Persons With Mental Retardation, Selected Locations Worldwide

Year	*Location*	*Ascertainment*	*M:F*
1890[80]	United States	Census	1.24:1
1938[9]	England (Colchester)	Institution	1.25:1
1966[18]	Australia (Victoria)	Institution	1.21:1
1966[14]	Scotland	Registry	1.31:1
1971[11]	United States (Massachusetts)	Institution	1.48:1
1973[46]	Canada (Quebec)	Multiple Sources	1.27:1
1976[12]	Denmark	Multiple Sources	1.23:1
1976[12]	England (London)	Registry	1.72:1
1977[35]	England (Hertfordshire)	Multiple Sources	1.47:1
1977[12]	Sweden (Uppsala)	Registry	1.23:1
1980[32]	Canada (Manitoba)	Institution	1.27:1
1981[30]	Sweden (Vasterbotten)	Registry	1.80:1
1981[12]	England (Cornwall)	Multiple Sources	1.38:1
1984[12]	Japan	Multiple Sources	2.28:1
1985[17]	Canada (British Columbia)	Registry	1.40:1
1993[71]	Kuwait	Institution	1.46:1
1996[82]	United States (South Carolina)	Multiple Sources	1.32:1
1997[18]	United States (Georgia)	All Sources	1.45:1

Table 2–8. XLMR in Era I: 1868–1942*

Year	*Authors*	*MIM #*	*Current Nomenclature*
1868	Duchenne[84]	310200	Duchenne muscular dystrophy
1885, 1909	Pelizaeus,[85] Merzbacher[86]	312080	Pelizaeus-Merzbacher syndrome
1908	Mendes de Costa and Van der Valk[87]	302000	X-linked hereditary bullous dystrophy
1910	Zinsser[88]	308310	Dyskeratosis congenita
1917	Hunter[89]	309900	Mucopolysaccharidosis II
1926, 1927	Bloch,[90] Sulzberger[91]	308310	Incontinentia pigmenti
1927	Norrie[92]	310600	Norrie panophthalmia syndrome
1927	Rud[93]	308200	XLMR-ichthyosis-hypogonadism
1942	Albright et al.[94]	300800	Albright hereditary osteodystrophy

*XLMR, X-linked mental retardation; MIM, Mendelian Inheritance in Man.

It is during this era that the understanding of the sex constitution of humans evolved.[95–97] Only in the latter years of the era was there general consensus regarding the XX sex chromosome constitution of females. The nature of the male sex chromosome constitution—X or XY—was still strongly debated at the close of the era. Nevertheless, early observations noted the marked distortion of the male:female ratio in the conditions listed in era I (Table 2–8). In most, there was exclusive or near exclusive occurrence in males. In contrast, incontinentia pigmenti affected only females.

Although Duchenne (1868) reported that his first patient (Joseph S.) with "pseudohypertrophic muscle paralysis" was intellectually dull, nearly 100 years would pass before systematic quantitation of cognitive function would be undertaken.[84,98] Cognitive impairment, presumably a pleiotrophic affect of the responsible gene, has been found in about 20% of affected males. Duchenne failed to focus attention initially on the limitation of the condition to males, although many cases must have been brought to his attention. Shortly after Duchenne's death in 1875, Gowers reviewed the 24 cases examined by him personally and 196 other cases, specifically noting the frequency of familial cases, the limitation to males, the absence of antecedent cases in the paternal linkage, and the transmission through normal females.[99]

The entity described by Pelizaeus (1885) and Merzbacher (1909) is characterized by nystagmus, mental retardation, and spastic paraplegia.[85,86] Trofatter et al. (1989) mapped the condition to Xq22 and found a mutation in the gene for myelin proteolipid protein (PLP) in affected males in one large family.[100] Simultaneously, Hudson et al. (1989) found another mutation in PLP in a second family.[101]

Hunter syndrome, initially described in 1917, has been shown to be a lysosomal storage disease with inadequate breakdown of mucopolysaccharides.[89] For many years, Hunter syndrome was combined with Hurler syndrome and other clinically similar lysosomal storage diseases. Njå distinguished the X-linked variety based on pedigree analysis and the absence of corneal clouding.[102] One subtype, mucopolysaccharidosis IIA, consistently has mental retardation. A deficiency of the enzyme iduronate sulfatase underlies this condition. The gene has been mapped to Xq28.[103,104]

Congenital blindness due to a panophthalmia was described in males in two families by Norrie in 1927.[92] He clearly recognized that only males were affected and that females who transmitted the condition had no expression. Eight males were affected in two generations of one family and five males in three generations of the second family. This entity was distinguished as a nosologic entity in 1961 by Warburg, who had occasion to see an additional affected relative of Norrie's second family, to update the pedigree, and to extend the clinical and pathological observations.[105]

Three entities with prominent cutaneous manifestations—hereditary bullous dystrophy, dyskeratosis congenita, and incontinentia pigmenti—were described during era I.[87,88,90,91] Incontinentia pigmenti occurs almost exclusively in females and two different loci have been identified, IP-1 in Xp11 based on chromosome rearrangements in sporadic cases, IP-2 in Xq28 based on linkage analysis of familial cases.[106–108]

Albright hereditary osteodystrophy and Rud syndrome are retained in the chronology of era I for historical purposes.[93,94] Until recently, Albright hereditary osteodystrophy was considered an example of X-linked dominant inheritance. Instances of male to male transmission and females affected as severely as males have called X-linkage into question. A gene on the X chromosome has not been localized. Most cases have mutations in the gene on 20q that codes for guanine nucleotide stimulatory (G_s) protein.[109] A quite similar phenotype has been associated with deletions of 2q37.[110] As yet there is no molecular evidence for a gene on the X chromosome. Neither of the patients described by Rud had mental retardation.[93] The syndrome of X-linked mental retardation (XLMR), ichthyosis, hypogonadotrophic hypogonadism, anosmia, and seizures often referred to as Rud syndrome probably represents a contiguous gene deletion syndrome in Xp22.3 rather than a single gene disorder.[111,112]

The genes for Duchenne muscular dystrophy, Pelizaeus-Merzbacher syndrome, mucopolysaccharidosis II, and Norrie panophthalmia have been cloned.[100,101,104,113,114] X-linked hereditary bullous dystrophy has been regionally mapped to Xq27.3-qter, dyskeratosis congenita to Xq28, and two forms of incontinentia pigmenti to Xp11 and Xq28.[106–108,115,116] As noted above, the existence of X-linked genes for Albright hereditary osteodystrophy and XLMR-ichthyosis-hypogonadism (Rud syndrome) has been called into question.

Era II: 1943–1968

Era II extended from 1943 to 1968, beginning with Martin and Bell's description of a family with "sex-linked" mental retardation, now known to be the fragile X syndrome (Table 2–9).[105,117–147] This was a formative period in which entities in which mental retardation was the exclusive or predominant manifestation attracted attention. It was a time as well when a number of syndromic entities (Renpenning, Börjeson-Forssman-Lehmann, Menkes, Lesch-Nyhan, Lowe, and Coffin-Lowry syndromes) which have now claimed important places in the field of XLMR were first recognized. This formative time culminated in the thesis of Lehrke in 1968 in which he proposed the concept of nonsyndromic X-linked mental retardation.[147]

Martin and Bell (1943) accepted "sex-linked" inheritance as the explanation for the presence of severe mental retardation in a family with 11 affected males in two generations.[117] This report constitutes the first entity with "sex-linked" inheritance in which mental retardation consistently appeared as the dominant manifestation. Affected males were described to be of sturdy build but without "any distinctiveness in shape of head or face . . . or other observed characteristic." Following Sutherland's (1977) demonstration of the association of the fragile site at Xq27.3 in other families with XLMR, this first family with XLMR was restudied by Richards et al. (1981) and shown to have the clinical features of this syndrome as well as the Xq27.3 fragile site.[148,149] It should be stated that Martin and Bell (1943) had noted that females could be affected, although less commonly and less severely than males. They also had predicted the occurrence of transmitting males: "All but one of the mothers concerned were the daugh-

TABLE 2–9. XLMR in Era II: 1943–1968

Year	*Authors*	*MIM*	*Current Nomenclature*
1943	Martin and Bell[117]	309550	Fragile X syndrome
1944	Allan et al.[118]	309600	Allan-Herndon-Dudley syndrome
1949	Bickers and Adams[119]	308840	X-linked hydrocephaly–MASA spectrum
1952	Lowe et al.[120]	309000	Lowe syndrome
1955	Lenz[121]	309800	Lenz microphthalmia syndrome
1959	van den Bosch[122]	314500	XLMR-choroideremia-ectodermal dysplasia
1960	Paine[123]	311400	Paine
1960, 1995	Mohr and Mageroy,[124] Tranebjaerg et al.[125]	304700	Mohr-Tranebjaerg syndrome
1961	Gorlin et al.[126]	311200	Oral-facial-digital I syndrome
1961	Losowsky[127]	309550	Fragile X syndrome
1961	Warburg[105]	310600	Norrie panophthalmia syndrome
1961	Warkany et al.[129]	308400	Warkany syndrome
1962	Renpenning et al.[128]	309500	Renpenning syndrome
1962	Börjeson et al.[130]	301900	Börjeson-Forssman-Lehmann syndrome
1962	Goltz et al.[131]	305600	Goltz syndrome
1962	Russell et al.[132]	311250	Ornithine transcarbamylase deficiency
1962–3	Dunn et al.[133]	309550	Fragile X syndrome
1962, 1964	Hoefnagal et al.,[134] Fanconi et al.[135]	300100	Adrenoleukodystrophy
1963	Menkes[136]	309400	Menkes syndrome
1964	Lesch and Nyhan[137]	308000	Lesch-Nyhan syndrome
1964	Plott[138]	308850	Plott syndrome
1964, 1982	Menkes et al.,[139] Kaplan[140]	304100	X-linked hydrocephaly—MASA* spectrum
1965	Åkesson[141]	304200	XLMR-thyroidaplasia-cutis verticis gyrata
1966	Baar and Gabriel[142]	312890	Baar-Gabriel syndrome
1966	Rett[143]	312250	Rett syndrome
1966, 1971	Coffin et al.,[144] Lowry and Miller[145]	303600	Coffin-Lowry syndrome
1967	Dudding et al.[146]	311300	Otopalatodigital I syndrome
1968	Lehrke[147]		Nonsyndromic XLMR

*MASA: *m*ental retardation, *a*phasia, *s*huffling gait, and *a*dducted thumbs.

ters of two brothers, the other being their sister; these two brothers are said to have been normal and the hypothesis is put forth that some controlling factor causes depression of the disease in them without affecting their liability to transmit it."[117]

Dunn et al. (1962–1963) noted a distinctive appearance with long face, prominent and malformed ears, and large mandible among 20 affected males in a Canadian family and published a photograph of the facial features in their report.[133] Later, Fox et al. (1980) found males in this family to have macroorchidism and demonstrated the fragile X chromosome.[150] Losowsky (1961) evaluated one male and one female in a family with severe mental retardation in 10 males and milder mental handicap in two females.[127] It is now known that this family represents the fragile X syndrome based on the demonstration of the Xq27.3 fragile site cytogenetically and a 500 bp expansion of the CGG repeat of the FMR1 gene in the only living affected female (Mueller 1996, personal communication).

A six-generation family with XLMR was described in 1944 by the pioneer American geneticists William Allan and Nash Herndon and their social worker associate Florence Dudley.[118] Twenty-four males were affected with global developmental delay, muscle weakness and atrophy, wide-based uncoordinated gait, depressed deep tendon reflexes, and severe mental retardation. Carrier females exhibited no abnormality. Stevenson et al. updated the pedigree in 1990 and noticed that with increased age affected males became spastic with dysarthria, ataxia, and hyperreflexia.[151] The condition was mapped to Xq21.[152] Additional families have been identified by Bialer et al. (1992) and Martin et al. (unpublished).[153] Other families reported as having X-linked spastic paraplegia (Malamud and Cohen 1958; Johnston and McKusick 1962; Baar and Gabriel 1966; Bundey and Griffiths 1977; Wieacker et al. 1985; and Apak et al. 1989) may represent the Allan-Herndon-Dudley syndrome or allelic entities.[142,154–158]

Perhaps the best known of the early XLMR reports is that of Renpenning et al. (1962).[128] While a medical student at the University of Saskachewan, Hans Renpenning identified a large family of Dutch Mennonite extraction in which 20 males in three generations had severe mental retardation. Affected males showed a tendency to small head circumference and prominent ears but other distinctive features were not described. The mothers had no distinctive features and normal intellect. Restudy of this family by Fox et al. (1980) and Stevenson et al. (1998) confirmed that affected males tended to have small head circumference, small testicular size, and short stature.[150,159] Linkage analysis placed the gene locus for Renpenning syndrome in the proximal short arm between Xp11.2 and Xp11.4.[159]

The first convincing demonstration of X-linked inheritance of hydrocephaly was made by Bickers and Adams in 1949.[119] They described a family with seven affected infants in two generations and gave detailed clinical and neuropathological findings in one infant. Hydrocephaly was shown to be caused by stenosis of the aqueduct of Sylvius. No mention was made of clasped thumb. X-linked hydrocephaly has since been linked to markers in Xq28 by Willems et al. (1990),[160] a location shared with MASA (*m*ental retardation, *a*phasia, *s*huffling gait, and *a*dducted thumbs) syndrome, clasped thumb syndrome, complicated spastic paraplegia[161,162] and agenesis of the corpus callosum.[163] Mutations in a candidate gene, L1CAM, have been reported for this complex of allelic conditions by Rosenthal et al. (1992) and Vits et al. (1994).[164,165]

Several noteworthy inborn errors of metabolism were recognized in the 1950s and 1960s. In Lowe syndrome, affected males have cataracts, glaucoma, growth failure, rickets, and mental retardation associated with aminoaciduria.[120] The disorder has been mapped to Xq26. The responsible gene coding for phosphatidylinositol biphosphate phosphatase (OCRL1), has been isolated, and mutations identified.[166,167] Lesch-Nyhan syndrome is caused by deficiency of hypoxanthine-guanine pyrophosphate ribosyl transferase (HPRT).[137] Clinical manifestations include choreoathetosis, severe mental impairment, and self-mutilation.[137,168] The gene, located at Xq26, was cloned by Jolly et al. (1983).[169] Menkes syndrome, a degenerative disease of the nervous system, was reported in 1962.[136] In addition to mental deterioration, affected males have growth impairment and kinky hair. The gene for Menkes syndrome (ATP7A) maps to Xq13 and is responsible for copper transport.[170–172]

Two of the more widely recognized XLMR syndromes—Borjeson-Forssman-Lehmann syndrome and Coffin-Lowry syndrome—were described in era II. Borjeson, Forssman, and Lehmann described three males with puffy face, large ears, short stature, obesity, hypogonadism, seizures, and mental impairment.[130] A number of additional families have been described and the entity has been regionally mapped to Xq26 by Turner et al. (1989) and Mathews et al. (1989).[173,174] Fibroblast growth factor homologous factor 2 (FHF2) has been proposed as a candidate gene on the basis of its localization at a duplication breakpoint in Xq26.3 in a male with a BFL-like phenotype.[175] Coffin and colleagues described two unrelated males with short stature, coarse facies, skeletal anomalies, and large soft hands.[144] Females had mild mental impairment and coarse facies. A three-generation pedigree with 10 affected males and females was reported several years later by Lowry and Miller.[145] For a time, the two reports were thought to represent two different syndromes. They were convincingly argued to be the same by Temtamy et al., who reported three additional families in 1975.[176] The responsible gene, RSK-2, a growth factor-related serine threonine kinase, has been mapped to Xp22.[177]

An intriguing syndrome in which girls who appear normal at birth and during the initial months of life but thereafter undergo multiphasic deterioration was described by Rett in 1966.[143] Developmental progress slows and stops in early childhood, growth rate decreases, and interaction with the environment wanes. Rapid loss of purposeful hand use, social skills, speech, and cognitive function ensues coincident with jerky limb and trunk movements, autistic mannerisms, disorganized respiratory efforts and seizures. After a variable period of less obvious deterioration, motor function worsens, eventually leading to muscle wasting, and cachexia, loss of mobility, hypertonicity, hyperreflexia, clonus, and vasomotor disturbances. Although Rett's publication went largely unnoticed for a number of years, the condition is now one of the most widely recognized of the X-linked conditions in which expression is limited to females.

Era II closes with the submission of a thesis by Lehrke in which he argued for the existence of major genes related to intellectual function located on the X chromosome.[147] Such genes, he hypothesized, affected brain structure or function and, if mutated, could lead to mental retardation. He culled five pedigrees from the literature (Martin and Bell 1943; Allan et al. 1944; Losowsky 1961; Renpenning et al. 1962; Dunn et al. 1963)[117,118,127,128,133] and added five pedigrees from the University of Wisconsin Genetic Counseling Center to illustrate the phenomenon, which he termed "nonspecific X-linked mental retardation."

Era III: 1969–1976

Era III encompassed the decade that began with the initial discovery of the Marker X syndrome by Lubs (1969) and may be best remembered as the time when the existence of this syndrome as an important cause of mental retardation could not be confirmed (Table 2–10).[76,178–193] As would be discovered later, this was due in large part to a coincidental change in the culture media commonly used to grow lymphocytes for chromosome analysis.[148,194,195] Prior to 1969, lymphocyte culture media lacked folic acid and it is in this folate-deficient environment that the Marker X was best manifested. Most cytogenetic laboratories began using folic-acid-supplemented media in the late 1960s and thus unknowingly precluded demonstration of the Marker X chromosome.

The pattern of somatic manifestations of a number of X-linked syndromes with mental retardation was recognized during era III. Among others, these included Aicardi syndrome, telecanthus-hypospadias syndrome (also know as Opitz BBB, Opitz G, and Opitz BBB/G syndromes), Aarskog-Scott syndrome, Opitz FG syndrome, and Pallister W syndrome. Of these, perhaps Aarskog-Scott syndrome has the greatest prevalence and poses the least diagnostic quandary. In 1970, Aarskog described a condition with growth impairment and distinct craniofacial, genital, and musculoskeletal abnormalities in seven males in one family.[182] Following his presentation of the family at the Third Conference on the Clinical Delineation of Birth Defects (1970), Scott showed a second family with nine affected males in four generations.[196] An X:8 translocation led to the localization of the gene, which was confirmed by linkage analysis.[197,198] The gene, FGD1, a

TABLE 2–10. XLMR in Era III: 1969–1976

Year	*Authors*	*MIM*	*Current Nomenclature*
1969	Lubs[178]	309550	Fragile X syndrome
1969	Aicardi et al.[179]	304050	Aicardi syndrome
1969	Opitz et al.[180]	300000	Telecanthus-hypospadias syndrome (G/BBB syndrome)
1969	Snyder and Robinson[181]	309583	Snyder-Robinson syndrome
1969	van Wijngaarden et al.[182]	310400	Myotubular myopathy
1970	Aarskog[183]	305400	Aarskog-Scott syndrome
1971	Juberg and Hellman[184]		XLMR-epilepsy
1972	AvRuskin et al.[185]		XLMR-TBG* deficiency
1974	Lehrke[76]		Nonsyndromic XLMR
1974	Cantú et al.[186]	308830	Cantú syndrome
1974	Max et al.[187]	305650	G_{M3} gangliosidosis (historical note only)
1974	Bianchine and Lewis[188]	303350	X-linked hydrocephaly-MASA spectrum
1974	Nance et al.[189]	302350	Nance-Horan syndrome
1974	Opitz and Kaveggia[190]	305450	Opitz FG syndrome
1974	Pallister et al.[191]	311450	Pallister W syndrome
1975	Went et al.[192]	311050	Optic atrophy-2, Went syndrome
1976	Fitch et al.[193]	304120	Otopalatodigitial II syndrome

*Thyroid-binding globulin.

rho rac guanine nucleotide exchange factor, has been identified and mutations have been demonstrated in several families.[199]

Two entities, Aicardi syndrome and XLMR-epilepsy, represent a group of X-linked disorders with mental retardation, now numbering seven, in which females are affected exclusively or nearly so.[179,184,200,201] Gestational lethality in males has been proposed to explain this phenomenon. Thomas has proposed that germline mutations in the father may better explain the limitation of the phenotype to females in these conditions.[201] He cites the absence of excess gestational loss of males as argument for this alternative explanation. Furthermore, the entities are generally short-lived since affected females often do not reproduce.

Bianchine and Lewis assigned the acronym MASA to a syndrome of mental retardation, aphasia, shuffling gait, and adducted thumbs that occurred in one family with six males and one female affected.[188] MASA syndrome is now known to be caused by mutations in the L1 cell adhesion molecule and is allelic to X-linked hydrocephaly, clasp thumb, complicated spastic paraplegia, and some cases of agenesis of the corpus callosum.[160–165,202]

An additional family with nine males in three generations considered to have nonspecific mental retardation was reported by Snyder and Robinson in 1969.[181] All were in their childhood years at the time of the initial description and manifested hypotonia, dysequilibrium, and mild mental retardation. Several had enlarged head circumferences. As adults, males have shown asthenic habitus, asymmetrical face, high-arched palate, muscle hypoplasia, scoliosis, and wide-based gait. This entity has been regionally mapped to Xp21.2 by Arena et al. (1996).[203]

Aside from Lubs's description of the fragile X syndrome, perhaps era III would be less memorable were it not for Lehrke's thesis becoming more widely available through publication in part in the *American Journal of Mental Deficiency* (1972) and redistribution as a monograph in the *Birth Defects: Original Article Series* (1974).[75,76,147,204–206] Lehrke put forth four hypotheses in support of his basic proposal that "there are cases of mental retardation or verbal disability, not easily identifiable individually on either an etiologic or clinical basis, that are totally or in part due to deleterious alleles of genes on the X chromosome":

1. Major genetic loci relating to human intellectual functioning are located on the X chromosome.
2. These genes, if mutated, can lead to subnormal intellectual functioning, including mental retardation, transmitted in an X-linked manner.
3. One or more of these major genes relates particularly to verbal functioning.
4. The deficit relates primarily to the central nervous system.

He cautioned that XLMR, although common, requires alertness to identify affected individuals and families.[76] Cases may be easily missed if family history is not pursued diligently, if the traceable family is small, if some carrier females have manifestations, if male gene carriers lack expression, if extraneous cases of mental retardation confuse the picture, and if the mutation is too recent to show the typical X-linked pedigree.

Lehrke's proposal, although widely accepted today, met with less than universal approval initially. Anastasi thought the evidence in favor of Lehrke's proposal was meager and at worst "irrelevant or misleading."[204] She doubted that nonspecific X-linked mental retardation could account for a large portion of the undiagnosed mental retardation (MR) but called for comprehensive evaluations of families in which XLMR appeared to be segregating. Nance and Engel questioned the basic premise that males were more commonly affected with MR than females and argued that pedigrees in which at least one female showed manifestations could not be readily attributed to an X-linked gene.[205]

Era IV: 1977–1987

Rediscovery of the fragile X syndrome marked the beginning of era IV and efforts to ascertain cases, delineate the clinical phenotype, and understand the epidemiology occupied the attention of physicians and scientists throughout the era (Table 2–11).[148,157,207–242] A place of prominence for the fragile X syndrome was claimed almost immediately with recognition that it accounted for 2%–6% of mental retardation in males and for 30%–40% of cases of XLMR. It was, in fact, quickly recognized as the most common of the specific heritable causes of mental retardation.

Numerous confounding aspects of the fragile X syndrome persisted through much of the era. Not the least of these was the quandary about the relationship between the syndrome and the fragile site at Xq27.3. Although cytogenetic expression of the fragile site was consistently present in males with mental retardation, it was never found in 100% of cells. The cytogenetic expression in obligate female carriers was even more perplexing. In some, no expression could be found; in others, expression was as high as that in males. A proportion, variously estimated at 30%–50% of females with cytogenetic expression, had significant learning disabilities, including frank cognitive impairment. The concept of transmitting or nonpenetrant males became necessary to explain transmission of the fragile X gene to all daughters of a male who had no clinical or cytogenetic evidence of the syndrome. In fairness, it should be noted that Martin and Bell (1943) and Dunn et al. (1963) predicted the existence of transmitting males on the basis of pedigree analysis of the two large families they evaluated.[117,133] Perhaps most intriguing was the observation—termed the Sherman Paradox—that daughters of transmitting males were more likely to have affected offspring than mothers of transmitting males. Explanations for most of these observations became obvious with the cloning of the FMR1 gene in 1991 and recognition that an unstable trinucleotide repeat segment was the site of virtually all mutations in the gene.[243–246]

Several XLMR entities described during era IV as distinct entities are now recognized or are suspected to be allelic to other XLMR entities delineated before or after (Table 2–11). Juberg and Marsidi described three males with intrauterine growth impairment, microcephaly, small palpebral fissures, strabismus, flat

TABLE 2–11. XLMR in Era IV: 1977–1987

Year	*Authors*	*MIM*	*Current Nomenclature*
1977	Harvey et al.,[207] Sutherland,[148] Giraud et al.[208]	309550	Fragile X syndrome
1977	Christian et al.[209]	309620	Christian skeletal dysplasia syndrome
1977	Feinberg and Leahy[210]	308350	West syndrome
1977	McCabe et al.[211]	307030	Glycerol kinase deficiency
1978	Riccardi and Marcus[212]		Hydrocephaly-cerebellar agenesis syndrome
1979	Urban et al.[213]		Urban syndrome
1979	Vasquez et al.[214]		Vasquez syndrome
1980	Juberg and Marsidi[215]	301040	Juberg-Marsidi syndrome (XLMR-hypotonic facies syndrome)
1980	Smith et al.[216]	309580	Smith-Fineman-Myers syndrome
1981	Jensen[217]	311150	Jensen syndrome (Mohr-Tranebjaerg syndrome)
1981	Say and Meyer[218]	314320	Say-Meyer syndrome
1982	Simpson et al.,[219] Golabi and Rosen,[220] Behmel et al.[221]	312870	Simpson-Golabi-Behmel syndrome
1982	Young and Hughes[222]		Young-Hughes syndrome
1983	Fitzsimmons et al.[223]	309560	Fitzsimmons syndrome
1984	Golabi et al.[224]		Golabi-Ito-Hall syndrome
1984	Gareis and Mason[225]	303350	X-linked hydrocephaly-MASA spectrum
1984	Holmes and Gang[226]		Holmes-Gang syndrome (XLMR-hypotonic facies syndrome)
1984	Livingstone et al.[227]	312170	Pyruvate dehydrogenase deficiency
1984	Lujan et al.[228]	309520	Lujan marfanoid habitus syndrome
1984	Schimke et al.[229]		Schimke syndrome
1984	Siber[230]		Cerebrooculogenital syndrome
1985	Atkin et al.[231]		Atkin-Flaitz syndrome
1985	Cowchock et al.[232]	310490	Charcot-Marie-Tooth, Cowchock variant
1985	Duker et al.[233]		Cerebrooculogenital syndrome
1985	Toriello et al.[234]	301950	X-linked branchial arch syndrome
1985	Wieacker et al.[157]		Wieacker-Wolff syndrome
1986	Bergia et al.[235]	309660	Bergia syndrome
1986	Kenwrick et al.[236]		X-linked hydrocephaly-MASA spectrum
1986	Fryns et al.[237]		XLMR-macroorchidism
1987	Hunter and MacMurray[238]	314390	VACTERL*-hydrocephalus syndrome
1987	Farlow et al.[239]	301840	Ataxia-dementia
1987	Goldblatt et al.[240]		XLMR-hypospadias
1987	Prieto et al.[241]	309610	Prieto syndrome
1987	Schmidley et al.[242]	301790	X-linked ataxia-deafness-dementia

*VACTERL: *v*ertebral, *a*nal, *c*ardiac, *t*racheal, *e*sophageal, *r*enal, and *l*imb anomalies.

nasal bridge, genital hypoplasia, and deafness.[215] This XLMR syndrome was shown to be due to a mutation in XNP, the gene responsible for XLMR-hypotonic facies syndrome (α-thalassemia mental retardation), an XLMR syndrome that was delineated clinically and molecularly during the 1990s.[247–249] Other XLMR entities that now have separate identities but are good candidates to be examples of XNP mutations include Holmes-Gang, Carpenter-Waziri, and Smith-Fineman-Myers syndromes.[216,222,226] Jensen described a syndrome with sensorineural deafness, progressive optic atrophy and vision loss, and adult-onset dementia in two brothers and their maternal nephew.[217] The syndrome has now been shown to be caused by a mutation in DDP, the gene responsible for the Mohr-Tranebjaerg syndrome, an entity described in 1960.[124,125,250] Schmidley syndrome, comprised of infancy-onset optic atrophy, sensorineural deafness, hypotonia, and progressive cerebellar signs and dementia, is another candidate for allelism.[243] Gareis and Mason reported six males with clasp thumb and mild mental retardation, an X-linked entity now known to be a part of the X-linked hydrocephaly-MASA spectrum, and due to mutation in the L1 cell adhesion molecule.[160–165,225]

Two variants of X-linked peripheral motor and sensory neuropathy were reported in era IV.[210,232] These two, the Cowchock and Ionasescu variants, have since been mapped to different regions of the X chromosome and have clinical manifestations which help to distinguish them from the more common CMTIA, CMTIB, and CMT2 types which map to 17p, 1q, and 1p, respectively.[251,252]

Some reservation must be maintained regarding the status of two entities listed as XLMR in Table 2–11. In Lujan marfanoid habitus syndrome, manifest by a long and narrow expressionless facies, large head, small mandible, general asthenia, pectus excavatum, joint hyperextensibility, and abnormal speech, only relatively small families have been identified, linkage analysis has not identified a gene location, and the condition may well be heterogeneous.[228,253,254] Glycerol kinase deficiency, described by McCabe in 1977, may not in itself cause mental retardation but instead may only do so when it is a part of a contiguous gene deletion syndrome.[211]

At the close of era IV, efforts to regionally map the XLMR syndromes were beginning to yield results. Certain gene localizations became possible through the fortuitous finding of X chromosome deletions or X:autosome translocations associated with an XLMR phenotype (see Chapter 1, Table 1–4).[255–263] In other cases, these early mapping successes utilized restriction fragment length polymorphisms (RFLPs) as markers to which candidate XLMR syndromes with large families available could be linked.[264,265]

Era V: 1988–Present

Early reports in era V set the standard for those to follow by including mapping information with the clinical delineation of XLMR (Table 2–12).[125,158,266–298] This became possible because of the availability of restriction fragment length polymorphisms distributed along the X chromosome which could be linked to XLMR disease loci. Two laboratories, one in Strasbourg headed by Jean-Louis Mandel and the other in Adelaide headed by Grant Sutherland, took the lead in these mapping efforts. Their initial successes were reported at the Third International Workshop on Fragile X and X-Linked Mental Retardation held in Torina, Sicily in 1987 and appeared in press in 1988.[299–302] The first mapping for nonsyndromic XLMR accompanied mapping of a number of XLMR syndromes in this wave.[270] Initially, these localizations were either very broad or reported only as linkages

TABLE 2–12. XLMR in Era V: 1988–Present

Year	*Authors*	*MIM #*	*Current Nomenclature*
1988	Carpenter et al.[266]	—	Carpenter-Waziri syndrome (XLMR-hypotonic facies syndrome)
1988	Chudley et al.[267]	309490	Chudley-Lowry syndrome
1988	Partington et al.[268]	309510	Partington syndrome
1988	Sutherland et al.[269]	309470	Sutherland-Haan syndrome
1988	Suthers et al.[270]	—	MRX1
1988	Tranebjaerg et al.[271]	309480	XLMR-psoriasis
1989	Apak et al.[158]	302500	Apak ataxia–spastic diplegia syndrome
1989	Goldblatt et al.[272]	312920	Goldblatt spastic paraplegia syndrome
1990	al-Gazali et al.[273]	309801	MIDAS syndrome*
1990	Graham et al.[274]	301590	Graham anophthalmia syndrome
1991	Wilkie et al.,[275] Gibbons et al.[276]	301040	XLMR-hypotonic facies (α-thalassemia mental retardation)
1991	Miles and Carpenter[277]	309605	Miles-Carpenter syndrome
1991	Pettigrew et al.[278]	304340	Pettigrew syndrome
1991	Stocco dos Santos et al.[279]	—	Stocco dos Santos syndrome
1991	Stoll et al.[280]	—	Stoll syndrome
1991	Wilson et al.[281]	309585	Wilson-Turner syndrome
1992	Arena et al.[282]	—	Arena spastic paraplegia syndrome
1992	Bertini et al.[283]	—	Bertini syndrome
1992	Hyde-Forster et al.[284]	—	Hyde-Forster syndrome
1992	Kang et al.[285]	—	Kang syndrome
1992	Porteous et al.[286]	—	Porteous syndrome
1992	Proud et al.[287]	—	Proud syndrome
1992	Tranebjaerg et al.[288]	—	XLMR-ataxia-apraxia
1993	Arts et al.[289]	301835	Arts syndrome
1993	Brunner et al.[290]	301850	Monoamine oxidase-A deficiency
1993	Gustavson et al.[291]	—	Gustavson syndrome
1994	Aldred et al.[292]	—	XLMR-retinitis pigmentosa
1994	Brooks et al.[293]	—	Brooks syndrome
1995	Tranebjaerg et al.[125]	—	Mohr-Tranebjaerg syndrome
1996	Hamel et al.[294]	—	XLMR-growth hormone deficiency
1996	Lindsay et al.[295]	—	PPM-X syndrome†
1996	Wittwer et al.[296]	—	Wittwer syndrome
1997	Stevenson et al.[297]	—	XLMR-arch fingerprints–hypotonia
1998	Armfield et al.[298]	—	Armfield syndrome

*MIDAS: microphthalmia, dermal aplasia, and sclerocornea.
†PPM-X: X-linked psychosis, pyramidal signs, and macroorchidism.

to a single DNA marker. For example, the Wieacker-Wolff and Carpenter-Waziri syndromes were reported as linked solely to DXYS1, a locus in the X-Y homology region of Xq21.3.[157,266] Because of the small number of RFLP markers and because these markers were often diallelic and relatively uninformative, mapping progressed slowly. Nonetheless, notable entities such as the Coffin-Lowry syndrome (CLS), Allan-Herndon-Dudley syndrome (AHD), Börjeson-Forssman-Lehmann syndrome (BFL), X-linked hydrocephaly spectrum, and XLMR-hypotonic facies syndrome (α-thalassemia X-linked mental retardation: ATR-X), were localized by 1992.[152,175,301–306]

Microsatellite or dinucleotide repeat markers became available in the early 1990s and greatly enhanced the mapping of XLMR conditions.[307,308] These markers, widely distributed along the X chromosome and, indeed, the entire genome, usually had a minimum of four alleles of varying frequencies, permitting linkage in most families with seven or more potentially informative meioses. Most investigators accepted a lod score of 2 to indicate linkage for X-linked disorders, although confounding results such as more than one region of linkage were found on occasion.[160,309] As a result, the pace of mapping of XLMR entities, both syndromic and nonsyndromic, quickened considerably so that by 1998, 120 XLMR syndromes and 58 families with nonsyndromic XLMR had been regionally localized (Fig. 2–2).[310]

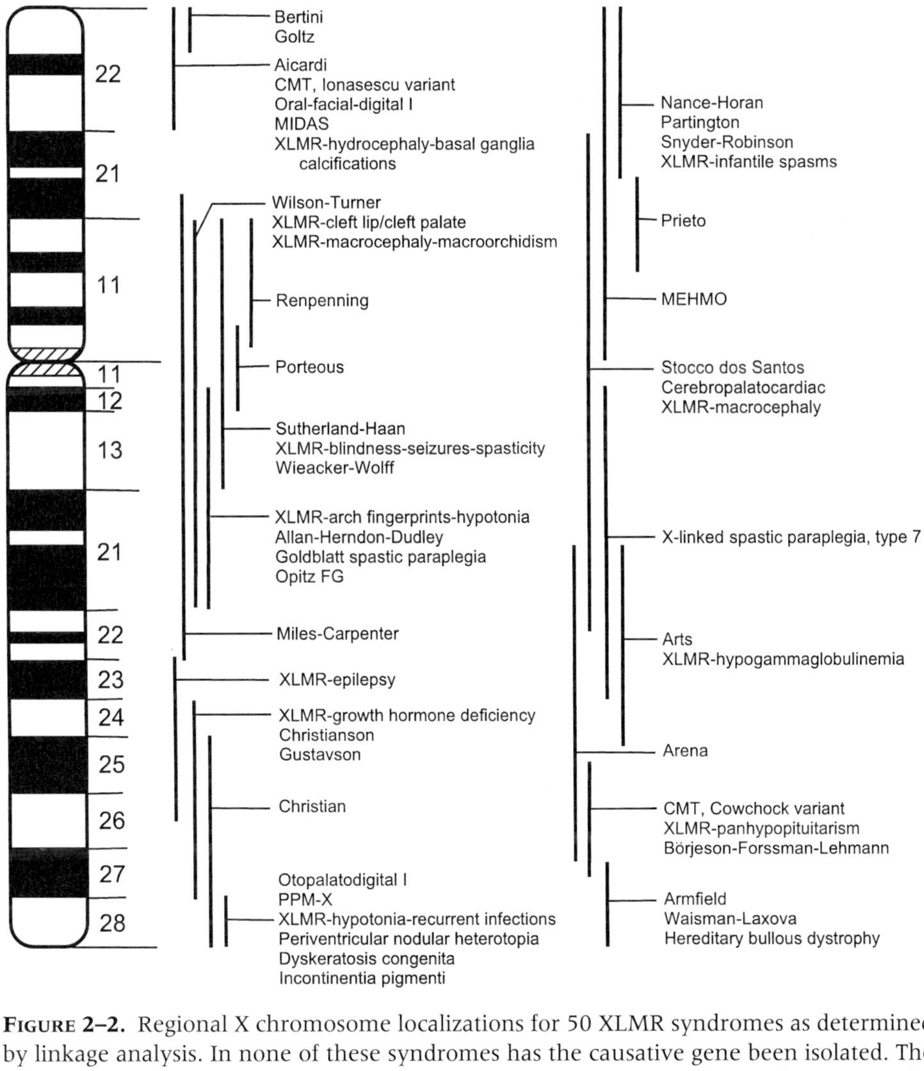

FIGURE 2–2. Regional X chromosome localizations for 50 XLMR syndromes as determined by linkage analysis. In none of these syndromes has the causative gene been isolated. The linkage limits are approximate, extending from the disease locus in each direction to the closest marker with recombination.

Nosologic considerations became more pressing with the rapid progress in mapping. One convention, the assignment of the acronym MRX (mental retardation, X-linked) and sequential numbers, was adopted for nonsyndromic XLMR.[311] Each family with nonsyndromic XLMR with lod score of ≥2 on linkage analysis was assigned an MRX number, in sequence as reported. MRX1–MRX58, mapped between 1988 and 1997, comprised at least 10 exclusive linkage groups (Fig. 2–3).[310–314] Hence, it is expected that many of the nonsyndromic XLMR families will have allelic mutations. To date, this has been demonstrated only for MRX41 and MRX48, each having a mutation in the Rab guanosine diphosphate (GDP)-dissociation inhibitor 1 gene (GDI1).[315] A number of families with nonsyndromic XLMR remain outside this system, however,

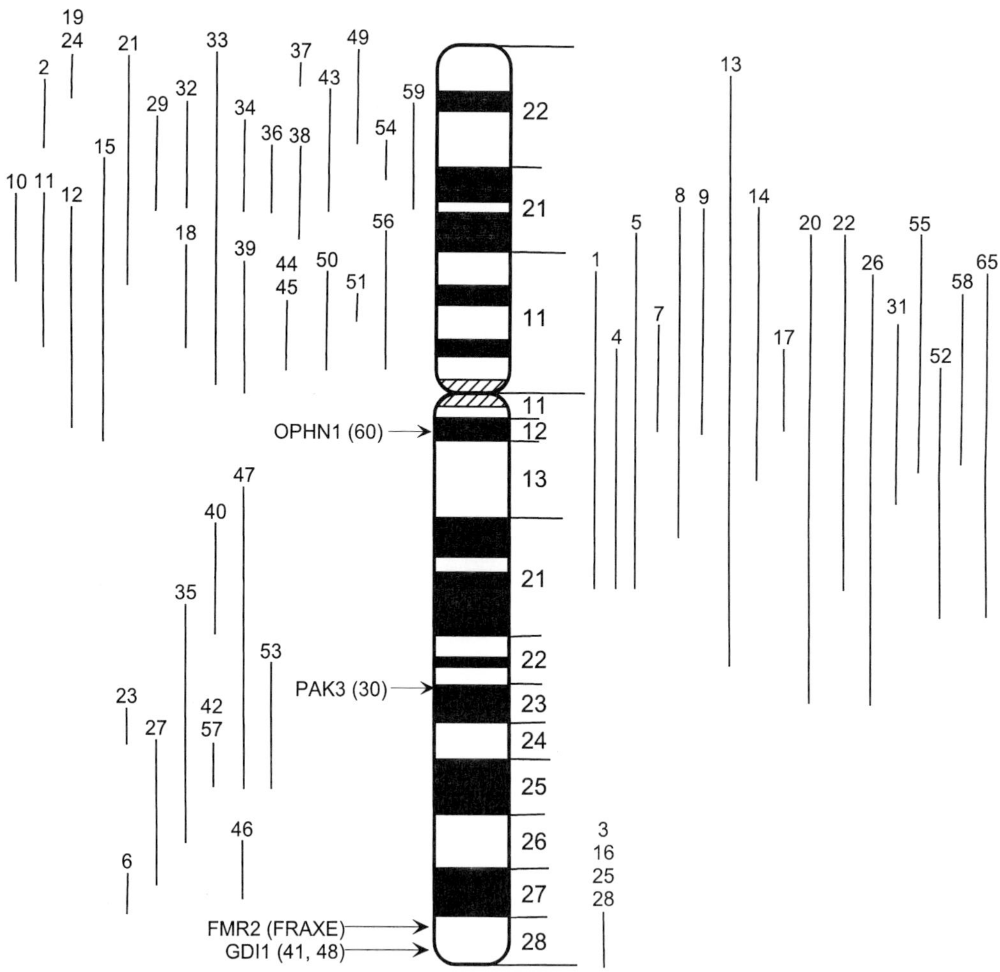

FIGURE 2–3. Approximate linkage limits for 56 families with nonsyndromic XLMR. Families are identified by their assigned MRX number (refer to Table 3.1). The arrows indicate the localizations of four genes that have been cloned: guanine diphosphate-dissociation inhibitor 1 (GDI1), responsible for MRX41 and MRX48; p21-activated kinase (PAK3), responsible for MRX30; oligophrenin 1 (OPHN1), responsible for MRX60; and familial mental retardation 2, responsible for the Fragile XE syndrome.

having been reported prior to adoption of the MRX convention or being of insufficient size or informativeness to achieve a lod score of ≥2.[76,77,316–320]

A similar system for the nomenclature of the XLMR syndromes was adopted in 1992.[311] It assigns an MRXS number to syndromes which have been linked (lod score ≥2) to X chromosome markers. However, the mixed system of nomenclature comprised of eponymic, descriptive, and acronymic designations already in place shows little sign of giving way to this suggested convention.

The other notable feature of era V was the cloning of genes responsible for XLMR (Fig. 2–4). Prior to era V, few genes—only those causing Lesch-Nyhan syndrome, Pelizaeus-Merzbacher syndrome, ornithine transcarbamylase deficiency, and Duchenne muscular dystrophy—had been isolated and mutations detected (Table 2–13).[101,102,104,113,114,164–167,169–172,177,199,244–246,249,250,290,317,321–328] Clearly, the success of three laboratories in cloning the fragile X gene in 1991 represented an

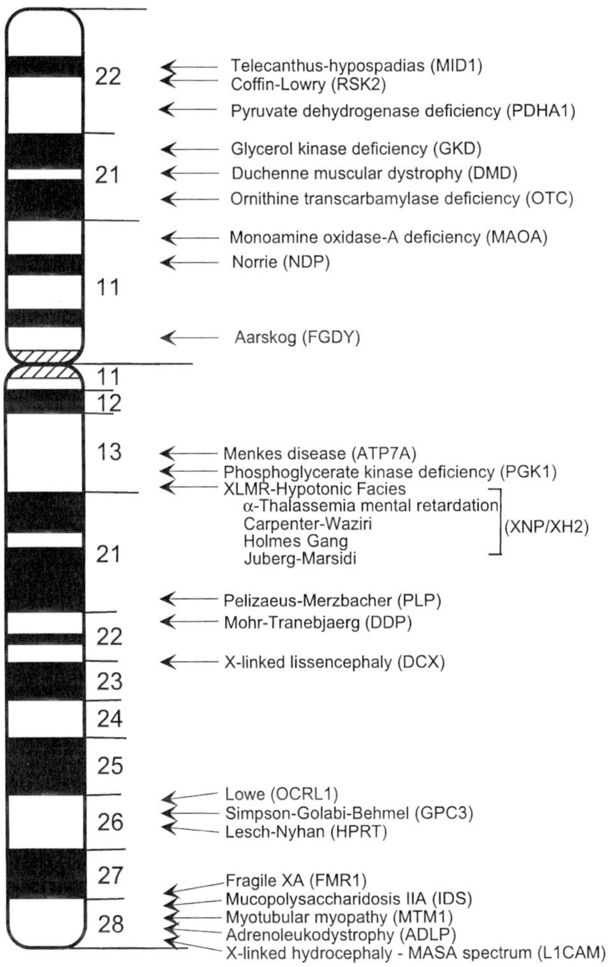

FIGURE 2–4. The gene localization for 23 syndromic types of X-linked mental retardation for which the gene has been cloned. The gene symbol is given in parentheses following the syndrome name.

Table 2–13. Progress in the Cloning of Genes Involved in X-Linked Mental Retardation

Year	*Gene Name*	*Gene Symbol*	*XLMR Entity*	*Function*
1983[169]	Hypoxanthine guanine phosphoribosyl transferase	HPRT	Lesch-Nyhan	Enzyme
1985[101, 102]	Proteolipid protein	PLP	PMP, SPG2	Myelination
1986[321]	Ornithine transcarbamylase	OTC	Ornithine transcarbamylase deficiency	Enzyme
1987[113]	Dystrophin	DMD	Duchenne	Structure of skeletal muscle membrane
1989[322]	Pyruvate dehydrogenase	PHDA1	Pyruvate dehydrogenase deficiency	Enzyme
1990[104]	Iduronate sulfatase	IDS	Mucopolysacchari-dosis II	Lysosomal enzyme
1991[244–246]	Fragile site mental retardation 1	FMR1	Fragile X	RNA-binding protein, gene regulation
1992[114]	Norrie	NDP	Norrie	Neuroectodermal cell interaction (?)
1992[116–167]	Oculorenal	OCRL1	Lowe	Enzyme
1992[164,165]	Cell adhesion molecule, L1	L1CAM	X-linked hydrocephaly, MASA, X-linked agenesis of the corpus callosum, X-linked spastic paraplegia, type 1	Neuronal migration, fascicle formation
1993[291]	Monoamine oxidase A	MAOA	Monoamine oxidase A deficiency	Enzyme
1993[323]	Adrenoleuko-dystrophy protein	ALDP	Adrenoleuko-dystrophy	Peroxisomal transport protein
1993[170–172]	Copper-transporting ATPase 7A	ATP7A	Menkes, occipital horn	Copper transport
1995[249]	X-linked nuclear protein, X-linked helicase 2	XNP, XH2	XLMR-hypotonic facies, α-thalassemia mental retardation, Juberg-Marsidi, Carpenter-Waziri, Holmes-Gang	Transcription factor, helicase activities
1996[199]	Faciogenital dysplasia	FGD1	Aarskog	Guanine nucleotide exchange factor
1996[324]	Fragile site mental retardation 2	FMR2	Fragile XE	Unknown

(continued)

TABLE 2–13. Continued

Year	*Gene Name*	*Gene Symbol*	*XLMR Entity*	*Function*
1996[250]	Dystonia-deafness peptide	DDP	Mohr-Tranebjaerg, Jensen	Transcription factor
1996[325]	Glypican 3	GPC3	Simpson-Golabi-Behmel	Cell adhesion, motility
1997[177]	Threonine-serine kinase 2	RSK2	Coffin-Lowry	Kinase signaling pathway
1997[317]	Rab GDP-dissociation inhibitor 1	GDI1	MRX41, MRX48	Stabilizes GDP-bound conformations
1997[326]	Midline 1	MID1	Opitz G/BBB	Zinc finger gene
1998[327]	Doublecortin	DCX	X-linked lissencephaly	Neuronal migration
1998[328]	Oligophrenin 1	OPHN1	MRX60	GTPase-activating protein

unrivaled benchmark.[244–246] Discovery that an unstable trinucleotide repeat in the 5′ untranslated region of the gene was the site of most mutations, study of the transgenerational dynamics of the repeat, and recognition that expansion beyond a certain limit (200–230 repeats) resulted in methylation and inactivation of the gene resolved many of the perplexing clinical and epidemiologic aspects of the fragile X syndrome. It heralded the discovery of other genes in which instability of a trinucleotide repeat was the usual mechanism of mutation.[329–332]

Typically, in families with the fragile X syndrome, the trinucleotide repeat was found to expand in each succeeding generation, proceeding from a premutation state (60–230 repeats) to full mutations (>230 repeats).[333] These observations helped to explain the Sherman paradox, a form of anticipation, which had been observed in fragile X families, and the existence of transmitting (nonpenetrant) males.[334–336] They also paved the way to understanding the phenomenon of anticipation in two classical autosomal dominant conditions: myotonic dystrophy and Huntington disease.[329,330]

Identification and cloning of other XLMR genes followed slowly (Table 2–13). Mutations in the L1CAM gene were identified in families with X-linked hydrocephalus in 1992.[164,165,202] The gene responsible for Menkes, ATP7A, was cloned in 1993 by multiple laboratories.[170–172] It is involved in the copper transport pathway as predicted from the clinical and biochemical findings associated with Menkes syndrome. Not until the latter years of era V was there a surge in the identification and cloning of XLMR genes. Undoubtedly, this was related directly to the progress of the Human Genome Project, which provided cloned material, sequence information, and ESTs (Expressed Sequence Tags) to the general community of researchers. All of this information facilitated the cloning and identification of the genes responsible for the Aarskog, Simpson-Golabi-Behmel, Mohr-Tranebjaerg, and fragile XE syndromes in 1996;[199,250,324,325] the Coffin-Lowry and Opitz G/BBB syndromes, and MRX41 and MRX48 in 1997;[177,317,326] and

X-linked lissencephaly/subcortical band heterotopia and MRX 60 in 1998 (Table 2–13).[327,328]

The cloning and identification of 17 XLMR genes from 1991 to early 1998 was instructive in two ways (Table 2–13). First, a majority of the genes, 10 of the 17, took advantage of cytogenetic translocations or fragile sites. For seven of these, the translocation occurred in females who exhibited either a syndromic phenotype or had only mental retardation. This latter point is critical since such female patients present one with the opportunity to clone an X-linked gene clearly involved in brain function. Thus far, two genes have been identified this way: oligophrenin, which is involved in MRX60,[328] and DXS16673E,[337] which has yet to be connected with a specific XLMR entity. More such genes are likely to be cloned since at least three other translocations have been identified in females,[338–340] and one breakpoint has been identified in a male with mental retardation and no somatic phenotype.[341]

The second instructive point derives from the function of many of the XLMR genes. Many of the genes appear to be involved in the regulation of gene transcription, cell motility, growth control, and membrane transport. Interestingly, three of the genes encode proteins involved in the regulation of the Ras superfamily of guanosine triphosphate (GTP)-binding proteins. The Aarskog gene, FGD1, is a guanine-nucleotide exchange factor (GEF) which enhances the exchange of bound GDP for GTP on Rho/Ras GTP.[199] Oligophrenin (OPHN1), implicated in MRX60, is a GTPase-activating protein (GAP) which increases the intrinsic rate of hydrolysis of bound GTP on Rho GTP.[328] GDI1, guanine-nucleotide dissociation inhibitor alpha, is responsible for MRX41 and MRX48.[317] It plays an important role in maintaining the balance between the GTP- and GDP-bound forms of Rab3. For these three genes, a model for their roles in neuronal process and synaptic transmission has been proposed.[340] Another gene, doublecortin (DCX), which is involved in X-linked lissencephaly, appears to have some role in calcium transport, which in turn may have a role in vesicle fusion at the synapses, a role similar to that played by Rab3.[327,341,342] This same gene plays a role in neuronal migration, as does the L1CAM gene which is responsible for the X-linked hydrocephalus–MASA syndrome–spastic paraplegia spectrum.[164,165,202] Based on its binding activities, glypican 3 (GLP3), which is involved in the Simpson-Golabi-Behmel syndrome, likely also plays a role in cell motility as well as cell growth.[325] Lastly, the Coffin-Lowry gene (Rsk-2) is a member of the serine-threonine protein kinase family of proteins, acts in the Ras-MAPK signaling pathway, and, as such, plays a role in many cellular functions.[177]

Two other XLMR genes act as transcription factors and provide another lesson. XNP, which was first shown to be responsible for the XLMR-hypotonic facies phenotype and is now known to be responsible for the Juberg-Marsidi, Carpenter-Waziri, and Holmes-Gang syndromes, has both zinc finger and helicase domains (Table 2–14).[215,249,266,343] As such, it can function as a transcription factor by either binding to DNA or by opening the helix of the DNA. As its expression is quite general, it is understandable how a mutation in the gene can give rise to a syndromic phenotype involving multiple organ systems (cerebro-facial-genital). Similarly, DDP, the gene involved in the Mohr-Tranebjaerg and

TABLE 2–14. Genes Implicated in Multiple XLMR Entities

L1CAM	X-linked hydrocephaly, MASA syndrome, X-linked agenesis of the corpus callosum, complicated spastic paraplegia type 1
XNP	XLMR-hypotonic facies (α-thalassemia mental retardation syndrome), Juberg-Marsidi syndrome, Carpenter-Waziri syndrome, Holmes-Gang syndrome
DDP	Mohr-Tranebjaerg syndrome, Jensen syndrome
GDI1	MRX41, MRX48
PLP	Pelizaeus-Merzbacher syndrome, complicated spastic paraplegia type 2

Jensen syndromes, is a member of a family of transcription factors.[124,125,217,250] Mutations in DDP give rise to a progressive neurological phenotype involving the special senses and central nervous system.

Thus, a common theme appears to be that defects in pathways that regulate gene transcription play a role in cognitive impairment. The extent of the phenotype, nonsyndromic vs. syndromic, may be dependent on the gene's location in the pathway, the nature of the mutation, the extent of its involvement in the regulation of multiple genes, and the partition of gene expression in different cell types or organ systems.

Prevalence of X-Linked Mental Retardation

Estimates of the prevalence of X-linked mental retardation may be made from three different lines of evidence: the male excess among persons with mental retardation, epidemiological studies on the causation of mental retardation, and the prevalence of recognized XLMR entities. Substantially different estimates are derived from the three sources.

Were genes on the X chromosome called upon to explain the 20% to 40% excess of males with mental retardation, such genes would cause approximately one in seven cases (~14%) of mental retardation.[9,76–82] Collectively, X-linked genes would be among the most common causes of mental retardation, comparable to the proportion of cases that can be attributed to chromosome aberrations (~12–15%) and substantially exceeding the proportion that could be attributed to autosomal genes (5%–8%) (Tables 2–2 and 2–3).

Surveys of various cohorts of persons with mental retardation for the purpose of assigning causation have found X-linked genes responsible for less than 5% of cases (Table 2–2 and 2–3).[11,12,28,32,34,35,70–72] Only Fryns et al. (1986) have found the frequency of XLMR among persons with mental retardation to be as high as 7.5%.[28] A number of factors may contribute to the shortfall between the estimated prevalence and the identifiable prevalence of X-linked mental retardation. Many XLMR entities may not have distinctive features which provide clues to clinical diagnosis. There are very few entities in which metabolic studies are diagnostic. If a significant percentage of cases represent new mutations, the pedigrees may not suggest X-linkage. Because females may be affected in many cases, the distinction between XLMR and culturofamilial mental retardation may be difficult.

Of the recognized forms of XLMR, the fragile X syndrome appears to be most common.[344–356] Recent molecular studies have shown the prevalence of fragile X syndrome to be one in 4000 to one in 6000 males and one in 8000 to one in 10,000 females. Assuming that this syndrome has an overall prevalence of 1.5 in 10,000 persons, and that it alone may account for 30%–40% of all X-linked mental retardation, X-linked genes would collectively account for 4.4 cases per 10,000 births or per 200 cases of mental retardation. This estimate (2.2% of cases of mental retardation) falls far below that necessary to explain the excess of males with mental retardation and somewhat below the percentage of cases with X-linked causes found in surveys of persons with mental retardation.

REFERENCES

1. Binet A, Simon T: Methodes nouvelles pour le diagnostic du niveau intellectuel des anormaux. Ann Psychol (Fr) 11:191, 1905.
2. Goddard HH: Four hundred feeble-minded children classified by the Binet method. J Psycho Asthenics 15:17, 1910.
3. Terman LM: The Measurement of Intelligence. An Explanation of and a Complete Guide for the Use of the Stanford Revision and Extension of the Binet-Simon Intelligence Scale. Houghton Mifflin, Boston, 1916.
4. Tredgold AF: A Textbook of Mental Deficiency (Amentia), Ed. 6. Bailliere, Tindall and Cox, London, 1937.
5. Doll EA: The essentials of an inclusive concept of mental deficiency. Am J Ment Defic 26:214, 1941.
6. Heber R: A manual on terminology and classification in mental retardation. Am J Med Defic (Monogr Suppl) 64:3, 1959.
7. Westling DL: Introduction to Mental Retardation. Prentice-Hall, Englewood Cliffs, NJ, 1986, pp. 2–21.
8. American Association on Mental Retardation: Mental Retardation: Definition, Classification and Systems of Support, Ed 9. American Association on Mental Retardation, Washington, DC, 1992.
9. Penrose LS: A clinical and genetic study of 1280 cases of mental defect. Special Report Series, Medical Research Council, No. 229. Her Majesty's Stationery Office, London, 1938.
10. Reed EW, Reed SC: Mental Retardation: A Family Study. WB Saunders, Philadelphia, 1965.
11. Moser HW, Wolf PA: The nosology of mental retardation: including the report of a survey of 1378 mentally retarded individuals at the Walter E. Fernald State School. Birth Defects Orig Art Series VII(1):117, 1971.
12. McLaren J, Bryson JE: Review of recent epidemiological studies of mental retardation: prevalence, associated disorders, and etiology. Am J Ment Retard 92:243, 1987.
13. Lewis EO: The Report of the Mental Deficiency Committee. Part IV—Report on an Investigation into the Incidence of Mental Deficiency in Six Areas, 1925–1927. His Majesty's Stationery Office, London, 1929.
14. Drillien CM, Jameson S, Wilkinson EM: Studies in mental handicap, part I: prevalence and distribution by clinical type and severity of defect. Arch Dis Child 41:528, 1966.
15. Kushlick A, Cox G: The epidemiology of mental handicap. Dev Med Child Neurol 15:748, 1973.

16. Hagberg B, Kyllerman M: Epidemiology of mental retardation: a Swedish survey. Brain Dev 5:441, 1983.
17. Baird PA, Sadovnick AD: Mental retardation in over half-a-million consecutive live-births: an epidemiological study. Am J Ment Defic 89:323, 1985.
18. Stoller A: Epidemiology of mental deficiency in Victoria. In: Proceedings of the Fourth Interstate Conference on Mental Deficiency. JD Van Zelt, ed. Australian Group for the Scientific Study of Mental Deficiency, Melbourne, Australia, 1965, pp. 18–28.
19. Yeargin-Allsopp M, Murphy CC, Cordero JF, et al.: Reported biomedical causes and associated medical conditions for mental retardation among 10-year-old children, metropolitan Atlanta, 1985 to 1987. Dev Med Child Neurol 39:142, 1997.
20. Wallin JEW: Prevalence of mental retardates. Sch Soc 86:55, 1958.
21. Calculations using data from US Department of Education, Office of Special Education Programs (Nov. 1993) and US Department of Education, National Center for Education Statistics (Feb. 1993).
22. Robinson HB, Robinson NM: The Mentally Retarded Child. A Psychological Approach. McGraw-Hill Book, New York, 1965, pp. 40–42.
23. Burt C: The distribution of intelligence. Br J Psychol 48:161, 1957.
24. Dingman HF, Tarjan G: Mental retardation and the normal distribution curve. Am J Ment Defic 64:991, 1960.
25. Opitz JM: Mental retardation: biologic aspects of concern to pediatricians. Pediatr Review 2:41, 1980.
26. Opitz JM, Kaveggia EG, Durkin-Stamm MV, et al.: Diagnostic/genetic studies in severe mental retardation. Birth Defects Orig Art Series XIV(6B):1, 1978.
27. Molteno CD, Roux A, Nelson MM, et al.: Causes of mental handicap in Cape Town. S Afr Med J 77:98, 1990.
28. Fryns JP, Kleczkowska A, Dereymaeker A, et al.: A genetic-diagnostic survey in an institutionalized population of 173 severely mentally retarded patients. Clin Genet 30:315, 1986.
29. McQueen PC, Spence MW, Winsor EJT, et al.: Causal origins of major mental handicap in the Canadian Maritime Provinces. Dev Med Child Neurol 28:697, 1986.
30. Blomquist HK, Gustavson K-H, Holmgren G: Mild mental retardation in children in a northern Swedish county. J Ment Defic Res 25:169, 1981.
31. Czeizel A, Lányi-Engelmayer A, Klujber L, et al.: Etiological study of mental retardation in Budapest, Hungary. Am J Ment Defic 85: 2:120, 1980.
32. Hunter AGW, Evans JA, Thompson DR, et al.: A study of institutionalized mentally retarded patients in Manitoba. I: Classification and preventability. Dev Med Child Neurol 22:145, 1980.
33. Morrison AA: The aetiology of mental retardation. N Z Med J 85:103, 1977.
34. Gustavson K-H, Hagberg B, Hagberg G, et al.: Severe mental retardation in a Swedish county. Acta Paediatr Scand 66:373, 1977.
35. Laxova R, Ridler MAC, Bowen-Bravery M: An aetiological survey of the severely retarded Hertfordshire children who were born between January 1, 1965 and December 31, 1967. Am J Med Genet 1:75, 1977.
36. Al-Ansari A: Etiology of mild mental retardation among Bahraini children: a community-based case control study. Ment Retard 31:140, 1993.
37. Asthana JC, Sinha S, Haslam JS et al.: Survey of adolescents with severe intellectual handicap. Arch Dis Child 65:1133, 1990.
38. Krishnan BR, Ramesh A, Kumari MP et al.: Genetic analysis of a group of mentally retarded children. Indian J Pediatr 56:249, 1989.
39. Kuo-Tai T: Mentally retarded persons in the People's Republic of China: review of epidemiological studies and services. Am J Ment Retard 93:193, 1988.
40. Lamont MA, Dennis NR: Aetiology of mild mental retardation. Arch Dis Child 63:1032, 1988.

41. Wendt L von, Rantakallio P: Mild mental retardation in Northern Finland. Ups J Med Sci Suppl 44:47, 1987.
42. Benassi G, Guarino M, Cammarata S, et al.: An epidemiological study on severe mental retardation among school children in Bologna, Italy. Dev Med Child Neurol 32:895, 1990.
43. Rantakallio P, Wendt L von: Risk factors for mental retardation. Arch Dis Child 60:946, 1985.
44. Costeff H, Cohen BE, Weller LE: Biological factors in mild mental retardation. Dev Med Child Neurol 25:580, 1983.
45. Proops R, Mayer M, Jacobs PA: A study of mental retardation in children in the Island of Hawaii. Clin Genet 23:81, 1983.
46. McDonald AD: Severely retarded children in Quebec: prevalence, causes, and care. Am J Ment Defic 78:205, 1973.
47. Wellesley D, Hockey A, Stanley F: The aetiology of intellectual disability in western Australia: a community-based study. Dev Med Child Neurol 33:963, 1991.
48. Turner G: An aetiological study of 1000 patients with an I.Q. assessment below 51. Med J Aust 2:927, 1975.
49. Sachs B: A family form of idiocy, generally fatal, associated with early blindness. J Nerv Ment Dis 21:475, 1896.
50. Sjögren T: Die juvenile amaurotische Idiotie. Klinische und erblichkeitsmedizinische Untersuchungen. Hereditas 14:197, 1931.
51. Laurence JZ, Moon RC: Four cases of retinitis pigmentosa occurring in the same family and accompanied by general imperfection of development. Ophthalmol Rev 2:32, 1866.
52. Bardet G: Sur un syndrome d'obesite infantile avec polydactylie et retinite pigmentaire, Thesis: Pairs, No 479, 1920. Contribution a l'etude des formes cliniques de l'obesite hypophysaire.
53. Folling A: Uber Ausscheidung von Phenylbrenztraubensaure in den Harn als Stoffwechselanomalie in Verbindung mit Imbezillitat. A Physiol Chem 277:169, 1934.
54. Roberts JAF: Sex-linked microphthalmia sometimes associated with mental deficiency. Br Med J 2:1213, 1937.
55. McKusick VA: Mendelian Inheritance in Man. A Catalog of Human Genes and Genetic Disorders, Ed. 12. Johns Hopkins University Press, Baltimore, 1998.
56. Tjio JH, Levan A: The chromosome number of man. Hereditas 42:1, 1956.
57. LeJeune J: Le mongolisme. Premier example d'aberration autosomique humaine. Ann Genet Semaine Hop 1:42, 1959.
58. Schinzel A: Catalogue of Unbalanced Chromosome Aberrations in Man. Walter de Gruyter, Berlin, 1984.
59. Pinkel D, Straume T, Gray JW: Cytogenetic analysis using quantitative, high-sensitivity, fluorescence hybridization. Proc Natl Acad Sci USA 83:294, 1986.
60. Speicher MR, Ballard SG, Ward DC: Karyotyping human chromosomes by combinatorial multi-fluor FISH. Nat Genet 12:368, 1996.
61. Schröck E, duManoir S, Veldman T, et al.: Multicolor spectral karyotyping of human chromosomes. Science 273:494, 1996.
62. Stevenson RE: The Fetus and Newly Born Infant. Influences of the Prenatal Environment, Ed. 2. CV Mosby, St. Louis, 1977.
63. Marine DM, Kimball OP: The prevention of simple goiter in man. J Lab Clin Med 3:40, 1917.
64. Goldstein L, Murphy DP: Etiology of ill-health in children born after maternal pelvic irradiation. Part II. Defective children born after postconception pelvic radiation. AJR Am J Roentgenol 22:322, 1929.
65. Levine P, Katzin EM, Burnham L: Isoimmunization in pregnancy, its possible bearing on the etiology of erythroblastosis fetalis. JAMA 116:825, 1941.

66. Gregg NM: Congenital cataract following German measles in the mother. Trans Ophthalmol Soc Australia 3:35, 1941.
67. Jones KL, Smith DW, Ulleland CN, et al.: Patterns of malformations in offspring of chronic alcoholic mothers. Lancet 1:1267, 1973.
68. Fanaroff AA, Martin RJ: Neonatal–Perinatal Medicine. Diseases of the Fetus and Infant, Ed. 5. Mosby Year Book, St. Louis, 1992, pp. 704–714.
69. Nelson KB, Leviton A: How much of neonatal encephalopathy is due to birth asphyxia? Am J Dis Child 145:1325, 1991.
70. Kaveggia EG, Durkin MV, Pendleton E: Diagnostic/genetic studies on 1,224 patients with severe mental retardation, Proceedings, 3rd Congress of the International Association for the Scientific Study of Mental Deficiency. Polish Medical, Warsaw, 1975, pp. 82–93.
71. Farag TI, Al-Awadi SA, El-Badramary MH, et al.: Disease profile of 400 institutionalized mentally retarded patients in Kuwait. Clin Genet 44:329, 1993.
72. Anderson G, Schroer RJ, Stevenson RE: Mental retardation in South Carolina II. Causation. Proc Greenwood Genet Center 15:32, 1996.
73. Rosanoff AJ: Sex-linked inheritance in mental deficiency. Am J Psychiatry 11:289, 1931.
74. Malzberg B: Sex differences in the prevalence of mental deficiency. Am J Ment Defic 58:301, 1953.
75. Lehrke R: A theory of X-linkage of major intellectual traits. Am J Ment Defic 76:611, 1972.
76. Lehrke RG: X-linked mental retardation and verbal disabilities. Birth Defects Orig Art Series X(1): 1, 1974.
77. Herbst DS, Miller JR: Non-specific X-linked mental retardation II: the frequency in British Columbia. Am J Med Genet 7:461, 1980.
78. DeBow JDB (Superintendent of the U.S. Census): Compendium of the Seventh Census: 1850. B. Tucker, Senate Printer, Washington, 1854, pp. 60, 78.
79. U.S. Department of the Interior: Census of the United States 1860 (Eight), 1870 (Ninth) and 1880 (Tenth). Government Printing Office, Washington, 1864, p. 647; 1872, pp. 492, 505; 1883, p. 926.
80. U.S. Department of the Interior: Compendium of the Eleventh Census: 1890. Part II. Government Printing Office, Washington, 1894, pp. 133–134.
81. Morton NE, Rao DC, Lang-Brown H, et al.: Colchester revisited: a genetic study of mental defect. J Med Genet 14:1, 1977.
82. Stevenson RE, Schroer RJ: Mental retardation in South Carolina. I. Characteristics of the study population. Proc Greenwood Genet Center 15:26, 1996.
83. Simensen RJ: Survey of sex ratio among students receiving special education services in public schools in the United States, 1993–1998, unpublished.
84. Duchenne GBA: Recherches sur la paralysie musculaire pseudo-hypertrophique, ou paralysie myosclérosique. Générales de Médecine 11:5, 1868. Translation in Arch Neurol 19:629, 1968.
85. Pelizaeus F: Ueber eine eigentumliche Form spastischer Lahmung mit Cerebralerscheinungen auf hereditarer Grundlage (multiple Sklerose). Arch Psychiatr Nervenkr 16:698, 1885.
86. Merzbacher L: Gesetzmaessigkeiten in der Vererbung und Verbreitung verschiedener hereditaer-familiaerer Erkrankungen. Arch Rass Ges Biol 6:172, 1909.
87. Mendes da Costa S, Van der Valk JW: Typus maculatus der bullosen hereditären dystrophie. Arch Dermatol Syph 91:1, 1908.
88. Zinsser F: Atrophia cutis reticularis cum pigmentatione, dystrophia unguim et leukoplakia oris. Ikonogr Dermatol 5:219, 1910.
89. Hunter C: A rare disease in two brothers. Proc R Soc Med 10:104, 1917.
90. Bloch B: Krankendemonstrationen aus der dermatologischen klinik Zürich. Schweiz Med Wochenschr 57:404, 1926.

91. Sulzberger MB: Über eine bisher nicht beschriebene congenitale Pigmentanomalie (Incontinentia pigmenti). Arch Dermatol Syph 154:19, 1927.
92. Norrie G: Causes of blindness in children. Acta Ophthalmol 5:7, 1927.
93. Rud E: Et Tilfaelde af Infantilisme med Tetani, Epilepsi, Polyneuritis, Ichthyosis og Anaemi of pernicios Type. Hospitalstidende 70:525, 1927.
94. Albright F, Burnett CH, Smith PH, et al.: Pseudo-hypoparathyroidism—an example of "Seabright-Bantam syndrome." Endocrinology 30:922, 1942.
95. McClung CE: The accessory-chromosome—sex determinant? Biol Bull 3:43, 1902.
96. Painter T: The sex chromosomes of man. Am Naturalist 58:506, 1924.
97. Koller PC: The genetical and mechanical properties of sex chromosomes. III. Man. Proc R Soc Edinb (Pt 2, Sec B) 57:194, 1937.
98. Emery AEH: Duchenne Muscular Dystrophy. Oxford University Press, Oxford, 1987, pp. 99–102.
99. Gowers WR: Pseudo-hypertrophic Muscular Paralysis—a Clinical Lecture. Churchill, London, 1879.
100. Trofatter JA, Dloughy SR, Demyer W, et al. : Pelizaeus-Merzbacher disease: tight linkage to proteolipid protein gene exon variant. Proc Natl Acad Sci USA 86:9247, 1989.
101. Hudson LD, Puckett C, Berndt J, et al.: Mutation of the proteolipid protein gene PLP in a human X chromosome-linked myelin disorder. Proc Natl Acad Sci USA 86:8128, 1989.
102. Njå R: A sex-linked type of gargoylism. Acta Paediatr 33:267, 1946.
103. Mossman J, Blunt S, Stephens S, et al.: Hunter's disease in a girl: association with X:5 chromosomal translocation disrupting the Hunter gene. Arch Dis Child 58:911, 1983.
104. Chase DS, Morris AH, Ballabio A, et al.: Genetics of Hunter syndrome: carrier detection, new mutations, segregation, and linkage analysis. Ann Hum Genet 50:349, 1986.
105. Warburg M: Norrie's disease. A new hereditary bilateral pseudotumour of the retina. Acta Ophthalmol 39:757, 1961.
106. Gilgenkrantz S, Tridon P, Pinel-Briquel N, et al.: Translocation X.9 in a girl with incontinentia pigmenti. Ann Genet (Paris) 20:90, 1985.
107. Hodgson SV, Neville B, Jones RWA, et al.: Two cases of X autosome translocation in females with incontinentia pigmenti. Hum Genet 75:98, 1985.
108. Sefiani A, Abel L, Heuertz S, et al.: The gene for incontinentia pigmenti is assigned to Xq28. Genomics 4:427, 1989.
109. Levine MA, Jap T-S, Mauseth RS, et al.: Activity of the stimulatory guanine nucleotide-binding protein is reduced in erythrocytes from patients with pseudohypoparathyroidism and pseudopseudohypoparathyroidism: biochemical, endocrine, and genetic analysis of Albright's hereditary osteodystrophy in 6 kindreds. J Clin Endocrinol Metab 62:497, 1986.
110. Phelan MC, Rogers RC, Clarkson KB, et al.: Albright hereditary osteodystrophy and del(2)(q37.3) in four unrelated individuals. Am J Med Genet 58:1, 1995.
111. Münke M, Kruse K, Goos M, et al.: Genetic heterogeneity of the ichthyosis, hypogonadism, mental retardation, and epilepsy syndrome. Eur J Pediatr 141:8, 1983.
112. Traupe H: The Ichthyoses. A Guide to Clinical Diagnosis, Genetic Counseling, and Therapy. Springer-Verlag, Berlin, 1989, p. 91.
113. Koenig M, Hoffman EP, Bertelson CJ, et al.: Complete cloning of the Duchenne muscular dystrophy (DMD) cDNA and preliminary genomic organization of the DMD gene in normal and affected individuals. Cell 50:509, 1987.
114. Chen Z-Y, Battinelli EM, Hendriks RW, et al.: Norrie disease gene: characterization of deletions and possible function. Genomics 16:533, 1993.
115. Wijker M, Ligtenberg MJL, Schoute F, et al.: The gene for hereditary bullous dystrophy, X-linked macular type, maps to the Xq27.3-qter region. Am J Hum Genet 56:1096, 1995.

116. Connor JM, Gatherer D, Gray FC, et al.: Assignment of the gene for dyskeratosis congenita to Xq28. Hum Genet 72:348, 1986.
117. Martin JP, Bell J: A pedigree of mental defect showing sex-linkage. J Neurol Psychiatry 6:154, 1943.
118. Allan W, Herndon CN, Dudley FC: Some examples of the inheritance of mental deficiency: apparently sex-linked idiocy and microcephaly. Am J Ment Defic 48:325, 1944.
119. Bickers DA, Adams RD: Hereditary stenosis of the aqueduct of Sylvius as a cause of congenital hydrocephalus. Brain 72:246, 1949.
120. Lowe CU, Terrey M, MacLachlan EA: Organic-aciduria, decreased renal ammonia production, hydrophthalmos, and mental retardation. Am J Dis Child 83:164, 1952.
121. Lenz W: Recessiv-geschlechtsgebundene mikrophthalmie mit multiplen miβbildungen. Z Kinderheil 77:384, 1955.
122. van den Bosch J: A new syndrome in three generations of a Dutch family. Ophthalmologica 137:422, 1959.
123. Paine RS: Evaluation of familial biochemically determined mental retardation in children, with special reference to aminoaciduria. N Engl J Med 262:658, 1960.
124. Mohr J, Mageroy K: Sex-linked deafness of a possibly new type. Acta Genet Stat Med 10:54, 1960.
125. Tranebjaerg L, Schwartz C, Eriksen H, et al.: A new X linked recessive deafness syndrome with blindness, dystonia, fractures, and mental deficiency is linked to Xq22. J Med Genet 32:257, 1995.
126. Gorlin RJ, Anderson VE, Scott CR: Hypertrophied frenuli, oligophrenia, familial trembling and anomalies of the hand. N Engl J Med 264:486, 1961.
127. Losowsky MS: Hereditary mental defect showing the pattern of sex influence. J Ment Defic Res 5:60, 1961.
128. Renpenning H, Gerrard JW, Zaleski WA, et al.: Familial sex-linked mental retardation. Can Med Assoc J 87:954, 1962.
129. Warkany J, Monroe BB, Sutherland BS: Intrauterine growth retardation. Am J Dis Child 102:249, 1961.
130. Börjeson M, Forssman H, Lehmann O: An X-linked recessively inherited syndrome characterized by grave mental deficiency, epilepsy and endocrine disorder. Acta Med Scand 171:13, 1962.
131. Goltz RW, Peterson WC, Gorlin RJ, et al.: Focal dermal hypoplasia. Arch Dermatol 86:52, 1962.
132. Russell A, Levin B, Oberholzer VG, et al.: Hyperammonaemia. A new instance of an inborn enzymatic defect of the biosynthesis of urea. Lancet II:699, 1962.
133. Dunn HG, Renpenning H, Gerrard JW, et al.: Mental retardation as a sex-linked defect. Am J Ment Defic 67:827, 1962–1963.
134. Hoefnagal D, Andrew ED, Mireault NG, et al.: Hereditary choreoathetosis, self-mutilation and hyperuricemia in young males. N Engl J Med 273:130, 1962.
135. Fanconi A, Prader A, Isler W, et al.: Morbus Addison mit Hirnswklerose im Kindesalter. Ein hereditaeres Syndrom mit X-chromosomaler Vererbung? Helv Paediatr Acta 18:480, 1964.
136. Menkes JH, Alter M, Steigleder GK, et al.: A sex-linked recessive disorder with retardation of growth, peculiar hair, and focal cerebral and cerebellar degeneration. Pediatrics 29:764, 1962.
137. Lesch M, Nyhan WL: A familial disorder of uric acid metabolism and central nervous system function. Am J Med 36:561, 1964.
138. Plott D: Congenital laryngeal-abductor paralysis due to nucleus ambiguus dysgenesis in three brothers. N Engl J Med 271:593, 1964.
139. Menkes JH, Philippart M, Clark DB: Hereditary partial agenesis of corpus callosum. Arch Neurol 11:198, 1964.
140. Kaplan P: X linked recessive inheritance of agenesis of the corpus callosum. J Med Genet 20:122, 1983.

141. Åkesson HO: Cutis verticis gyrata thyroaplasia and mental deficiency. Acta Genet Med Gemellol 14:200, 1965.
142. Baar HS, Gabriel AM: Sex-linked spastic paraplegia. Am J Ment Defic 71:13, 1966.
143. Rett A: Uber ein eigenartiges hirnatrophisches syndrom bei hyperammonämie im kindesalter. Wien Med Wochenschr 116:723, 1966.
144. Coffin GS, Siris E, Wegienka LC: Mental retardation with osteocartilaginous anomalies. Am J Dis Child 112:205, 1966.
145. Lowry B, Miller JR: A new dominant gene mental retardation syndrome. Am J Dis Child 121:496, 1971.
146. Dudding BA, Gorlin RJ, Langer LO Jr: The oto-palato-digital syndrome: a new symptom-complex consisting of deafness, dwarfism, cleft palate, characteristic facies, and a generalized bone dysplasia. Am J Dis Child 113:214, 1967.
147. Lehrke RG: Sex-linked mental retardation and verbal disability (thesis). University Microfilms, Ann Arbor, MI, 1968.
148. Sutherland GR: Fragile sites on human chromosomes. III. Detection of Fra(X)(q27) in males with X-linked mental retardation and their female relatives. Hum Genet 53:23, 1977.
149. Richards BW, Sylvester PE, Brooker C: Fragile X-linked mental retardation: the Martin-Bell syndrome. J Ment Defic Res 25:253, 1981.
150. Fox P, Fox D, Gerrard JW: X-linked mental retardation: Renpenning revisited. Am J Med Genet 7:491, 1980.
151. Stevenson RE, Goodman HO, Schwartz CE, et al.: Allan-Herndon syndrome. I. Clinical studies. Am J Hum Genet 47:446, 1990.
152. Schwartz CE, Ulmer J, Brown A, et al.: Allan-Herndon syndrome. II. Linkage to DNA markers in Xq21. Am J Hum Genet 47:454, 1990.
153. Bialer MG, Lawrence L, Stevenson RE, et al.: Allan-Herndon-Dudley syndrome: clinical and linkage studies on a second family. Am J Med Genet 43:491, 1992.
154. Malamud N, Cohen P: Unusual form of cerebellar ataxia with sex-linked inheritance. Neurology 8:261, 1958.
155. Johnston AW, McKusick VA: A sex-linked recessive form of spastic paraplegia. Am J Hum Genet 14:83, 1962.
156. Bundey S, Griffiths MI: Recurrence risks in families of children with symmetrical spasticity. Dev Med Child Neurol 19:179, 1977.
157. Wieacker P, Wolff G, Wienker TF, et al.: A new X-linked syndrome with muscle atrophy, congenital contractures, and oculomotor apraxia. Am J Med Genet 20:597, 1985.
158. Apak S, Yüksel M, Özmen M, et al.: Heterogeneity of X-linked recessive (spino)cerebellar ataxia with or without spastic diplegia. Am J Med Genet 34:155, 1989.
159. Stevenson RE, Arena JF, Ouzts E, et al.: Renpenning syndrome maps to Xp11. Am J Hum Genet 62:1092, 1998.
160. Willems PJ, Dijkstra I, Van der Auwera BJ, et al.: Assignment of X-linked hydrocephalus to Xq28 by linkage analysis. Genomics 8:367, 1990.
161. Winter RM, Davies KE, Bell MV, et al.: MASA syndrome: further clinical delineation and chromosomal localisation. Hum Genet 82:367, 1989.
162. Fryns JP, Spaepen A, Cassiman JJ, et al.: X-linked complicated spastic paraplegia, MASA syndrome, and X-linked hydrocephalus owing to congenital stenosis of the aqueduct of Sylvius: variable expression of the same mutation at Xq28. J Med Genet 28:429, 1991.
163. Boyd E, Schwartz CE, Schroer RJ, et al.: Agenesis of the corpus callosum associated with MASA syndrome. Clin Dysmorphol 2:332, 1993.
164. Rosenthal A, Jouet M, Kenwrick S: Aberrant splicing of neural cell adhesion molecule L1 mRNA in a family with X-linked hydrocephalus. Nat Genet 2:107, 1992.
165. Vits L, Van Camp G, Coucke P, et al.: MASA syndrome is due to mutations in the neural cell adhesion gene L1CAM. Nat Genet 7:408, 1994.

166. Reilly DS, Lewis RA, Nussbaum RL: Genetic and physical mapping of Xq24-q26 markers flanking the Lowe oculocerebrorenal syndrome. Genomics 8:62, 1990.
167. Attree O, Olivos IM, Okabe I, et al.: The Lowe's oculocerebrorenal syndrome gene encodes a protein highly homologous to inositol polyphosphate-5-phosphatase. Nature 358:239, 1992.
168. Hoefnagel D, Andrew ED, Mireault NG, et al.: Hereditary choreoathetosis, self-mutilation and hyperuricemia in young males. N Engl J Med 273:130, 1965.
169. Jolly DJ, Okayama H, Berg P, et al.: Isolation and characterization of a full-length expressible cDNA for human hypoxanthine phosphoribosyltransferase. Proc Natl Acad Sci USA 80:477, 1983.
170. Vulpe C, Levinson B, Whitney S, et al.: Isolation of a candidate gene for Menkes disease and evidence that it encodes a copper transporting ATPase. Nat Genet 3:7, 1993.
171. Chelly J, Tümer Z, Tønnesen T, et al.: Isolation of a candidate gene for Menkes disease that encodes a potential heavy metal binding protein. Nat Genet 3:14, 1993.
172. Mercer JFB, Livingston J, Hall B, et al.: Isolation of a partial candidate gene for Menkes disease by positional cloning. Nat Genet 3:20, 1993.
173. Turner G, Gedeon A, Mulley J, et al.: Borjeson-Forssman-Lehman syndrome: clinical manifestations and gene localization to Xq26-27. Am J Med Genet 34:463, 1989.
174. Mathews KD, Ardinger HH, Nishimura DY, et al.: Linkage localization of Börjeson-Forssman-Lehmann syndrome. Am J Med Genet 34:470, 1989.
175. Gecz J, Baker E, Donnelly A, et al.: Fibroblast growth factor homologous factor 2 (FHF2): gene structure, expression and mapping to the Börjesen-Forssman-Lehmann syndrome region in Xq26 delineated by a duplication breakpoint in a BFLS-like patient. Hum Genet 104:56, 1999.
176. Temtamy SA, Miller JD, Hussels-Maumenee I: The Coffin-Lowry syndrome: an inherited faciodigital mental retardation syndrome. Pediatrics 86:724, 1975.
177. Trivier E, DeCesare D, Jacquot S, et al.: Mutations in the kinase Rsk-2 associated with Coffin-Lowry syndrome. Nature 384:567, 1996.
178. Lubs HA: A marker X chromosome. Am J Hum Genet 21:231, 1969.
179. Aicardi J, Chevrie J-J, Rousselie F: Le syndrome spasmes en flexion, agenesie calleuse, anomalies chorio-retiniennes. Arch Fr Pediatr 26:1103, 1969.
180. Opitz JM, Summitt RL, Smith DWG: The BBB syndrome. Familial telecanthus with associated congenital anomalies. Birth Defects Orig Art Series V(2):86, 1969.
181. Snyder RD, Robinson A: Recessive sex-linked mental retardation in the absence of other recognizable abnormalities. Clin Pediatr 8:669, 1969.
182. Wijngaarden GK van, Fleury P, Bethlem J, et al.: Familial myotubular myopathy. Neurology 19:901, 1969.
183. Aarskog D: A familial syndrome of short stature associated with facial dysplasia and genital anomalies. J Pediatr 77:856, 1970.
184. Juberg RC, Hellman CD: A new familial form of convulsive disorder and mental retardation limited to females. J Pediatr 79:726, 1971.
185. AvRuskin TW, Braverman LE, Crigler JF: Thyroxine-binding globulin deficiency and associated neurological deficit. Pediatrics 50:638, 1972.
186. Cantú J-M, Hernandez A, Larracilla J, et al.: A new X-linked recessive disorder with dwarfism, cerebral atrophy, and generalized keratosis follicularis. J Pediatr 84:564, 1974.
187. Max SR, Maclaren NK, Brady RO, et al.: GM_3 (hematoside) sphingolipodystrophy. N Engl J Med 291:929, 1974.
188. Bianchine JW, Lewis RC: The MASA syndrome: a new heritable mental retardation syndrome. Clin Genet 5:298, 1974.
189. Nance WE, Warburg M, Bixler D, et al.: Congenital X-linked cataract, dental anomalies and brachymetacarpalia. Birth Defects Orig Art Series X(4):285, 1974.
190. Opitz JM, Kaveggia EG: Studies of malformation syndromes of man XXXIII: the FG syndrome. An X-linked recessive syndrome of multiple congenital anomalies and mental retardation. Z Kinderkeilk 117:1, 1974.

191. Pallister PD, Herrmann J, Spranger JW, et al.: The W syndrome. Studies of malformation syndromes of man XXVIII. Birth Defects Orig Art Series X(7):51, 1974.
192. Went LN, De Vries-De Mol EC, Völker-Dieben HJ: A family with apparently sex-linked optic atrophy. J Med Genet 12:94, 1975.
193. Fitch N, Jequier S, Papageorgiou A: A familial syndrome of cranial, facial, oral and limb anomalies. Clin Genet 10:226, 1976.
194. Sutherland GR: Fragile sites on human chromosomes: demonstration of their dependence on the type of tissue culture medium. Science 197:265, 1977.
195. Glover TW: FUdR induction of the X-chromosome fragile site: evidence for the mechanism of folic acid and thymidine inhibition. Am J Hum Genet 33:234, 1981.
196. Scott CI, Jr: Unusual facies, joint hypermobility, genital anomaly and short stature: a new dysmorphic syndrome. New York: Alan R Liss, for the National Foundation–March of Dimes. Birth Defects Orig Art Series VII(6):240, 1971.
197. Bawle E, Tyrkus M, Lipman S, et al.: Aarskog syndrome: full male and female expression associated with an X-autosome translocation. Am J Med Genet 17:595, 1984.
198. Stevenson RE, May M, Arena JF, et al.: Aarskog-Scott syndrome: confirmation of linkage to the pericentromeric region of the X chromosome. Am J Med Genet 52:339, 1994.
199. Pasteris NG, Cadle A, Logie LJ, et al.: Isolation and characterization of the faciogenital dysplasia (Aarskog-Scott syndrome) gene: a putative rho/rac guanine nucleotide exchange factor. Cell 79:669, 1994.
200. Ryan SG, Chance PF, Zou C-H, et al.: Epilepsy and mental retardation limited to females: an X-linked dominant disorder with male sparing. Nat Genet 17:92, 1997.
201. Thomas GE: High male:female ratio of germ-line mutations: an alternative explanation for postulated gestational lethality in males in X-linked dominant disorders. Am J Hum Genet 58:1364, 1996.
202. Jouet M, Rosenthal A, Armstrong G, et al.: X-linked spastic paraplegia (SPG1), MASA syndrome and X-linked hydrocephalus result from mutations in the L1 gene. Nat Genet 7:402, 1994.
203. Arena JF, Schwartz CE, Ouzts L, et al.: X-linked mental retardation with thin habitus, asymmetric face and prominent lower lip: linkage to Xp22.12-p21.3. Am J Med Genet 64:50, 1996.
204. Anastasi A: Four hypotheses with a dearth of data: response to Lehrke's "A theory of X-linkage of major intellectual traits." Am J Ment Defic 76:620, 1972.
205. Nance WE, Engel E: One X and four hypotheses: response to Lehrke's "A theory of X-linkage of major intellectual traits." Am J Ment Defic 76:623, 1972.
206. Lehrke R: Response to Dr. Anastasi and to the Drs. Nance and Engel. Am J Ment Defic 76:626, 1972.
207. Harvey J, Judge C, Wiener S: Familial X-linked mental retardation with an X chromosome abnormality. J Med Genet 14:46, 1977.
208. Giraud F, Ayme S, Mattei JF, et al.: Constitutional chromosomal breakage. Hum Genet 34:125, 1976.
209. Christian JC, DeMeyer W, Franken EA, et al.: X-linked skeletal dysplasia with mental retardation. Clin Genet 11:128, 1977
210. Feinberg AP, Leahy WR: Infantile spasms: case report of sex-linked inheritance. Dev Med Child Neurol 19:524, 1977.
211. McCabe ERB, Fennessey PV, Guggenheim MA, et al.: Human glycerol kinase deficiency with hyperglycerolemia and glyceroluria. Biochem Biophys Res Commun 78:1327, 1977.
212. Riccardi VM, Marcus ES: Congenital hydrocephalus and cerebellar agenesis. Clin Genet 13:443, 1978.
213. Urban MD, Rogers JG, Meyer WJ: Familial syndrome of mental retardation, short stature, contractures of the hands, and genital anomalies. J Pediatr 94:52, 1979.
214. Vasquez SB, Hurst DL, Sotos JF: X-linked hypogonadism, gynecomastia, mental retardation, short stature, and obesity—a new syndrome. J Pediatr 94:56, 1979.

215. Juberg RC, Marsidi I: A new form of X-linked mental retardation with growth retardation, deafness, and microgenitalism. Am J Hum Genet 32:714, 1980.
216. Smith RD, Fineman RM, Myers GG: Short stature, psychomotor retardation, and unusual facial appearance in two brothers. Am J Med Genet 7:5, 1980.
217. Jensen PKA: Nerve deafness, optic nerve atrophy and dementia: a new X-linked recessive syndrome? Am J Med Genet 9:55, 1981.
218. Say B, Meyer J: Familial trigonocephaly associated with short stature and developmental delay. Am J Dis Child 135:711, 1981.
219. Simpson JL, Landey S, New M, et al.: A previously unrecognized X-linked syndrome of dysmorphia. Birth Defects Orig Art Ser XI(2):18, 1975.
220. Golabi M, Rosen L: A new X-linked mental retardation-overgrowth syndrome. Am J Med Genet 17:345, 1984.
221. Behmel A, Plöchl E, Rosenkranz W: A new X-linked dysplasia gigantism syndrome: Identical with the Simpson dysplasia syndrome? Hum Genet 67:409, 1984.
222. Young ID, Hughes HE: Sex-linked mental retardation, short stature, obesity and hypogonadism: report of a family. J Ment Defic Res 26:153, 1982.
223. Fitzsimmons JS, Fitzsimmons EM, McLachlan JI, et al.: Four brothers with mental retardation, spastic paraplegia and palmoplantar hyperkeratosis. A new syndrome? Clin Genet 23:329, 1983.
224. Golabi M, Ito M, Hall BD: A new X-linked multiple congenital anomalies/mental retardation syndrome. Am J Med Genet 17:367, 1984.
225. Gareis FJ, Mason JD: X-linked mental retardation associated with bilateral clasp thumb anomaly. Am J Med Genet 17:333, 1984.
226. Holmes LB, Gang DL: Brief clinical report: an X-linked mental retardation syndrome with craniofacial abnormalities, microcephaly and club foot. Am J Med Genet 17:375, 1984.
227. Livingstone IR, Gardner-Medwin D, Pennington RJT: Familial intermittent ataxia with possible X-linked recessive inheritance. J Neurol Sci 64:89, 1984.
228. Lujan JE, Carlin ME, Lubs HA: A form of X-linked mental retardation with Marfanoid habitus. Am J Med Genet 17:311, 1984.
229. Schimke RN, Horton WA, Collins DL, et al.: A new X-linked syndrome comprising progressive basal ganglion dysfunction, mental and growth retardation, external ophthalmoplegia, postnatal microcephaly and deafness. Am J Med Genet 17:323, 1984.
230. Siber M: X-linked recessive microencephaly, microphthalmia with corneal opacities, spastic quadriplegia, hypospadias and cryptorchidism. Clin Genet 26:453, 1984.
231. Atkin JF, Flaitz K, Patil S, et al.: A new X-linked mental retardation syndrome. Am J Med Genet 21:697, 1985.
232. Cowchock FS, Duckett SW, Streletz LJ, et al.: X-linked motor-sensory neuropathy type-II with deafness and mental retardation: a new disorder. Am J Med Genet 20:307, 1985.
233. Duker JS, Weiss JS, Siber M, et al.: Ocular findings in a new heritable syndrome of brain, eye, and urogenital abnormalities. Am J Ophthalmol 88:51, 1985.
234. Toriello HV, Higgins JV, Abrahamson J, et al.: X-linked syndrome of branchial arch and other defects. Am J Med Genet 21:137, 1985.
235. Bergia B, Sybers HD, Butler IJ: Familial lethal cardiomyopathy with mental retardation and scapuloperoneal muscular dystrophy. J Neurol Neurosurg Psychiatry 49:1423, 1986.
236. Kenwrick S, Ionasescu V, Ionasescu G, et al.: Linkage studies of X-linked recessive spastic paraplegia using DNA studies. Hum Genet 73:264, 1986.
237. Fryns JP, Dereymaeker A, Hoefnagels M, et al.: Partial fragile(X) phenotype with megalotestes in fragile(X)-negative patients with acquired lesions of the central nervous system. Am J Med Genet 23:213, 1986.
238. Hunter AGW, MacMurray B: Malformations of the VATER association plus hydrocephalus in a male infant and his maternal uncle. Proc Greenwood Genet Center 6:146, 1987.

239. Farlow MR, DeMyer W, Dlouhy SR, et al.: X-linked recessive inheritance of ataxia and adult-onset dementia: clinical features and preliminary linkage analysis. Neurology 37:602, 1987.
240. Goldblatt J, Wallis C, Viljoen D: A new hypospadias—mental retardation syndrome in three brothers. Am J Dis Child 141:1168, 1987.
241. Prieto F, Badia L, Mulas F, et al.: X-linked dysmorphic syndrome with mental retardation. Clin Genet 32:326, 1987.
242. Schmidley JW, Levinsohn MW, Manetto V: Infantile X-linked ataxia and deafness: a new clinicopathologic entity. Neurology 37:1344, 1987.
243. Oberle I, Rousseau F, Heitz D, et al.: Instability of a 550-base pair DNA segment and abnormal methylation in fragile X syndrome. Science 252:1097, 1991.
244. Bell MV, Hirst MC, Nakahori Y, et al.: Physical mapping across the fragile X: Hypermethylation and clinical expression of the fragile X syndrome. Cell 64:861, 1991.
245. Yu S, Pritchard M, Kremer E, et al.: Fragile X genotype characterized by an unstable region of DNA. Science 252:1179, 1991.
246. Verkerk AJMH, Pieretti M, Sutcliffe JS, et al.: Identification of a gene (FMR-1) containing a CGG repeat coincident with a breakpoint cluster region exhibiting length variation in fragile X syndrome. Cell 65:905, 1991.
247. Villard L, Gecz J, Mattei JF, et al.: XNP mutation in a large family with Juberg-Marsidi syndrome. Nat Genet 12:359, 1996.
248. Gibbons RJ, Picketts DJ, Villard L, et al.: Mutations in a putative global transcriptional regulator cause X-linked mental retardation with α-thalassemia (ATR-X syndrome). Cell 80:837, 1995.
249. Gibbons RJ, Breuton L, Buckle VJ, et al.: Clinical and hematologic aspects of the X linked α-thalassemia/mental retardation syndrome (ATR-X). Am J Med Genet 55:288, 1995.
250. Jin H, May M, Tranebjaerg L, et al.: A novel X-linked gene, DDP, shows mutations in families with deafness (DFN-1), dystonia, mental deficiency and blindness. Nat Genet 14:177, 1996.
251. Cowchock FS, Duckett SW, Streletz LJ, et al.: X-linked motor-sensory neuropathy type-II with deafness and mental retardation: a new disorder. Am J Med Genet 20:307, 1985.
252. Ionasescu VV, Trofatter J, Haines JL, et al.: Heterogeneity in X-linked recessive Charcot-Marie-Tooth neuropathy. Am J Hum Genet 48:1075, 1991.
253. Fryns J-P, Buttiens M: X-linked mental retardation with Marfanoid habitus. Am J Med Genet 28:267, 1987.
254. Lalatta F, Livini E, Selicorni A, et al.: X-linked mental retardation with Marfanoid habitus: first report of four Italian patients. Am J Med Genet 38:228, 1991.
255. Greenstein RM, Reardon MP, Chan TS: An X-autosome translocation in a girl with Duchenne muscular dystrophy (DMD): evidence for DMD gene localization. (Abstract) Pediatr Res 11:457, 1977.
256. Tyrkus M, Bawle E, Lipman S, et al.: Aarskog-Scott syndrome inherited as an X-linked dominant with full male-female expression. (Abstract) Am J Hum Genet 32:134A, 1980.
257. Ropers HH, Zuffardi O, Bianchi E, et al.: Agenesis of corpus callosum, ocular, and skeletal anomalies (X-linked dominant Aicardi's syndrome) in a girl with balanced X/3 translocation. Hum Genet 61:364, 1982.
258. Mossman J, Blunt S, Stephens R, et al.: Hunter's disease in a girl: association with X:5 chromosomal translocation disrupting the Hunter gene. Arch Dis Child 58:911, 1983.
259. Hodgson SV, Neville B, Jones RWA, et al.: Two cases of X/autosome translocation in females with incontinentia pigmenti. Hum Genet 71:231, 1985.
260. Hodgson SV, Heckmatt JZ, Hughes E, et al.: A balanced de novo X/autosome translocation in a girl with manifestations of Lowe syndrome. Am J Med Genet 23:837, 1986.

261. Kapur S, Higgins JV, Delp K, et al.: Menkes syndrome in a girl with X-autosome translocation. Am J Med Genet 26:503, 1987.
262. Journel H, Melki J, Turleau C, et al.: Rett phenotype with X/autosome translocation: possible mapping to the short arm of chromosome X. Am J Med Genet 35:142, 1990.
263. Berger W, Meindl A, van de Pol TJR, et al.: Isolation of a candidate gene for Norrie disease by positional cloning. Nat Genet 1:199, 1992.
264. Botstein D, White RL, Skolnick M, et al.: Construction of a genetic linkage map in man using restriction fragment length polymorphisms. Am J Hum Genet 32:314, 1980.
265. Schwartz CE: Genetic markers. Tumor Biol 8:170, 1987.
266. Carpenter NJ, Waziri M, Liston J, et al.: Studies on X-linked mental retardation: evidence for a gene in the region Xq11-q22. Am J Hum Genet 43:A139, 1988.
267. Chudley AE, Lowry RB, Hoar DI: Mental retardation, distinct facial changes, short stature, obesity, and hypogonadism. A new X-linked mental retardation syndrome. Am J Med Genet 31:741, 1988.
268. Partington MW, Mulley JC, Sutherland GR, et al.: X-linked mental retardation with dystonic movements of the hands. Am J Med Genet 30:251, 1988.
269. Sutherland GR, Gedeon AK, Haan EA, et al.: Linkage studies with the gene for an X-linked syndrome of mental retardation, microcephaly and spastic diplegia. Am J Med Genet 30: 493, 1988.
270. Suthers GK, Turner G, Mulley JC: A non-syndromal form of X-linked mental retardation (XLMR) is linked to *DXS14*. Am J Med Genet 30:485, 1988.
271. Tranebjaerg L, Svejgaard A, Lykkesfeldt G: X-linked mental retardation associated with psoriasis: a new syndrome? Am J Med Genet 30:263, 1988.
272. Goldblatt J, Ballo R, Sachs B, et al.: X-linked spastic paraplegia: evidence for homogeneity with a variable phenotype. Clin Genet 35:116, 1989.
273. Al-Gazali LI, Mueller RF, Caine A, et al.: Two 46,XX,t(X;Y) females with linear skin defects and congenital microphthalmia: a new syndrome at Xp22.3. J Med Genet 27:59, 1990.
274. Graham CA, Redmond RM, Nevin NC: X-linked clinical anophthalmos: localization of the gene to Xq27-Xq28. Ophthalmic Paediatr Genet 12:43, 1990.
275. Wilkie AOM, Gibbons RJ, Higgs DR, et al.: X-linked α-thalassaemia/mental retardation: spectrum of clinical features in three related males. J Med Genet 28:738–741, 1991.
276. Gibbons RJ, Wilkie AOM, Weatherall DJ, et al.: A newly defined X-linked mental retardation syndrome associated with alpha thalassaemia. J Med Genet 28:729, 1991.
277. Miles JH, Carpenter NJ: Unique X-linked mental retardation syndrome with fingertip arches and contractures linked to Xq21.31. Am J Med Genet 38:215, 1991.
278. Pettigrew AL, Jackson LG, Ledbetter DH: New X-linked mental retardation disorder with Dandy-Walker malformation, basal ganglia disease, and seizures. Am J Med Genet 38:200, 1991.
279. Stocco dos Santos RC, Barretto OCO, Nonoyama K, et al.: X-linked syndrome: mental retardation, hip luxation, and G6PD variant [Gd(+) butantan]. Am J Med Genet 39:133, 1991.
280. Stoll C, Géraudel A, Chauvin A: New X-linked syndrome of mental retardation, short stature, and hypertelorism. Am J Med Genet 39:474, 1991.
281. Wilson M, Mulley J, Gedeon A, et al.: New X-linked syndrome of mental retardation, gynecomastia, and obesity is linked to DXS255. Am J Med Genet 40:406, 1991.
282. Arena JF, Schwartz C, Stevenson R, et al.: Spastic paraplegia with iron deposits in the basal ganglia: a new X-linked mental retardation syndrome. Am J Med Genet 43:479, 1992.
283. Bertini E, Cusmai R, de Saint Basile G, et al.: Congenital X-linked ataxia, progressive myoclonic encephalopathy, macular degeneration and recurrent infections. Am J Med Genet 43:443, 1992.

284. Hyde-Forster I, McCarthy G, Berry AC: A new X linked syndrome with mental retardation and craniofacial dysmorphism? J Med Genet 29:736, 1992.
285. Kang W-M, Huang C-C, Lin S-J: X-linked recessive inheritance of dysgenesis of corpus callosum in a Chinese Family. Am J Med Genet 44:619, 1992.
286. Porteous MEM, Johnson H, Burn J, et al.: A new mental retardation syndrome mapping to the pericentromeric region of the X-chromosome. Am J Hum Genet 51: A106, 1992.
287. Proud VK, Levine C, Carpenter NJ: New X-linked syndrome with seizures, acquired microencephaly, and agenesis of the corpus callosum. Am J Med Genet 43:458, 1992.
288. Tranebjaerg L, Lou H, Andresen J: New X-linked syndrome with apraxia, ataxia, and mental deficiency: clinical, cytogenetic and neuropsychological studies in two Danish families. Am J Med Genet 43:498, 1992.
289. Arts WFM, Loonen MCB, Sengers RCA, et al.: X-linked ataxia, weakness, deafness, and loss of vision in early childhood with a fatal course. Ann Neurol 33:535, 1993.
290. Brunner HG, Nelen M, Breakefield XO, et al.: Abnormal behavior associated with a point mutation in the structural gene for monoamine oxidase A. Science 262:578, 1993.
291. Gustavson K-H, Annerén G, Malmgren H, et al.: New X-linked syndrome with severe mental retardation, severely impaired vision, severe hearing defect, epileptic seizures, spasticity, restricted joint mobility, and early death. Am J Med Genet 45:654, 1993.
292. Aldred MA, Dry KL, Knight-Jones EB, et al.: Genetic analysis of a kindred with X-linked mental handicap and retinitis pigmentosa. Am J Hum Genet 55:916, 1994.
293. Brooks SS, Wisniewski K, Brown WT: New X-linked mental retardation (XLMR) syndrome with distinct facial appearance and growth retardation. Am J Med Genet 51:586, 1994.
294. Hamel CJ, Smits APT, Otten BJ, et al.: Familial X-linked mental retardation and isolated growth hormone deficiency. Am J Med Genet 64:35, 1996.
295. Lindsay S, Splitt M, Edney S, et al.: PPM-X: A new X-linked mental retardation syndrome with psychosis, pyramidal signs, and macroorchidism maps to Xq28. Am J Hum Genet 58:1120, 1996.
296. Wittwer B, Kircheisen R, Leutelt J, et al.: New X-linked mental retardation syndrome with the gene mapped tentatively in Xp22.3. Am J Med Genet 64:42, 1996.
297. Stevenson RE, Häne B, Arena JF, et al.: Arch fingerprints, hypotonia, and areflexia associated with X linked mental retardation. J Med Genet 34:465, 1997.
298. Armfield K, Nelson R, Lubs HA, et al.: An XLMR syndrome with short stature, small hands and feet, seizures, cleft palate, and glaucoma is linked to Xq28. Am J Med Genet 85:236, 1998.
299. Arveiler B, Alembik Y, Hanauer A, et al.: Linkage analysis suggests at least two loci for X-linked non specific mental retardation. Am J Med Genet 30:473, 1988.
300. Sutherland GR, Gedeon AK, Haan EA, et al.: Linkage studies with the gene for an X-linked syndrome of mental retardation, microcephaly and spastic diplegia (*MRX2*). Am J Med Genet 30: 493, 1988.
301. Partington MW, Mulley JC, Sutherland GR, et al.: A family with the Coffin-Lowry syndrome revisited: localization of CLS to Xp21-pter. Am J Med Genet 30:509, 1988.
302. Hanauer A, Alembik Y, Gilgenkrantz S: Probably localisation of the Coffin-Lowry locus in Xp22.2-p22.1 by multipoint linkage analysis. Am J Med Genet 30:523, 1988.
303. Schrander-Stumpel C, Legius E, Fryns JP, et al.: MASA syndrome: new clinical features and linkage analysis using DNA probe. J Med Genet 22:688, 1990.
304. Mathews KD, Beutow K, Turner G, et al.: Börjeson-Forssman-Lehmann syndrome localization. (Letter) Am J Med Genet 34:475, 1989.
305. Turner G, Gedeon A, Mulley J, et al.: Börjeson-Forssman-Lehmann syndrome: clinical manifestations and gene localization to Xq26-27. Am J Med Genet 34:463, 1989.

fragile XE syndrome in a special education needs population. Am J Med Genet 64:428, 1996.
350. Slaney SF, Wilkie AO, Hirst MC, et al.: DNA testing for fragile X syndrome in schools for learning difficulties. Arch Dis Child 72:33, 1995.
351. Van den Ouweland AM, de Vries BB, Bakker PL, et al.: DNA diagnosis of the fragile X syndrome in a series of 236 mentally retarded subjects and evidence for a reversal of mutation in the FMR-1 gene. Am J Med Genet 41:482, 1994.
352. Hagerman RJ, Wilson P, Staley LW, et al.: Evaluation of school children at high risk for fragile X syndrome utilizing buccal cell FMR-1 testing. Am J Med Genet 51:474, 1994.
353. Jacobs PA, Bullman H, Macpherson J, et al.: Population studies of the fragile X: a molecular approach. J Med Genet 30:454, 1993.
354. Kahkonen M, Alitalo T, Airaksinen E, et al.: Prevalence of the fragile X syndrome in four birth cohorts of children of school age. Hum Genet 77:85, 1987.
355. Webb TP, Bundey S, Thake A, et al.: The frequency of the fragile X chromosome among school children in Coventry. J Med Genet 23:396, 1986.
356. Gustavson KH, Blomquist HK, Holmgren G: Prevalence of the fragile-X syndrome in mentally retarded boys in a Swedish country. Am J Med Genet 23:581, 1986.

3

Nonsyndromic XLMR

Mental retardation caused by mutations of genes on the X chromosome without accompanying somatic, neurologic, biochemical, or behavioral manifestations which permit distinction from nonaffected male siblings or from other males with mental retardation is designated nonsyndromic XLMR. The term nonspecific XLMR has been used with the same meaning.

Mutations of X-linked genes that impair cognitive and adaptive function exclusively or almost exclusively account for a substantial portion of the cases of mental retardation in males. Collectively, such gene mutations may cause more cases of mental retardation than Down syndrome or the fragile X syndrome, the two most common specific types of genetic mental retardation. There is, however, no contemporary study that provides a reliable prevalence for nonsyndromic XLMR. Using a 30% excess of males among persons with mental retardation, attributing all of the male excess to XLMR, and disregarding the small number of females with mental retardation due to X-linked genes, one may calculate that XLMR makes up 13% of all mental retardation (formula: $2a + b = 1$, where a = the number of females with non X-linked MR, $+a$ = the number of males with non-X-linked mental retardation (MR), $+b$ = the number of males with X-linked MR, and $a + b = 1.3a$). If nonsyndromic XLMR accounts for half of all XLMR, it would explain 6%–7% of all mental retardation.

Lehrke proposed that nonsyndromic XLMR could explain all of the excess of males among persons with mental retardation.[1–3] Since most of the syndromic forms of XLMR have been described since Lehrke's report, it is presumed that these forms should be included in his nonsyndromic XLMR numbers. Indeed, he cited as nonsyndromic XLMR the families reported by Martin and Bell (1943), Allan et al. (1944), Losowsky (1961), Renpenning et al. (1962), and Dunn et al. (1963).[4–8] These families are now considered to have syndromic forms of XLMR, three of the five representing the fragile X syndrome.

Turner and associates have also found that nonsyndromic XLMR contributes substantially to the excess of males with mental retardation and to the preponderance of males among mentally retarded siblings.[9–12] They calculated the prevalence of nonsyndromic XLMR in New South Wales to be 0.55 cases/1000 males in the population. Parenthetically, it may be noted that Turner and colleagues used the term *Renpenning syndrome* for nonsyndromic XLMR and argued for inclusion of only those cases lacking macrocephaly or microcephaly, epilepsy, major malformations or more than one minor malformation, and neurological signs. Although the somatic phenotype of Renpenning syndrome is indeed mild, consisting of microcephaly, short stature, and microorchidism, it is treated in this monograph as an XLMR syndrome (see Chapters 4 and 5).

A higher prevalence for nonsyndromic XLMR, 1.83 cases/1000 males in the population, has been calculated by Herbst and Miller.[13] They included the fragile X syndrome among the nonsyndromic XLMR numbers and presumably included other less well-defined syndromes as well. They concluded that seven to 19 X-linked genes may be responsible for nonsyndromic XLMR.

A number of characteristics of nonsyndromic XLMR can be set forth. Affected males lack morphologic, neuromuscular, or behavioral manifestations that distinguish them from unaffected brothers or from other males with mental retardation.[14–17] They also lack diagnostic findings on cranial imaging, biochemical studies, or cytogenetic analysis. The diagnosis requires at least three affected males related in a fashion consistent with X-linked inheritance. Optimally, observations will be available on affected individuals of different ages which confirm that syndromic manifestations do not become apparent with age. Carrier females may experience less severe learning problems.

Caution must be taken in designating an XLMR entity as nonsyndromic. The designation implies that growth, morphological features, neuromuscular development and function, behavior, brain imaging, and laboratory testing are normal. One example will suffice to illustrate that entities considered on initial evaluation to be nonsyndromic may be shown subsequently to be syndromic. In 1943, Martin and Bell described a "sex-linked" entity affecting 11 males in two generations which they described as nonspecific.[4] They stated, "No peculiar features, either mental or physical, have been recognized which would serve to distinguish the disease. . . . Physically the affected members are not abnormal. They are in general of sturdy build, but they do not show any distinctions in shape of head or face, colour of eyes, dentition, bodily proportions, or other observed physical character. . . . Their sexual development appears to be normal." When the family was restudied in Richards et al. in 1981, affected males were found to have prognathism, large ears, and macroorchidism, clinical features typical of the fragile X syndrome.[18] Chromosome analysis documented the fragile site on Xq27.3 in the affected males.

Because of the lack of distinctive clinical features, patients with nonsyndromic XLMR pose a great diagnostic challenge. How does one decide if a male with mental retardation and no other feature harbors a detrimental gene on the X chromosome or has some other undetected environmental or genetic insult? A conclusion should only be reached after thorough investigation of the patient and then with considerable reservation. The absence of historical information, clinical manifestations, and laboratory evidence implicating a specific insult and the presence of additional similarly affected males related through females provide the strongest evidence in support of XLMR. The more males affected the stronger the support for XLMR. Less severe learning difficulty might occur in female carriers.

Localization of Genes for Nonsyndromic XLMR

Before the availability of polymorphic molecular markers, no nonsyndromic XLMR entity had been mapped. A major advance in understanding nonsyndromic XLMR came in 1988 when Suthers et al. utilized restriction fragment length polymorphisms (RFLPs) to regionally map a mental retardation condition to the pericentromeric region of the X chromosome (Xp11.3-q12).[19] This allowed distinction of this family with nonsyndromic XLMR, designated MRX1, from all other XLMR families who could be shown to have nonoverlapping linkage limits. Additional families were to be mapped in the years to follow using RFLPs.[20–22,24–30] A convention established in 1990 has assisted in the systematic study of families with nonsyndromic XLMR.[15] Those families in which linkage analysis produced lod scores of greater than 2 were assigned MRX numbers. The subsequent development of microsatellite markers in the early 1990s has greatly quickened the pace of regional mapping of these conditions.[30–71] To date, over 60 MRX numbers have been assigned (Table 3–1). These families form at least eight exclusive linkage groups, and four genes have been identified (Fig. 3–1). These are certain to be partitioned further as linkage limits are refined and as new families with linkage data are added.

In addition, there are numerous other families with apparent XLMR which have not been available for linkage analysis or which are too small or in which available family members have not been informative.[3,9,12,72–77] As a larger battery of genes that cause nonsyndromic XLMR becomes available, mutational analysis may prove informative in these families.

Although criteria for nonsyndromic XLMR have been established for some time, a not insignificant number of families who have received MRX designation do have clinical manifestations which might permit distinction of affected males from nonaffected siblings (Table 3–1). By and large, these manifestations have not been sufficiently distinct to convince the authors that clinical diagnosis could be consistently accomplished and hence the assignment of MRX numbers to some entities with neuromuscular, behavioral, or somatic manifestations.

There is a similar group of families among the XLMR syndromes (see Chapter 4) in which there exist neuromuscular, somatic, or behavioral manifestations that are inconsistent but occur with sufficient frequency so that the authors have decided on a syndromic designation. There may in fact be a greater tendency, for publication or perhaps other reasons, to designate an entity as syndromic.

Genes That Cause Nonsyndromic XLMR

In four instances, the genes for nonsyndromic XLMR have been isolated and mutations identified.[45,46,58,62,71,78–80] FMR2, the gene that causes the FRAXE syn-

Table 3–1. Nonsyndromic X-Linked Mental Retardation*

Designation	Reference	Regional Localization	Remarks
MRX1	Suthers et al. 1988[19] Kerr et al. 1992[20]	Xp11.4-q21.31	Moderate MR
MRX2	Proops et al. 1983[21] Arveiller et al. 1988[22] Hu et al. 1994[23]	Xp22.1-p22.3	Mild–moderate MR, distinctive facies, short hands and feet, macroorchidism, heterozygote manifestation
MRX3	Gedeon et al. 1991[24]	Xq28-qter	Mild–moderate MR, behavior problems, brachycephaly, increased limb span
MRX4	Arveiller et al. 1988[22] Hu et al. 1994[23]	Xp11.22-q21.31	Moderate MR
MRX5	Samanns et al. 1991[25]	Xp21.1-q21.3	Deviant behavior, hyperactivity
MRX6	Kondo et al. 1991[26]	Xq27	Moderate MR, short stature, coarse facies, broad nasal tip, short hands and feet, heterozygote manifestation
MRX7	Jedele et al. 1992[27]	Xp11.23-q12	Mild MR, behavioral problems
MRX8	Schwartz et al. 1992[28]	Xp21-q21.1	Moderate–severe MR
MRX9	Willems et al. 1993[29]	Xp21.2-q12	Moderate MR
MRX10	Kerr et al. 1992[20]	Xp11.4-p21.3	Variable MR, heterozygote manifestation
MRX11	Kerr et al. 1992[20]	Xp11.22-p21.3	Moderate-severe MR, heterozygote manifestation
MRX12	Kerr et al. 1992[20]	Xp21.2-q12	Mild–moderate MR, prematurity/low birth weight, large ears, hypotelorism, short stature
MRX13	Kerr et al. 1992[20]	Xp22.3-q22	Mild–moderate MR, heterozygote manifestation
MRX14	Gendrot et al. 1994[30]	Xp21.2-q13	Moderate–severe MR, inconsistent phenotypic abnormalities
MRX15	Moraine et al. 1995[31]	Xp22.1-Xq12	Severe MR, hypotonia
MRX16	Moraine et al. 1995[31]	Xp27.3-qter	Moderate MR, hyperactive deep tendon reflexes, variable short stature and microcephaly
MRX17	Gedeon et al. 1994[32]	Xp11.22-q12	Moderate MR
MRX18	Gedeon et al. 1994[32]	Xp11.22-p21.1	Mild–severe MR, heterozygote manifestation
MRX19	Donnelly et al. 1994[33]	Xp22.2-p22.3	Moderate MR
MRX20	Lazzarini et al. 1995[34]	Xp21.1-q23	Mild–moderate MR, large ears, obesity, dysarthria
MRX21	Kozak et al. 1993[35]	Xp11.4-pter	Moderate MR, heterozygote manifestation
MRX22	Passos-Bueno et al. 1993[36]	Xp21.1-q21.31	Severe MR, generalized muscle atrophy
MRX23	Gregg et al. 1996[37]	Xq23-q24	
MRX24	Martinez et al. 1995[38]	Xp22.2-p22.3	Moderate–severe MR, "slightly coarse facies," small head circumference
MRX25	Nordstrom et al. 1992[39]	Xq27.3	Severe MR, heterozygote manifestation

(continued)

Table 3–1. Nonsyndromic X-Linked Mental Retardation—Continued

Designation	*Reference*	*Regional Localization*	*Remarks*
MRX26	Robledo et al. 1991[40]	Xp11.4-q23	
MRX27	Glass et al. 1991[41] Gedeon et al. 1995[42]	Xq24-q27.1	
MRX28	Holinski-Feder et al. 1995[43]	Xq27.3-qter	
MRX29	Häne et al. 1996[44]	Xp21.2-p22	Severe MR
MRX30	Donnelly et al. 1995[45] Allen et al. 1998[46]	Xq22.3-q23	Mild MR, below average OFC and height, gene cloned: PAK3
MRX31	Donnelly et al. 1995[45]	Xp11.23-q13.3	Moderate MR, slightly above average OFC, height, weight
MRX32	Howard-Peebles et al. 1979 (Family C)[47] Häne et al. 1999[48]	Xp21-p22.2	Variable MR
MRX33	Holinski-Feder et al. 1995[43]	Xp11.1-pter	
MRX34	Raeymaekers et al. 1995[49] Marynen et al. 1995[50]	Xp21.3	Microdeletion
MRX35	Gu et al. 1996[51]	Xq21.3-q26	Heterozygote manifestations
MRX36	Claes et al. 1996[52]	Xp21-p22.1	
MRX37	Bar-David et al. 1996[53]	Xp22.31-p22.32	
MRX38	Schutz et al. 1996[54]	Xp21.1-p22.13	Macrocephaly, seizures
MRX39	Teboul et al. 1989[55]	Xp11	Sporadic cases with X/autosome translocations
MRX40	May et al. 1995[56]	Xq21	Microdeletion
MRX41	D'Adamo et al. 1998[57] Bienvenu et al. 1998[58]	Xq28	Gene cloned: GDI1
MRX42	Holinski-Feder et al. 1997[59]	Xq24-q25?	Clinical and linkage details not yet published
MRX43	Hamel et al. 1999[60,61]	Xp21.2-p22.31	Moderate–severe MR, obesity, large head, wide palpebral fissures, periorbital fullness
MRX44	Hamel et al. 1999[60,61]	Xp11.21-p11.3	Moderate–severe MR, behavioral aberrations
MRX45	Hamel et al. 1999[60,61]	Xp11.21-p11.3	Variable MR, large ears and hands
MRX46	Hamel et al. 1999[61] Yntema et al. 1998[62]	Xq26-q27	Variable MR, behavioral disturbances
MRX47	des Portes et al. 1997[63]	Xq13-q25	Moderate–severe MR
MRX48	D'Adamo et al. 1998[57] Bienvenu et al. 1998[58]	Xq28	Gene cloned: GDI1, heterozygote manifestation
MRX49	Claes et al. 1997[64]	Xp22.1-pter	Mild–moderate MR, possible heterozygote manifestation
MRX50	Claes et al. 1997[64]	Xp11.21-p11.4	Moderate–severe MR, macrocephaly, short stature
MRX51	Claes et al. 1999[65]	Xp11.23-p11.3	Mild MR
MRX52	Hamel et al. 1999[60,61]	Xp11.21-q21.33	Moderate–severe MR, down-slanting palpebral fissures, midface hypoplasia
MRX53	Ahmad et al. 1997[66]	Xq22.2-q25	
MRX54	Ben Jemaa et al. 1999[67]	Xp21.3-p22.1	Variable MR, long face, thin lips, large ears
MRX55	Deqaqi et al. 1998[68]	Xp21.1-q13	

(continued)

TABLE 3–1. Continued

Designation	Reference	Regional Localization	Remarks
MRX56	Holinski-Feder et al. 1997[59]	Xp11.21-p21.1?	Clinical and linkage details not yet published
MRX57	Holinski-Feder et al. 1997[59]	Xq24-q25?	Clinical and linkage details not yet published
MRX58	Holinski-Feder et al. 1999[59]	Xp11.3-q13.1?	Clinical and linkage details not yet published
MRX59	Carpenter et al. 1999	Xp21.2-p22.2	Variable MR and craniofacial findings, aggressive behavior
MRX60	Billuart et al. 1998[71]	Xq12	Gene cloned: Oligophrenin-1
MRX61			
MRX62			
MRX63			
MRX64			
MRX65	Yntema et al. 1999[69]	Xp11.4-q21.33	Mild–moderate MR, obesity, small testes, behavioral disturbances
MRX66			
MRX67			
MRX68			

*Other families with nonsyndromic XLMR have been reported by Opitz et al. (1965),[72] Turner et al. (1971),[11] Yarbrough and Howard-Peebles (1976),[76] Wilson et al. (1992),[77] Gedeon et al. (1994),[32] Herbst et al. (1980, 1981),[13,73,74] Lehrke (1974),[3] and others.

drome, was cloned in 1993, allowing distinction from FMR1, the gene that causes FRAXA syndrome.[78] Like FMR1, the FMR2 gene is a gene in which an unstable trinucleotide (CGG) repeat occurs in the 5′ untranslated region. The usual number of CGG repeats in the general population is 16 with a range of two to 38 repeats. Individuals with premutations have 39 to 230 repeats; those with full mutations have in excess of 230 repeats. Methylation accompanies full mutations, resulting in cessation of transcription. Males with full mutations do not have a distinctive somatic phenotype but may have mild mental impairment. In childhood, this is manifest to a greater degree in speech delay.

Billuart et al. were directed to a gene in Xq12 that was transected in a balanced X:12 translocation and was associated with mild mental retardation.[71] They found a 1 bp deletion in the gene in a nonsyndromic XLMR family, MRX60. The gene, mutations of which encode a Rho-GTPase-activating protein termed *oligophrenin-1* (OPHN-1), may affect cell migration and axon outgrowth during brain morphogenesis.

Two families with nonsyndromic XLMR (MRX41 and MRX48) have been shown to have mutations in GDI1, a gene that encodes a Rab GDP-dissociation inhibitor protein.[57,58] Members of this family of proteins control the recycling of Rab GTPases involved in membrane traffic and may thus play a role in neurotransmission. The mutation in MRX48 led to a truncated GDI protein; the mutation in MRX41 caused a protein substitution resulting in an altered Rab binding site.

A mutation in the PAK3 gene, which encodes a serine-threonine kinase, has been found in MRX30, which maps to Xq22.[45,46] The PAK3 protein is highly ex-

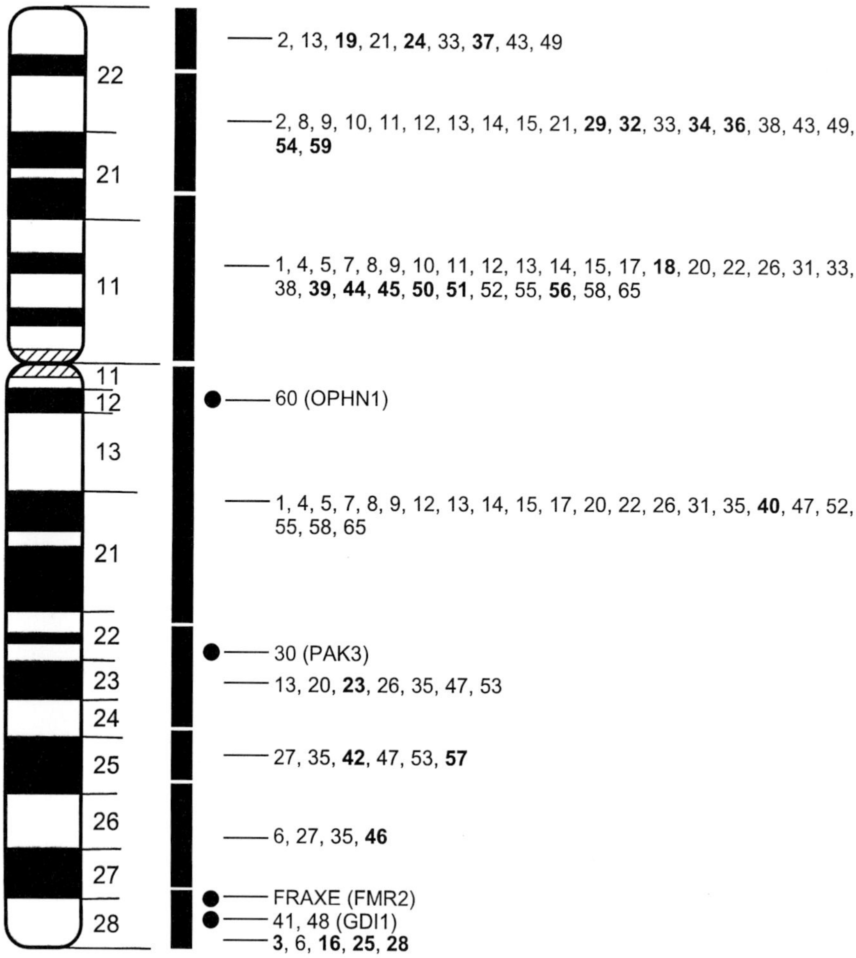

FIGURE 3–1. Provisional map of nonsyndromic types of XLMR showing eight exclusive linkage groups (bars) and four specific gene locations (circles). The MRX families that map to each of the lingage groups are indicated. Those families with mapping limits within a single linkage group are shown in bold, those with mapping limits that overlap two or more linkage groups are not bold.

pressed in the cerebral cortex and hippocampus. The mutation suppresses kinase activity.

Numerous deletions of contiguous genes on the X chromosome have been described and in some instances the deletions are presumed to include genes that cause nonsyndromic XLMR. Deletions in Xq13-q21 are typical.[56,81] In several cases, deletions in this region extend from the deafness gene (DFN3) proximally to the choroideremia gene (CHM) distally and in the process eliminate an intervening gene for nonsyndromic XLMR. In other instances, microdeletions have interrupted a gene for nonsyndromic XLMR but have not extended into adjacent genes.[49,50,82,83]

Counseling

In the absence of a specific diagnosis for affected male siblings or affected males related through females, it is not unreasonable to give recurrence risks as appropriate for X-linked inheritance. It is equally appropriate to qualify all counseling by acknowledgment of the incomplete understanding of XLMR and the inability to specifically diagnose most nonsyndromic entities and to distinguish them from one another. Of the many families with nonsyndromic XLMR that have been described and the 60 families for which regional gene mapping has been successful, the underlying gene has been cloned in only four instances. Hence a specific diagnosis can be made only for these nonsyndromic types of XLMR by molecular methods. Linkage and haplotype analysis may be beneficial for families in which the gene has not been isolated, as a means of providing carrier identification, prenatal detection, and postnatal diagnosis.

REFERENCES

1. Lehrke RG: Sex-linked mental retardation and verbal disability (thesis). University Microfilms, Ann Arbor, MI, 1968.
2. Lehrke R: A theory of X-linkage of major intellectual traits. Am J Ment Defic 76:611, 1972.
3. Lehrke RG: X-linked mental retardation and verbal disabilities. Birth Defects Orig Art Series X(1):1, 1974.
4. Martin JP, Bell J: A pedigree of mental defect showing sex-linkage. J Neurol Psychiatry 6:154, 1943.
5. Allan W, Herndon CN, Dudley FC: Some examples of the inheritance of mental deficiency: apparently sex-linked idiocy and microcephaly. Am J Ment Defic 48:325, 1944.
6. Losowsky MS: Hereditary mental defect showing the pattern of sex influence. J Ment Defic Res 5:60, 1961.
7. Renpenning H, Gerrard JW, Zaleski WA, et al.: Familial sex-linked mental retardation. Can Med Assoc J 87:954, 1962.
8. Dunn HG, Renpenning H, Gerrard JW, et al.: Mental retardation as a sex-linked defect. Am J Ment Defic 67:827, 1962–63.
9. Turner G, Engisch B, Lindsay DG, et al.: X-linked mental retardation without physical abnormality (Renpenning's syndrome) in sibs in an institution. J Med Genet 9:324, 1972.
10. Turner G, Turner B, Collins E: Renpenning's syndrome—X-linked mental retardation. Lancet 2:365, 1970.
11. Turner G, Turner B, Collins E: X-linked mental retardation without physical abnormality: Renpenning's syndrome. Dev Med Child Neurol 13:71, 1971.
12. Turner G, Turner B: X-linked mental retardation. J Med Genet 11:109, 1974.
13. Herbst DS, Miller JR: Nonspecific X-linked mental retardation II: the frequency in British Columbia. Am J Med Genet 7:461, 1980.
14. Kerr B, Turner G, Mulley J, et al.: Non-specific X linked mental retardation. J Med Genet 28:378, 1991.
15. Mulley JC, Kerr B, Stevenson R, et al.: Nomenclature guidelines for X-linked mental retardation. Am J Med Genet 43:383, 1992.
16. Gedeon AK, Donnelly AJ, Mulley JC, et al.: How many X-linked genes for non-specific mental retardation (MRX) are there? Am J Med Genet 64:158, 1996.

17. Schwartz CE: Invited editorial: X-linked mental retardation: in pursuit of a gene map. Am J Med Genet 52:1025, 1993.
18. Richards BW, Sylvester PE, Brooker C: Fragile X-linked mental retardation: the Martin-Bell syndrome. J Ment Defic Res 25:253, 1981.
19. Suthers GK, Turner G, Mulley JC: A non-syndromal form of X-linked mental retardation (XLMR) is linked to *DXS14*. Am J Med Genet 30:485, 1988.
20. Kerr B, Gedeon A, Mulley J, et al.: Localization of non-specific X-linked mental retardation genes. Am J Med Genet 43:392, 1992.
21. Proops R, Mayer M, Jacobs PA: A study of mental retardation in children in the island of Hawaii. Clin Genet 23:81, 1983.
22. Arveiler B, Alembik Y, Hanauer A, et al.: Linkage analysis suggests at least two loci for X-linked non-specific mental retardation. Am J Med Genet 30:473, 1988.
23. Hu L-J, Blumenfeld-Heyberger S, Hanauer A, et al.: Non-specific X-linked mental retardation: linkage analysis in MRX2 and MRX4 families revisited. Am J Med Genet 51:569, 1994.
24. Gedeon A, Kerr B, Mulley J, et al.: Localisation of the MRX3 gene for non-specific X linked mental retardation. J Med Genet 28:372, 1991.
25. Samanns C, Albrecht R, Neugebauer M, et al.: Gene for non-specific X-linked mental retardation maps in the pericentromeric region. Am J Med Genet 38:224, 1991.
26. Kondo I, Tsukamoto K, Niikawa N, et al.: A new form of X-linked mental retardation (XLMR) linked to DXS369(RN1). Cytogenet Cell Genet 58:2071, 1991.
27. Jedele KB, Michels VV, Schaid DJ, et al.: Linkage of nonspecific X-linked mental retardation to Xq21.31. Am J Med Genet 43:436, 1992.
28. Schwartz CE, May M, Huang T, et al.: MRX8: An X-linked mental retardation condition with linkage to Xq21. Am J Med Genet 43:467, 1992.
29. Willems P, Vits L, Buntinx I, et al.: Localization of a gene responsible for nonspecific mental retardation (MRX9) to the pericentromeric region of the X chromosome. Genomics 18:290, 1993.
30. Gendrot C, Ronce N, Toutain A, et al.: X-linked mental retardation exhibiting linkage to DXS255 and PGKP1: a new MRX family (MRX14) with localization in the pericentromeric region. Clin Genet 45:145, 1994.
31. Moraine C, Gendrot C, Dourlens J, et al.: Non-specific non-fragile X mental deficiency: clinical and molecular study in ten families. Fifth International Workshop on Fragile X and X-Linked Mental Retardation. Strasbourg, 1991.
32. Gedeon A, Kerr B, Mulley J, et al.: Pericentromeric genes for non-specific X-linked mental retardation (MRX). Am J Med Genet 51:553, 1994.
33. Donnelly AJ, Choo KHA, Kozman HM, et al.: Regional localisation of a non-specific X-linked mental retardation gene (MRX19) to Xp22. Am J Med Genet 51:581, 1994.
34. Lazzarini A, Stenroos ES, Lehner T, et al.: Short tandem repeat polymorphism linkage studies in a new family with X-linked mental retardation (MRX20). Am J Med Genet 57:552, 1995.
35. Kozak L, Chiurazzi P, Genuardi M, et al.: Mapping of a gene for non-specific X linked mental retardation: evidence for linkage to chromosomal region Xp21.1-Xp22.3. J Med Genet 30:866, 1993.
36. Passos-Bueno MR, Byth BC, Rosenberg S, et al.: Severe nonspecific X-linked mental retardation caused by a proximally Xp located gene: intragenic heterogeneity or a new form of X-linked mental retardation? Am J Med Genet 46:172, 1993.
37. Gregg RG, Palmer C, Kirkpatrick S, et al.: Localization of a non-specific X-linked mental retardation gene, MRX23, to Xq23-q24. Hum Mol Genet 5:411, 1996.
38. Martinez F, Gal A, Palau F, Prieto F: Localization of a gene for X-linked nonspecific mental retardation (MRX24) in Xp22.2-p22.3. Am J Med Genet 55:387, 1995.
39. Nordstrom A-M, Penttinen M, von Koskull H: Linkage to Xq28 in a family with nonspecific X-linked mental retardation. Hum Genet 90:263, 1992.
40. Robledo R, Melis P, Laficara F, et al.: Further linkage evidence for localization of mu-

tational sites for nonsyndromic types of X-linked mental retardation at the pericentromeric region. Am J Med Genet 64:107, 1996.

41. Glass IA, White EM, Pope MJ, et al.: Linkage analysis in a large family with nonspecific X-linked retardation. Am J Med Genet 38:240, 1991.
42. Gedeon AK, Glass IA, Connor JM, et al.: Genetic localization of MRX27 to Xq24-26 defines the sixth discrete gene for non-specific X-linked mental retardation. Am J Med Genet 64:121, 1996.
43. Holinski-Feder E, Golla A, Rost I, et al.: Regional localization of two MRX genes to Xq28 (MRX28) and to Xp11.4-Xp22.12 (MRX33). Am J Med Genet 64:125, 1996.
44. Häne B, Schroer RJ, Arena JF, et al.: Nonsyndromic X-linked mental retardation: review and mapping of MRX29 to Xp21. Clin Genet 50:176, 1996.
45. Donnelly AJ, Partington MW, Ryan AK, et al.: Regional localisation of two nonspecific X-linked mental retardation genes (MRX30 and MRX31). Am J Med Genet 64:113, 1996.
46. Allen KM, Gleeson JG, Bagrodia S, et al.: PAK3 mutation in nonsyndromic X-linked mental retardation. Nat Genet 20:25, 1998.
47. Howard-Peebles PN, Stoddard GR, Mims MG: Familial X-linked mental retardation, verbal disability, and marker X chromosomes. Am J Hum Genet 31:214, 1979.
48. Häne B, Stevenson RE, Arena JF, et al.: Gene for nonsyndromic X-linked mental retardation (MRX32) maps to a 18 Mb region of Xp21.2-p22. Am J Med Genet, in press, 1999.
49. Raeymaekers P, Lin J, Gu XX, et al.: Nonspecific mental retardation is probably caused by a microdeletion in a Belgian family. Seventh International Workshop on Fragile X and X-Linked Mental Retardation. Tromso, Norway, 1995.
50. Marynen P, Gu XX, Soekarman D, et al.: A microdeletion of the X chromosome is the probable cause of non-specific mental retardation in a Belgian family. Am J Hum Genet 57:A263, 1995.
51. Gu XX, Decorte R, Marynen P, et al.: Localization of a new gene for non-specific mental retardation to Xq22-q26 (MRX35). J Med Genet 33:52, 1996.
52. Claes S, Gu XX, Legius E, et al.: Linkage analysis in three families with nonspecific X-linked mental retardation. Am J Med Genet 64:137, 1996.
53. Bar-David S, Lerer I, Sarfaty CK, et al.: Localization of two X-linked mental retardation (XLMR) genes to Xp: MRX37 gene at Xp22.31-p22.32 and a putative MRX gene on Xp22.11-p22.2. Am J Med Genet 64:83, 1996.
54. Schutz CK, Ives EJ, Chalifoux M, et al.: Regional localization of an X-linked mental retardation gene to Xp21.1-Xp22.13. Am J Med Genet 64:89, 1996.
55. Teboul M, Mujica P, Chery M, et al.: Translocations X-autosomes equilibrees et retard mental. Contribution a la cartographie des retards mentaux lies a l'X. J Genet Hum 37:179, 1989.
56. May M, Colleaux L, Murgia A, et al.: Molecular analysis of four males with mental retardation and deletions of Xq21 places the putative MR region in Xq21.1 between DXS233 and CHM. Hum Mol Genet 4:1465, 1995.
57. D'Adamo P, Menegon A, Lo Nigro C, et al.: Mutations in *GDI1* are responsible for X-linked non-specific mental retardation. Nat Genet 19:134, 1998.
58. Bienvenu T, des Portes V, Saint Martin A, et al.: Non-specific X-linked semidominant mental retardation by mutations in a Rab GDP-dissociation inhibitor. Hum Mol Genet 7:1311, 1998.
59. Holinski-Feder E, Charockh-Zadeh S, Golla A, et al.: Non-syndromic X-linked mental retardation: mapping of four novel MRX families. Eighth International Workshop on Fragile X and X-Linked Mental Retardation. Picton, Canada, 1997.
60. Hamel BCJ, Smits APT, van den Helm B, et al.: Four families (MRX43, 44, 45, 52) with nonspecific X-linked mental retardation: clinical and psychometric data and results of linkage analysis. Am J Med Genet 85:290, 1999.
61. Hamel BCJ, Smits APT, van Roosmalen T, et al.: Nonspecific X-linked mental retardation in 5 families (MRX43, 44, 45, 46 and 52): clinical, psychometric and molecu-

lar data. Eight International Workshop on Fragile X and X-Linked Mental Retardation. Picton, Canada, 1997.
62. Yntema HG, Hamel BC, Smits AP, et al.: Localisation of a gene for non-specific X linked mental retardation (MRX46) to Xq25-q26. J Med Genet 35:801, 1998.
63. des Portes V, Soufir N, Carrie A, et al.: Gene for nonspecific X-linked mental retardation (MRX47) is located in Xq22.3-q24. Am J Med Genet 72:324, 1997.
64. Claes S, Vogels A, Holvoet M, et al.: Regional localization of two genes for nonspecific X-linked mental retardation to Xp22.3-p22.2 (MRX49) and Xp11.3-p11.21 (MRX50). Am J Med Genet 73:474, 1997.
65. Claes S, Volcke P, Devriendt K, et al.: Regional localization of a gene for nonspecific XLMR to Xp11.3-p11.23 (MRX51) and tentative localization of a MRX gene to Xp23-q26.1. Am J Med Genet 85:283, 1999.
66. Ahmad W, Fusco MD, Haque MF, et al.: Mapping of three new loci for X-linked mental retardations. Am J Hum Genet 61:A265, 1997.
67. Ben Jemaa L, des Portes V, Zemni R, et al.: A refined 2.7 centimorgan locus in Xp21.3-22.1 for a nonspecific X-linked mental retardation gene (MRX54). Am J Med Genet 85:276, 1999.
68. Deqaqi SC, N'Guessan M, Forner J, et al.: A gene for non-specific X-linked mental retardation (MRX55) is located in Xp11. Ann Genet 41:11, 1998.
69. Yntema HG, van den Helm B, Knoers NVAM, et al.: X-linked mental retardation: Evidence for a recent mutation in a five-generation family (MRX65) linked to the pericentromeric region. Am J Med Genet 85:305, 1999.
70. Carpenter NJ, Brown WT, Qu Y, et al.: Regional localization of a non-specific X-linked mental retardation gene (MRX59) to Xp21.2-p22.2. Am J Med Genet 85:266, 1999.
71. Billuart P, Bienvenu T, Ronce N, et al.: Oligophrenin-1 encodes a rhoGAP protein involved in X-linked mental retardation. Nature 392:923, 1998.
72. Optiz JM, Segal AT, Kl ve H, et al.: X-linked mental retardation: study of a large kindred with 20 affected members. Midw Res Soc Ped Res, Winnipeg meeting. J Pediatr 67:713, 1965.
73. Herbst DS: Nonspecific X-linked mental retardation I: a review with information from 24 new families. Am J Med Genet 7:443, 1980.
74. Herbst DS, Dunn HG, Dill FJ, et al.: Further delineation of X-linked mental retardation. Hum Genet 58:366, 1981.
75. Tariverdian G, Weck B: Nonspecific X-linked mental retardation—a review. Hum Genet 62:95, 1982.
76. Yarbrough KM, Howard-Peebles PN: X-linked nonspecific mental retardation. Report of a large kindred. Clin Genet 9:125, 1976.
77. Wilson GN, Richards CS, Katz K, et al.: Non-specific X linked mental retardation with aphasia exhibiting genetic linkage to chromosomal region Xp11. J Med Genet 29:629, 1992.
78. Knight SJL, Flannery AV, Hirst MC, et al.: Trinucleotide repeat amplification and hypermethylation of a CpG island in *FRAXE* mental retardation. Cell 74:127, 1993.n
79. Hamel BCJ, Smits APT, de Graaff E, et al.: Segregation of FRAXE in a large family: clinical, psychometric, cytogenetic, and molecular data. Am J Hum Genet 55:923, 1994.
80. Mulley JC, Yu S, Loesch DZ, et al.: FRAXE and mental retardation. J Med Genet 32:162, 1995.
81. van der Maarel SM, Scholten IHJM, Maat-Kievit JA, et al.: Yeast artificial chromosome cloning of the Xq13.3-q21.31 region and fine mapping of a deletion associated with choroideremia and nonspecific mental retardation. Eur J Hum Genet 3:207, 1995.
82. Billuart P, Vient MC, des Portes V, et al.: Identification by STS PCR screening of a microdeletion in Xp21.3-22.1 associated with non-specific mental retardation. Hum Mol Genet 5:977, 1996.
83. des Portes V, Carrié A, Billuart P, et al.: Inherited microdeletion in Xp21.3-22.1 involved in non-specific mental retardation. Clin Genet 53:136, 1998.

4

Syndromic XLMR

Clinical and laboratory studies have permitted delineation of numerous syndromes in which mental retardation is but one manifestation of a mutant gene on the X chromosome. In the most recent XLMR update, Lubs et al. (1999) identified 120 such types of syndromic XLMR.[1] Associated manifestations may be malformations or other structural anomalies, neuromuscular signs, metabolic derangements, or behavioral disturbances. One syndromic subgroup has expression primarily in females.

Because of the combination of certain disorders, separation of others, and elimination of those with insufficient evidence to justify designation as an XLMR syndrome, the listing of XLMR syndromes to follow in this chapter differs slightly from that of Lubs et al. (1999). For example, Vles syndrome in the Lubs et al. listing appears to be the same as X-linked hydrocephaly–MASA spectrum.[2] Carpenter-Waziri and Holmes-Gang syndromes are now known to be the same as XLMR–hypotonic facies syndrome (α-thalassemia mental retardation).[3] Clark-Baraitser syndrome is considered to be different from Atkin-Flaitz syndrome.[4,5] Although there is insufficient evidence to support designation of Albright hereditary osteodystrophy, G_{M3} gangliosidosis, and Rud syndrome as XLMR syndromes, they are included for historical reasons.

Deletions of contiguous genes may masquerade as single gene mutations with pleiotropic effects and variable expression. When the evidence appears strong that a phenotype is produced by a contiguous gene deletion, that phenotype is excluded from the syndrome section of this chapter (e.g., XLMR–choroideremia–ectodermal dysplasia).[6] When the evidence for a contiguous gene deletion is less, the syndrome is retained (e.g., XLMR–retinitis pigmentosa, glycerol kinase deficiency, X-linked optic atrophy).[7–9]

A prevalence for most of the XLMR syndromes has not been determined. Duchenne muscular dystrophy and fragile X syndrome are most common, with a birth prevalence of 1:3500–4500 males in the former and 1:4000–6000 males and 1:8000–10,000 females in the latter.[10–12] X-linked hydrocephaly–MASA spectrum and XLMR–hypotonic facies syndrome (α-thalassemia mental retardation)

Table 4–1. XLMR Syndromes With Malformations or Distinctive Craniofacial Findings

Aarskog Syndrome
Short stature, hypertelorism, downslanting palpebral fissures, ptosis, cupped ears, anteverted nares, brachydactyly, horizontal palmar crease, midfoot varus, joint laxity, shawl scrotum, cryptorchidism, inguinal hernias

Armfield Syndrome
Short stature, cataracts or glaucoma, dental anomalies, small hands and feet, hydrocephaly, joint stiffness, seizures

Atkin-Flaitz Syndrome
Macrocephaly, short stature, hypertelorism, downslanting palpebral fissures, broad nasal tip, thick lower lip, brachydactyly, seizures

Börjeson-Forssman-Lehmann Syndrome
Obesity, hypotonia, hypogonadism, short stature, microcephaly, coarse facies, large ears, gynecomastia, narrow sloped shoulders, visual impairment, tapered digits

Brooks Syndrome
Microcephaly, short stature, deep-set eyes, blepharophimosis, cupped ears, bulbous nose, small mouth, thin upper lip, pectus excavatum, flexion contractures, dysgenesis of corpus callosum

Cantu Syndrome
Short stature, microcephaly, alopecia, hyperpigmented lesions, follicular keratosis, cortical atrophy, seizures, pancytopenia

Carpenter-Waziri Syndrome
Microcephaly, short stature, open mouth, tented upper lip, brachydactyly, allelic to XLMR-hypotonic facies (α-thalassemia mental retardation) Holmes-Gang and Juberg-Marsidi syndromes

Cerebrooculogenital Syndrome
Short stature, microcephaly, microphthalmia, ptosis, clubfoot, hydrocephaly, agenesis of corpus callosum, spasticity, hypospadias, cryptorchidism

Cerebropalatocardiac Syndrome
Microcephaly, short stature, cleft palate, cupped ears, bulbous nose, short philtrum, tented upper lip, complex cardiac defect, childhood death

Christian Syndrome
Vertebral anomalies, abducens palsy, metopic ridge

Chudley Hypogammaglobulinemia Syndrome
Prominent glabella, synophrys, prognathism, hirsutism, weakness, gait disturbance, seizures, hypogammaglobulinemia

Chudley-Lowry Syndrome
Short stature, bitemporal narrowing, almond-shaped eyes, depressed nasal bridge, tented upper lip, open mouth, hypogonadism, hypotonia, obesity

Clark-Baraitser Syndrome
Macrocephaly, large stature, obesity, dental abnormalities, broad nasal tip, thick lower lip, macroorchidism

Coffin-Lowry Syndrome
Short stature, microcephaly, hypertelorism, anteverted nares, tented upper lip, prominent lips and large mouth, large ears, soft hands with tapered digits, pectus carinatum, hypotonia

(continued)

TABLE 4–1. Continued

Cranioorodigital Syndrome
Undergrowth, hearing impairment, prominent forehead, flat/broad nasal bridge, ocular hypertelorism, downslanting palpebral fissures, flat midface, cleft palate, blunted, flexed, overlapping fingers, rockerbottom feet, hypoplastic fibulae, subluxed/dislocated joints

Dyskeratosis Congenita
Short stature, alopecia, hyperpigmented lesions, palmar and plantar hyperkeratosis, mucosal leucoplakia, nail ridging or splitting, pancytopenia, premalignant skin and mucosal lesions

Fragile X Syndrome
Normal or excessive growth, macrocephaly, prominent forehead, long face, midface hypoplasia, large ears, prominent mandible, macroorchidism

Golabi-Ito-Hall Syndrome
Microcephaly, short stature, telecanthus, high nasal root, cupped ears, cardiac malformation, thoracic asymmetry, sacral dimple, dry/brittle/sparse hair, cutis marmorata, nail hypoplasia

Goltz Syndrome
Cataracts, ocular dysgenesis, linear areas of dermal aplasia, cutaneous adipose herniations, dystrophic nails, abnormal teeth and hair, vertebral anomalies, limb reduction defects, genitourinary anomalies

Graham Anophthalmia Syndrome
Anophthalmia, ankyloblepharon, shallow orbits, short eyebrows and eyelids

Holmes-Gang Syndrome
Short stature, microcephaly, hypertelorism, epicanthus, short nose, anteverted nares, tented upper lip, clubfeet, allelic to XLMR-hypotonic facies (α-thalassemia mental retardation), Carpenter-Waziri, and Juberg-Marsidi syndromes

Hyde-Forster Syndrome
Brachycephaly, plagiocephaly, coarse facial features (status as a unique XLMR syndrome not certain)

Incontinentia Pigmenti
Cutaneous vesicles, verrucous lesions, and irregular hyperpigmentation, microcephaly, ocular anomalies, oligodontia, abnormally shaped teeth, spasticity, seizures

Juberg-Marsidi Syndrome
Short stature, microcephaly, cupped ears, tented upper lip, deafness, allelic to XLMR-hypotonic facies (α-thalassemia mental retardation), Carpenter-Waziri and Holmes-Gang syndromes

Kang Syndrome
Microcephaly, frontal prominence, telecanthus, small nose, short hands, dysgenesis of corpus callosum, seizures, downslanted mouth, brachydactyly

Lenz Microphthalmia Syndrome
Microcephaly, microphthalmia, ocular dysgenesis, malformed ears, cleft lip/palate, cardiac and genitourinary anomalies, thumb duplication or hypoplasia, narrow shoulders

Lujan Syndrome
Marfanoid habitus, asthenic build, long face, prominent forehead, high palate, micrognathia, long digits, pectus excavatum, joint hyperextensibility, seizures, hyperactivity

MIDAS Syndrome
Microphthalmia, ocular dysgenesis, corneal opacification, dermal aplasia, dysgenesis of corpus callosum, cardiac defects, cardiomyopathy

(continued)

Table 4–1. XLMR Syndromes With Malformations or Distinctive Craniofacial Findings—Continued

Miles-Carpenter Syndrome
Microcephaly, short stature, ptosis, small palpebral fissures, open mouth, pectus excavatum, scoliosis, long hands, camptodactyly, rockerbottom feet, arch fingerprints, spasticity, unsteady gait

Nance-Horan Syndrome
Microcornea, cataracts, nystagmus, cupped ears, dental anomalies, short fourth metacarpals

Otopalatodigital I
Short stature, conductive hearing impairment, prominent brow, broad nasal root, apparent ocular hypertelorism, downslanting palpebral fissures, cleft palate, blunted distal phalanges, irregular curvature and spacing of digits, limitation of elbow movement

Opitz FG Syndrome
Macrocephaly, broad forehead, downslanted palpebral fissures, everted lower lip, dysgenesis of corpus callosum, cardiac defects, imperforate anus, constipation, broad flat thumbs and great toes, hypotonia

Pallister W Syndrome
Short stature, prominent forehead, wide nasal tip, incomplete cleft lip/palate, spasticity, contractures

Porteous Syndrome
Short stature, high forehead, receding hairline

Prieto Syndrome
Ventricular enlargement, facial asymmetry, hypertelorism, prominent eyes, ptosis, long narrow nose, micrognathia, inquinal hernia, cryptorchidism

Proud Syndrome
Microcephaly, hearing loss, vision loss, agenesis of corpus callosum, cryptorchidism, inguinal hernias, ataxia, spasticity, seizures

Renpenning Syndrome
Microcephaly, short stature, upslanting palpebral fissures, small testes

Say-Meyer Syndrome
Short stature, microcephaly, craniosynostosis, hypotelorism

Simpson-Golabi-Behmel Syndrome
Somatic overgrowth, supernumerary nipples, polydactyly

Smith-Fineman-Myers Syndrome
Microcephaly, ptosis, flat philtrum, scoliosis, midfoot varus, narrow feet, seizures, hypotonia

Snyder-Robinson Syndrome
Asthenic build, high or cleft palate, prominent lower lip, kyphoscoliosis, long great toes, nasal speech, hypotonia in childhood

Stoll Syndrome
Short stature, forehead prominence, hypertelorism, depressed nasal root, anteverted nares

Sutherland-Haan Syndrome
Microcephaly, short stature, upslanting palpebral fissures, asthenic habitus, pectus excavatum, scoliosis, stiff joints, pes cavus, small testes, spasticity

Telecanthus-Hypospadias Syndrome
High broad nasal root, dysplastic ears, cleft lip/palate, abnormal cranial contour or symmetry

(continued)

Table 4–1. Continued

Urban Syndrome Short stature, small hands and feet, digital contractures, osteoporosis
VACTERL-Hydrocephalus Syndrome Vertebral anomalies, hydrocephaly, radial limb defect, tracheal and esophageal anomalies, renal malformations, anal anomalies
Vasquez Syndrome Short stature, microcephaly, gynecomastia, obesity, hypotonia, hypogonadism
Warkany Syndrome Intrauterine growth retardation, short stature, microcephaly, ptosis, cupped ears
Wilson-Turner Syndrome Normal growth, small hands and feet, obesity, tapered digits, hypogonadism, gynecomastia, hypotonia, emotional lability
Wittwer Syndrome Growth deficiency, microcephaly, microphthalmia, hearing loss, vision loss, hypertelorism, genitourinary anomalies, hypotonia, seizures
X-Linked Branchial Arch Syndrome Microcephaly, branchial arch defects, micrognathia, facial and limb asymmetry
X-Linked Hereditary Bullous Dystrophy Microcephaly, short stature, upslanting palpebral fissures, protruding ears, digits short and tapered, cardiac defects, bullous dystrophy, small testes, early death from pulmonary infections
XLMR–Arch Fingerprints–Hypotonia Hypotonic facies, tapered fingers, arch fingerprints, genu valgum, areflexia, hypotonia
XLMR-Hypospadias Microcephaly, trigonocephaly, synophrys, beaked nose, hypotonia, hypospadias
XLMR–Hypotonia–Recurrent Infections Hypotonic facies, hypertelorism, downslanting palpebral fissures, gastroesophageal reflux, recurrent infections, seizures, developmental regression, childhood death
XLMR–Hypotonic Facies (α-thalassemia mental retardation, Carpenter-Waziri syndrome, Holmes-Gang syndrome, Juberg-Marsidi syndrome) Microcephaly, short stature, small testes, telecanthus, small triangular nose, tented upper lip, open mouth, spacing of teeth, genital anomalies, musculoskeletal anomalies, hemoglobin H inclusions in erythrocytes
XLMR-Macrocephaly Macrocephaly, downslanting palpebral fissures, obesity, elbow limitation
XLMR-Macrocephaly-Macroorchidism Elongated face, prominent mandible, macroorchidism, clumsiness, repetitive movements
XLMR-Psoriasis Hypertelorism, open mouth, large ears, hypotonia, seizures, psoriasis
XLMR–Retinitis Pigmentosa Microcephaly, bone spicule type retinitis pigmentosa
Young-Hughes Syndrome Short stature, small palpebral fissures, cupped ears, ichthyosiform scaling

may have similar high birth prevalence. In contrast, a number of XLMR syndromes are represented by a single family.

XLMR Syndromes with Malformations or Distinctive Craniofacial Findings

Somatic manifestations in the form of malformations or other structural anomalies, distinctive craniofacial characteristics, and cutaneous findings occur in many of the XLMR syndromes (Table 4–1). These manifestations, individually and in recognizable patterns, provide substantial clues to diagnosis. In small families and in individuals with new mutations the somatic features may be of greater importance to the diagnosis than the pedigree. Somatic manifestations are of sufficient benefit to the clinician that they have been utilized in some diagnostic schemes as the first classification criterion. Opitz et al., Moser, and others have used as the two major categories of mental retardation those with malformations and those without malformations.[13,14] Others prefer not to use this hierarchy but nonetheless find malformations helpful as diagnostic clues.

The concurrence of somatic manifestations offers the researcher additional assistance in localization and identification of the responsible gene. Small families or families in which only a few members are available may be combined when the diagnosis is certain on the basis of physical features. Hence, the necessary numbers for linkage analysis may be obtained. Further, identification of the tissues in which gene expression is manifest may, in theory at least, assist in the selection of candidate genes for investigation.

No generalization can be made regarding manifestations in carriers. Although one might anticipate that there would be a greater likelihood of manifestations among carriers of syndromic XLMR than among carriers of nonsyndromic XLMR, that is, in fact, not the case. Mild mental retardation and minor somatic findings are common among carriers of nonsyndromic XLMR.[1,15] So far as somatic manifestations among carriers, one may point to XLMR syndromes in which carriers nearly always have somatic findings (e.g., Coffin-Lowry syndrome),[16] those in which carriers rarely show somatic findings (XLMR–hypotonic facies syndrome),[17] and those with an intermediate prevalence of carrier expression (fragile XA syndrome).[12] Preferential inactivation of the mutation-bearing X chromosome precludes carrier expression in some XLMR syndromes, e.g., XLMR–hypotonic facies syndrome.

Certain diagnostic motifs emerge from consideration of the somatic manifestations found in syndromic XLMR. For example, one group of syndromic XLMR shares hypotonia, obesity, and hypogonadism as common features. These shared manifestations form the basis of the differential matrices which accompany the clinical descriptions of syndromes in the following chapter.

Malformations and XLMR

Major structural malformations do not occur commonly among the XLMR syndromes (Table 4–2). Disruptions (structural defects resulting from a destructive

Table 4–2. Malformations Associated with XLMR Syndromes

Central Nervous System
Aicardi
Bertini
Brooks
Cerebrooculogenital
Hydrocephaly–cerebellar agenesis
Gustavson
Kang
Lujan
MIDAS
Myotubular myopathy
Opitz FG
Oral-facial-digital I
Periventricular nodular heterotopia
Pettigrew
Proud
Pyruvate dehydrogenase
VACTERL-Hydrocephalus
X-linked agenesis of corpus callosum
X-linked hydrocephaly-basal ganglia calcification
X-linked hydrocephaly–MASA
X-linked lissencephaly

Ocular
Aicardi
Cerebrooculo-genital
Goltz
Graham
Incontinentia pigmenti
Lenz
MIDAS
Nance-Horan
Norrie
Wittwer

Dental
Golabi-Ito-Hall
Goltz
Incontinentia pigmenti
Nance-Horan
Oral-facial-digital I
Pallister W

Facial Clefting
Aicardi
Armfield
Cerebropalatocardiac
Cranioorodigital
Goltz
Lenz
Oral-facial-digital I
Otopalatodigital I
Pallister W
Simpson-Golabi-Behmel
Snyder-Robinson
Telecanthus-hypospadias
VACTERL-hydrocephalus
XLMR-hypotonic facies

Cardiac
Cerebropalatocardiac
Golabi-Ito-Hall
Lenz
Lujan
MIDAS
Simpson-Golabi-Behmel
Telecanthus-hypospadias
X-linked hereditary bullous dystrophy
XLMR-hypotonic facies

Ectodermal
Cantu
Dyskeratosis congenita
Fitzsimmons
Golabi-Ito-Hall
Goltz
Incontinentia pigmenti
Menkes
MIDAS
Oral-facial-digital I
X-linked hereditary bullous dystrophy
XLMR-psoriasis
Young-Hughes

Gastrointestinal
Armfield
MIDAS
Opitz FG
Prieto
Simpson-Golabi-Behmel
Sutherland-Haan
VACTERL-hydrocephalus

Genitourinary
Aarskog
Armfield
Börjeson-Forssman-Lehmann
Cerebrooculogenital
Chudley-Lowry
Dyskeratosis congenita
Goltz
Holmes-Gang
Lenz
Myotubular myopathy
Opitz FG
Oral-facial-digital I
Opitz FG
Prieto
Proud
Simpson-Golabi-Behmel
Telecanthus-hypospadias
Urban
VACTERL-hydrocepalus
Wilson-Turner
Wittwer
X-linked branchial arch
X-linked hereditary bullous dystrophy
XLMR-hypospadias
XLMR-hypotonic facies

Skeletal
Aarskog
Aicardi
Albright hereditary osteodystrophy
Apak
Atkin-Flaitz
Börjeson-Forssman-Lehmann
Brooks
Christian
Christianson
Chudley-Lowry
Coffin-Lowry
Cranioorodigital
Fitzsimmons
Goltz
Gustavson
Holmes-Gang
Kang
Lenz
Lujan
Miles-Carpenter
Nance-Horan
PPM-X
Opitz FG
Oral-facial-digital I
Otopalatodigital I
Pallister W
Pettigrew
Prieto
Proud
Say-Meyer
Simpson-Golabi-Behmel
Smith-Fineman-Myers
Snyder-Robinson
Sutherland-Haan
Urban
VACTERL-hydrocephalus
Wieacker-Wolff
X-linked branchial arch
X-linked hereditary bullous dystrophy
X-linked hydrocephaly–basal ganglia Calcification
XLMR-hypotonic facies
XLMR-psoriasis

process during or following embryogenesis) have not been described although a disruptive process might be considered in some cases of dermal aplasia (Goltz and MIDAS syndromes).[18,19] Deformations (positional abnormalities resulting from mechanical forces on normally formed structures) are common, the consequence of neuromuscular impairments.

Although the mental impairment is usually the disability of greatest significance in syndromic XLMR, recognition of malformations may be important in management. Hydrocephalus, facial clefting, cardiac malformations, and genitourinary anomalies are among those most likely to require medical and surgical management. Yet, only a few examples of XLMR syndromes may be given in which the somatic manifestations pose the major problem in management.

Gross malformations of the central nervous system can be found in only a few XLMR syndromes and hence cannot be called upon to explain the impaired cognitive function or neurologic manifestations. The most common of the central nervous system malformations, dysgenesis of the corpus callosum, may have little or nothing to do with neurological manifestations since it has been found in individuals with normal neurological function. That lesser malformations of nervous system structures, which escape detection by imaging or direct examination, may contribute to the impaired neurologic–cognitive function cannot be excluded.

Early lethality, while not uncommon among the XLMR syndromes, appears more related to the severity of neurologic dysfunction and susceptibility to infections than to malformations. Death during childhood is typical in several syndromes (Table 4–3) and is seen occasionally in others. Only rarely has early death been attributed to malformations. Gestational lethality of males is believed to occur in certain XLMR syndromes in which expression is limited to females. The basis for male lethality in these conditions is not known.

TABLE 4–3. XLMR Syndromes With Early Childhood Lethality

Adrenoleukodystrophy
Arts syndrome
Bertini syndrome
Gustavson syndrome
Holmes-Gang syndrome (XLMR-hypotonic facies syndrome)
Hydrocephaly–cerebellar agenesis syndrome
Menkes syndrome
Myotubular myopathy
Ornithine transcarbamylase deficiency
Paine syndrome
Pyruvate dehydrogenase deficiency
VACTERL-hydrocephalus syndrome
X-linked hydrocephaly–MASA spectrum
X-linked lissencephaly
XLMR–hypotonia–recurrent infections
X-linked infantile spasms

XLMR Syndromes with Neuromuscular Manifestations

Thirty-five XLMR syndromes have been described in which neuromuscular manifestations are prominent (Table 4–4). Twenty-three of these syndromes have been regionally mapped and six have been cloned. Neuromuscular manifestations also occur among the other XLMR categories, those in which malformations or other structural anomalies, metabolic derangements, behavioral disturbances, and female-limited expression are more notable.

The XLMR syndromes with prominent neuromuscular manifestations include myopathies (e.g., Duchenne muscular dystrophy, myotubular myopathy) and neuropathies (Charcot-Marie-Tooth—Cowchock and Ionasescu variants). More commonly, however, the specific basis for the neuromuscular manifestations remains obscure. Presumably, the hypotonia or spastic paraplegia found in many of the XLMR syndromes results from a developmental insult to the central nervous system.

TABLE 4–4. XLMR Syndromes with Prominent Neuromuscular Manifestations

Allan-Herndon-Dudley Syndrome
Large ears with cupping or abnormal architecture, muscle hypoplasia, childhood hypotonia, contractures, dysarthria, athetosis, ataxia, spastic paraplegia

Apak Ataxia–Spastic Paraplegia Syndrome
Short stature, clubfoot, muscle hypoplasia, ataxia, spastic paraplegia

Arena Syndrome
Muscle hypoplasia, clubfoot, iron deposits in basal ganglia, ataxia, spastic paraplegia, rigidity, dystonia

Arts Syndrome
Growth deficiency, paucity of muscles, hypotonia, areflexia, ataxia, deafness, vision loss, seizures, childhood death

Bergia Cardiomyopathy
Scapuloperoneal muscle atrophy, wasting of distal muscles, hypertrophic cardiomyopathy, limited exercise tolerance, arrhythmias

Bertini Syndrome
Macular degeneration, hypotonia, ataxia, seizures, childhood death, hypoplasia of cerebellar vermis and corpus callosum, developmental delays and regression, postnatal growth impairment

Charcot-Marie-Tooth Neuropathy, Cowchock Variant
Peripheral motor and sensory neuropathy, deafness, pes cavus, weakness, areflexia

Charcot-Marie-Tooth Neuropathy, Ionasescu Variant
Peripheral motor and sensory neuropathy, weakness, areflexia, wasting of intrinsic hand muscles, enlarged ulnar nerves, pes cavus

Christianson Syndrome
Short stature, microcephaly, general asthenia, contractures, seizures, ophthalmoplegia

Duchenne Muscular Dystrophy
Hypertrophy of calf muscles, elevated muscle enzymes, progressive weakness, loss of reflexes, muscle wasting, contractures

(continued)

TABLE 4–4. XLMR Syndromes with Prominent Neuromuscular Manifestations Continued

Fitzsimmons Syndrome
Pes cavus, hyperkeratosis of palms and soles, dystrophic nails, spastic paraplegia

Goldblatt Spastic Paraplegia Syndrome
Optic atrophy, exotropia, nystagmus, ataxia, spastic paraplegia, dysarthria, muscle hypoplasia, contractures

Gustavson Syndrome
Microcephaly, short stature, optic atrophy with blindness, large ears, deafness, joint contractures, rockerbottom feet, brain undergrowth, hydrocephaly, cerebellar hypoplasia, spasticity, seizures

Hydrocephaly-Cerebellar Agenesis Syndrome
Hydrocephaly, absent cerebellar hemispheres, hypotonia, seizures

Mohr-Tranebjaerg Syndrome and Jensen Syndrome
Hearing loss, vision loss, neurologic deterioration with childhood onset, dystonia, spasticity

Myotubular Myopathy
Hypotonic facies, open mouth, tented upper lip, hydrocephaly, long digits, cryptorchidism, hypotonia, weakness, areflexia

Norrie Disease
Ocular dysplasia and degeneration, adult onset hearing loss

Paine Syndrome
Microcephaly, short stature, optic atrophy, vision and hearing loss, spasticity, seizures

Partington Syndrome
Scoliosis, flexed posture, dysarthria, dystonia, seizures

Pelizaeus-Merzbacher Syndrome
Optic atrophy, nystagmus, hypotonia, spasticity, ataxia, dystonia, central nervous system dysmyelination

Pettigrew Syndrome
Dandy-Walker malformation, spasticity, seizures, microcephaly or hydrocephaly, long face with macrostomia, small testes, contractures, choreoathetosis, iron deposits in basal ganglia

Plott Syndrome
Expressionless face, respiratory stridor, laryngeal abductor paralysis

PPM-X
Macroorchidism, spastic paraplegia, psychosis, parkinsonian features

Schimke Syndrome
Microcephaly, sunken eyes, downslanting palpebral fissures, narrow nose, spacing of teeth, cupped ears, hypotonia, abducens palsy, hearing loss, vision loss, spasticity, choreoathetosis, contractures

Waisman-Laxova Syndrome
Spasticity

Wieacker-Wolff Syndrome
Weakness, distal muscle atrophy, contractures, dysarthria, oculomotor apraxia

X-Linked Agenesis of the Corpus Callosum
Dysgenesis of the corpus callosum, hydrocephaly or microcephaly, seizures (most cases may represent X-linked hydrocephaly–MASA spectrum or other XLMR syndromes)

(continued)

TABLE 4–4. Continued

X-Linked Ataxia-Deafness-Dementia
Optic atrophy, vision loss, hearing loss, spastic paraplegia, ataxia, hypotonia, seizures, childhood death

X-Linked Ataxia-Dementia
Ataxia, spastic paraplegia, adult-onset dementia

X-Linked Hydrocephaly–MASA Spectrum
Hydrocephaly, adducted thumbs, spastic paraplegia, dysgenesis of corpus callosum

X-Linked Lissencephaly
Defect in neuronal migration resulting in frontal pachygyria in males and subcortical band heterotopia in carrier females, dysgenesis of corpus callosum, hypotonia, spasticity, seizures, genital hypoplasia

X-Linked Spastic Paraplegia, Type 7
Nystagmus, reduced vision, absent speech and ambulation, bowel and bladder dysfunction, spastic tetraplegia

XLMR-Ataxia-Apraxia
Prominent forehead, large ears, uncoordinated movement, hypotonia, seizures, tremors

XLMR–Hydrocephaly–Basal Ganglia Calcifications
Hydrocephaly, calcifications of basal ganglia, muscle hypoplasia, sensory impairment, spasticity

XLMR–Infantile Spasms
Developmental regression, seizures, electroencephalogram hypsarrhythmia pattern, early childhood death

XLMR–Spastic Paraplegia–Athetosis
Nystagmus, weakness, dysarthria, spastic paraplegia, muscle wasting, contractures

XLMR with Metabolic Derangements

Fourteen syndromes have been delineated in which an X-linked inborn error of metabolism is associated with mental retardation (Table 4–5). Two other syndromes, Albright hereditary osteodystrophy and G_{M3} gangliosidosis, once considered XLMR syndromes, have been removed from this category.

In 10 of the 14 XLMR syndromes with metabolic derangements, the gene has been cloned. Mutational analysis permits prenatal and postnatal diagnosis to be performed with precision in these cases.

XLMR with Behavioral Disturbances

Although behavioral disturbances may be noted in many of the XLMR syndromes, in two of these syndromes, monoamine oxidase A deficiency and Rett syndromes, the behavioral manifestations predominate (Table 4–6).[20,21] There are few somatic findings in these two conditions. Neurological findings in the form of ataxia, involuntary movements, and seizures do occur in most cases of Rett syndrome.

TABLE 4–5. XLMR Syndromes with Metabolic Derangements

Adrenoleukodystrophy
Adrenal insufficiency, diffuse skin pigmentation, spastic paraplegia, progressive neurologic deterioration and dementia, elevated long chain fatty acids in plasma

Glycerol Kinase Deficiency
Short stature, hypogonadotrophic hypogonadism, osteoporosis, fractures, muscle weakness, spasticity and seizures when a part of GKD contiguous gene syndrome. Isolated GKD may be asymptomatic.

Lesch-Nyhan Syndrome
Spasticity, choreoathetosis, self-mutilation, hyperuricemia

Lowe Syndrome
Short stature, cataracts, hypotonia, aminoaciduria, progressive renal disease

Menkes Syndrome
Growth deficiency, sparse kinky hair, hypothermia, pallor, limited movement, hypertonicity, seizures, metaphyseal widening and spurs, arterial tortuosity, childhood death

Monoamine Oxidase-A Deficiency
Aggressive behavior, repetitive hand movements

Mucopolysaccharidosis IIA
Macrocephaly, short stature, coarse facies, hepatosplenomegaly, hernias, joint stiffness, thick skin, hirsutism, behavioral disturbance

Ornithine Transcarbamylase Deficiency
Chronic or intermittent hyperammonemia, microcephaly, protein induced vomiting and lethargy, ataxia, seizures

Phosphoglycerate Kinase Deficiency
Expressionless face, weakness, decreased deep tendon reflexes, seizures, myoglobinuria, hemolytic anemia

Pyruvate Dehydrogenase Deficiency
Lactic acidosis, microcephaly, hypotonia, ataxia, dysarthria, CNS anomalies

XLMR–Isolated Growth Hormone Deficiency
Short stature, gynecomastia, growth hormone deficiency

XLMR-Panhypopituitarism
Short stature, hypogenitalism, small sella turcica, deficiency of pituitary, thyroid, adrenal, and gonadal hormones

XLMR–Thyroidaplasia–Cutis Verticis Gyrata
Short stature, cutis gyrata of scalp, myxedema due to thyroid aplasia, diastasis rectus, ulnar deviation of hands, aphasia

XLMR With Thyroxine-Binding Globulin Deficiency
Short stature, TBG deficiency

*Albright hereditary osteodystrophy and G_{M3} gangliosidosis, previously considered XLMR syndromes, have been removed from this listing.

TABLE 4–6. XLMR Syndromes with Prominent Behavioral Manifestations

Monoamine Oxidase-A Deficiency
Aggressive behavior, repetitive hand movements

Rett Syndrome
Acquired microcephaly, developmental regression, truncal ataxia, repetitive hand movements, autistic features

XLMR Syndromes with Expression Predominantly in Females

A remarkable subgroup of X-linked syndromes have expression exclusively, or nearly so, in females. The majority have associated mental retardation (Table 4–7). Lenz suggested that gestational lethality in males would explain the apparent female-limited expression.[22] Females, having a normal allele on their second X chromosome active in half of the body's cells, would have less severe expression permitting survival. Males, having no such modifying influence would suffer the full brunt of the disease gene, resulting in prenatal lethality. Certain pedigrees with a paucity of males and an increase in spontaneous abortions have been reported. This explanation has received wide acceptance during the past four decades.

TABLE 4–7. X-Linked Syndromes Expressed Predominantly in Females

Aicardi Syndrome (MIM 304050)
Ocular dysgenesis, lacunar retinopathy, costovertebral anomalies, agenesis of corpus callosum, seizures

Goltz Syndrome (MIM 305600)
Cataracts, ocular dysgenesis, linear areas of dermal aplasia, cutaneous adipose herniations, dystrophic nails, abnormal teeth and hair, vertebral anomalies, limb reduction defects, genitourinary anomalies

Incontinentia Pigmenti (MIM 308310)
Cutaneous vesicles, verrucous lesions, and irregular hyperpigmentation, microcephaly, ocular anomalies, oligodontia, abnormally shaped teeth, spasticity, seizures

MIDAS Syndrome (MIM 309801)
Microphthalmia, ocular dysgenesis, corneal opacification, dermal aplasia, dysgenesis of corpus callosum, cardiac defects, cardiomyopathy

Oral-Facial-Digital Syndrome I (MIM 311200)
Sparse scalp hair, dystopia canthorum, flat midface, hypoplastic alae nasi, hypertrophic and aberrant oral frenuli, intraoral clefts and pseudoclefts, lingual hamartomas, brachydactyly, syndactyly, clinodactyly, structural brain anomalies, polycystic kidneys

Periventricular Nodular Heterotopias (MIM 300049)
Bilaterial subependymal nodular heterotopias, seizures

Rett Syndrome (MIM 321750)
Acquired microcephaly, developmental regression, truncal ataxia, repetitive hand movements, autistic features

XLMR-Epilepsy (MIM 300088)
Developmental regression, repetitive stereotypic hand movements, seizures

Entities Without Mental Retardation
CHILD (Unilateral ichthyosiform erythroderma with ipsilateral malformations, MIM 308050)
CODAS (cerebral, ocular, dental, auricular, skeletal abnormalities, MIM 600373)
Congenital cataract with microcornea or slight microphthalmia (MIM 302300)
Conradi-Hunermann or Happle (chondrodysplasia punctata, X-linked dominant, MIM 302960)
Kobberling-Dunnigan (lipodystrophy, familial partial, MIM 308980)
SFPK (serpentine fibula–polycystic kidney, MIM 600330)
Wildervanck (Cervicooculoacoustic, MIM 314600)

Thomas has offered an alternative explanation for the female excess among these disorders.[23] Females with these syndromes, he suggested, arise in virtually all cases from de novo mutations in the father's germline. The absence or paucity of males is thus explained by two factors: Males do not inherit their X chromosome from their fathers and females affected with these syndromes in most cases do not reproduce.

The model proposed by Thomas predicts:

- Affected individuals will be exclusively females.
- Almost all cases (except MZ twins) will be sporadic.
- MZ twins will be concordant.
- Almost all DZ twins will be discordant.
- Affected families will show no increase in spontaneous abortions.
- Affected families will show no increase in male lethality.
- Mothers and fathers of the patients will be noncarriers in somatic tissues
- The de novo mutations will be found on the paternally derived X chromosome.
- An affected female will have a 50% chance of having an affected (male or female) offspring in the unlikely event of a pregnancy.

Evidence in favor of this concept is the higher rate of mutations in male meiosis than in female meiosis. It is possible that both mechanisms—excessive gestational lethality of males in some families and new mutations in the father's germline in other families—may contribute as causes of X-linked conditions with expression predominantly in females.

Private Syndromes

There is a tendency to keep potentially distinct syndromes separate until they are shown convincingly by phenotype, laboratory testing, linkage, or mutational analysis to represent a previously recognized syndrome. Fully one-half of the X-linked syndromes are private in the sense that they are represented in the literature as single families. It is anticipated that further molecular studies will show that certain of these families are, in fact, variants of other XLMR syndromes.

Jensen syndrome, a previously named XLMR syndrome, has been shown to have a mutation in the deafness dystonia protein (DDP) and hence is allelic to Mohr-Tranebjaerg syndrome.[24,25] Similarly, mutations in the X nuclear protein (XNP) have been found in Juberg-Marsidi, Carpenter-Waziri, and Holmes-Gang syndromes,[3,26] thus adding these families to the phenotypic spectrum of the XLMR–hypotonic facies (α-thalassemia mental retardation) syndrome. Review of the craniofacial phenotype in the Chudley-Lowry, Brooks, Proud, XLMR-psoriasis, XLMR–arch fingerprints–hypotonia syndromes suggests that these XLMR syndromes are candidates for allelism with the XLMR–hypotonic facies syndrome as well.[27–33]

An Atlas of XLMR syndromes appears in Chapter 5. Details of the clinical phenotype, neurologic manifestations, brain imaging, and laboratory findings are given for each syndrome. Gene localization and gene identification are provided when available. A differential matrix compares each syndrome to other XLMR syndromes with overlapping manifestations.

REFERENCES

1. Lubs H, Chiurazzi P, Arena J, et al.: XLMR genes: updated 1998. Am J Med Genet 83:237, 1999.
2. Vles JSH, Fryns JP, Folmer K, et al.: Corpus callosum agenesis, spastic quadriparesis and irregular lining of the lateral ventricles on CT-scan. A distrinct X-linked mental retardation syndrome? Genet Counsel 38:97, 1990.
3. Abidi F, Schwartz CE, Carpenter NJ, et al.: The Carpenter-Waziri syndrome results from a mutation in XNP. Am J Med Genet 85:249, 1999.
4. Clark RD, Baraitser M: Letter to the editor: a new X-linked mental retardation syndrome. Am J Med Genet 26:13, 1987.
5. Atkin JF, Flaitz K, Patil S, et al.: A new X-linked mental retardation syndrome. Am J Med Genet 21:697, 1985.
6. van den Bosch J: A new syndrome in three generations of a Dutch family. Ophthalmologica 137:422, 1959.
7. Aldred MA, Dry KL, Knight-Jones EB, et al.: Genetic analysis of a kindred with X-linked mental handicap and retinitis pigmentosa. Am J Hum Genet 55:916, 1994.
8. McCabe ERB, Guggenheim MA, Fennessey PV, et al.: Glyceroluria, psychomotor retardation, spasticity dystrophic myopathy, and osteoporosis in a sibship. Pediatr Res 11:527, 1977.
9. Went LN, De Vries-De Mol EC, Völker-Dieben HJ: A family with apparently sex-linked optic atrophy. J Med Genet 12:94, 1975.
10. Duchenne GBA: Recherches sur la paralysie musculaire pseudo-hypertrophique, ou paralysie myosclérosique. Gén Méd 11:5, 1868. Translation in Arch Neurol 19:629, 1968.
11. Turner G, Webb T, Wake S, et al.: Prevalance of fragile X syndrome. Am J Med Genet 64:196, 1996.
12. de Vries BBA, Halley DJJ, Oostra BA, Niermeijer MF: The fragile X syndrome. J Med Genet 35:579–589, 1998.
13. Opitz JM, Kaveggia EG: Studies of malformation syndromes of man XXXIII: the FG syndrome. An X-linked recessive syndrome of multiple congenital anomalies and mental retardation. Z Kinderheilk 117:1, 1974.
14. Moser HW, Wolf PA: The nosology of mental retardation: including the report of a survey of 1378 mentally retarded individuals at the Walter E. Fernald State School. Birth Defects Orig Art Series VII(1):117, 1971.
15. Häne B, Schroer RJ, Arena JF, et al.: Nonsyndromic X-linked mental retardatiom: review and mapping of MRX29 to Xp21. Clin Genet 50:176, 1996.
16. Lowry B, Miller JR: A new dominant gene mental retardation syndrome. Am J Dis Child 121:496, 1971.
17. Gibbons RJ, Brueton L, Buckle VJ, et al.: Clinical and hematologic aspects of the X-linked α-thalassemia/mental retardation syndrome (ATR-X). Am J Med Genet 55:288, 1995.
18. Goltz RW: Focal dermal hypoplasia syndrome. An update. Arch Dermatol 128:1108, 1992.
19. Al-Gazali LI, Mueller RF, Caine A, et al.: Two 46,XX,t(X;Y) females with linear skin defects and congenital microphthalmia: a new syndrome at Xp22.3. J Med Genet 27:59, 1990.

20. Brunner HG, Nelen MR, van Zandvoort P, et al.: X-linked borderline mental retardation with prominent behavioral disturbance: phenotype, genetic localization, and evidence for disturbed monoamine metabolism. Am J Hum Genet 52:1032, 1993.
21. Moeschler JB, Charman CE, Berg SZ, et al.: Rett syndrome: natural history and management. Pediatrics 82:1, 1988.
22. Lenz W: Half chromatid mutations may explain incontinentia pigmenti in males. (Letter) Am J Hum Genet 27:690, 1975.
23. Thomas GE: High male:female ratio of germ-line mutations: an alternative explanation for postulated gestational lethality in males in X-linked dominant disorders. Am J Hum Genet 58:1364, 1996.
24. Jensen PKA: Nerve deafness, optic nerve atrophy and dementia: a new X-linked recessive syndrome? Am J Med Genet 9:55, 1981.
25. Tranebjaerg L, Schwartz C, Eriksen H, et al.: A new X linked recessive deafness syndrome with blindness, dystonia, fractures, and mental deficiency is linked to Xq22. J Med Genet 32:257, 1995.
26. Juberg RC, Marsidi I: A new form of X-linked mental retardation with growth retardation, deafness, and microgenitalism. Am J Hum Genet 32:714, 1980.
27. Chudley AE, Lowry RB, Hoar DI: Mental retardation, distinct facial changes, short stature, obesity, and hypogonadism. A new X-linked mental retardation syndrome. Am J Med Genet 31:741, 1988.
28. Brooks SS, Wisniewski K, Brown WT: New X-linked mental retardation (XLMR) syndrome with distinct facial appearance and growth retardation. Am J Med Genet 51:586, 1994.
29. Holmes LB, Gang DL: Brief clinical report: an X-linked mental retardation syndrome with craniofacial abnormalities, microcephaly and club foot. Am J Med Genet 17:375, 1984.
30. Proud VK, Levine C, Carpenter NJ: New X-linked syndrome with seizures, acquired microencephaly, and agenesis of the corpus callosum. Am J Med Genet 43:458, 1992.
31. Tranebjaerg L, Svejgaard A, Lykkesfeldt G: X-linked mental retardation associated with psoriasis: a new syndrome? Am J Med Genet 30:263, 1988.
32. Stevenson RE, Häne B, Arena JF, et al.: Arch fingerprints, hypotonia, and areflexia associated with X linked mental retardation. J Med Genet 34:465, 1997.

5

Atlas of XLMR Syndromes

Aarskog Syndrome

(Aarskog-Scott Syndrome, Faciogenital Dysplasia, Faciodigitogenital Syndrome, MIM 305400)

Definition. XLMR with short stature, hypertelorism, downslanting palpebral fissures, joint hyperextensibility, and shawl scrotum. The gene (FGD1) has been mapped to Xp11.21 and mutations have been described.

Somatic Features. Prominent forehead, widow's peak, hypertelorism, downslanting palpebral fissures, ptosis, short nose with anteverted nares, cupped ears, wide upper lip, indistinct philtral pillars, and small chin comprise the facial phenotype. In adults the face elongates and the prominent forehead and hypertelorism may not be apparent. When extended, the fingers are held in flexion at the metacarpophalangeal joints, hyperextension at the proximal interphalangeal joints, and flexion at the distal interphalangeal joints, presumably because of shortening of the flexor tendons. Other musculoskeletal findings include brachydactyly, horizontal palmar crease, varus foot, and generalized joint hyperextensibility. The scrotum tends to surround the penis, giving the "shawl scrotum" appearance. Protruding umbilicus, cryptorchidism, and inguinal hernias may occur.

Growth and Development. From birth, linear growth follows the lower centiles. Head circumference is normal.

Cognitive Features. Intelligence is usually normal but is quite variable from normal into the mildly impaired range.

Neurological Findings. Hypermobility of the cervical spine may lead to cord impingement.

Heterozygote Expression. Carrier females tend to be shorter than noncarriers and have subtle facial features.

Comment. Aarskog syndrome has one of the distinctive recognizable somatic phenotypes with which very few conditions are likely to be mistaken. Noonan

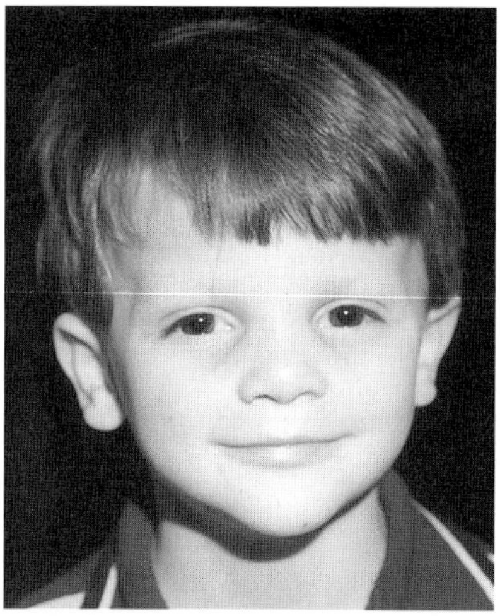

A

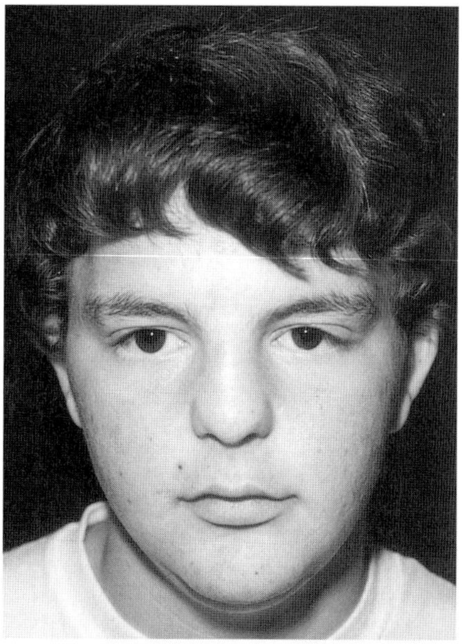

B

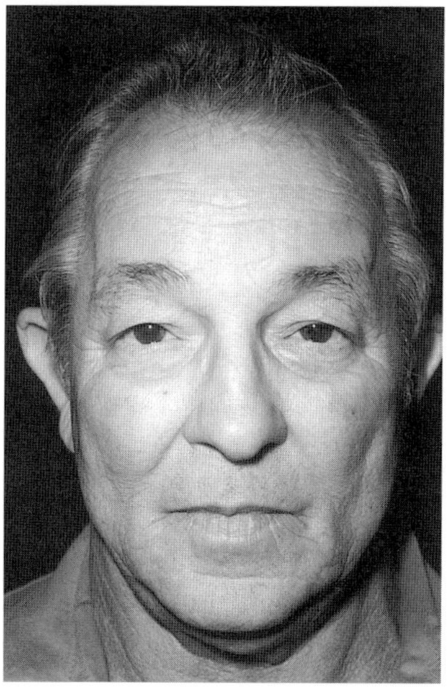

C

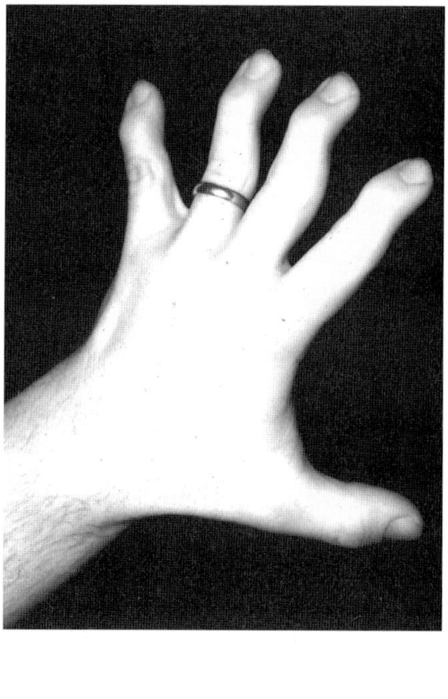

D

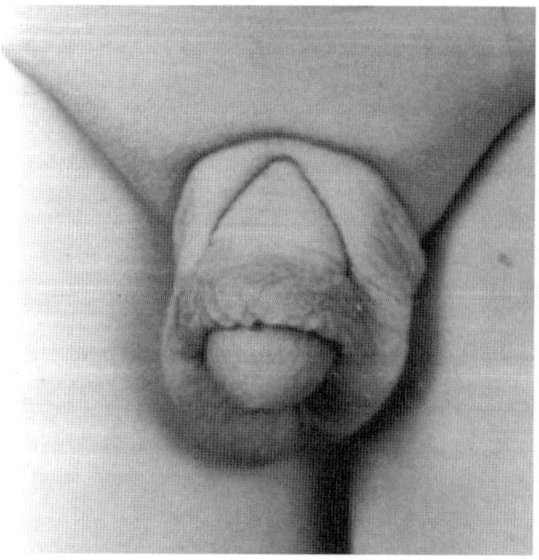

E

Aarskog Syndrome. Four-year-old with hypertelorism, downslanting palpebral fissures, and prominent forehead (A); 17-year-old with prominent forehead, ptosis, and cupped ears (B); 60-year-old with balding and cupped ears, but less apparent widening of the midface (C); characteristic posturing of extended fingers (D); shawl scrotum (E).

syndrome shares ptosis, downslanting palpebral fissures, short stature, and pectus excavatum. However, patients with Noonan syndrome often have a broad and webbed neck and a cardiac defect; patients with Aarskog syndrome often have shawl scrotum. These findings serve as distinguishing but not pathognomonic findings. An X:8 translocation led to the mapping (Xp11.21) and cloning of the Aarskog syndrome gene, a Rho/Rac guanine nucleotide exchange factor. Only a few mutations, however, have been found and mutations have not been demonstrated in the two original families reported by Aarskog (1970) and Scott (1971).

REFERENCES

Aarskog D: A familial syndrome of short stature associated with facial dysplasia and genital anomalies. J Pediatr 77:856, 1970.

Pasteris NG, Cadle A, Logie LJ, et al.: Isolation and characterization of the faciogenital dysplasia (Aarskog-Scott syndrome) gene: a putative Rho/Rac guanine nucleotide exchange factor. Cell 79:669, 1994.

Porteous MEM, Goudie DR: Aarskog syndrome. J Med Genet 28:44, 1991.

Porteous MEM, Curtis A, Lindsay S, et al.: The gene for Aarskog syndrome is located between DXS255 and DXS566 (Xp11.2-Xq13). Genomics 14:298, 1992.

Scott CI, Jr: Unusual facies, joint hypermobility, genital anomaly and short stature: a new dysmorphic syndrome. Birth Defects Orig Art Ser VII(6):240, 1971.

Stevenson RE, May M, Arena JF, et al.: Aarskog-Scott syndrome: confirmation of linkage to the pericentromeric region of the X chromosome. Am J Med Genet 52:339, 1994.

Differential Matrix

Syndrome	Telecanthus/ Hypertelorism	Brachy-dactyly	Genital Anomaly	Comments
Aarskog	+	+	+	Short stature, downslanting palpebral fissures, ptosis, cupped ears, anteverted nares, horizontal palmar crease, midfoot varus, joint laxity, shawl scrotum, cryptorchidism, inguinal hernias
Atkin-Flaitz	+	+	+	Macrocephaly, short stature, downslanting palpebral fissures, broad nasal tip, thick lower lip, macroorchidism, seizures
Simpson-Golabi-Behmel	+	+	+	Somatic overgrowth, supernumerary nipples, polydactyly
XLMR-hypotonic facies (Carpenter-Waziri) (Holmes-Gang) (Juberg-Marsidi)	+	+	+	Short stature, microcephaly, small triangular nose, tented upper lip, open mouth, spacing of teeth, musculoskeletal anomalies, hemoglobin H inclusions in erythrocytes
Kang	+	+	0	Microcephaly, frontal prominence, downturned angles of mouth
Otopalatodigital I	+	+	0	Cleft palate, hearing impairment, short stature, skeletal dysplasia, mild cognitive impairment
X-linked hereditary bullous dystrophy	0	+	+	Microcephaly, short stature, upslanting palpebral fissures, protruding ears, short and tapered digits, cardiac defects, bullous dystrophy, small testes, early death from pulmonary infection
Opitz FG	+	0	+	Macrocephaly, broad forehead, downslanted palpebral fissures, everted lower lip, dysgenesis of corpus callosum, cardiac defects, imperforate anus, constipation, broad flat thumbs and great toes, hypotonia
Proud	+	0	+	Microcephaly, hearing loss, vision loss, agenesis or corpus callosum, cryptorchidism, inguinal hernias, ataxia, spasticity, seizures
Telecanthus-hypospadias	+	0	+	High broad nasal root, dysplastic ears, cleft lip/palate, abnormal cranial contour or symmetry
Wittwer	+	0	+	Growth deficiency, microcephaly, microphthalmia, hearing loss, vision loss, hypotonia, seizures
XLMR-psoriasis	+	0	+	Open mouth, large ears, hypotonia, seizures, psoriasis

Adrenoleukodystrophy

(Addison Disease and Cerebral Sclerosis, Adrenomyeloneuropathy, Siemerling-Creutzfeldt Disease, Bronze Schilder Disease, Melanodermic Leukodystrophy, MIM 300100)

Definition. XLMR with variable and progressive vision and hearing loss, spasticity, and neurological deterioration associated with demyelination of the central nervous system and adrenal insufficiency. The gene for adrenoleukodystrophy protein (ALD) is located in Xq28. The product is a peroxisomal membrane ATP-binding cassette (ABC) protein.

Somatic Features. Malformations are not features of this peroxisomal disorder. With elevated melanocyte-stimulating hormone (MSH) in overt or covert adrenal insufficiency, the skin may become diffusely darkened.

Growth and Development. In childhood onset adrenoleukodystrophy, normal growth and development for the first several years are followed by developmental stagnation or regression and growth failure.

Cognitive Features. Cerebral demyelination during childhood results in cognitive arrest and in adulthood results in dementia.

Neurological Findings. X-linked adrenoleukodystrophy usually presents with neurologic features. The neurologic presentation, age of onset, and progression

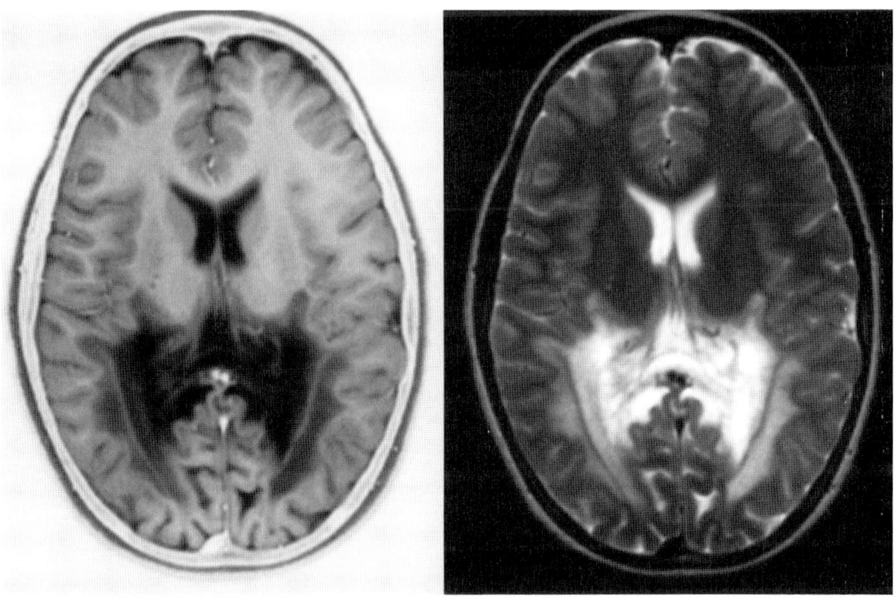

Adrenoleukodystrophy. T-2 axial images of the brain (image on the left is video-inverted) showing bilateral, symmetric abnormal signal in the occipital lobe white matter, and splenium of the corpus callosum due to dysmyelination/demyelination. Courtesy of Dr. G. Shashidhar Pai, Medical University of South Carolina, Charleston.

are variable. Cerebral involvement predominates in childhood. Spinal cord presentation is more common in adulthood. At any age, cerebral demyelination has a more rapid progression.

NATURAL HISTORY. Cerebral adrenoleukodystrophy usually presents at 4 to 8 years of age but may present in adolescence. Slowing and then arrest of motor, mental, and social development, with behavioral changes, is followed by spasticity, vision and hearing impairments, and, in a matter of years, death in an extremely debilitated state. The adult-onset cerebral presentation includes dementia and psychosis and is also rapidly progressive. More commonly, however, adults present with more slowly progressive spastic paraparesis (adrenomyeloneuropathy). They may develop sphincter incompetence and impotence. About half will develop cerebral involvement.

By the time of neurologic manifestations, frank adrenal insufficiency or, more commonly, compromise of adrenal reserve may be found. About 15% of childhood-onset adrenoleukodystrophies present with adrenal insufficiency. About 40% of adrenomyeloneuropathy patients have clinical adrenal insufficiency before the onset of neurologic symptoms. Of those with neurologic presentation, 85% have compromise of adrenal reserve by adrenocorticotropic hormone (ACTH) provocative testing. Variable presentation within families is commonplace.

HETEROZYGOTE EXPRESSION. Heterozygotes may be affected in this condition, most commonly with adrenomyeloneuropathy, but sometimes with cerebral involvement. One-half or more of carriers show some mild neurologic manifestation and about 20% have adrenomyeloneuropathy. Adrenal insufficiency is very rare in heterozygotes.

NEUROPATHOLOGY. Brain demyelination commences in the parietooccipital region and progresses anteriorly in 85% of cerebral cases. The demyelination is accompanied by an inflammatory response. Spinal cord pathology is that of a distal axonopathy fiber loss with minimal or no inflammatory response. Adrenal pathology is characterized initially by cellular edema followed by atrophy.

LABORATORY. Very long chain fatty acids are increased in blood and other tissues. Cortisol may be low or decreased cortisol reserve may be detected with provocative tests.

TREATMENT. Cortisol replacement is indicated for adrenal insufficiency. Evaluation of intervention for neurologic features is complicated by the variability of presentation. Dietary therapy with GTO-GTE oils (glyceryl trioleate–glyceryl trierucate) normalizes very long chain fatty acid levels but does not alter the progression of preexisting neurologic impairment. The efficacy of the diet in preventing the onset of neurologic symptoms is under investigation. Also under study are bone marrow transplantation and antiinflammatory interventions.

COMMENT. The existence of a modifier gene has been proposed because the severity of the neurologic involvement does not correlate with gene mutations, very long chain fatty acid levels, or adrenal insufficiency. It is proposed that the modifier gene may affect the cerebral inflammatory response.

REFERENCES

Dodd A, Rowland SA, Hawkes SLJ, et al.: Mutations in the adrenoleukodystrophy gene. Hum Mutat 9:500, 1997.

Gartner J, Braun A, Holzinger A, et al.: Clinical and genetic aspects of X-linked adrenoleukodystrophy. Neuropediatrics 29:3, 1998.

Moser HW: Adrenoleukodystrophy: phenotype, genetics, pathogenesis and therapy. Brain 120:1485, 1997.

Mosser J, Lutz Y, Stoeckel ME, et al.: The gene responsible for adrenoleukodystrophy encodes a peroxismal membrane protein. Hum Mol Genet 3:265, 1994.

Differential Matrix

Syndrome	Spastic Paraplegia	Vision Loss	Hearing Loss	Comments
Adrenoleukodystrophy	+	+	+	Adrenal insufficiency, diffuse skin pigmentation, progressive neurological deterioration and dementia, elevated very long chain fatty acids in plasma
Gustavson	+	+	+	Microcephaly, short stature, optic atrophy with blindness, large ears, joint contractures, rockerbottom feet, brain undergrowth, hydrocephaly, cerebellar hypoplasia, seizures
Mohr-Tranebjaerg (Jensen)	+	+	+	Neurologic deterioration with childhood onset, dystonia
Schimke	+	+	+	Microcephaly, sunken eyes, downslanting palpebral fissures, narrow nose, spacing of teeth, cupped ears, hypotonia, abducens palsy, choreoathetosis, contractures
Paine	+	+	+	Microcephaly, short stature, optic atrophy, seizures
Proud	+	+	+	Microcephaly, agenesis of corpus callosum, cryptorchidism, inguinal hernias, ataxia, seizures
XLMR-ataxia-deafness-dementia	+	+	+	Optic atrophy, ataxia, hypotonia, seizures, childhood death
Cerebrooculogenital	+	+	0	Short stature, microcephaly, hydrocephaly, agenesis of corpus callosum, microphthalmia, ptosis, hypospadias, cryptorchidism, clubfoot
Goldblatt spastic paraplegia	+	+	0	Optic atrophy, exotropia, nystagmus, ataxia, dysarthria, muscle hypoplasia, contractures
Pelizaeus-Merzbacher	+	+	0	Optic atrophy, nystagmus, hypotonia, ataxia, dystonia, CNS dysmyelination
XLMR-blindness-seizures-spasticity	+	+	0	Poor growth, postnatal microcephaly, clubfoot, seizures, contractures, scoliosis, hypomyelination
X-linked spastic parapleglia, type 7	+	+	0	Nystagmus, reduced vision, absent speech and ambulation, bowel and bladder dysfunction, spastic quadriplegia
Wittwer	0	+	+	Growth deficiency, microcephaly, microphthalmia, hypertelorism, genitourinary anomalies, hypotonia, seizures

Aicardi Syndrome

(Agenesis of Corpus Callosum–Lacunar Chorioretinopathy syndrome, MIM 304050)

Definition. XLMR with agenesis of the corpus callosum, lacunar chorioretinopathy, costovertebral anomalies, and seizures in females. The gene has been tentatively localized to Xp22 based on an X:3 translocation with the X breakpoint at p22.2-22.3.

Somatic Features. More than any other manifestation, lacunar chorioretinopathy serves to distinguish Aicardi syndrome from other conditions with agenesis of the corpus callosum and seizures. Bilateral punched out areas of pigment epithelium occur near the optic disc, appear yellow-white, and have little surrounding pigment deposition. Microphthalmia, iris synechiae, optic atrophy, and colobomas may occur as well. Cranial size varies depending upon whether enlarged ventricles are present. Cortical heterotopias occur in half of cases.

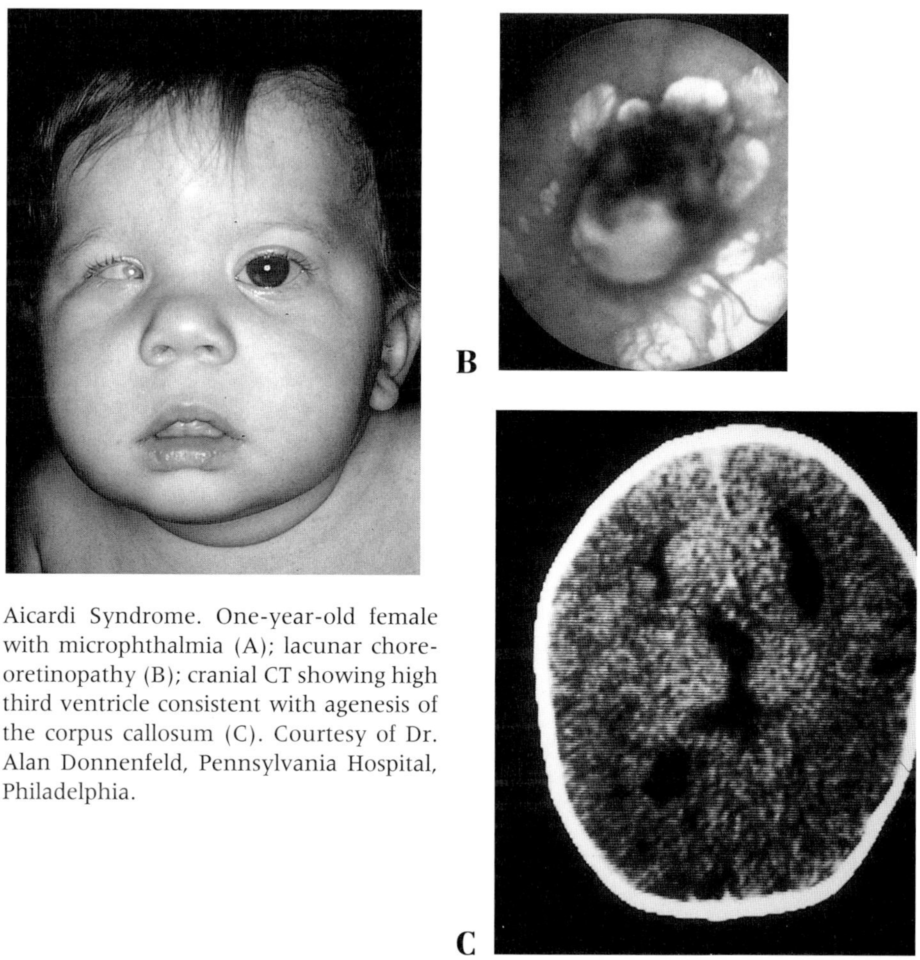

A

B

C

Aicardi Syndrome. One-year-old female with microphthalmia (A); lacunar choreoretinopathy (B); cranial CT showing high third ventricle consistent with agenesis of the corpus callosum (C). Courtesy of Dr. Alan Donnenfeld, Pennsylvania Hospital, Philadelphia.

Hemivertebrae, scoliosis and absent or malformed ribs are found in one-third. Cleft lip and cleft palate, hiatal hernia, and hip dysplasia have been described in a few cases.

GROWTH AND DEVELOPMENT. Normal intrauterine and postnatal growth is the rule but developmental milestones are globally delayed.

COGNITIVE FEATURES. Severe impairment.

NEUROLOGICAL FINDINGS. Severe impairment of neurologic function is obvious from early infancy. Seizures of a wide variety (infantile spasms, generalized seizures, staring spells) occur, in some cases beginning as early as the first day of life. The EEG shows the characteristic burst–suppression pattern of hypsarrhythmia, other seizure discharges, and asynchrony between the cerebral hemispheres.

IMAGING. Agenesis of the corpus callosum, enlarged lateral ventricles, cerebellar hypoplasia, and posterior fossa cysts may be demonstrated.

COMMENT. Microcephaly, chorioretinopathy, seizures, and developmental delay call to mind prenatal infection, especially prenatal toxoplasmosis. The distinctive lacunar retinopathy serves best to distinguish Aicardi syndrome from these infections. As a rule, Aicardi syndrome occurs in females and in sporadic fashion. No affected female has reproduced. Consideration that the syndrome is X-linked dominant with expression in females and gestational lethality in males is based on the increased abortions and decreased male:female ratio in at-risk sibships.

REFERENCES

Aicardi J, Lefebvre J, Lerique A: Spasms in flexion, callosal agenesis, ocular abnormalities: a new syndrome. Electroencephalogr Clin Neurophysiol 19:609, 1965.

Aicardi J, Chevrie J-J, Rousselie F: Le syndrome spasmes en flexion, agenesie calleuse, anomalies chorio-retiniennes. Arch Fr Pediatr 26:1103, 1969.

Donnenfeld AE, Packer RJ, Zackai EH, et al.: Clinical, cytogenetic, and pedigree findings in 18 cases of Aicardi syndrome. Am J Med Genet 32:461, 1989.

Willis J, Rosman NP: The Aicardi syndrome versus congenital infection: diagnostic considerations. J Pediatr 96:235, 1980.

Differential Matrix

Syndrome	Ocular Abnormality	CNS Anomalies	Vertebral or Rib Defects	Comments
Aicardi	+	+	+	Lacunar retinopathy, costovertebral anomalies, agenesis of corpus callosum, seizures
Goltz	+	+	+	Cataracts, linear areas of dermal aplasia, cutaneous adipose herniations, dystrophic nails, abnormal teeth and hair, limb reduction defects, genitourinary anomalies
Cerebrooculogenital	+	+	0	Short stature, microcephaly, hydrocephaly, agenesis of corpus callosum, microphthalmia, ptosis, hypospadias, cryptorchidism, clubfoot, spasticity
MIDAS	+	+	0	Microphthalmia, corneal opacification, dermal aplasia, dysgenesis of corpus callosum, cardiac defects, cardiomyopathy
Lenz microphthalmia	+	0	+	Microcephaly, microphthalmia, malformed ears, cleft lip/palate, cardiac and genitourinary anomalies, thumb duplication or hypoplasia, narrow shoulders
Wittwer	+	+	0	Growth deficiency, microcephaly, microphthalmia, hearing loss, vision loss, hypertelorism, genitourinary anomalies, hypotonia, seizures

ALBRIGHT HEREDITARY OSTEODYSTROPHY

(Pseudohypoparathyroidism, Pseudopseudohypoparathyroidism, MIM 300800)

DEFINITION. XLMR with short stature, brachydactyly, and obesity associated with end organ resistance to parathyroid hormone. Genetic heterogeneity exists with two known autosomal loci. Although a gene on the X chromosome has not been identified or localized, the entity is included for historical reasons. Most cases have a mutation of the G_s protein of adenyl cyclase (20q) or a deletion of distal 2q.

SOMATIC FEATURES. The facies are rounded with short neck but have no other distinguishing characteristics. Skeletal manifestations include generalized shortening of the long bones resulting in short stature and variable brachydactyly. Commonly, the shortest segment is the distal phalanx, the shortest rays are the lateral three rays due to shortening of the third, fourth, and fifth metacarpals

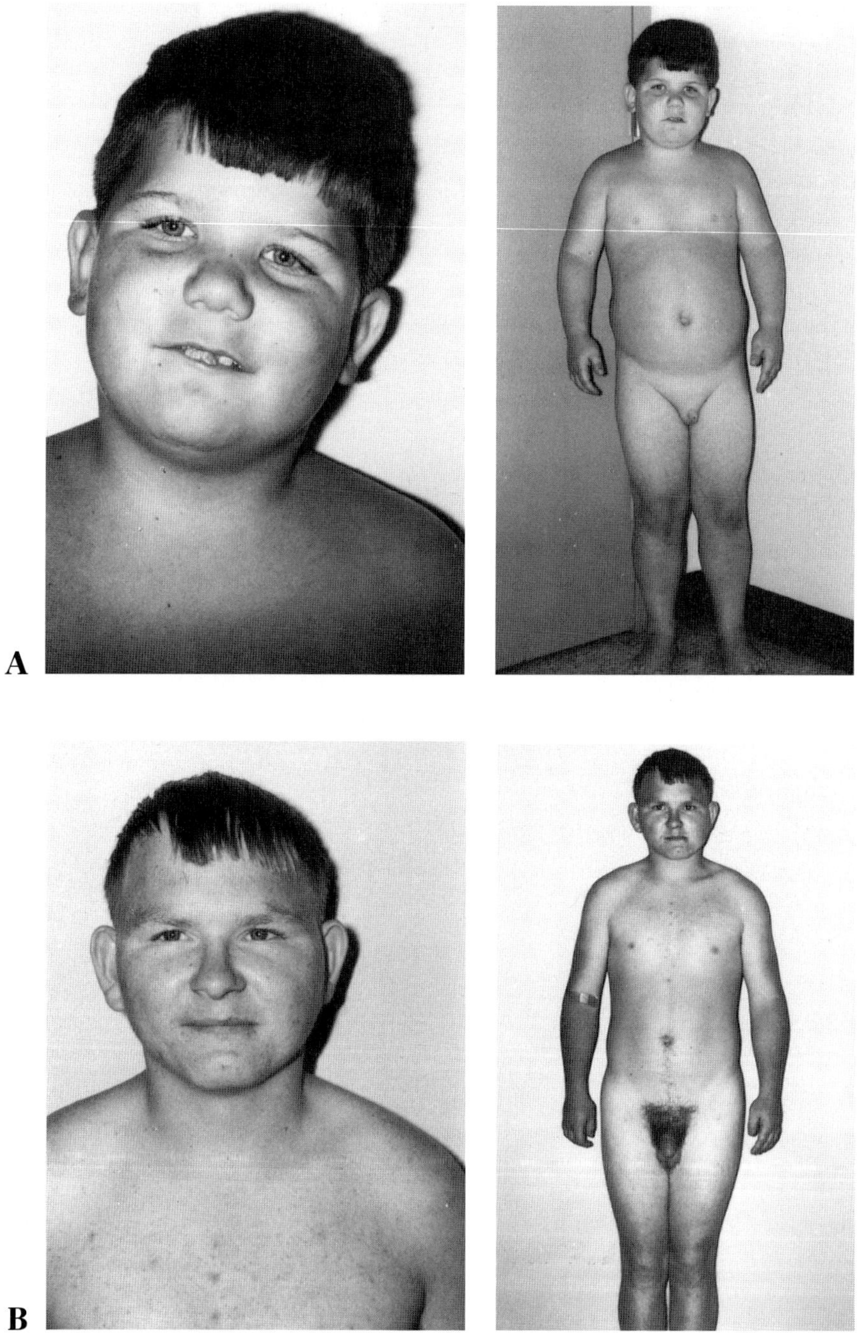

Albright Hereditary Osteodystrophy. Nine year-old boy with round face, depressed nasal bridge, short stature, brachydactyly and obesity (A); 14-year-old boy with round face and short stature (B).

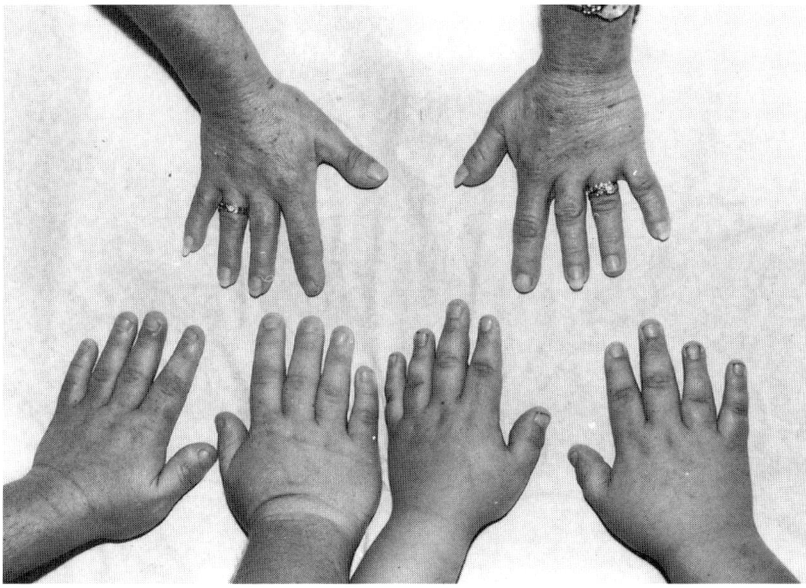

C

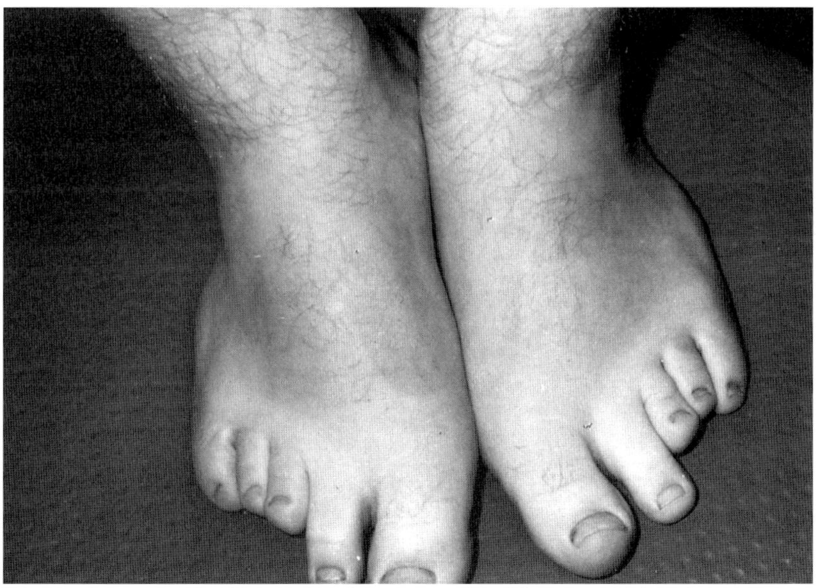

D

Albright Hereditary Osteodystrophy. (continued) Brachydactyly in mother and two sons (C); short toes secondary to short metatarsals (D).

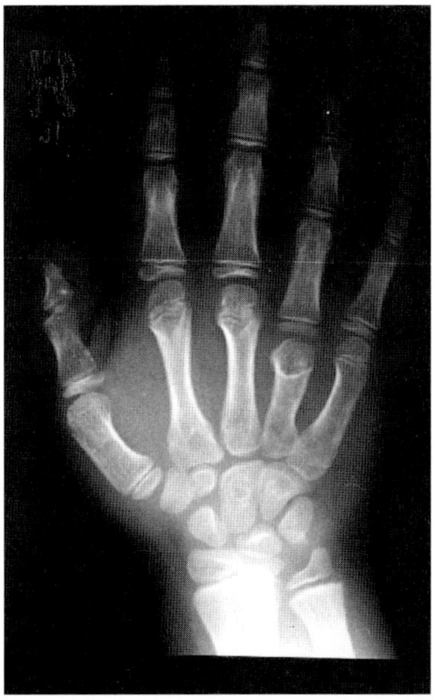

E

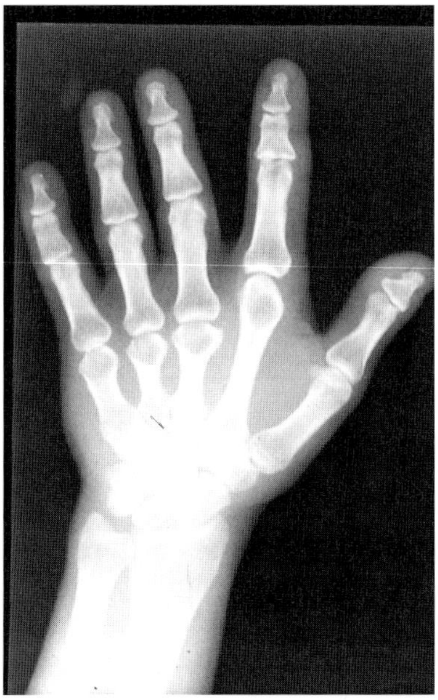

F

Albright Hereditary Osteodystrophy. (continued) Short fourth metacarpal in a 9 year old (E); short third, fourth, and fifth metacarpals in adult female (F).

and metatarsals, and the middle finger is often shorter than the index finger. Excessive weight for height is typical. Cataracts are the most common ocular finding but microphthalmia, unequal pupils, malformed or atrophic optic discs, macular degeneration, nystagmus, and other abnormalities have been noted. Ectopic calcification in soft tissues occurs in about half of patients. Fibrous dysplasia, exostoses, osteochondromas, cystic lesions, and decreased bone density have been described. Advanced bone age is often found in early childhood.

Growth and Development. Although weight tends to be excessive for height, even at birth, a wide distribution of weight, including some below −2 SD, can be found in most series. In similar fashion, the height tends toward shortness. This is particularly so in adults: The majority measure below −2 SD and few measure above the 15th centile. Height typically exceeds span. Head circumference tends to be in the upper centiles. Developmental delay predicts mental retardation and occurs in the majority of those with hypocalcemia.

Cognitive Features. Cognitive impairment is inconstant, occurring in 70% of those with hypocalcemia and in less than half of those without hypocalcemia.

Neurological Findings. Seizures commonly occur, especially among those with hypocalcemia.

Imaging. Calcification of the basal ganglia has been commonly described.

Laboratory. Patients with Albright hereditary osteodystrophy have end organ resistance to parathyroid hormone. Those with hypocalcemia and hyperphosphatemia are designated pseudohypoparathyroid; those with normal calcium and phosphate levels in serum are designated pseudopseudohypoparathyroid. Both variants may be seen in the same family. Most patients will have reduced activity of the α subunit of the G_s protein of adenyl cyclase. Thyroid dysfunction, particularly hypothyroidism, is common.

COMMENT. Although the familial nature of Albright hereditary osteodystrophy has long been recognized, the type of genetic transmission has been problematic. A lack of male to male transmission in early reports and the 1:2 male to female sex ratio led to the notion that it was an X-linked disorder. A number of lines of evidence, however, have called this into doubt. Male-to-male transmission has now been documented in a number of instances. Females tend to be as severely affected or more so than males. A majority of individuals have reduced expression of the α subunit of the G_s (guanine nucleotide stimulatory) protein of adenyl cyclase. Mutations have been demonstrated in the G_s α gene (GNAS1), which is located in 20q12-13.2. A minority of patients, those with normal G_s α activity, have been found to have a deletion of 2q37. Finally, to date, an X chromosome locus has not been identified.

REFERENCES

Albright F, Burnett CH, Smith PH, et al.: Pseudo-hypoparathyroidism—an example of "Seabright-Bantam syndrome." Endocrinology 30:922, 1942.

Fitch N: Albright's hereditary osteodystrophy: a review. Am J Med Genet 11:11, 1982.

Levine MA, Ahn TG, Klupt SF, et al.: Genetic deficiency of the α subunit of the guanine nucleotide-binding protein G_s, as the molecular basis for Albright hereditary osteodystrophy. Proc Natl Acad Sci USA 85:617, 1988.

Phelan MC, Rogers RC, Clarkson KB, et al.: Albright hereditary osteodystrophy and del(2)(q37.3) in four unrelated individuals. Am J Med Genet 58:1, 1995.

Weinberg AG, Stone RT: Autosomal dominant inheritance in Albright's hereditary osteodystrophy. J Pediatr 79:996, 1971.

Differential Matrix

Syndrome	Short Stature	Obesity	Brachy-dactyly	Comments
Albright hereditary osteodystrophy	+	+	+	Short metacarpals and metatarsals, ectopic calcifications
Chudley-Lowry	+	+	+	Bitemporal narrowing, almond-shaped eyes, depressed nasal bridge, tented upper lip, open mouth, hypogonadism, hypotonia
Aarskog	+	0	+	Hypertelorism, downslanting palpebral fissures, ptosis, cupped ears, anteverted nares, horizontal palmar crease, midfoot varus, joint laxity, shawl scrotum, cryptorchidism, inguinal hernias
XLMR-hypotonic facies (Carpenter-Waziri) (Holmes-Gang) (Juberg-Marsidi)	+	0	+	Microcephaly, telecanthus, small triangular nose, tented upper lip, open mouth, spacing of teeth, genital anomalies, musculoskeletal anomalies, hemoglobin H inclusions in erythrocytes
Börjeson-Forssman-Lehmann	+	+	0	Hypotonia, hypogonadism, microcephaly, coarse facies, large ears, gynecomastia, narrow sloped shoulders, visual impairment, tapered digits

ALLAN-HERNDON-DUDLEY SYNDROME

(Allan-Herndon Syndrome, MIM 309600)

DEFINITION. XLMR with generalized muscle hypoplasia, childhood hypotonia, ataxia, athetosis, dysarthria, and spastic paraplegia. The gene is located between DXS983 (Xq13) and DXS995 (Xq21), lod score (three families) of 9.22 at DXS566 (Xq13).

SOMATIC FEATURES. Marked hypotonia and paucity of skeletal muscle mass permits diagnosis in infancy. While the facies do not appear distinctive in childhood, there is a tendency in adult life toward elongation of the face, cupping or abnormal folding of the ears, and large ears. In one family bitemporal narrowness and midface hypoplasia were noted. No malformations have been noted. Spastic paraplegia and contractures of the small and large joints become evident in adult life. Shallow pectus excavatum, ulnar deviation of the hand, scoliosis, and valgus position of the great toe may be seen. Excessive drooling and dysarthria continue into adult life, deep tendon reflexes are hyperactive, and clonus and Babinski signs may be seen. Fungal infections appear to be common.

GROWTH AND DEVELOPMENT. Some affected males never develop speech or independent ambulation. Adult stature and head circumference are normal. Puberty occurs at the usual age and external genitalia are normal.

COGNITIVE FEATURES. Severe impairment.

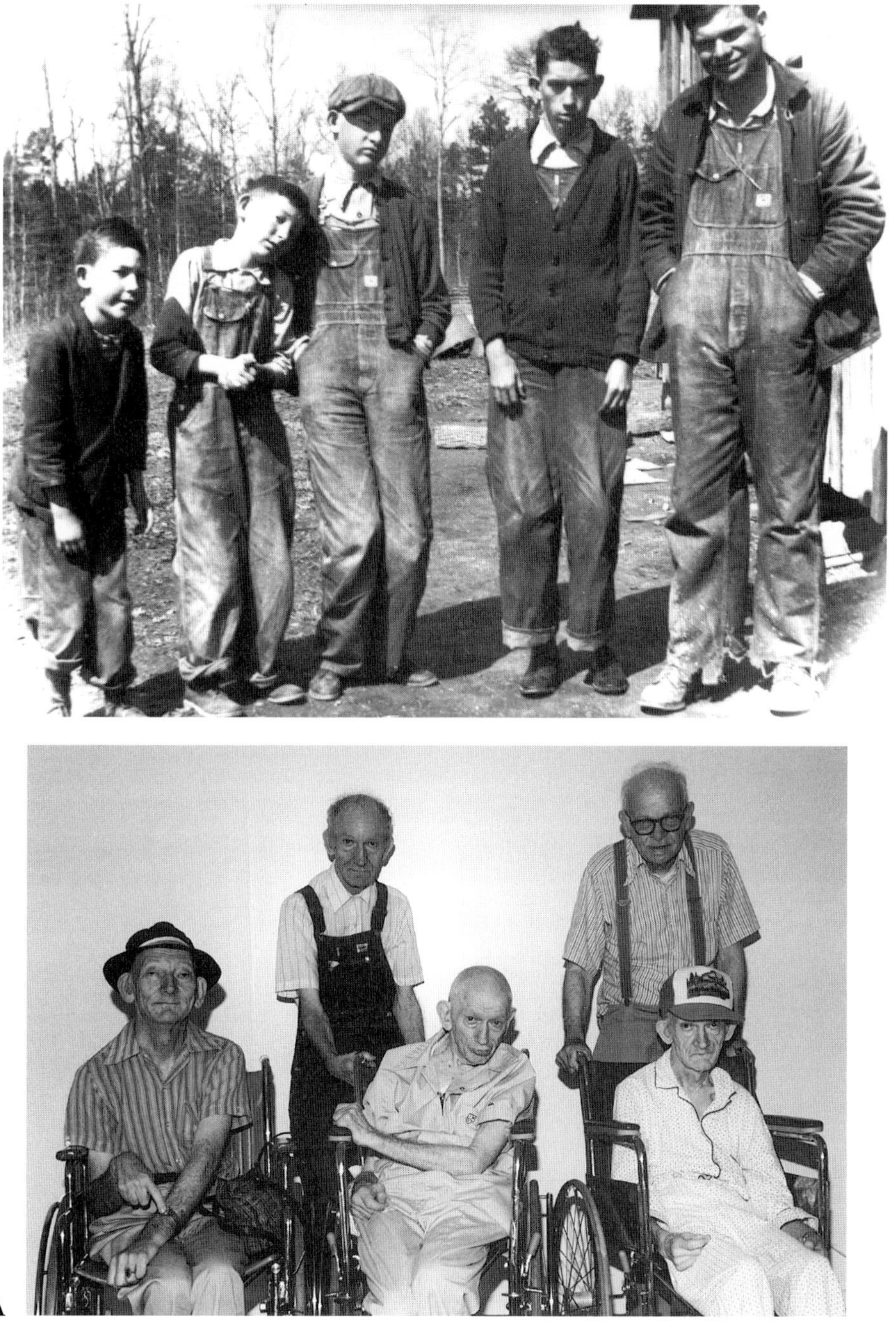

A

Allan-Herndon-Dudley Syndrome. Five affected males in childhood and late adult life (A).

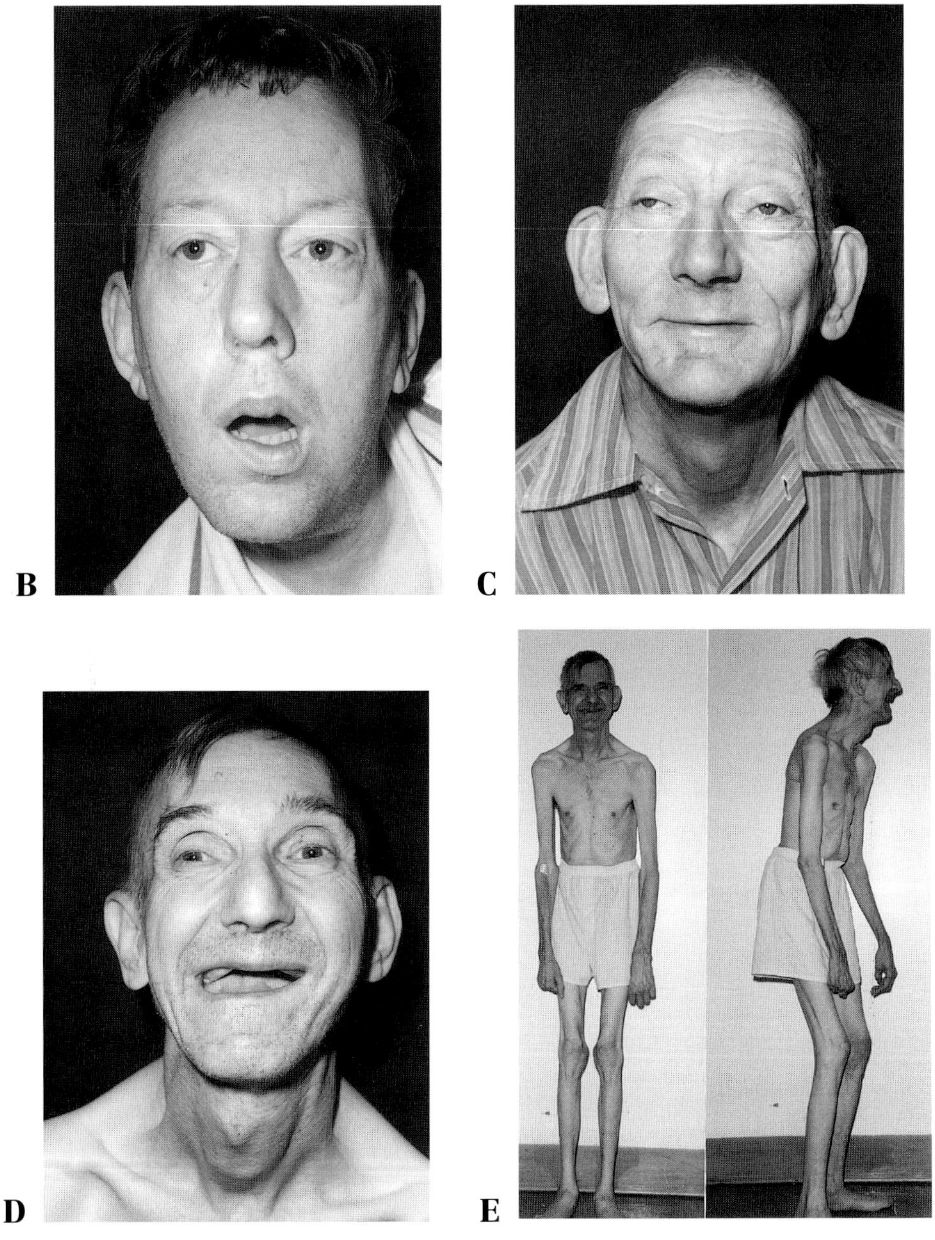

Allan-Herndon-Dudley Syndrome. (continued) 49-year-old with long face, bitemporal narrowing, flat midface, and myopathic appearance (B); 61-year-old with bitemporal narrowing, midface hypoplasia, and simple cupped ears (C); 65-year-old with bitemporal narrowing, cupped ears, and marked hypoplasia of musculature (D, E).

HETEROZYGOTE EXPRESSION. None

IMAGING. Magnetic resonance imaging of the brain in a 1-year-old was normal; in a 58-year-old it showed prominence of the cortical sulci and mild dilation of the ventricular system.

LABORATORY. Peripheral nerve (peroneal) conduction in one affected male was mildly impaired and showed some spontaneous motor potentials, but muscle microscopy showed no pathologic changes.

COMMENT. Three large families with the Allan-Herndon-Dudley syndrome have been studied. There is some interfamilial variability which calls into question whether or not they represent mutations of the same gene. This syndrome represents the numerous, heterogeneous, and overlapping X-linked ataxias and spastic paraplegias which have long taxed the clinician and discouraged the laboratory. Molecular studies may bring some insight into the developmental and functional aberrations which underly the clinical variability.

REFERENCES

Allan W, Herndon CN, Dudley FC: Some examples of the inheritance of mental deficiency: apparently sex-linked idiocy and microcephaly. Am J Ment Defic 48:325, 1944.

Bialer MG, Lawrence L, Stevenson RE, et al.: Allan-Herndon-Dudley syndrome: clinical and linkage studies on a second family. Am J Med Genet 43:491, 1992.

Schwartz CE, Ulmer J, Brown A, et al.: Allan-Herndon syndrome. II. Linkage to DNA markers in Xq21. Am J Hum Genet 47:454, 1990.

Stevenson RE, Goodman HO, Schwartz CE, et al.: Allan-Herndon syndrome. I. Clinical studies. Am J Hum Genet 47:446, 1990.

Differential Matrix

Syndrome	Ataxia	Spastic Paraplegia	Muscle Hypoplasia	Comments
Allan-Herndon-Dudley	+	+	+	Childhood hypotonia, dysarthria, athetosis, large ears with cupping or abnormal architecture, contractures
Apak ataxia-spastic diplegia	+	+	+	Short stature, clubfoot, dysarthria, nystagmus
Arena	+	+	+	Clubfoot, iron deposits in basal ganglia, rigidity, dystonia
Goldblatt spastic paraplegia	+	+	+	Optic atrophy, exotropia, nystagmus, dysarthria, contractures
XLMR-spastic paraplegia-athetosis	+	+	+	Nystagmus, weakness, dysarthria, muscle wasting, contractures
Adrenoleukodystrophy	+	+	0	Adrenal insufficiency, diffuse skin pigmentation, progressive neurologic deterioration and dementia, elevated very long chain fatty acids in plasma
Pelizaeus-Merzbacher	+	+	0	Optic atrophy, nystagmus, hypotonia, dystonia, CNS dysmyelination
Pettigrew	+	+	0	Microcephaly or hydrocephaly, long face with macrostomia and prognathism, Dandy-Walker malformation, small testes, contractures, choreoathetosis, iron deposits in basal ganglia
X-linked ataxia-deafness-dementia	+	+	0	Optic atrophy, deafness, hypotonia, hyperreflexia, recurrent episodes of choking and vomiting, seizures, childhood death
X-linked ataxia-dementia	+	+	0	adult-onset dementia
X-linked hydrocephaly-MASA spectrum	+	+	0	Ophthalmoplegia, lack of speech and ambulation, incontinence
X-linked spastic paraplegia, type 7	+	+	0	Nystagmus, reduced vision, absent speech and ambulation, bowel and bladder dysfunction
Fitzsimmons	0	+	+	Pes cavus, hyperkeratosis of palms and soles, dystrophic nails
Arts	+	0	+	Growth deficiency, paucity of muscles, hypotonia, areflexia, seizures, childhood death
Christianson	+	0	+	Microcephaly, short stature, long narrow face, contractures, seizures

APAK ATAXIA-SPASTIC DIPLEGIA SYNDROME

DEFINITION. XLMR with short stature, muscle hypoplasia, nystagmus, ataxia, and spasticity. The gene has not been mapped.
SOMATIC FEATURES. The head circumference is normal and facial abnormalities are not described. The musculature, especially the peroneal muscles, are hypoplastic; clubfoot and other foot contractures occur.
GROWTH AND DEVELOPMENT. Short stature is obvious in childhood.
COGNITIVE FEATURES. Specific testing is not available, but comprehension appears better than limited speech and motor skills suggest.
NEUROLOGICAL FINDINGS. Males never learn to walk and speech is dysarthric. Ataxia is manifest as head and truncal instability, nystagmus, dysmetria, and adiadochokinesis. The ability to sit may be gained by age 2 years but is lost within a few years. Spasticity is manifest by impaired fine motor skills, increased deep tendon reflexes, Babinski signs, and contractures of the joints. Sensation appears normal. Neurological signs appear early with nystagmus in early months, spasticity by the end of the first year, truncal ataxia at 2–3 years, and dysarthric speech at 3–4 years. Death from infections occurs in the third or fourth decade.
HETEROZYGOTE EXPRESSION. One carrier female had hyperactive deep tendon reflexes.
IMAGING. Computed tomography was normal in one case at age 9 years.

A

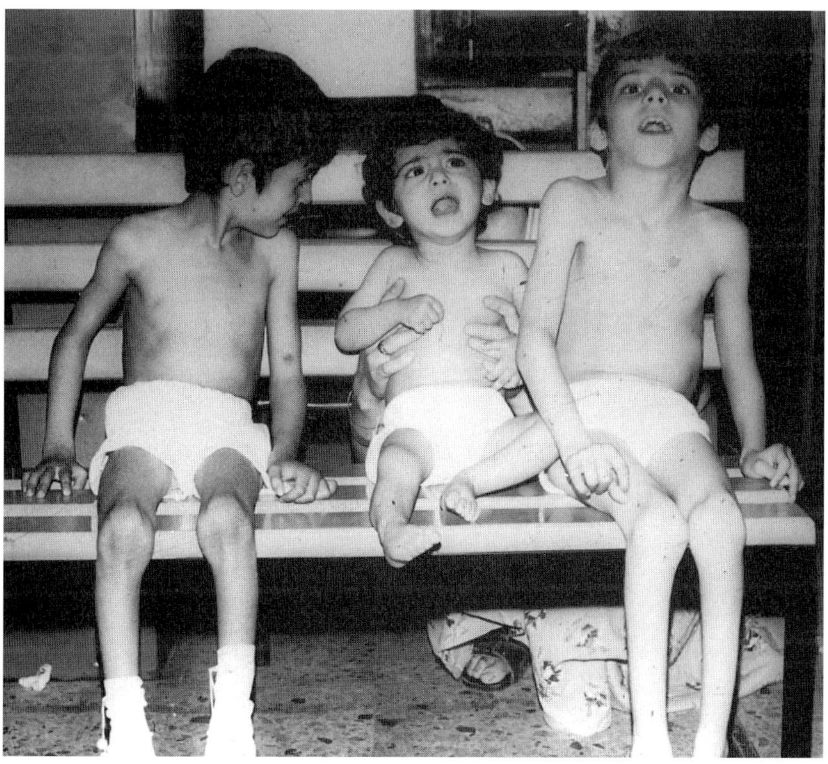

Apak–Ataxia–Spastic Diplegia Syndrome. Affected brothers at ages 6, 2, and 8 years (A).

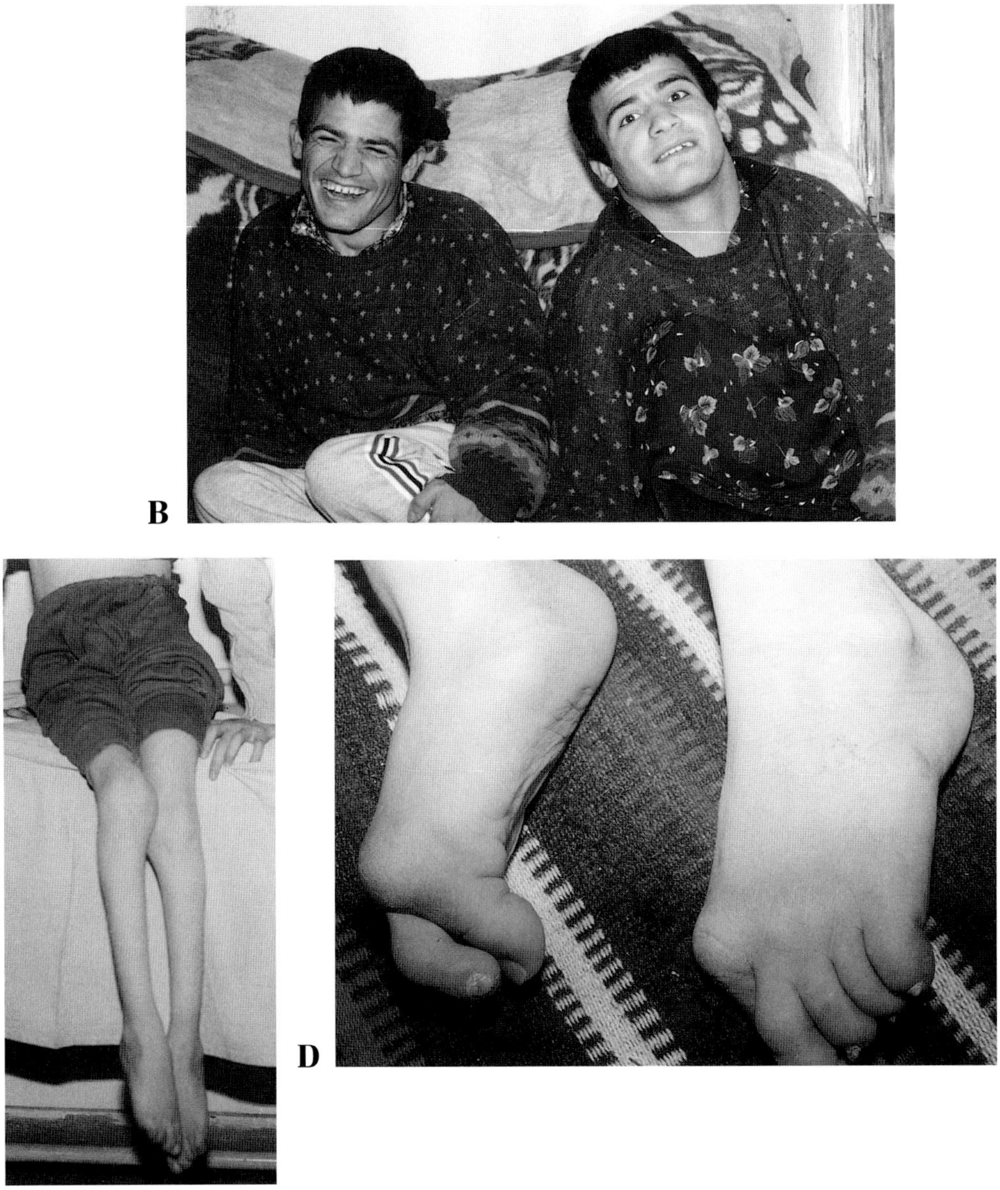

B C D

Apak–Ataxia–Spastic Diplegia Syndrome. (continued) Maternal uncles as young adults (B); muscle hypoplasia of lower limbs in an 8-year-old (C); foot contractures in a young adult (D). Courtesy of Dr. Selcuk Apak, Institute of Child Health, University of Istanbul, Turkey.

LABORATORY. Electroencephalogram, electromyogram, and nerve conduction velocity were normal in one case.

COMMENT. Apak syndrome, represented by a single family, is set aside as a distinct syndrome because it differs in some respects from other X-linked cerebellar ataxias and spastic diplegias. Cerebellar and pyramidal signs become obvious in the initial years of life, cognitive function is impaired, neurological dysfunction progresses to total disability in the teen years, and lifespan is shortened. Linkage studies were not successful in mapping the gene location.

REFERENCE

Apak S, Yüksel M, Özmen M, et al.: Heterogeneity of X-linked recessive (spino)cerebellar ataxia with or without spastic diplegia. Am J Med Genet 34:155, 1989.

Differential Matrix

Syndrome	Ataxia	Spastic Paraplegia	Muscle Hypoplasia	Comments
Apak ataxia-spastic diplegia	+	+	+	Short stature, nystagmus, dysarthria, contractures
Allan-Herndon-Dudley	+	+	+	Childhood hypotonia, dysarthria, athetosis, large ears with cupping or abnormal architecture, contractures
Arena	+	+	+	Clubfoot, rigidity, dystonia, iron deposits in basal ganglia
Goldblatt spastic paraplegia	+	+	+	Optic atrophy, exotropia, nystagmus, dysarthria, contractures
XLMR-spastic paraplegia-athetosis	+	+	+	Nystagmus, weakness, dysarthria, muscle wasting, contractures
Adrenoleukodystrophy	+	+	0	Adrenal insufficiency, diffuse skin pigmentation, progressive neurologic deterioration and dementia, elevated very long chain fatty acids in plasma
Pelizaeus-Merzbacher	+	+	0	Optic atrophy, nystagmus, hypotonia, dystonia, CNS dysmyelination
Pettigrew	+	+	0	Microcephaly or hydrocephaly, long face with macrostomia and prognathism, Dandy-Walker malformation, small testes, contractures, choreoathetosis, iron deposits in basal ganglia
X-linked ataxia-deafness-dementia	+	+	0	Optic atrophy, vision loss, hearing loss, hypotonia, seizures, childhood death
X-linked ataxia-dementia	+	+	0	adult-onset dementia
X-linked hydrocephaly-MASA spectrum	+	+	0	Hydrocephaly, adducted thumbs, dysgenesis of corpus callosum
X-linked spastic paraplegia, type 7	+	+	0	Nystagmus, reduced vision, absent speech and ambulation, bowel and bladder dysfunction
Fitzsimmons	0	+	+	Pes cavus, hyperkeratosis of palms and soles, dystrophic nails
Arts	+	0	+	Growth deficiency, paucity of muscles, hypotonia, areflexia, seizures, childhood death

ARENA SYNDROME

(XLMR–Spastic Paraplegia—Iron Deposition)

DEFINITION. XLMR with muscle hypoplasia of lower limbs, clubfoot, spasticity, ataxia, dystonia, rigidity, and iron deposition in the basal ganglia. The gene maps to the large area between DXS3 (Xq21.3) and DXS425 (Xq26), lod score 1.86.

SOMATIC FEATURES. Apart from the neuromuscular system, malformations or other distinctive somatic characteristics do not occur. The face appears normal. Underdevelopment of musculature in the lower limbs and clubfoot are obvious from birth. The pelvis is small and scoliosis is present.

GROWTH AND DEVELOPMENT. Stature is probably short although measurement is compromised by scoliosis and spasticity.

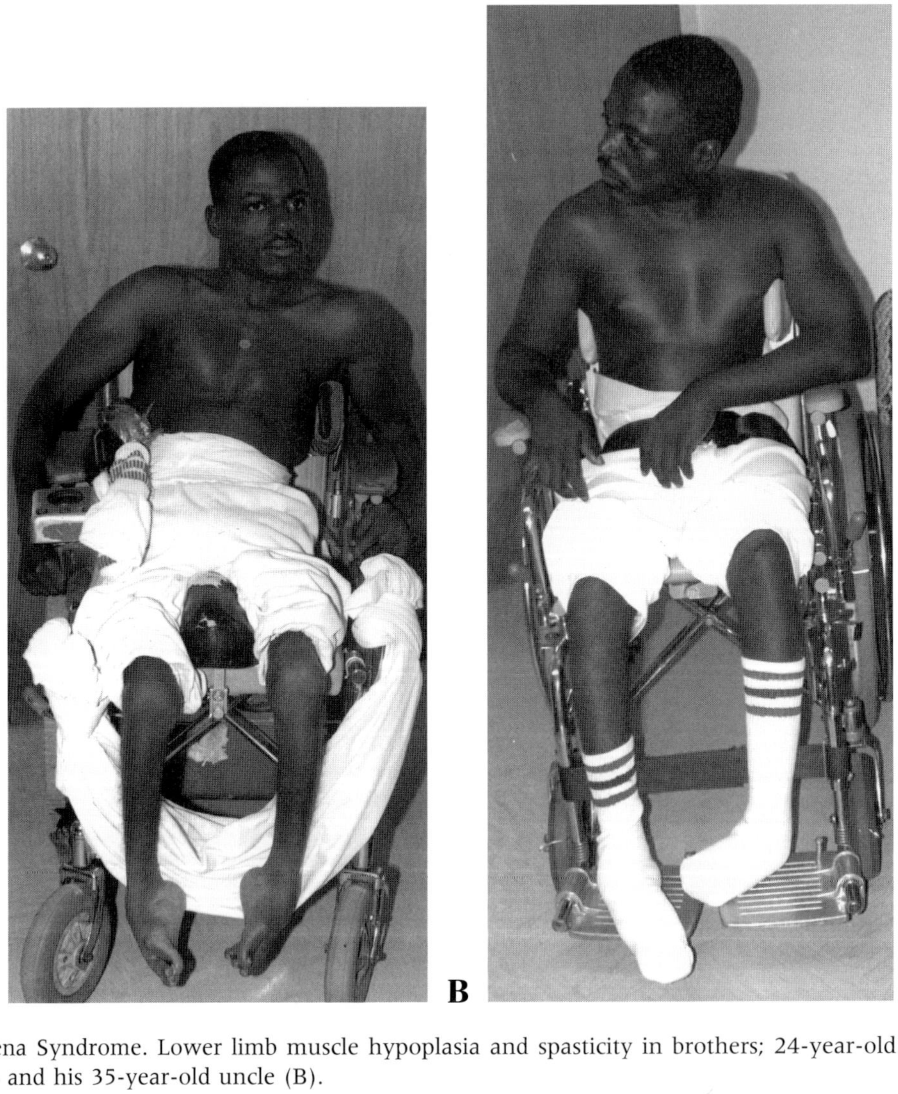

A B

Arena Syndrome. Lower limb muscle hypoplasia and spasticity in brothers; 24-year-old (A) and his 35-year-old uncle (B).

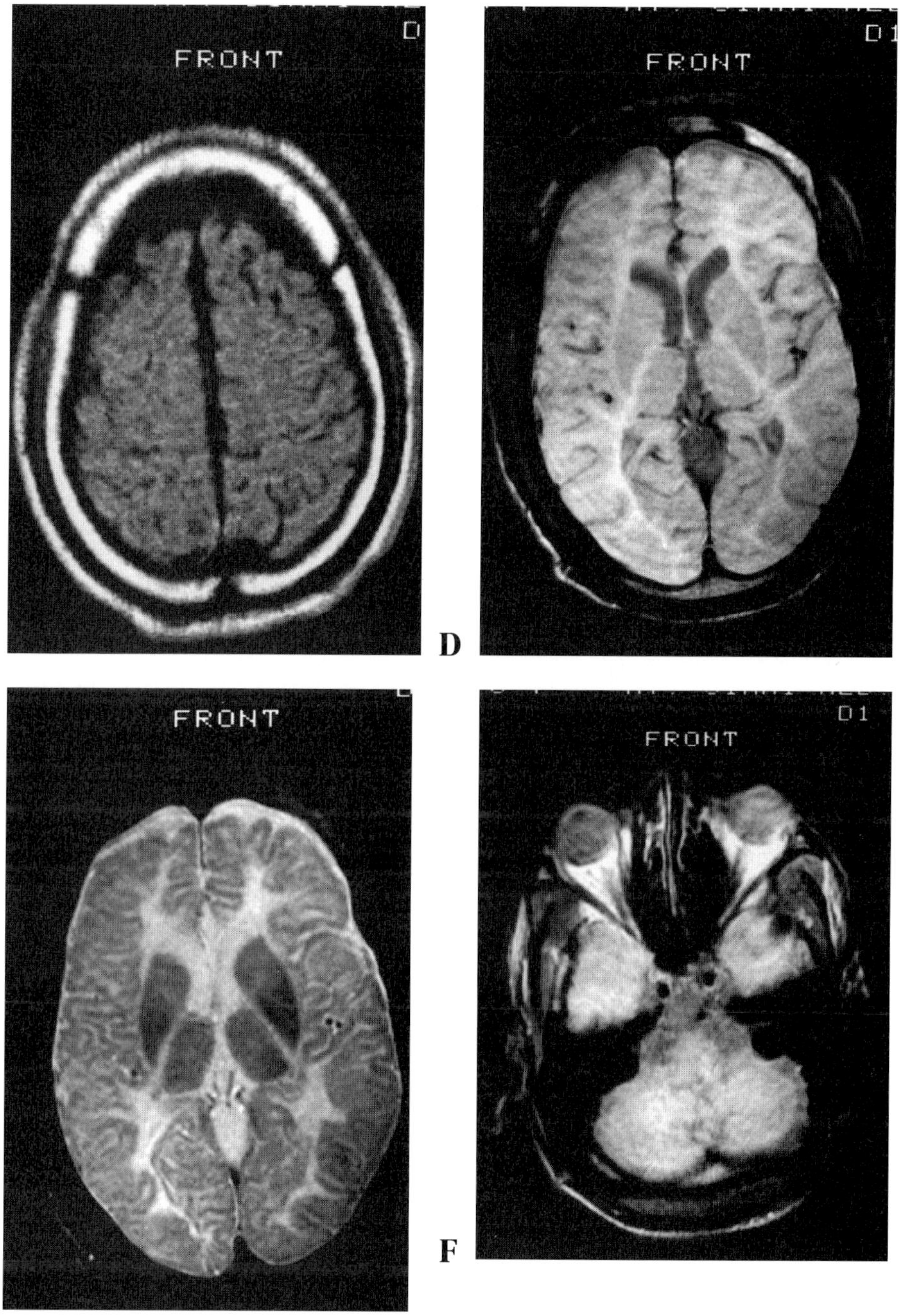

C D E F

Arena Syndrome. (continued) Cranial MRIs showing macrogyria (C); hypoplastic white matter (D); hypoplastic white matter and evidence suggesting iron accumulation in basal ganglia and thalamus (E); hypoplastic cerebellum and brain stem (F).

COGNITIVE FEATURES. Severe impairment.

NEUROLOGICAL FINDINGS. Severe neuromuscular impairment prevents independent ambulation. Stability and movement are disturbed by dystonic and ataxic movements, rigidity, and spasticity. Bowel and bladder continence are not achieved. Speech, if present at all, is limited to short phrases with indistinct and nasal quality. Sensation appears normal.

IMAGING. Magnetic resonance imaging documents small brain, macrogyria, diffuse white matter hypoplasia, small brain stem and cerebellum, and evidence for iron deposits in the thalamus and basal ganglia.

COMMENT. Arena syndrome shares many features—microcephaly, contractures, truncal ataxia, absent or limited speech, absent ambulation, and hypoplasia of the cerebellum and brain stem—with Christianson syndrome, which maps to the same region. However, Arena syndrome has normal facial appearance, lacks seizures, and has MRI changes suggesting iron deposits in the basal ganglia and thalamus. By virtue of similar features and overlapping linkage limits, Gustavson syndrome must also be considered as a candidate for allelism. Profound developmental failure, blindness, deafness, and seizures become apparent soon after birth and lead to death in infancy or early childhood. Other XLMR syndromes with overlapping mapping limits appear quite different.

REFERENCES

Arena JF, Schwartz C, Stevenson R, et al.: Spastic paraplegia with iron deposits in the basal ganglia: a new X-linked mental retardation syndrome. Am J Med Genet 43:479, 1992.

Christianson AL, Stevenson RE, van der Meuden CH, et al.: X-linked mental retardation, mild craniofacial dysmorphology, epilepsy, ophthalmoplegia, and cerebral atrophy in a large South African kindred, J Med Genet, in press, 1999.

Gustavson K-H, Annerén G, Malmgren H, et al.: New X-linked syndrome with severe mental retardation, severely impaired vision, severe hearing defect, epileptic seizures, spasticity, restricted joint mobility, and early death. Am J Med Genet 45:654, 1993.

Differential Matrix

Syndrome	Absent Speech, Ambulation and Continence	Truncal Ataxia	Cerebellar and Brain Stem Hypoplasia	Comments
Arena	+	+	+	Muscle hypoplasia, clubfoot, iron deposits in basal ganglia, spastic paraplegia, rigidity, dystonia
Christianson	+	+	+	Short stature, microcephaly, general asthenia, contractures, seizures, ophthalmoplegia
Bertini	+	+	+	Macular degeneration, hypotonia, seizures, childhood death, developmental delays and regression, postnatal growth impairment
Gustavson	+	+	+	Microcephaly, short stature, optic atrophy with blindness, large ears, deafness, joint contractures, rockerbottom feet, brain undergrowth, hydrocephaly, spasticity, seizures
Schimke	+	+	+	Microcephaly, sunken eyes, downslanting palpebral fissures, narrow nose, spacing of teeth, cupped ears, hypotonia, abducens palsy, hearing loss, vision loss, spasticity, choreoathetosis, contractures
Paine	+	0	+	Microcephaly, short stature, vision and hearing loss, optic atrophy, spasticity, seizures
Pettigrew	0	+	+	Dandy-Walker malformation, spasticity, seizures, microcephaly or hydrocephaly, long face with macrostomia and prognathism, small testes, contractures, myoglobinuria, hemolytic anemia

ARMFIELD SYNDROME

(XLMR-Glaucoma-Clefting)

DEFINITION. XLMR with short stature, small hands and feet, glaucoma, cleft palate, and seizures. The gene maps to Xq28 distal to DXS1113, lod score 2.11. **SOMATIC FEATURES.** Facial characteristics include prominent forehead, epicanthus, downslanting palpebral fissures, midface hypoplasia, large ears, cleft palate, and micrognathia. Cataracts and glaucoma may develop in adult life. The head circumference is quite variable, from below the third centile to above the 97th centile, the latter probably secondary to hydrocephaly. Short stature is typical. The hands and feet are small and there is stiffness of large and small joints. Other variable features include facial asymmetry, cupped ears, inguinal hernias, and undescended testes.

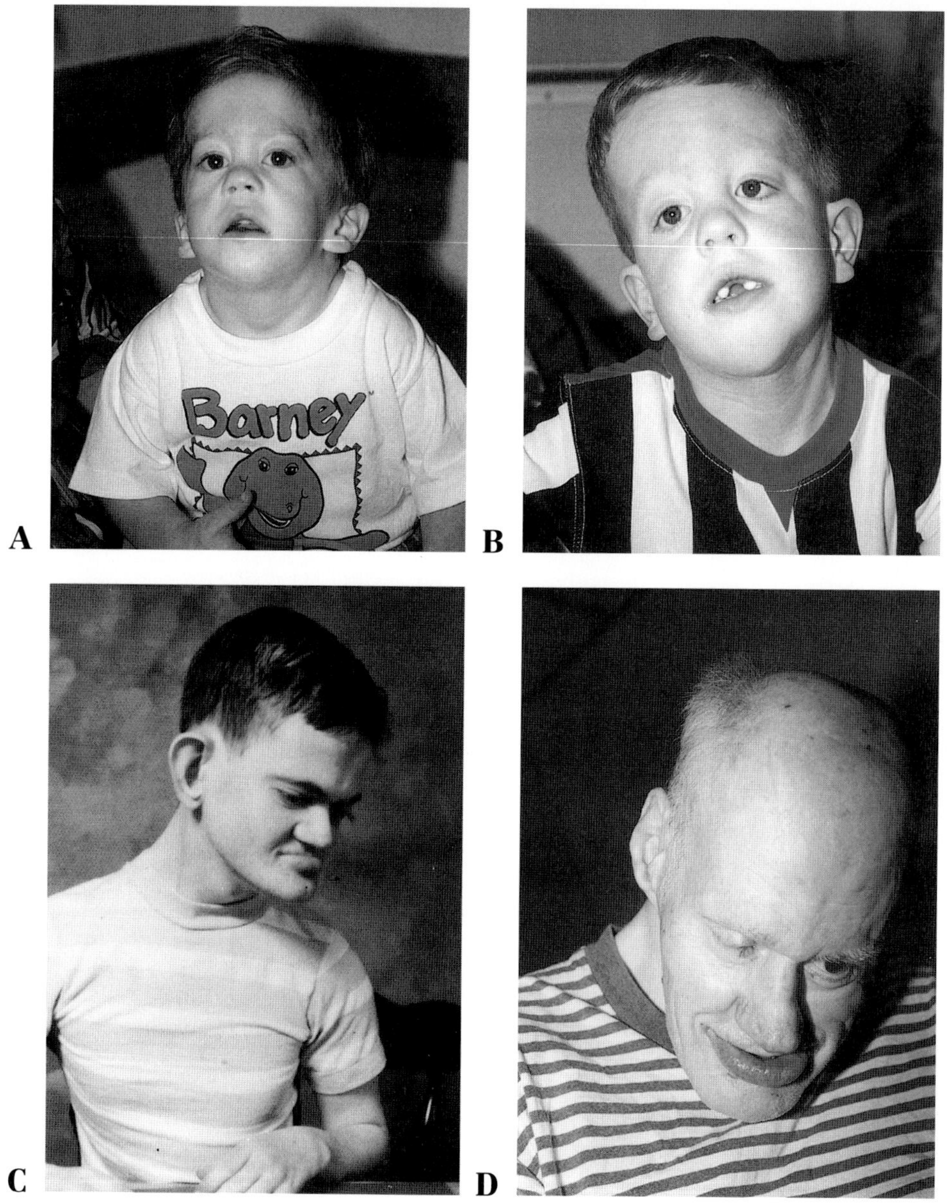

Armfield Syndrome. Brothers at age 4 years (A) and 8 years (B) showing macrocephaly, ptosis, hypertelorism, downslanting palpebral fissures, and upfolded earlobes; uncles age 25 years (C) and 62 years (D) showing tall forehead, cupped ears, depressed midface, short philtrum, and patulous lower lip.

GROWTH AND DEVELOPMENT. Short stature with onset prenatally.
COGNITIVE FEATURES. Severe impairment with IQs 20–50.
NEUROLOGICAL FINDINGS. Seizures, with onset in infancy or early childhood, are a consistent sign.
HETEROZYGOTE EXPRESSION. None.

IMAGING. Hydrocephaly was documented in two males, one of whom also had a cystic fourth ventricle.

LABORATORY. Low somatomedin C was found in two patients.

COMMENT. Xq28 is the most densely mapped region of the human genome. Fourteen XLMR syndromes, exhibiting a broad spectrum of clinical phenotypes, have been mapped there, as have FRAXE mental retardation and six families with non-syndromic XLMR. Cleft palate and adult-onset glaucoma or cataracts serve to distinguish Armfield syndrome from the others.

REFERENCE

Armfield K, Schwartz CE, Lubs HA, et al.: An XLMR syndrome with short stature, small hands and feet, seizures, cleft palate, and glaucoma is linked to Xq28. Am J Med Genet, in press, 1999.

Differential Matrix

Syndrome	Ocular Abnormality	Facial Clefting	Seizures	Comments
Armfield	+	+	+	Short stature, cataracts or glaucoma, dental anomalies, small hands and feet, hydrocephaly, joint stiffness
Oral-facial-digital I	0	+	+	Sparse scalp hair, dystopia canthorum, flat midface, hypoplastic alae nasi, lingual hamartomas, syndactyly, clinodactyly, structural brain anomalies, polycystic kidneys
Pallister W	0	+	+	Short stature, prominent forehead, wide nasal tip, incomplete cleft lip/palate, spasticity, contractures
Cerebrooculogenital	+	0	+	Short stature, microcephaly, hydrocephaly, agenesis of corpus callosum, microphthalmia, ptosis, hypospadias, cryptorchidism, clubfoot, spasticity
Incontinentia pigmenti	+	0	+	Cutaneous vesicles, verrucous lesions, irregular hyperpigmentation, microcephaly, oligodontia, abnormally-shaped teeth, spasticity
Lowe	+	0	+	Short stature, cataracts, hypotonia, aminoaciduria, progressive renal disease
Wittwer	+	0	+	Growth deficiency, microcephaly, microphthalmia, hearing loss, vision loss, hypertelorism, genitourinary anomalies, hypotonia

ARTS SYNDROME

(Lethal XLMR–Ataxia–Deafness, MIM 301835)

DEFINITION. XLMR with impaired growth, paucity of muscles, and progressive neurological deterioration with ataxia, deafness, vision loss, seizures, and areflexia. The gene is located between markers DXS1231 (Xq21.33) and DXS1001 (Xq24), lod score 6.97.

SOMATIC FEATURES. No craniofacial features have been described. Neuromuscular findings predominate. There is a generalized paucity of muscles. From birth, males are hypotonic, weak, and areflexic. Motor development appears to worsen following respiratory infection in early childhood. In particular, truncal and limb ataxia develop and progressively worsen. Hearing appears severely impaired, in some cases from birth. None developed speech. Vision may be normal initially, but, if so, it deteriorates with pallor of the discs and nystagmus within the first few years. Seizures, tonic-clonic or complex types, further complicate the childhood course.

NEUROLOGICAL FINDINGS. A relentless neuromuscular deterioration leads to death in early childhood (newborn–5 years). Neurological findings appear to accentuate following childhood infection. Generalized muscle underdevelopment is reflected in hypotonia and weakness. Reflexes are absent. Truncal and limb ataxia are present from infancy. Deafness, loss of vision, and seizures are further manifestations of the deterioration.

A

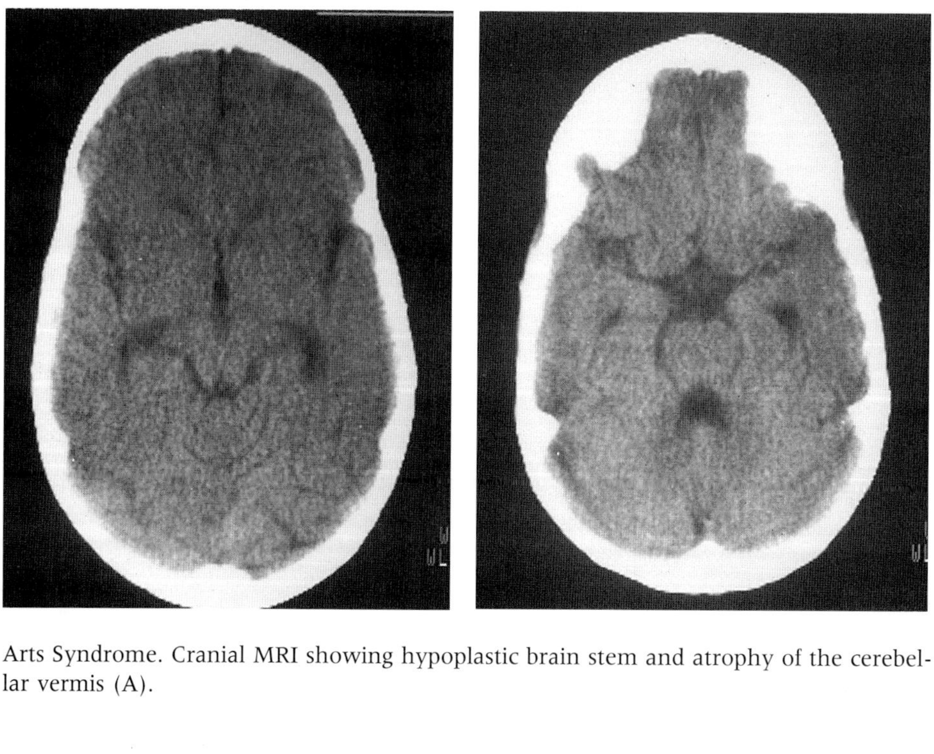

Arts Syndrome. Cranial MRI showing hypoplastic brain stem and atrophy of the cerebellar vermis (A).

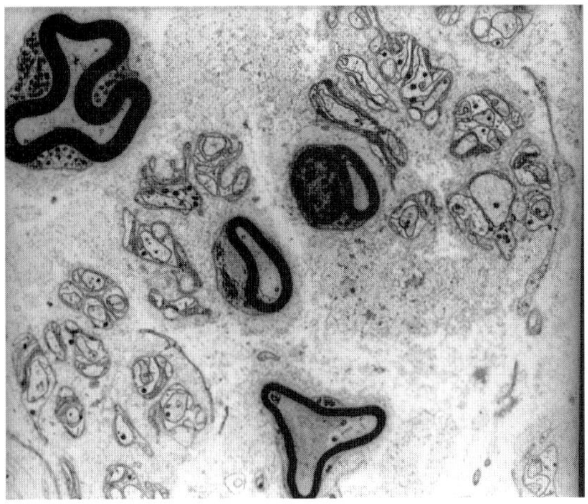

B

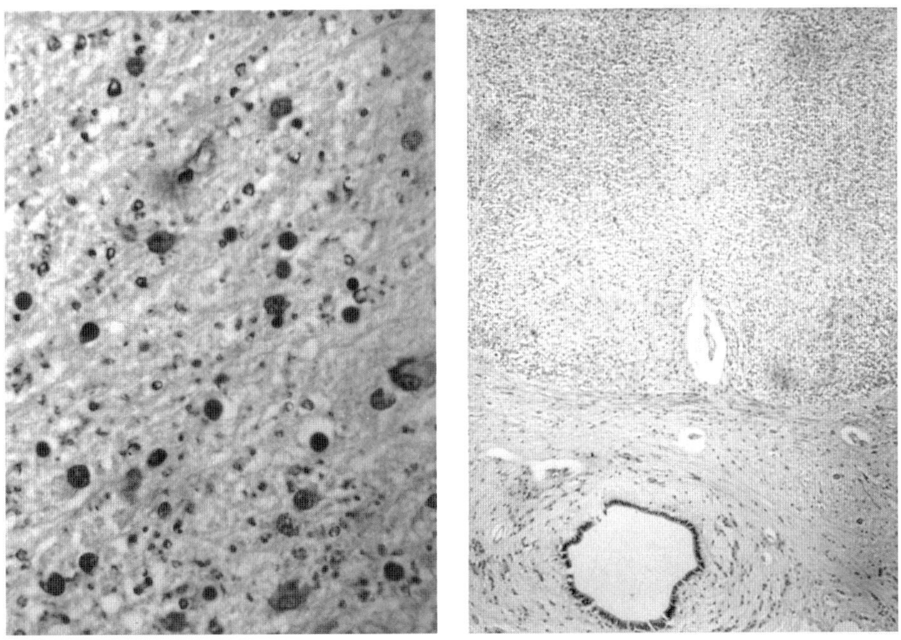

C

Arts Syndrome. (continued) Electron microscopy of sural nerve showing reduced number of myelinated fibers and evidence of remyelinization (B); sections of spinal cord with absence of myelinated fibers in the posterior column but presence of myelinated fibers in the anterior cortical spinal tract (C). Courtesy of Dr. Willem Arts, Sophia Children's Hospital, Rotterdam, The Netherlands.

HETEROZYGOTE EXPRESSION. Carrier females frequently have perceptive hearing impairment in early adulthood. One obligate carrier had clubfoot, ataxia, hypotonia, hyperreflexia, and Babinski signs. Two other possible carriers had similar findings.

NEUROPATHOLOGY. Diffuse slowing or seizure discharges were present on EEG. The EMG and muscle histology show signs of denervation (usually with grouping of type 1 fibers). Visual stimulation showed increased transmission latency in one case and absence of occipital response in another. On postmortem examination of one case, the brain stem, cerebrum, and cerebellum were normal. The dorsal columns and dorsal nerve roots lacked axonal myelination, a finding similar to that seen in Friedreich ataxia.

LABORATORY. A wide range of studies were normal, including renal function, thyroid hormones, serum and cerebrospinal fluid pyruvate and lactate, carnitine, very long chain fatty acids, phytanic acid, cranial MRI, and lysosomal enzymes. Serum immunoglobulins were normal but with low-normal IgA. No mutation has been found in DDP (dystonia deafness peptide).

COMMENT. Childhood lethality may serve as a measure of the overall severity of the biological insult resulting from mutation of X-linked genes. Lethality in the XLMR syndromes appears more commonly associated with impaired nervous system function than with specific malformations or malfunction of essential organs such as the heart or kidneys. XLMR syndromes with severely impaired nervous system function and childhood lethality include Arts, Bertini, Gustavson, Holmes-Gang, hydrocephaly–cerebellar agenesis, hereditary bullous dystrophy, Paine, VACTERL-hydrocephalus, XLMR-ataxia-deafness-dementia, and X-linked lissencephaly. Childhood lethality may also be associated with metabolic insults (e.g., ornithine transcarbamylase deficiency, pyruvate dehydrogenase deficiency, adrenoleukodystrophy).

REFERENCES

Arts WFM, Loonen MCB, Sengers RCA, et al.: X-linked ataxia, weakness, deafness, and loss of vision in early childhood with a fatal course. Ann Neurol 33:535, 1993.

Kremer H, Hamel BCJ, van den Helm B, et al.: Localization of the gene (or genes) for a syndrome with X-linked mental retardation, ataxia, weakness, hearing impairment, loss of vision and a fatal course in early childhood. Hum Genet 98:513, 1996.

Differential Matrix

Syndrome	Ataxia	Hearing Loss	Vision Loss	Comments
Arts	+	+	+	Growth deficiency, paucity of muscles, hypotonia, areflexia, seizures, childhood death
Mohr-Tranebjaerg (Jensen)	+	+	+	Neurologic deterioration with childhood onset, dystonia, spasticity
X-linked ataxia-deafness-dementia	+	+	+	Optic atrophy, spastic paraplegia, hypotonia, seizures, childhood death
Gustavson	0	+	+	Microcephaly, short stature, optic atrophy with blindness, large ears, joint contractures, rockerbottom feet, brain undergrowth, hydrocephaly, cerebellar hypoplasia, spasticity, seizures
Norrie	0	+	+	Ocular dysplasia and degeneration, adult-onset hearing loss
Paine	0	+	+	Microcephaly, short stature, optic atrophy, spasticity, seizures
Proud	0	+	+	Spasticity, seizures, short stature, microcephaly, agenesis of corpus callosum, cryptorchidism, inguinal hernias
Schimke	0	+	+	Microcephaly, sunken eyes, downslanting palpebral fissures, narrow nose, spacing of teeth, cupped ears, hypotonia, abducens palsy, spasticity, choreoathetosis, contractures
Wittwer	0	+	+	Growth deficiency, microcephaly, microphthalmia, hypertelorism, genitourinary anomalies, hypotonia, seizures
Bertini	+	0	+	Macular degeneration, hypotonia, seizures, childhood death, hypoplasia of cerebellar vermis and corpus callosum, developmental delays and regression, postnatal growth impairment
Goldblatt spastic paraplegia	+	0	+	Optic atrophy, exotropia, nystagmus, spastic paraplegia, dysarthria, muscle hypoplasia, contractures
X-linked optic atrophy	+	0	+	Optic atrophy, tremors, areflexia, emotional lability

ATKIN-FLAITZ SYNDROME

(Atkin Syndrome)

DEFINITION: XLMR with short stature, macrocephaly, coarse facial features, broad short hands with tapered fingers, macroorchidism, and seizures. The gene has not been mapped.

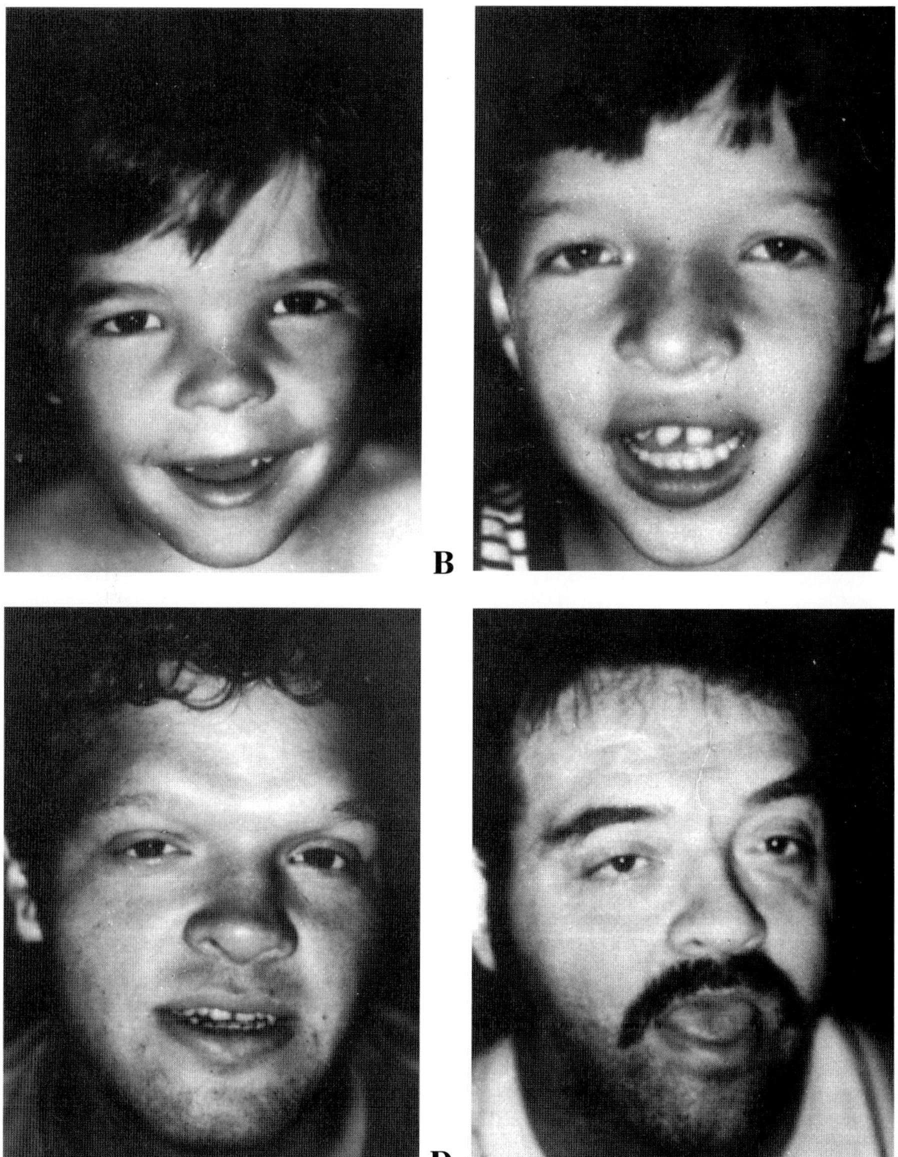

A B C D

Atkin-Flaitz Syndrome. Coarse facial features with macrocephaly, hypertelorism, broad nasal tip, and prominent lips in affected males at ages 6, 8, 21, and 39 years (A, B, C, D).

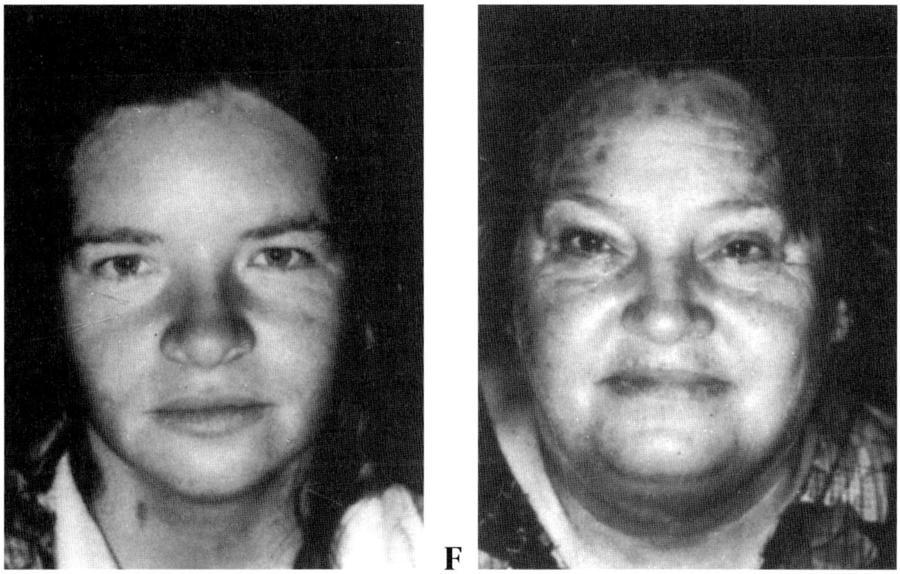

E F

Atkin-Flaitz Syndrome. (continued) And in carrier females at ages 28 and 53 years (E, F). Courtesy of the *American Journal of Medical Genetics,* Copyright © 1985, Alan R. Liss, Inc.

Somatic Features. Macrocephaly, large forehead, prominent supraorbital ridges, hypertelorism, broad nasal tip with anteverted nostrils, and thick lower lip give the distinctive facial appearance. Large ears, downslanted palpebral fissures, and micrognathia may also be present. Intraoral findings include an upper midline diastema, small upper lateral incisors, palatal torus or prominent raphe, and prominent median furrow of the tongue. The former two findings as well as macrocephaly and micrognathia may represent familial characteristics within the first reported family. Other than short stature, short hands, and a tendency to postpubertal obesity, there are no musculoskeletal findings. The hands, although short and broad with tapered fingers, do not have the doughy consistency found in the Coffin-Lowry syndrome. The testes are large, a finding noted also in nonaffected male relatives. Seizures occur in a minority.

Cognitive Features. Mental retardation of moderate degree is usual.

Neurological Findings. Seizures occur in a minority. Although facial structures suggest muscular hypotonia, it has not been described.

Heterozygote Expression. Carrier females are less severely affected, having mild cognitive impairment, large forehead with prominent supraorbital ridges, hypertelorism, broad nasal tip, and thick lower lip. They are short and tend to be obese.

Comment. Although the facial coarseness suggests the Coffin-Lowry syndrome, the presence of macrocephaly and macroorchidism and the absence of soft doughy hands and skeletal abnormalities should provide easy distinction. Clark and Baraitser have described a mother and two sons with similar features except that they lacked hypertelorism and short stature.

REFERENCES

Atkin JF, Flaitz K, Patil S, et al.: A new X-linked mental retardation syndrome. Am J Med Genet 21:697, 1985.

Clark RD, Baraitser M: Letter to the editor: a new X-linked mental retardation syndrome. Am J Med Genet 26:13, 1987.

Baraitser M, Reardon W, Vijeratnam S: Nonspecific X-linked mental retardation with macrocephaly and obesity. Am J Med Genet 57:380, 1995.

Differential Matrix

Syndrome	Short Stature	Coarse Facial Features	Obesity	Comments
Atkin-Flaitz	+	+	+	Macrocephaly, hypertelorism, downslanting palpebral fissures, broad nasal tip, thick lower lip, brachydactyly, seizures
Börjeson-Forssman-Lehmann	+	+	+	Hypotonia, hypogonadism, microcephaly, large ears, gynecomastia, narrow sloped shoulders, visual impairment, tapered digits
Coffin-Lowry	+	+	0	Microcephaly, hypertelorism, anteverted nares, tented upper lip, prominent lips and large mouth, large ears, soft hands with tapered digits, pectus carinatum, hypotonia
Mucopolysaccharidosis II	+	+	0	Macrocephaly, hepatosplenomegaly, hernias, joint stiffness, thick skin, hirsutism, behavioral disturbance
Clark-Baraitser	0	+	+	Macrocephaly, large stature, dental abnormalities, broad nasal tip, thick lower lip, macroorchidism

Bergia Cardiomyopathy

(X-Linked Familial Lethal Cardiomyopathy)

Definition. XLMR with myopia, slowly progressive scapuloperoneal muscular dystrophy and hypertrophic cardiomyopathy. The gene has not been mapped.

Somatic Features. Major malformations or distinctive craniofacial characteristics do not occur. There is a slowly progressive muscular dystrophy with predominant humeroperoneal weakness. The clinical course is dominated by the cardiomyopathy, manifested by subendocardial and patchy subepicardial fibrosis, vacuolization, and fatty deposition in myocytes, which leads to limited exercise tolerance, syncope, heart failure, arrhythmias, and death by early adult life. Marked myopia may be a feature.

Growth and Development. Childhood growth proceeds normally. Muscle hypertrophy does not occur; rather, muscles show progressive wasting. Early childhood developmental milestones may be achieved at the usual times.

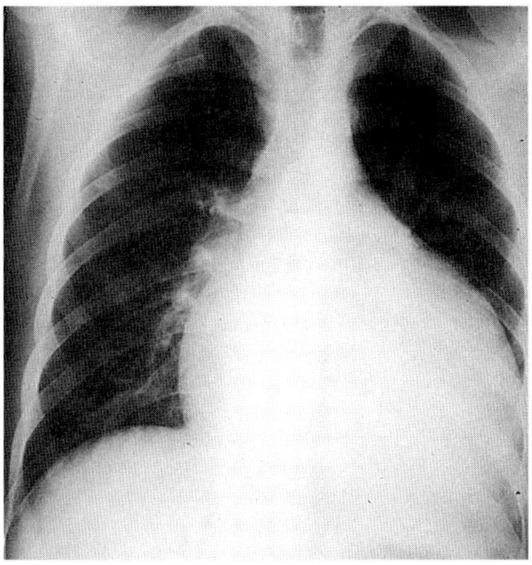

A

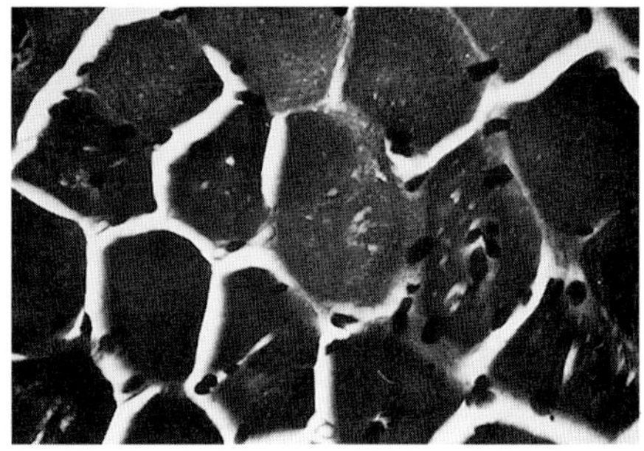

B

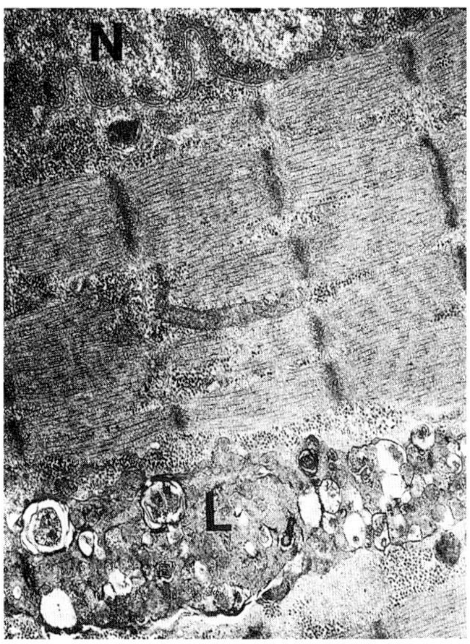

C

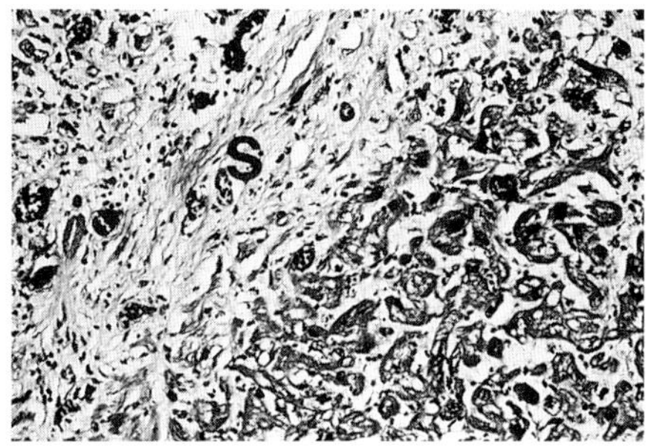

D

Bergia Cardiomyopathy. Chest radiograph of 17-year-old male showing cardiomegaly (A). Light microscopy of quadriceps biopsy revealing variable fiber size and shape and internalization of nuclei (B); electron microscopy of quadriceps showing increased lysosomes[L] containing necrotic fibers (C); light microscopy of left ventricle with increased interstitial connective tissue and fibrosis[s] (D). Courtesy of Dr. Ian Butler, University of Texas Health Science Center, Houston.

COGNITIVE FEATURES. Impairment of cognitive function is first noted at 5–6 years of age and may be progressive.

NEUROLOGICAL FINDINGS. Incoordination becomes notable as ambulation is acquired. Deep tendon reflexes are normal. Weakness is best demonstrated in humeral and peroneal muscles. Incoordination may be secondary to the weakness. Distal muscle wasting and winging of the scapulae may be present. Nerve conduction appears normal. Electromyography is consistent with a myopathy. Electroencephalography, brain stem auditory evoked responses, and visual evoked responses may be abnormal.

HETEROZYGOTE EXPRESSION. Dilation and poor function of the left ventricle has been described in one carrier female. There was no evidence for dystrophy of skeletal muscles or impairment of cognitive function.

LABORATORY. Muscle biopsy shows a dystrophic process with variation in fiber size, internalization of nuclei, and slight increase in fibrosis and fatty infiltration.

Although increased glycogen may be present in muscle cells, enzymes involved in glycogen metabolism have been normal. Creatine kinase and other muscle enzymes are elevated.

COMMENT. Cardiac disease occurs uncommonly among the XLMR syndromes and even more rarely is responsible for childhood demise. Structural heart defects have been described in cerebrofaciogenital, hereditary bullous dystrophy, Opitz FG, telecanthus-hypospadias, Golabi-Ito-Hall, Lenz, MIDAS, and Simpson-Golabi-Behmel syndromes.

REFERENCES

Bergia B, Sybers HD, Butler IJ: Familial lethal cardiomyopathy with mental retardation and scapuloperoneal muscular dystrophy. J Neurol Neurosurg Psychiatry 49:1423, 1986.

Differential Matrix

Syndrome	Cardio-myopathy	Muscular Wasting	Childhood Death	Comments
Bergia cardiomyopathy	+	+	+	Scapuloperoneal muscle atrophy, limited exercise tolerance, arrhythmias
Duchenne muscular dystrophy	+	+	+	Hypertrophy of calf muscles, elevated muscle enzymes, progressive weakness, loss of reflexes, contractures
Myotubular myopathy	+	+	+	Hypotonic facies, open mouth, tented upper lip, hydrocephaly, long digits, cryptorchidism, hypotonia, weakness, areflexia

BERTINI SYNDROME

(Bertini-des Portes Syndrome, XLMR–Myoclonus–Macular Degeneration)

DEFINITION. XLMR with hypotonia, ataxia, myoclonus, macular degeneration. The gene maps to markers distal to DXS1060 (Xp22.33) near or in the pseudoautosomal region.

SOMATIC FEATURES. Facial or musculoskeletal features are not described; imaging studies document hypoplasia of the cerebellar vermis and of the corpus callosum.

GROWTH AND DEVELOPMENT. Intrauterine growth is normal or nearly so but slow statural and cephalic growth becomes obvious postnatally. Development skills are acquired slowly and are lost during late childhood.

COGNITIVE FEATURES. Development is globally delayed and cognitive function markedly impaired.

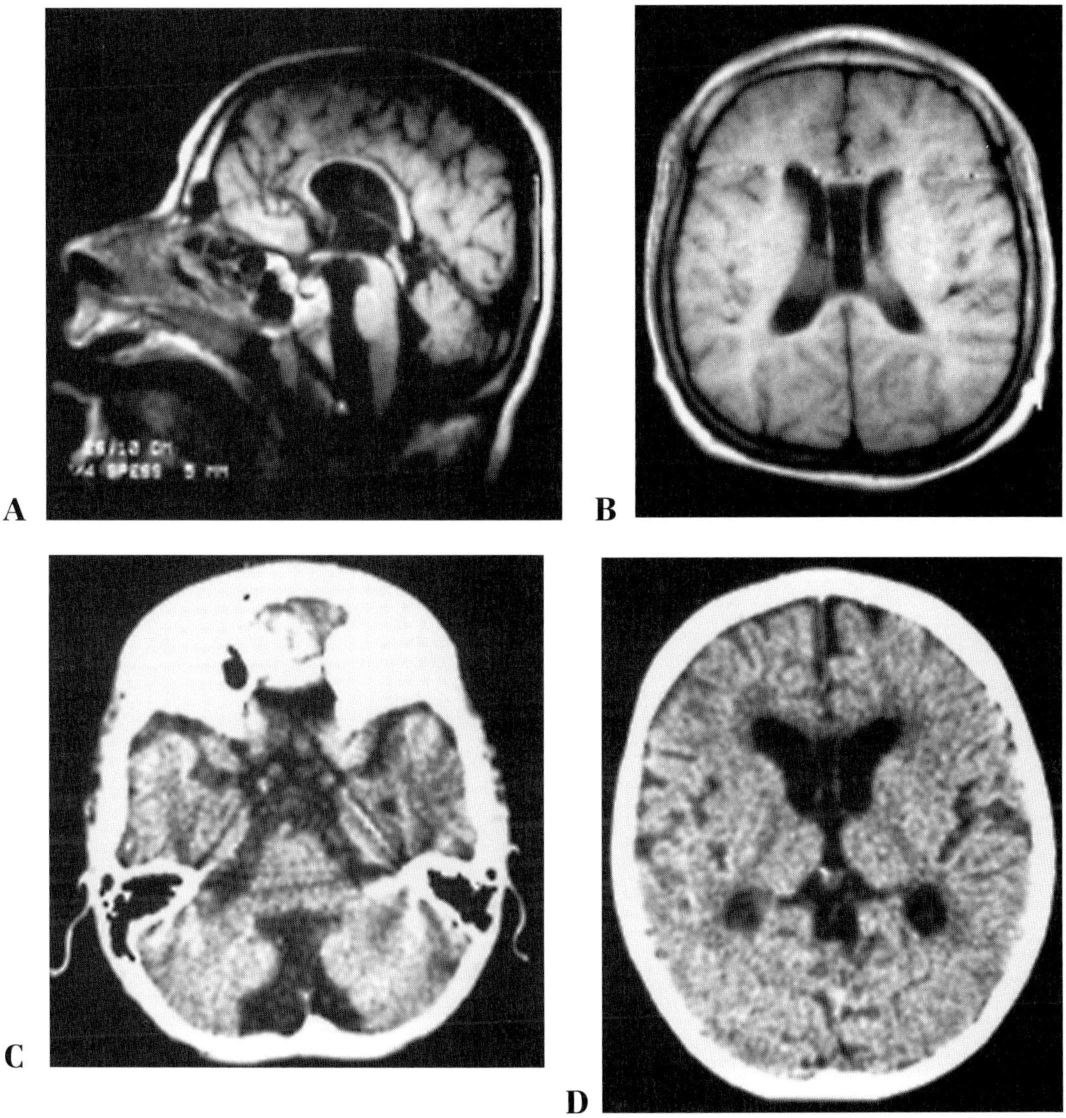

Bertini Syndrome. MRI of 10-year-old male showing hypoplasia of cerebellar vermis, hypoplasia of corpus callosum, and septum pellucidum cyst (A, B); cranial tomography of 10-year-old cousin showing hypoplasia of cerebellar vermis, cyst of the septum pellucidum, and persistent cavum vergae (C, D). Courtesy of the *American Journal of Medical Genetics*, Copyright © 1992, Wiley-Liss, Inc.

NEUROLOGICAL FINDINGS. Males appear severely affected from birth with hypotonia and ataxia. They suck poorly and development progresses slowly. Death often occurs from infections in infancy and survivors follow a relentless course of deterioration with seizures, macular degeneration, and death by late childhood.

NEUROPATHOLOGY. Partial brain examination in one case showed no neuronal loss or storage products.

COMMENT. Although the course mimics storage disease, extensive search has not identified such an underlying disorder. Several other XLMR syndromes with hypoplasia of the cerebellum and agenesis of the corpus callosum have been recognized but none map to the same region of Xp.

REFERENCES

Bertini E, Cusmai R, de Saint Basile G, et al.: Congenital X-linked ataxia, progressive myoclonic encephalopathy, macular degeneration and recurrent infections. Am J Med Genet 43:443, 1992.

des Portes V, Bachner L, Brüls T, et al.: X-linked neurodegenerative syndrome with congenital ataxia, late-onset progressive myoclonic encephalopathy and selective macular degeneration, linked to Xp22.33-pter. Am J Med Genet 64:69, 1996.

Differential Matrix

Syndrome	Ataxia	Cerebellar Hypoplasia	Hypotonia	Comments
Bertini	+	+	+	Developmental delays and regression, postnatal growth impairment, macular degeneration, seizures
Pettigrew	+	+	+	Dandy-Walker malformation, spasticity, seizures, microcephaly or hydrocephaly, long face with macrostomia and prognathism, small testes, contractures, choreoathetosis, iron deposits in basal ganglia
Christianson	+	+	0	Short stature, microcephaly, general asthenia, contractures, seizures, ophthalmoplegia
Arena	+	+	0	Muscle hypoplasia, clubfoot, iron deposits in basal ganglia, spastic paraplegia, rigidity, dystonia
Schimke	0	+	+	Microcephaly, sunken eyes, downslanting palpebral fissures, narrow nose, spacing of teeth, cupped ears, abducens palsy, hearing loss, vision loss, spasticity, choreoathetosis, contractures

BÖRJESON-FORSSMAN-LEHMANN SYNDROME

(BFL Syndrome, MIM 301900)

DEFINITION. XLMR with short stature, microcephaly, angular face with prominent cheekbones, deep-set eyes, large and thick ears, gynecomastia, small testes, obesity, and hypotonia. The gene is localized between DXS10 (Xp26) and DXS105 (Xq27), lod score 4.1.

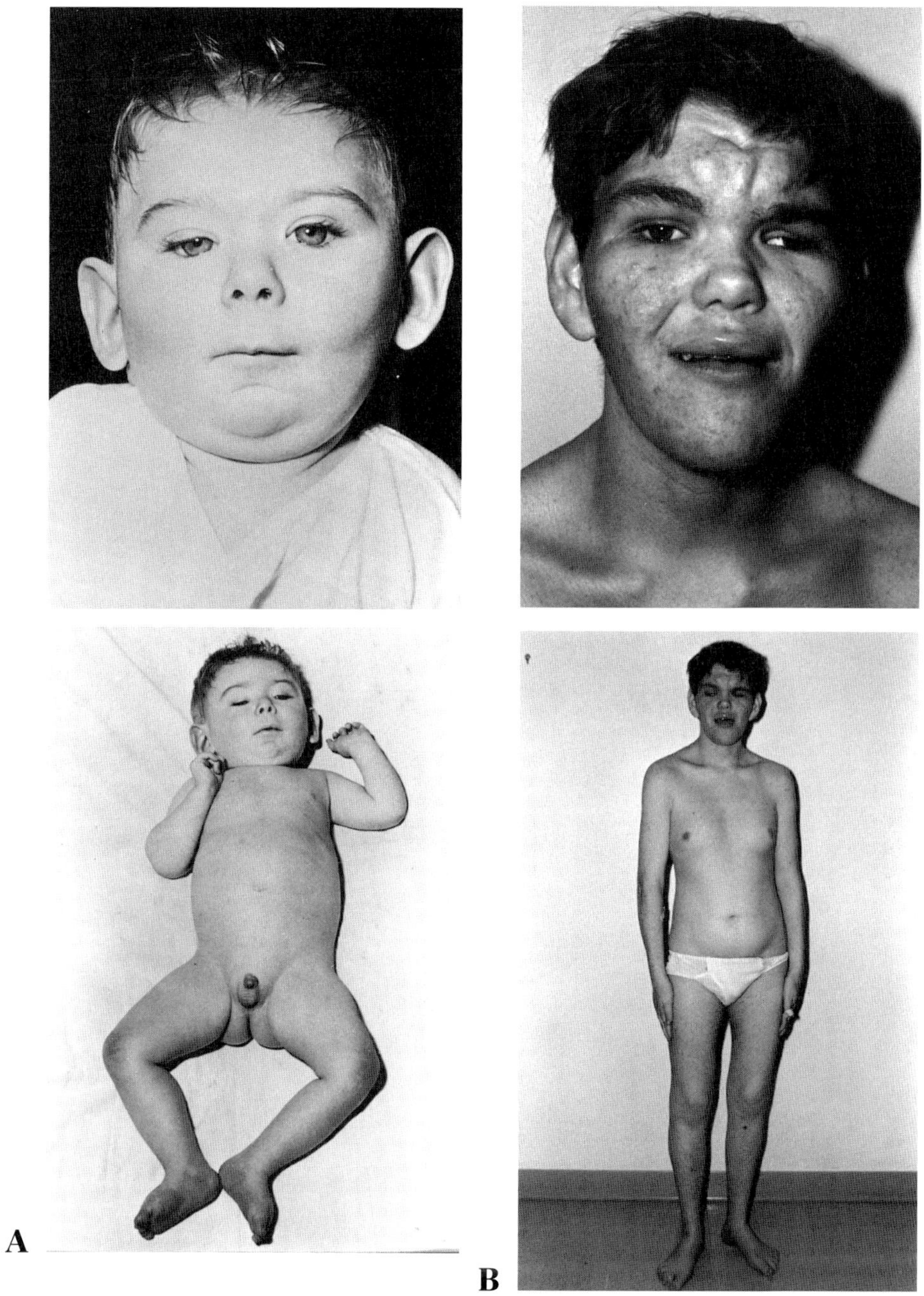

Börjeson-Forssman-Lehmann Syndrome. Ten-month-old male with microcephaly, large ears, depressed nasal bridge, ptosis, and hypotonia (A); 24-year-old male with coarse facies and short stature (B).

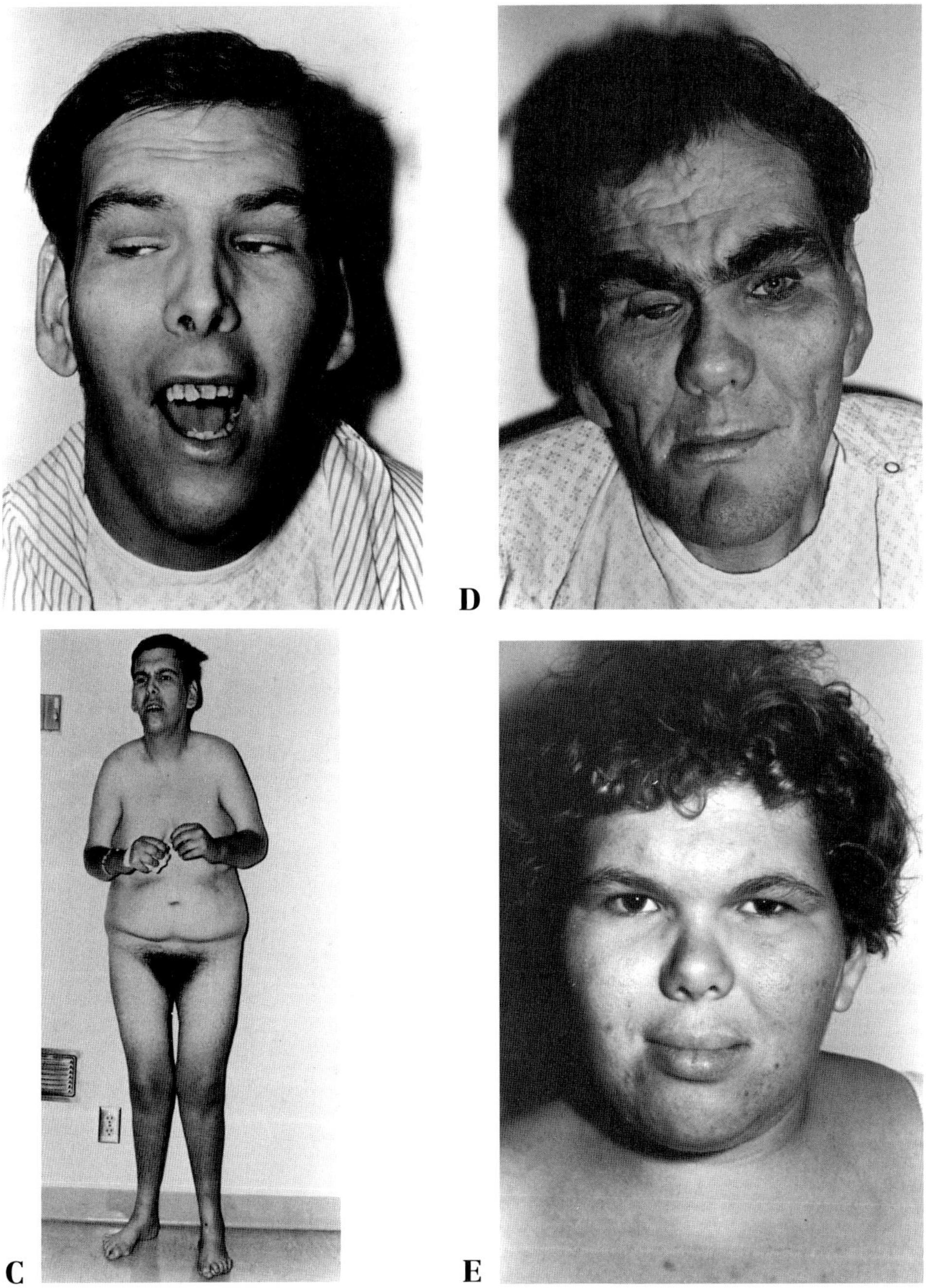

Börjeson-Forssman-Lehmann Syndrome, (continued) 27-year-old male with ptosis, large ears, short stature, obesity, and hypogenitalism (C); 40-year-old male with heavy cheekbones and sculpted facies (D); 23-year-old female carrier with coarse facies, prominent supraorbital ridges, and large ears (E). Courtesy of Dr. Holly Hutchison Ardinger, University of Iowa Hospitals and Clinics, Iowa City.

SOMATIC FEATURES. The midface is most characteristic, the face appearing heavy and angular with prominent supraorbital ridges and cheekbones, dense eyebrows, deeply set eyes, ptosis, epicanthus, and large fleshy ears. There is a tendency to visual impairment with pale optic discs, hyperopia, nystagmus, and cataract formation. The nose is small and triangular with anteverted nares. The mouth may have a tented upper lip. The angular nature of the face may be softened to a variable degree by fat deposition and hypotonia. Shoulders are narrow and may be excessively sloped. The fingers taper and have hyperextensible joints. There is shortness and spading of the toes, some of which may be flexed. Otherwise, patients have short stature, microcephaly, generalized obesity with notable fat deposition in the breasts, hypotonia, small genitalia with hypogonadism, and seizures. The skin feels soft and doughy and acne is common. A milder phenotype with normal head circumference, normal stature, and mild to moderate mental retardation which links to the same region may represent allelic heterogeneity.

GROWTH AND DEVELOPMENT. Birth weight is normal, but generalized obesity appears early in childhood. Other growth parameters show considerable variability, but microcephaly and short stature are typical. All developmental milestones lag.

COGNITIVE FEATURES. Cognitive function parallels the somatic phenotype with those having the most pronounced somatic manifestations having the most severe cognitive impairment.

NEUROLOGICAL FINDINGS. Hypotonia is notable and evidenced during pregnancy by poor fetal movement. Some cases have vision loss with nystagmus and pale optic discs. Hyperreflexia occurs in many cases.

HETEROZYGOTE EXPRESSION. Carrier females tend to be short and heavy with broad midface, large ears, and mild cognitive impairment. Some have impaired vision, hypotonia and soft skin, tapered digits, and short, flexed, and widely spaced toes.

IMAGING. Mild ventricular dilation.

LABORATORY. Both hypogonadotropic and hypergonadotropic hypogonadism have been documented. The EEG shows generalized low voltage with diminished α activity. Ardinger et al. have stressed radiographic features, thick calvarium, narrow cervical spinal cord, Scheuermann-like vertebral changes, and epiphyseal dysplasia with delayed bone maturation, short distal phalanges, and small proximal heads of the femora and humeri.

COMMENT. Börjeson-Forssman-Lehmann is the prototypic XLMR syndrome with hypotonia, hypogonadism, and obesity. The considerable interfamilial variability, particularly in regard to growth and cognitive function, has not been explained.

REFERENCES

Ardinger HH, Hanson JW, Zellweger HU: Börjeson-Forssman-Lehmann syndrome. Am J Med Genet 19:653, 1984.

Börjeson M, Forssman H, Lehmann O: An X-linked recessively inherited syndrome characterized by grave mental deficiency, epilepsy and endocrine disorder. Acta Med Scand 171:13, 1962.

Dereymaeker AM, Fryns JP, Hoefnagels M, et al.: The Börjeson-Forssman-Lehmann syndrome. Clin Genet 29:317, 1986.

Gedeon AK, Kozman HM, Robinson H, et al.: Refinement of the background genetic map of Xq26-q27 and gene localisation for Börjeson-Forssman-Lehmann syndrome. Am J Med Genet 64:63, 1996.

Mathews KD, Ardinger HH, Nishimura DY, et al.: Linkage localization of Börjeson-Forssman-Lehmann syndrome. Am J Med Genet 34:470, 1989.

Robinson LK, Jones KL, Culler F, et al.: The Börjeson-Forssman-Lehmann syndrome. Am J Med Genet 15:457, 1983.

Turner G, Gedeon A, Mulley J, et al.: Börjeson-Forssman-Lehmann syndrome: clinical manifestations and gene localization to Xq26-27. Am J Med Genet 34:463, 1989.

Weber FT, Frias JL, Julius RL, et al.: Primary hypogonadism in the Börjeson-Forssman-Lehmann syndrome. J Med Genet 15:63, 1978.

Differential Matrix

Syndrome	Obesity	Hypotonia	Hypo-gonadism	Comments
Börjeson-Forssman-Lehmann	+	+	+	Short stature, microcephaly, coarse face, large ears, gynecomastia, narrow sloped shoulders, visual impairment, tapered digits
Chudley-Lowry	+	+	+	Short stature, bitemporal narrowing, almond-shaped eyes, depressed nasal bridge, tented upper lip, open mouth
Vasquez	+	+	+	Short stature, microcephaly, gynecomastia
Wilson-Turner	+	+	+	Normal growth, small hands and feet, tapered digits, gynecomastia, emotional lability
XLMR-hypotonic facies (Carpenter-Waziri) (Holmes-Gang) (Juberg-Marsidi)	0	+	+	Short stature, microcephaly, telecanthus, small triangular nose, tented upper lip, open mouth, spacing of teeth, genital anomalies, musculoskeletal anomalies, hemoglobin H inclusions in erythrocytes
Urban	+	0	+	Short stature, small hands and feet, digital contractures, osteoporosis
Young-Hughes	+	0	+	Short stature, small palpebral fissures, cupped ears, ichthyosiform scaling

BROOKS SYNDROME

(Sklower-Brooks Syndrome, Brooks-Wisniewski-Brown Syndrome)

DEFINITION. XLMR with short stature, microcephaly, blepharophimosis, cupped ears, bulbous nose, small mouth, flexion contractures, hydrocephaly, seizures, and spasticity. The gene has not been localized.

Somatic Features. Abnormalities in all regions of the face contribute to the distinctive appearance. Bifrontal narrowing, deeply set eyes, blepharophimosis, epicanthus inversus, and, in some cases, hypotelorism characterize the upper face. A full or bulbous nose and low-set, retroverted, and cupped ears punctuate a flattened midface. An overall triangular lower face is further distinguished by a small mouth and mandible and a thin, tented upper lip. The neck appears short and the posterior hairline low. Although microcephalic, the cerebral ventricles are enlarged and dysgenesis of the corpus callosum may be present. Undergrowth and decreased muscle bulk give the appearance of generalized frailness. Pectus excavatum, contractures at the elbows and knees, and finger 5 clinodactyly also occur.

Growth and Development. Intrauterine growth is retarded, some infants weighing less than 2000 g at birth. All parameters of postnatal growth are markedly slow. Development lags far behind. Speech is limited, if present at all. Some cases never achieve independent ambulation or continence.

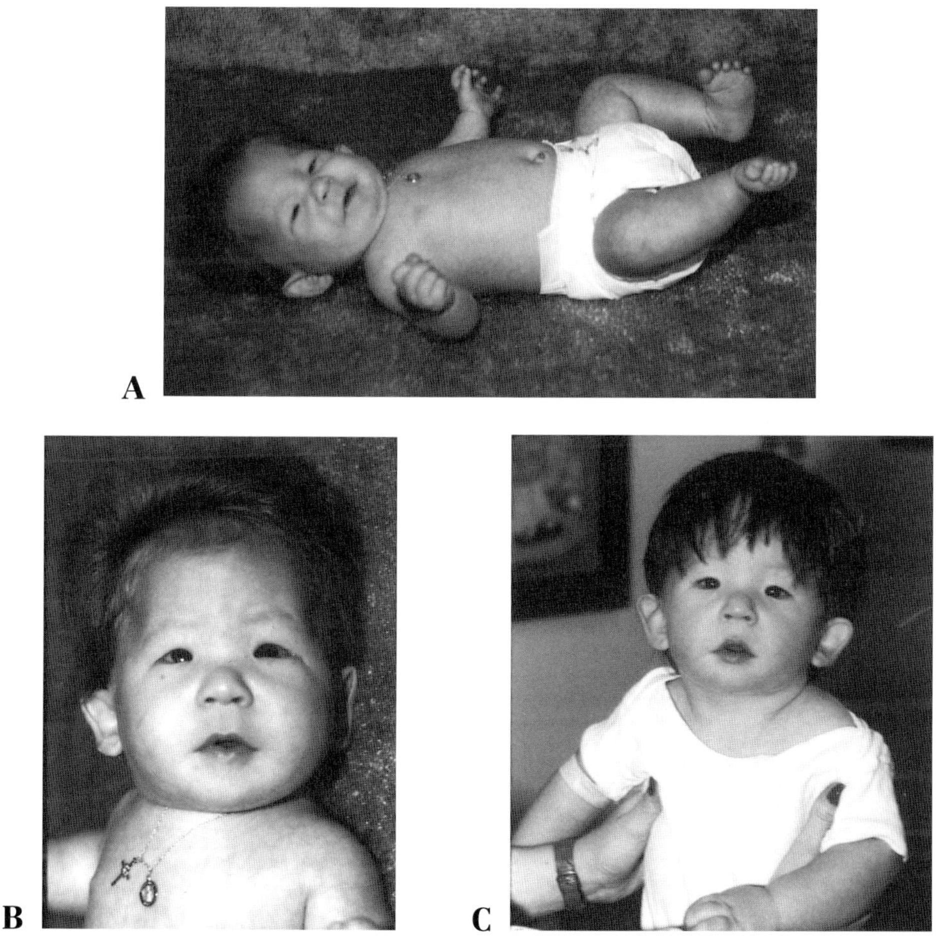

Brooks Syndrome. Microcephaly, blepharophimosis, depressed nasal bridge, simple cupped ears, bulbous nose, and deep-set eyes in an affected male at 4 months (A, B), 2 years (C).

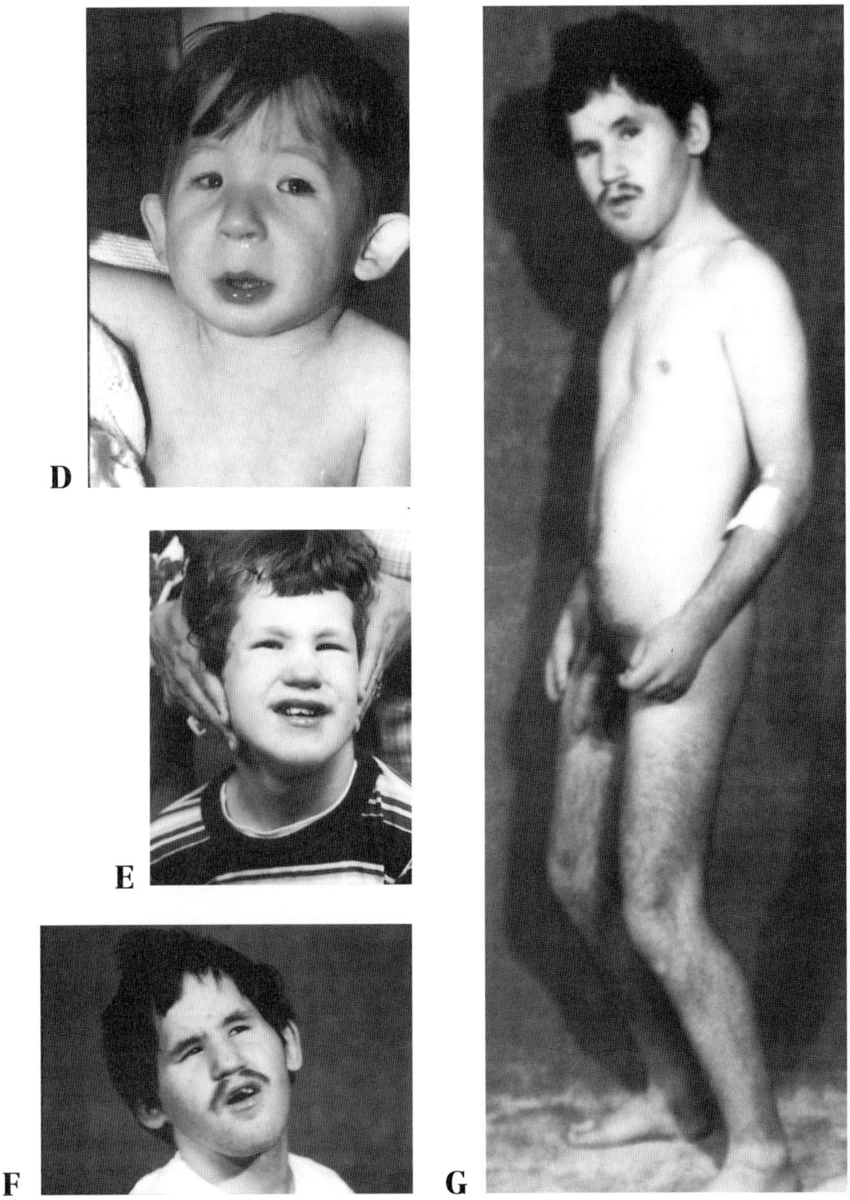

Brooks Syndrome. (continued) And 4 years (D); affected uncle at age 14 years (E) and 22 years (F, G). (C) Courtesy of Dr. Susan Sklower Brooks, New York State Institute for Basic Research in Developmental Disabilities, Staten Island.

COGNITIVE FEATURES. Severe impairment.
NEUROLOGICAL FINDINGS. Hypotonia is notable from infancy. Hyperreflexia and spasticity, especially of the lower limbs, become evident in infancy as well. Poor vision is associated with strabismus, nystagmus, myopia, and optic atrophy. Hearing loss occurs in some cases. Generalized seizures occasionally begin in infancy.
HETEROZYGOTE EXPRESSION. None.

IMAGING. Cranial CT and MRI show enlarged ventricles and dysgenesis of the corpus callosum.

COMMENT. Microcephaly in the presence of hydrocephaly attests to the marked underdevelopment of the brain. This is reflected in the general frailness, slow growth, and profound developmental failure in this syndrome. In these aspects and others, Brooks syndrome is similar to Gustavson, Pettigrew, and Schimke syndromes.

REFERENCES

Brooks SS, Wisniewski K, Brown WT: New X-linked mental retardation (XLMR) syndrome with distinct facial appearance and growth retardation. Am J Med Genet 51:586, 1994.

Morava E, Storcz J, Kosztolányi G: X-linked mental retardation syndrome: three brothers with the Brooks-Wisniewski-Brown syndrome. Am J Med Genet 64:59, 1996.

Differential Matrix

Syndrome	Microcephaly and Hydrocephaly	Spasticity	Seizures	Comments
Brooks	+	+	+	Short stature, deep-set eyes, blepharophimosis, cupped ears, bulbous nose, small mouth, thin upper lip, pectus excavatum, flexion contractures, dysgenesis of corpus callosum
Gustavson	+	+	+	Short stature, optic atrophy with blindness, large ears, deafness, joint contractures, rockerbottom feet, brain undergrowth, cerebellar hypoplasia
Pettigrew	+	+	+	Dandy-Walker malformation, microcephaly or hydrocephaly, long face with macrostomia and prognathism, small testes, contractures, choreoathetosis, iron deposits in basal ganglia
Schimke	+	+	0	Sunken eyes, downslanting palpebral fissures, narrow nose, spacing of teeth, cupped ears, hypotonia, abducens palsy, hearing loss, vision loss, choreoathetosis, contractures

CANTU SYNDROME

(XLMR–Alopecia–Short Stature, XLMR–Keratosis Follicularis, MIM 308830)

DEFINITION. XLMR with short stature, microcephaly, alopecia, and seizures. The gene has not been localized.

SOMATIC FEATURES. From birth, males are distinguished by near total absence of scalp hair, eyebrows, and eyelashes. The teeth erupt late. A generalized follicular keratosis occurs with greater prominence on the scalp, back, and limbs. Head growth is slow due to cortical atrophy. The face appears round and the mandible is small.

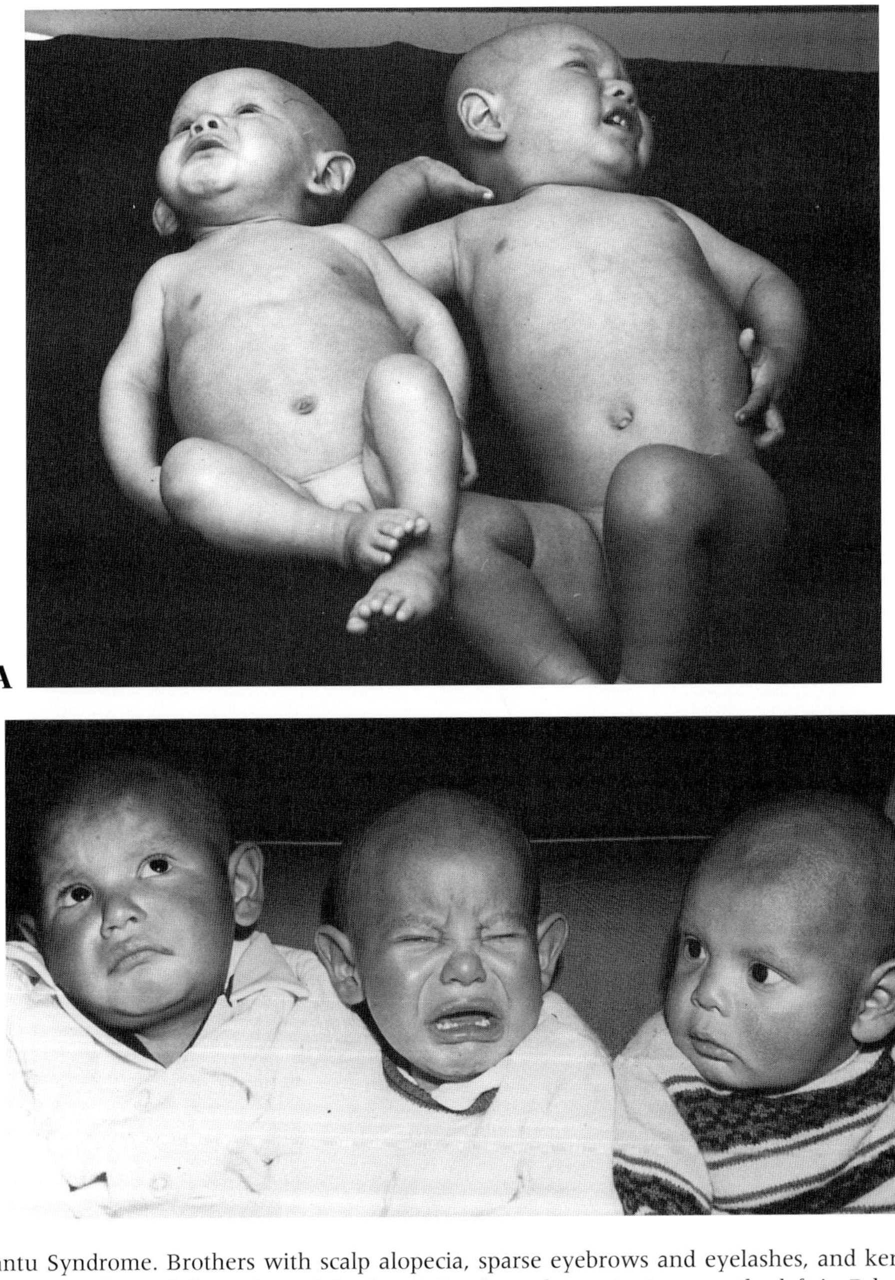

A

B

Cantu Syndrome. Brothers with scalp alopecia, sparse eyebrows and eyelashes, and keratosis follicularis of the scalp and forehead. Brothers shown in A are to the left in B but in reversed position. Courtesy of Dr. Jose Maria Cantu, Latin American Human Genome Program, Guadalajara, Mexico.

GROWTH AND DEVELOPMENT. Intrauterine and postnatal growth are moderately impaired.
NEUROLOGICAL FINDINGS. Seizures, beginning in early childhood, occurred in three of the four cases described.
HETEROZYGOTE EXPRESSION. None.
LABORATORY. Microscopy of scalp and skin biopsies shows normal dermis and keratosis follicularis. Hair appears normal.
IMAGING. Pneumoencephalography demonstrated severe cortical atrophy.
COMMENT. Among XLMR syndromes, near total alopecia is unique to Cantu syndrome and X-linked hereditary bullous dystrophy. Linkage studies have not been conducted in the single family with Cantu syndrome reported to date.

REFERENCE

Cantu J-M, Hernandez A, Larracilla J, et al.: A new X-linked recessive disorder with dwarfism, cerebral atrophy, and generalized keratosis follicularis. J Pediatr 84:564, 1974.

Differential Matrix

Syndrome	Alopecia	Micro-cephaly	Seizures	Comments
Cantu	+	+	+	Short stature, follicular keratosis, cortical atrophy
X-linked hereditary bullous dystrophy	+	+	0	Short stature, bullous dystrophy, upslanting palpebral fissures, protruding ears, short and tapered digits, cardiac defects, small testes, early death from pulmonary infection

CARPENTER-WAZIRI SYNDROME

DEFINITION. XLMR with short stature, small head, hypotonic facies, and brachydactyly. A mutation in the gene XNP (Xq13) has been documented; hence, the Carpenter-Waziri syndrome is allelic to XLMR-hypotonic facies (α-thalassemia mental retardation), Juberg-Marsidi, and Holmes-Gang syndromes.
SOMATIC FEATURES. Small cranium, thick eyebrows, depressed nasal bridge, wide nasal tip, small ears, open mouth with prominent lips, and widely spaced teeth form a distinctive facial appearance. An upsweep of the frontal hair and epicanthus have also been described. Short stature is apparent in childhood. The hands are short with widened distal phalanges, and the thumbs are proximally placed. Hyperextension at the elbow, fifth finger clinodactyly, and syndactyly of toes 2–4 may occur. Genital abnormalities have not been described. Gallstones have occurred during childhood in one case.

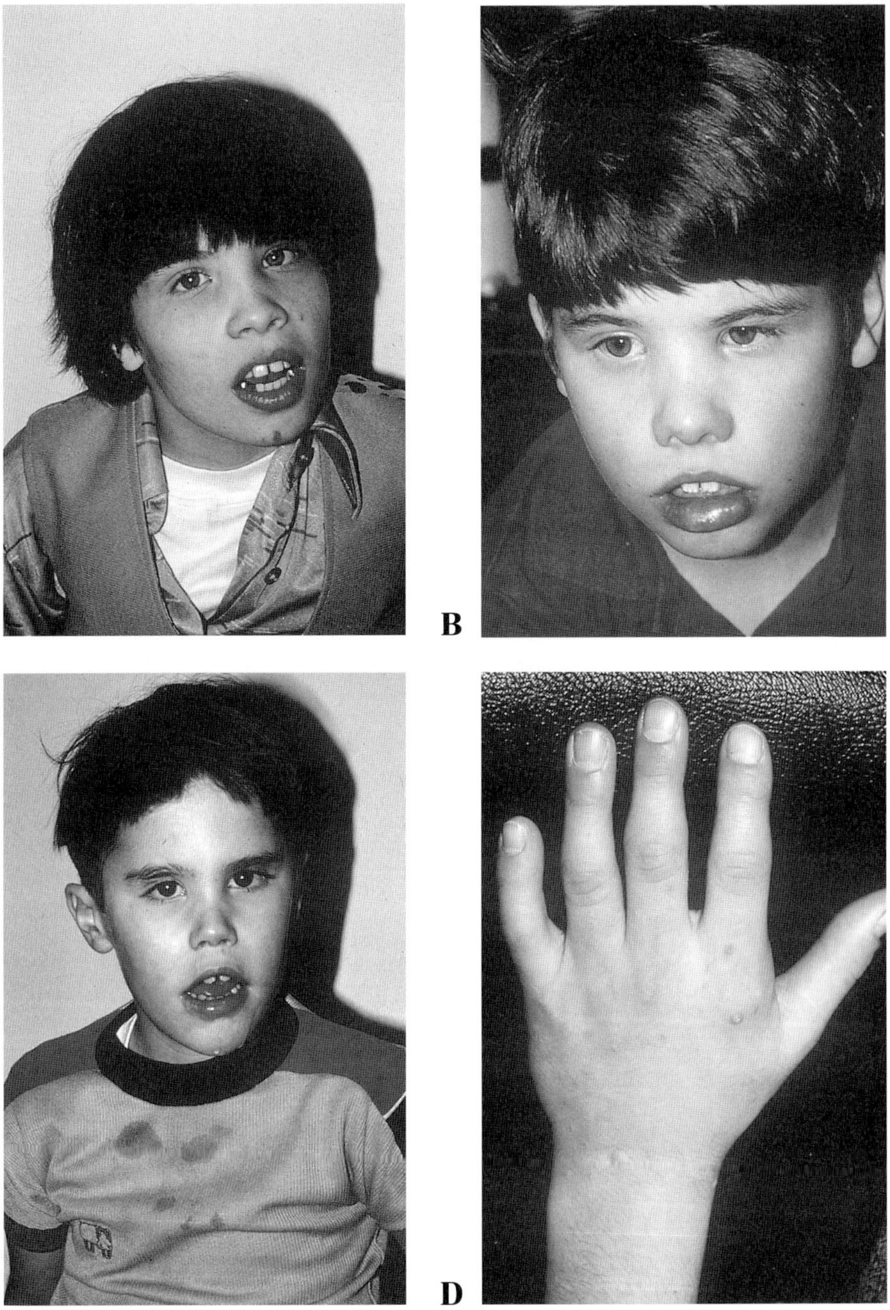

A B C D

Carpenter-Waziri Syndrome. Microcephaly, depressed nasal bridge, tented upper lip, open mouth, prominent lower lip, and spacing of the teeth in brothers at ages 10 and 11 years (A, B); thick eyebrows, tented upper lip, open mouth, and prominent lower lip in 7-year-old maternal cousin of children shown in A and B (C); brachydactyly affecting all digits (D).

GROWTH AND DEVELOPMENT. Although birth weight may be normal, short stature and microcephaly are usually present during childhood.

NEUROLOGICAL FINDINGS. None.

HETEROZYGOTE EXPRESSION. None.

IMAGING. None.

COMMENT. Phenotypic similarities to XLMR–hypotonic facies syndrome (α-thalassemia mental retardation) and the pericentromeric localization have led to documentation of a missense mutation (I2056T) in helicase IV domain of the XNP gene.

REFERENCES

Abidi F, Carpenter NJ, Villard L, et al.: The Carpenter-Waziri syndrome results from a mutation in XNP. Am J Med Genet, in press, 1999.

Carpenter NJ, Waziri M, Liston J, et al.: Studies on X-linked mental retardation: evidence for a gene in the region Xq11-q22. Am J Hum Genet 43:A139, 1988.

Carpenter NJ, Qu Y, Curtis M, et al.: An XLMR syndrome with coarse facies, wide distal phalanges, and short stature maps to the proximal region of Xq. Am J Med Genet, in press, 1999.

Differential Matrix

Syndrome	Micro-cephaly	Hypotonic Facies	Brachy-dactyly	
Carpenter-Waziri (Holmes-Gang) (Juberg-Marsidi) (XLMR-hypotonic facies)	+	+	+	Short stature, telecanthus, small triangular nose, tented upper lip, open mouth, spacing of teeth, genital anomalies, musculoskeletal anomalies, hemoglobin H inclusions in erythrocytes
Coffin-Lowry	+	+	0	Short stature, hypertelorism, anteverted nares, tented upper lip, prominent lips and large mouth, large ears, soft hands with tapered digits, pectus carinatum
Miles-Carpenter	+	+	0	Short stature, ptosis, small palpebral fissures, open mouth, pectus excavatum, scoliosis, long hands, camptodactyly, rockerbottom feet, arch fingerprints, spasticity, unsteady gait
Proud	+	+	0	Hearing loss, vision loss, agenesis of corpus callosum, cryptorchidism, inguinal hernias, ataxia, spasticity, seizures
Smith-Fineman-Myers	+	+	0	Ptosis, flat philtrum, scoliosis, midfoot varus, narrow feet, seizures, hypotonia

CEREBROOCULOGENITAL SYNDROME

(Siber Microphthalmia, Duker Microphthalmia, Siber-Duker Microphthalmia)

DEFINITION. XLMR with microcephaly, short stature, microphthalmia, agenesis of the corpus callosum, hypospadias or other genital anomalies, and spastic quadriplegia. The gene has not been localized.

SOMATIC FEATURES. Blepharoptosis, corneal clouding with fibrovascular dysgenesis of the stroma, uveal hypoplasia, cataracts, retinal dysplasia, and optic nerve hypoplasia accompany the microphthalmia. Aniridia has been described. The eyes move through the full range and have nystagmus. Agenesis of the corpus callosum may be demonstrated on cranial imaging. Microcephaly is constant and low-set ears and micrognathia may be present. Small penis, hypospadias, undescended testes, finger V clinodactyly, joint limitation, and clubfoot complete the somatic phenotype.

GROWTH AND DEVELOPMENT. At birth, weight is normal but microcephaly or hydrocephaly is present in all cases.

COGNITIVE FEATURES. Severe impairment.

NEUROLOGICAL FINDINGS. Spastic quadriplegia.

HETERZYGOTE EXPRESSION. No cognitive impairment and no ocular or other somatic manifestations have been described.

NEUROPATHOLOGY. In one case, the brain was extremely small with a cerebral cyst which communicated with the ventricle system, absent corpus callosum, and small optic nerves. The other case showed severe hydrocephalus with aqueductal stenosis; hypoplasia of the cerebral hemispheres, cerebellum and brain stem; absent olfactory, optic, and oculomotor nerves; and macrogyria.

IMAGING. Absence of corpus callosum.

A

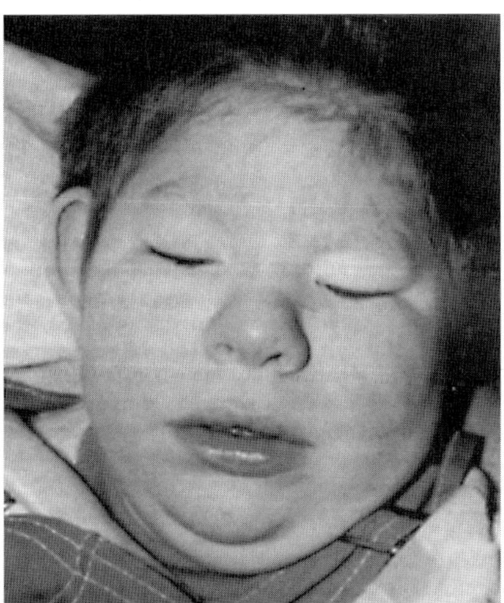

Cerebrooculogenital Syndrome. Five-year-old with microcephaly, blepharophimosis, and microphthalmia (A).

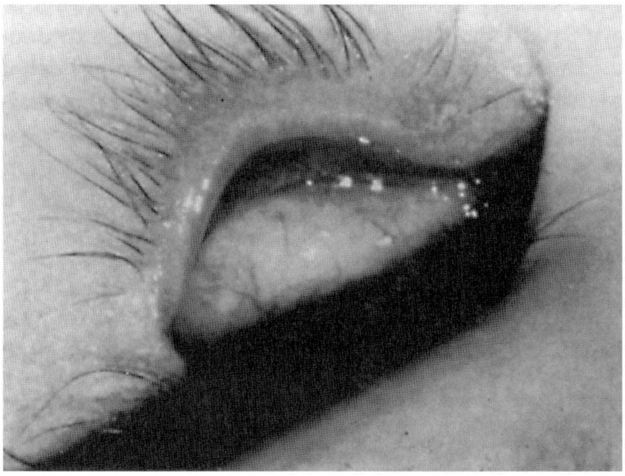

B

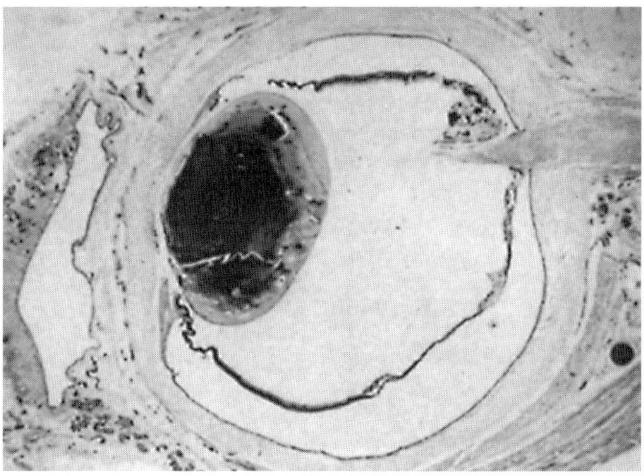

C

Cerebrooculogenital Syndrome. (continued) Microphthalmia with cornea obscured by fibrovascular membrane (B); cross section of fetal cornea showing absent Bowman's layer and Descemet's membrane (C). Courtesy of Dr. Frederick Bieber, Brigham and Women's Hospital and Massachusetts General Hospital, Boston.

COMMENT. Ocular disorders of a great variety are caused by genes distributed along the entirety of the X chromosome. These genes alter visual acuity by influencing structural development of the eyes, by interfering with ocular movement, by obstructing the ocular medium, and by disturbing the reception and transmission of images to the occipital cortex. They are distributed from distal Xp (Aicardi, Bertini, Goltz, MIDAS, Nance-Horan and Wittwer syndromes) to distal Xq (Graham syndrome) with a number of important loci in between (Norrie dysplasia—Xp11.3, XLMR-choroideremia—Xq21, Mohr-Tranebjaerg syndrome—Xq22, Arts syndrome–Xq21-q24, Lowe syndrome—Xq26). Other syndromes with vision loss have yet to be mapped (XLM–retinitis pigmentosa, Schimke syndrome, Proud syndrome). The nature of the ocular anomaly, the presence of nonocular manifestations, and the gene localizations are helpful in differentiating the XLMR entities with ocular abnormalities.

REFERENCE

Duker JS, Weiss JS, Siber M, et al.: Ocular findings in a new heritable syndrome of brain, eye, and urogenital abnormalities. Am J Ophthalmol 99:51, 1985.
Siber M: X-linked recessive microencephaly, microphthalmia with corneal opacities, spastic quadriplegia, hypospadias and cryptorchidism. Clin Genet 26:453, 1984.

Differential Matrix

Syndrome	Micro-cephaly	Ocular Anomaly	Genito-urinary Anomaly	Comments
Cerebrooculogenital	+	+	+	Short stature, hydrocephaly, agenesis of corpus callosum, microphthalmia, ptosis, hypospadias, cryptorchidism, clubfoot, spasticity
Lenz microphthalmia	+	+	+	Malformed ears, cleft lip/palate, cardiac anomalies, thumb duplication or hypoplasia, narrow shoulders
Wittwer	+	+	+	Growth deficiency, hearing loss, vision loss, hypertelorism, hypotonia, seizures
MIDAS	+	+	0	Dermal aplasia, dysgenesis of corpus callosum, cardiac defects, cardiomyopathy
Goltz	0	+	+	Linear areas of dermal aplasia, cutaneous adipose herniations, dystrophic nails, abnormal teeth and hair, vertebral anomalies, limb reduction defects
Lowe	0	+	+	Short stature, hypotonia, aminoaciduria, progressive renal disease

CEREBROPALATOCARDIAC SYNDROME

(Hamel Syndrome, XLMR–Cleft Palate–Cardiac Defect Syndrome)

DEFINITION. XLMR with microcephaly, short stature, cupped ears, bulbous nose, highly arched or cleft palate, short philtrum, tented upper lip, malar hypoplasia, cardiac defect, and slender hands and feet. Multipoint linkage analysis suggests that the gene locus may be in the pericentromeric region.

SOMATIC FEATURES. Microcephaly, broad nasal bridge, bulbous nose, malar hypoplasia, dysplastic cupped ears, short philtrum, tented upper lip, and small mouth contribute to a distinctive craniofacial appearance. The initially oval facial configuration elongates with age. Highly arched or cleft palate occurs consistently. Complex cardiac defects, tetralogy of Fallot in one case, atrial and ven-

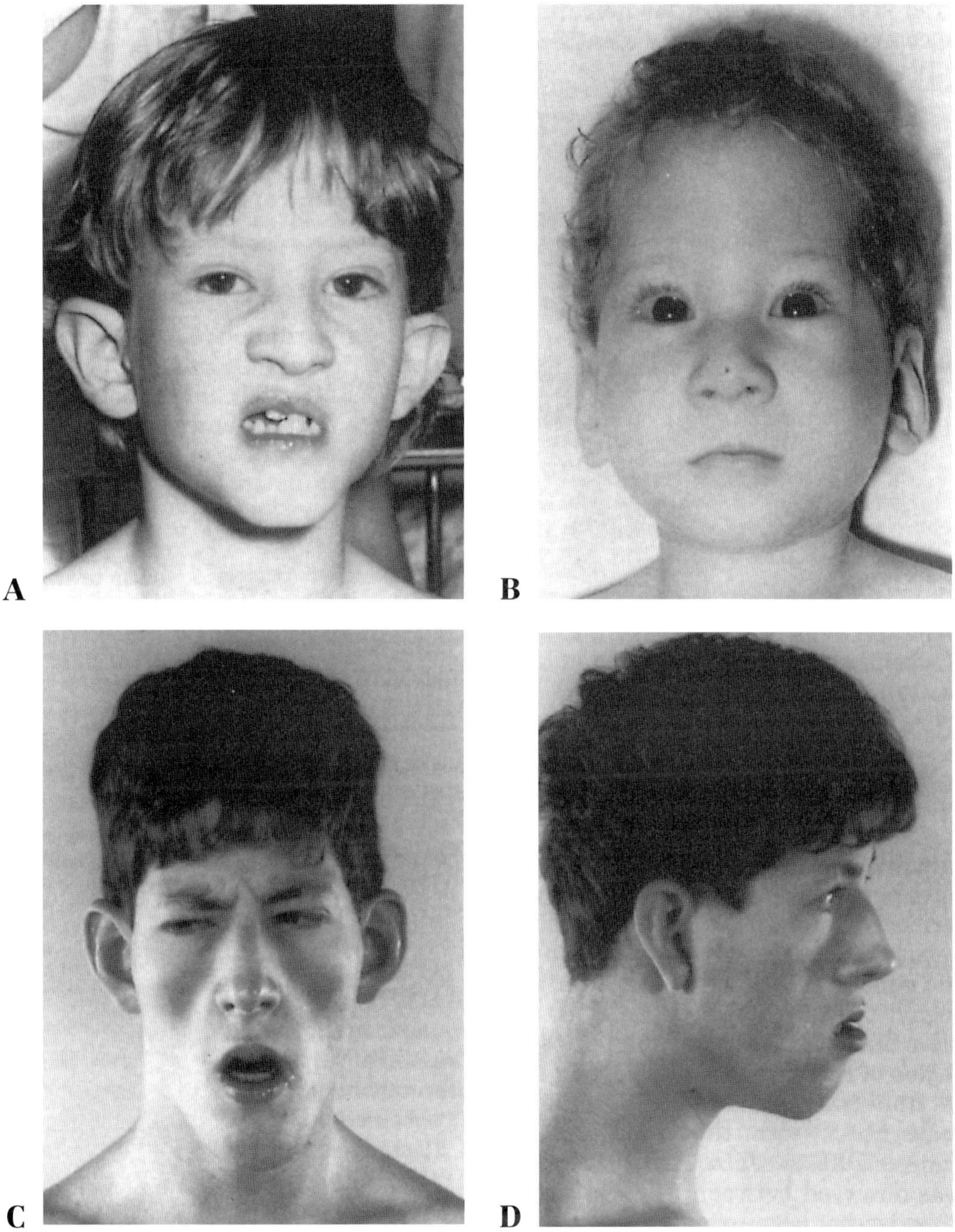

Cerebropalatocardiac Syndrome. Long narrow face, broad nasal bridge, bulbous nose, prominent mandible, cupped ears and short philtrum at age 8 years (A); long narrow face, broad nasal bridge, bulbous nose, malar hypoplasia, cupped ears, and small mouth in brother at ages 7 months (B) and 20 years (C,D). Courtesy of Dr. Ben Hamel, University Hospital, Nijmegen, The Netherlands and the *American Journal of Medical Genetics,* Copyright © 1994, Wiley-Liss, Inc.

tricular septal defects and overriding aorta in another, and undiagnosed defects in two others are symptomatic in all cases. Only minor skeletal anomalies occur, including long slender hands and feet, finger 5 clinodactyly, and contractures at the elbows and knees. Hypospadias was present in one case.

GROWTH AND DEVELOPMENT. All parameters of growth are retarded prenatally and postnatally. Delay of developmental milestones becomes obvious in infancy.

NEUROLOGICAL FINDINGS. Hypertonicity was noted in one case.

HETEROZYGOTE EXPRESSION. The carrier mother of two affected males had an atrial septal defect but no other manifestation.

IMAGING. Small brain without structural malformation was found in the single case so studied.

COMMENT. The cerebropalatocardiac syndrome seems to be an exception to the generalization that XLMR syndromes do not have lethal malformations. In three of the four cases described in the original family, death occurred during infancy or childhood, their cardiac defect being the principal contributor.

REFERENCES

Hamel BCJ, Mariman ECM, van Beersum SEC, et al.: Mental retardation, congenital heart defect, cleft palate, short stature, and facial anomalies: a new X-linked multiple congenital anomalies/mental retardation syndrome: clinical description and molecular studies. Am J Med Genet 51:591, 1994.

Differential Matrix

Syndrome	Cardiac Defect	Facial Clefting	Distinctive Facial Features	Comments
Cerebropalatocardiac	+	+	+	Microcephaly, short stature, cleft palate, cupped ears, bulbous nose, short philtrum, tented upper lip, childhood death
Lenz microphthalmia	+	+	+	Microcephaly, microphthalmia, ocular dysgenesis, malformed ears, cleft lip/palate, cardiac and genitourinary anomalies, thumb duplication or hypoplasia, narrow shoulders
Simpson-Golabi-Behmel	+	+	+	Somatic overgrowth, supernumerary nipples, polydactyly
Telecanthus-hypospadias	+	+	+	High broad nasal root, dysplastic ears, cleft lip/palate, abnormal cranial contour or symmetry
Cranioorodigital	0	+	+	Undergrowth, hearing impairment, prominent forehead, flat/broad nasal bridge, ocular hypertelorism, downslanting palpebral fissures, flat midface, cleft palate, blunted flexed overlapping fingers, rockerbottom feet, hypoplastic fibulae, subluxed/dislocated joints
Oral-facial-digital I	o	+	+	Sparse scalp hair, dystopia canthorum, flat midface, hypoplastic alae nasi, hypertrophic and aberrant oral frenuli, intraoral clefts and pseudoclefts, lingual hamartomas, brachydactyly, syndactyly, clinodactyly, structural brain anomalies, polycystic kidneys
Otopalatodigital I	0	+	+	Short stature, conductive hearing impaiment, prominent brow, broad nasal root, apparent ocular hypertelorism, downslanting palpebral fissures, cleft palate, blunted distal phalanges, irregular curvature and spacing of digits, limitation of elbow movement
Pallister W	0	+	+	Short stature, prominent forehead, wide nasal tip, incomplete cleft lip/palate, spasticity, contractures
Opitz FG	+	0	+	Macrocephaly, broad forehead, downslanted palpebral fissures, everted lower lip, dysgenesis of corpus callosum, imperforate anus, constipation, flat thumbs and great toes, hypotonia
X-linked hereditary bullous dystrophy	+	0	+	Microcephaly, short stature, upslanting palpebral fissures, protruding ears, short and tapered digits, bullous dystrophy, small testes, early death from pulmonary infection

Charcot-Marie-Tooth Neuropathy, Cowchock Variant

(XLMR–Motor-Sensory Neuropathy–Deafness, Cowchock Syndrome, MIM 310490)

Definition. XLMR associated with infancy-onset peripheral motor and sensory neuropathy and deafness. The gene has been linked to markers in Xq26.

Somatic Features. Affected males are profoundly weak and areflexic from birth. Pes cavus and hammer toes become obvious with age. Malformations or craniofacial manifestations do not occur.

Growth and Development. Growth impairment has not been described. Global developmental delay occurs, although delay of motor milestones may be more notable.

Cognitive Features. Impairment of cognitive function is inconsistent, being present in less than half of cases.

Neurological Findings. From birth, infants are areflexic and weak, so much so as to be considered affected by spinal muscular atrophy. Slow motor development may be attributed in part to muscle weakness but is too severe to be explained by this alone. Affected males eventually walk alone. Weakness appears most notable in the distal muscles of the lower limbs but is demonstrably generalized in adults. Fasciculations of the tongue and deltoid muscles may be seen in some cases. Sensorineural hearing loss has been found in most cases.

Heterozygote Expression. Clinical abnormalities have not been reported in obligate carrier females, although prolongation in sural nerve latency was documented in two.

Laboratory. Electromyography shows denervation and occasional fibrillation; median motor nerve conduction velocity is moderately slowed in some patients; sensory conduction is markedly slowed in median and sural nerves; nerve biopsy shows a paucity of myelinated nerve fibers and an increase in connective tissue; muscle biopsy shows muscle atrophy of neurogenic type.

Comment. Peripheral neuropathies constitute a heterogenous group of genetic disorders with both autosomal (17p and 1q) and X chromosome gene loci. Only the X-linked Cowchock and Ionasescu variants have associated mental retardation and the mental impairment does not affect all patients. Cowchock variant may be distinguished clinically by sensorineural hearing loss and by gene localization in Xq26. Both variants have onset in infancy.

REFERENCES

Cowchock FS, Duckett SW, Streletz LJ, et al.: X-linked motor-sensory neuropathy type-II with deafness and mental retardation: a new disorder. Am J Med Genet 20:307, 1985.

Fischbeck KH, ar-Rushdi N, Pericak-Vance M, et al.: X-linked neuropathy: gene localization with DNA probes. Ann Neurol 20:527, 1986.

Priest JM, Fischbeck KH, Nouri N, et al.: A locus for axonal motor-sensory neuropathy with deafness and mental retardation maps to Xq24–q26. Genomics 29:409, 1995.

Differential Matrix

Syndrome	Peripheral Motor-Sensory Neuropathy	Hearing Loss	Areflexia	Comments
Charcot-Marie-Tooth neuropathy, Cowchock variant	+	+	+	Pes cavus, weakness
Charcot-Marie-Tooth neuropathy, Ionasescu variant	+	0	+	Weakness, wasting of intrinsic hand muscles, enlarged ulnar nerves, pes cavus

CHARCOT-MARIE-TOOTH NEUROPATHY, IONASESCU VARIANT

(XLMR–Charcot-Marie-Tooth Neuropathy, X-Linked Recessive Charcot-Marie-Tooth Disease Type 2, MIM 302801)

DEFINITION. XLMR associated with onset of peripheral motor and sensory neuropathy in infancy. Linkage of the disease locus with markers DXS16–DXS43 in Xp22.2 (maximal multipoint lod score 3.48) provides the basis for separation from other X-linked and autosomal forms of Charcot-Marie-Tooth (CMT) neuropathy.

SOMATIC FEATURES. Musculoskeletal findings are secondary to the peripheral neuropathy and include atrophy of distal leg muscles and pes cavus. Malformations and distinctive craniofacial manifestations do not occur.

GROWTH AND DEVELOPMENT. Growth abnormalities have not been described.

COGNITIVE FEATURES. Impairment of cognitive function is found in less than half of cases.

NEUROLOGICAL FINDINGS. Areflexia and weakness of the distal leg muscles are present from birth or early infancy. Foot drop or steppage gait results from atrophy of the tibialis anterior and peroneal muscles. Wasting of the intrinsic muscles of the hands and mild to moderate sensory loss in the distal limbs may also be demonstrated. Typically the ulnar nerve is enlarged and pes cavus becomes progressively more notable.

HETEROZYGOTE EXPRESSION. Carrier females do not have muscle weakness or other clinical signs of the disorder. Electromyography and nerve conduction velocity are normal although muscle biopsy may show evidence of mild neurogenic muscle atrophy.

LABORATORY. Electromyography shows denervation; median nerve conduction velocity shows mild to moderate slowing.

COMMENT. In addition to gene loci for CMT neuropathy in 1q and 17p, at least three gene loci may be present on the X chromosome (Xp22, Xp11–q21, Xq24–q26). Mental retardation occurs only in the Ionasescu and Cowchock variants and in these variants is not found in all males with peripheral neuropathy. The Ionasescu and Cowchock variants both have onset in infancy and lack clinically significant carrier manifestations but may be distinguished by the presence of deafness in the Cowchock variant and by gene localization (Xp22.2 in Ionasescu variant; Xq26 in Cowchock variant).

REFERENCES

Ionasescu VV, Trofatter J, Haines JL, et al.: Heterogeneity in X-linked recessive Charcot-Marie-Tooth neuropathy. Am J Hum Genet 48:1075, 1991.

Differential Matrix

Syndrome	Peripheral Motor-Sensory Neuropathy	Areflexia	Distal Leg Muscle Atrophy/ Hypoplasia	Comments
Charcot-Marie-Tooth neuropathy, Ionasescu variant	+	+	+	Weakness, wasting of intrinsic hand muscles, enlarged ulnar nerves, pes cavus
Charcot-Marie-Tooth neuropathy, Cowchock variant	+	+	+	Deafness, pes cavus, weakness

CHRISTIAN SYNDROME

(X-Linked Skeletal Dysplasia–Mental Retardation, MIM 309620)

DEFINITION. XLMR with short stature, metopic ridge, vertebral anomalies, abducens palsy and glucose intolerance. The gene localizes distal to DXS100 (Xq25), lod score 3.27.

SOMATIC FEATURES. Multiple abnormalities occur in the axial skeleton, including occipitalization of the atlas, odontoid hypoplasia, fusion of the bodies and neural arches of other cervical vertebrae, thoracic hemivertebrae with scoliosis, and hypoplasia of the sacrum. Appendicular anomalies are limited to general shortening of the bones and clinodactyly of the fifth fingers. The cranium has normal circumference, typically has a prominent metopic ridge, and may have asymmetry and slight platybasia. The interorbital measurement is reduced, the palpebral fissures slant downward, and epicanthus and abducens palsy are present. Flattening of the superior helices or cupped ears may recur. All hand bones are short, the middle phalanges tending to be shorter than the others. Imperforate anus occurred in one case and constipation in another. Glucose intolerance is manifest by melituria and excessive increase in blood glucose after oral loading.

GROWTH AND DEVELOPMENT. Intrauterine growth appears normal. Postnatally, head growth continues to be normal, but linear growth is impaired, resulting in short stature.

COGNITIVE FEATURES. Borderline normal to mild impairment.

HETEROZYGOTE EXPRESSION. Carrier females may have fusion of the cervical vertebrae, short middle phalanges, and diabetes mellitus or intolerance to oral glucose loading but have normal cognitive function.

IMAGING. Pneumoencephalogram was performed on one child, showing dilation of the lateral and third ventricles.

COMMENT. Only two other XLMR syndromes (Christianson syndrome, Schimke syndrome) have abducens palsy as a manifestation. Christian syndrome and Christianson syndrome have overlapping linkage limits but are phenotypically different. Schimke syndrome has not been mapped.

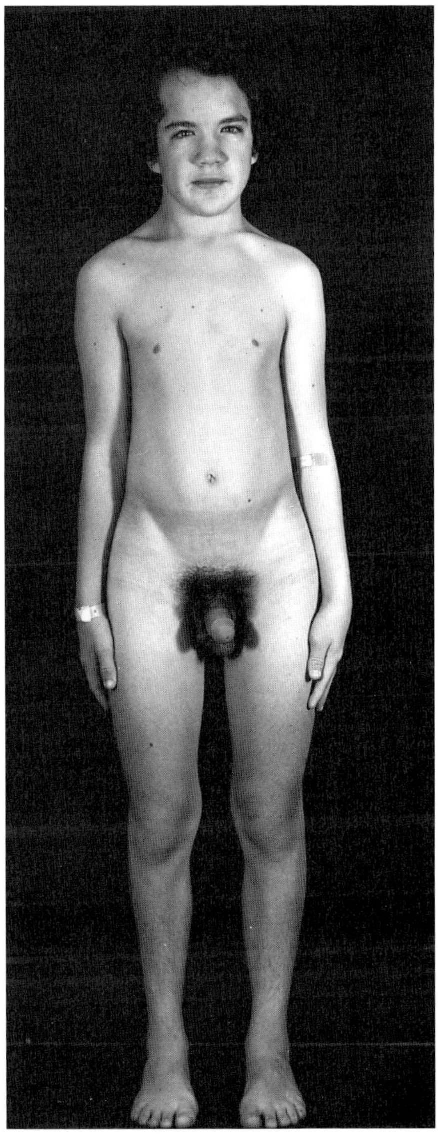

A

Christian Syndrome. Sixteen-year-old male with short stature (A).

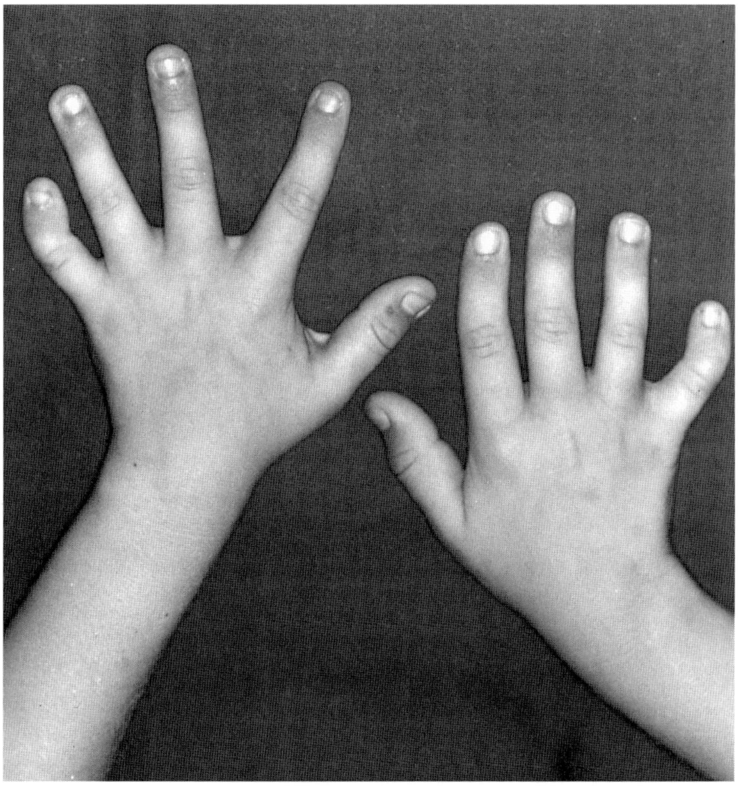

B

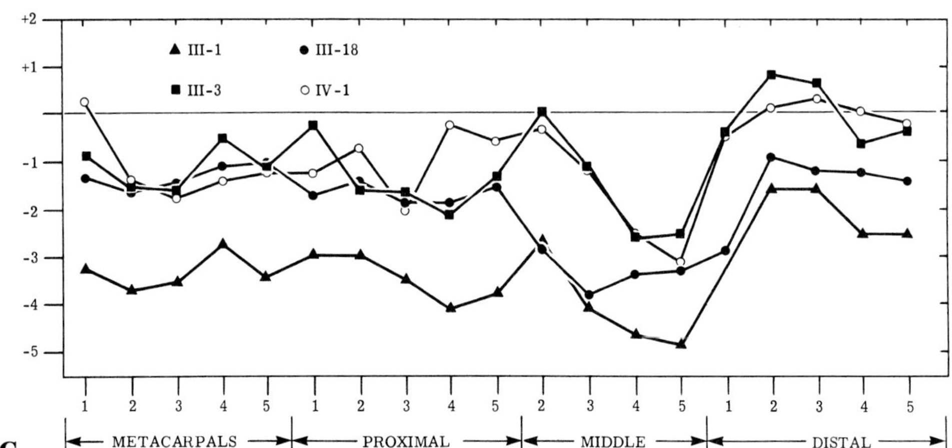

C

Christian Syndrome. (continued) Clinodactyly of fifth fingers (B); metacarpal phalangeal profile showing predominant shortening of the middle phalanges for affected males (C). Courtesy of Dr. Joe C. Christian, Indiana University School of Medicine, Indianapolis.

REFERENCES

Christian JC, DeMeyer W, Franken EA, et al.: X-linked skeletal dysplasia with mental retardation. Clin Genet 11:128, 1977.

Dlouhy SR, Christian JC, Haines JL, et al.: Localization of the gene for a syndrome of X-linked skeletal dysplasia and mental retardation to Xq27-qter. Hum Genet 75:136, 1987.

Differential Matrix

Syndrome	Short Stature	Abducens Palsy	Vertebral Anomalies	Comments
Christian	+	+	+	Metopic ridge
Christianson	+	+	0	Microcephaly, general asthenia, contractures, seizures, ophthalmoplegia
Schimke	+	+	0	Microcephaly, sunken eyes, downslanting palpebral fissures, narrow nose, spacing of teeth, cupped ears, hypotonia, hearing loss, vision loss, spasticity, choreoathetosis, contractures
Aarskog	+	0	+	Hypertelorism, downslanting palpebral fissures, ptosis, cupped ears, anteverted nares, brachydactyly, horizontal palmar crease, midfoot varus, joint laxity, shawl scrotum, cryptorchidism, inguinal hernias
Goltz	+	0	+	Cataracts, ocular dysgenesis, linear areas of dermal aplasia, cutaneous adipose herniations, dystrophic nails, abnormal teeth and hair, vertebral anomalies, limb reduction defects, genitourinary anomalies
Otopalatodigital 1	+	0	+	Conductive hearing impairment, prominent brow, broad nasal root, apparent ocular hypertelorism, downslanting palpebral fissures, cleft palate, blunted distal phalanges, irregular curvature and spacing of digits, limitation of elbow movement
Stoccos dos Santos	+	0	+	Heavy eyebrows, strabismus, short palpebral fissures, short philtrum, thin upper lip, prominent nasal tip, hip dislocation, hirsutism, kyphosis, precocious puberty, recurrent respiratory infections
Sutherland-Haan	+	0	+	Microcephaly, upslanting palpebral fissures, asthenic habitus, pectus excavatum, scoliosis, stiff joints, pes cavus, small testes, spasticity

CHRISTIANSON SYNDROME

DEFINITION. XLMR with short stature, microcephaly, long narrow face, large ears, long straight nose, prominent mandible, general asthenia, narrow chest, long thin digits, adducted thumbs, contractures, seizures, autistic features, truncal ataxia, ophthalmoplegia, mutism, incontinence, and hypoplasia of the cerebellum and brain stem. Linkage analysis places the gene between DXS424 (Xq23) and DXS548 (Xq27), lod score 2.81.

SOMATIC FEATURES. Profound disability with absence of speech, failure or loss of ambulation, incontinence, seizures, and cognitive deficiency is paralleled by somatic frailty with general asthenia, microcephaly and short stature, narrow chest, long thin digits, and contractures. The long narrow face is further defined by large ears, straight thin nose, squint and prominent square mandible. Major malformations do not occur. Genitalia including testicular volume are normal.

GROWTH AND DEVELOPMENT. Birth weight is normal, but during childhood weight falls below the third centile. Head circumference and height measure in the lower centiles or slightly below.

COGNITIVE FEATURES. Profound impairment is the rule with inability to speak and assist in the rudiments of self-care.

NEUROLOGICAL FINDINGS. Affected males never achieve basic skills for self care. They never develop speech, although hearing appears intact. Incontinence of bowel and bladder persists throughout life. Ophthalmoplegia, due to abducens nerve dysfunction, contributes to strabismus. Muscle tone appears normal. Deep tendon reflexes are usually normal, although brisk reflexes at the knees and equivocal plantar responses were noted in several patients. Clonus has not been described. Truncal ataxia occurs even in childhood. Generalized seizures begin in infancy. Nerve conduction and EMG are normal.

NEUROPATHOLOGY. The brain is undergrown generally, but with hypoplasia or atrophy of the cerebellar vermis and brain stem particularly. Cerebellar morphology is characterized by loss of neurons in the granular and Purkinje cell layers, microcystic changes in the molecular layer, and depletion of myelin.

HETEROZYGOTE EXPRESSION. Two of eight carrier females had learning impairments or mild mental retardation and during childhood had behavior problems and aggressiveness.

IMAGING. An MRI in one patient has shown undergrowth of the cerebellum and brain stem in the company of prominent cerebellar cisterns and fourth ventricle but normal lateral ventricles.

→

Christianson Syndrome. Ten-year-old male with incompletely folded helices, strabismus, long straight nose, and square jaw (A); 19-year-old cousin with long narrow face, bushy eyebrows, strabismus, long straight nose, large ears, and square jaw (B); 24-year-old cousin with bushy eyebrows, long straight nose, square jaw, and decreased muscle mass (C); profile of maternal uncle showing deeply-set eyes, long straight nose, prominent jaw, and large ears (D); and 35-year-old carrier female with large ears and long straight nose (E). Courtesy of Professor Arnold Christianson, Department of Human Genetics and Developmental Biology, University of Pretoria, Republic of South Africa.

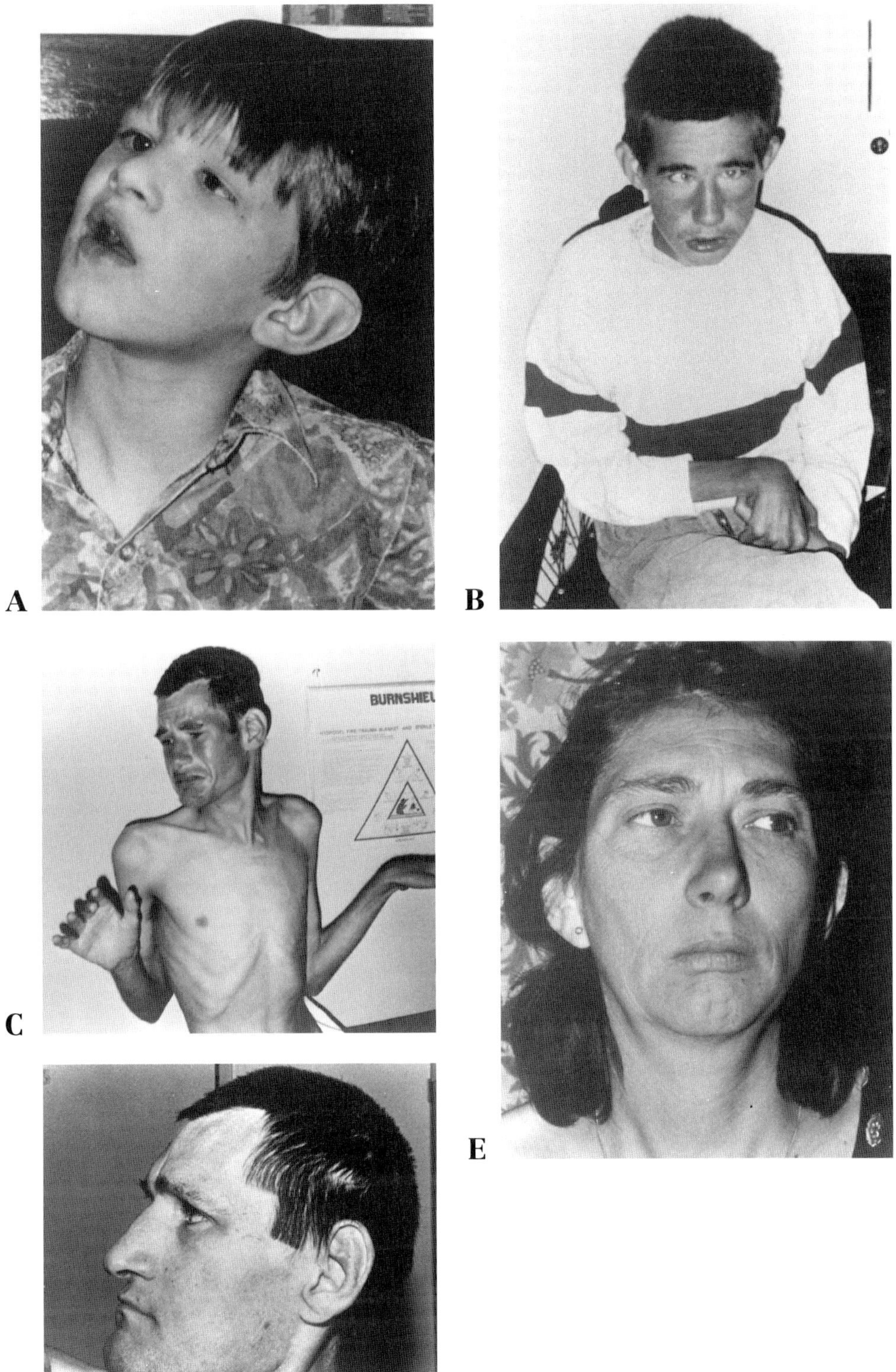
A
B
C
D
E

COMMENT. Christianson syndrome maps to Xq23–q27, an area least populated with genes that cause X-linked mental retardation. There are many features—microcephaly, absent speech, absent ambulation, incontinence, truncal ataxia, contractures, and hypoplasia of the cerebellum and brain stem—in common with Arena syndrome, which maps to the same region. Arena syndrome has normal facial appearance, lacks seizures, and has MRI changes in the basal ganglia suggesting iron deposition. Another candidate for allelism, Gustavson syndrome, has overlapping linkage limits, cerebellar hypoplasia, microcephaly, short stature, profound developmental failure, blindness, deafness, and seizures. Severe impairments are obvious from birth and death occurs in infancy or early childhood. Other XLMR syndromes with overlapping mapping limits include Arts, Miles-Carpenter, Hamel, Börjesson-Forssman-Lehmann, hereditary bullous dystrophy, and XLMR-hypogammaglobulinemia syndromes, none of which is similar in phenotype to Christianson syndrome. Schimke syndrome, as yet not mapped, should be considered in the differential because of microcephaly, short stature, abducens palsy, and progressive basal ganglia dysfunction.

REFERENCE

Arena JF, Schwartz C, Stevenson R, et al.: Spastic paraplegia with iron deposits in the basal ganglia: a new X-linked mental retardation syndrome. Am J Med Genet 43:479, 1992.

Christianson AC, Stevenson RE, van der Meyden CH, et al.: X linked mental retardation, mild craniofacial dysmorphology, epilepsy, ophthalmoplegia, and cerebellar atrophy in a large South African kindred. J Med Genet, in press, 1999.

Gustavson K-H, Annerén G, Malmgren H, et al.: New X-linked syndrome with severe mental retardation, severely impaired vision, severe hearing defect, epileptic seizures, spasticity, restricted joint mobility, and early death. Am J Med Genet 45:654, 1993.

Differential Matrix

Syndrome	Absent Speech, Ambulation and Continence	Truncal Ataxia	Cerebellar and Brain Stem Hypoplasia	Comments
Christianson	+	+	+	Short stature, microcephaly, general asthenia, contractures, seizures, ophthalmoplegia
Arena	+	+	+	Muscle hypoplasia, clubfoot, iron deposits in basal ganglia, spastic paraplegia, rigidity, dystonia
Bertini	+	+	+	Macular degeneration, hypotonia, seizures, childhood death, developmental delays and regression, postnatal growth impairment
Gustavson	+	+	+	Microcephaly, short stature, optic atrophy with blindness, large ears, deafness, joint contractures, rockerbottom feet, brain undergrowth, hydrocephaly, spasticity, seizures
Schimke	+	+	+	Microcephaly, sunken eyes, downslanting palpebral fissures, narrow nose, spacing of teeth, cupped ears, hypotonia, abducens palsy, hearing loss, vision loss, spasticity, choreoathetosis, contractures
Paine	+	0	+	Microcephaly, short stature, vision and hearing loss, optic atrophy, spasticity, seizures
Pettigrew	0	+	+	Dandy-Walker malformation, spasticity, seizures, microcephaly or hydrocephaly, long face with macrostomia and prognathism, small testes, contractures, myoglobinuria, hemolytic anemia

CHUDLEY-LOWRY SYNDROME

(XLMR-Hypotonia-Hypogonadism, MIM 309490)

DEFINITION. XLMR with short stature, hypotonic facies, obesity, and hypogenitalism. Molecular studies have excluded distal Xp and Xq as the gene location. **SOMATIC FEATURES.** Narrow bitemporal diameter, almond shaped eyes, depressed nasal bridge, and large open mouth with arched upper lip, short philtrum, and high palate contribute to a facial appearance that suggests intrauterine and early developmental hypotonia. Only in one case, however, was hypotonia specifically noted. Skeletal manifestations include short neck, mild brachydactyly, tapering of the digits, finger 5 camptodactyly, and genu valgum. An excess number of arch fingerprints and low total ridge count were documented. Although the testes were small or incompletely descended, sex hormone levels and secondary sexual characteristics were normal.

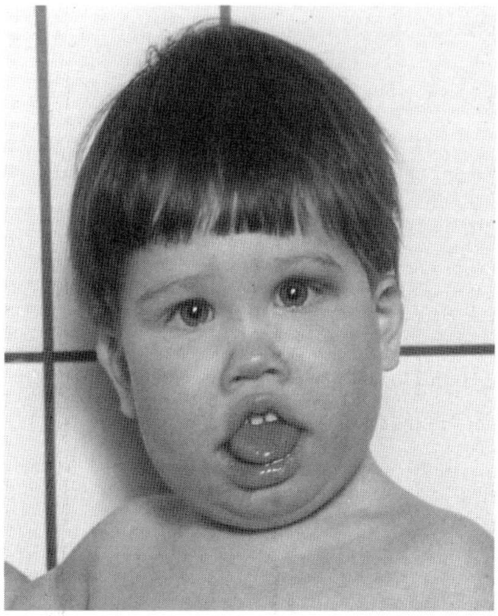
A

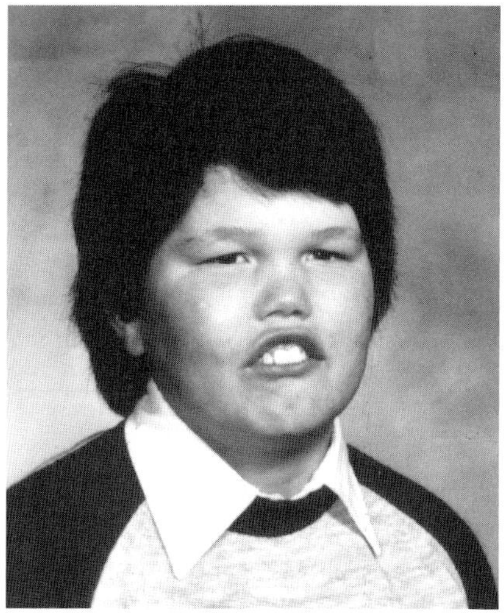
B

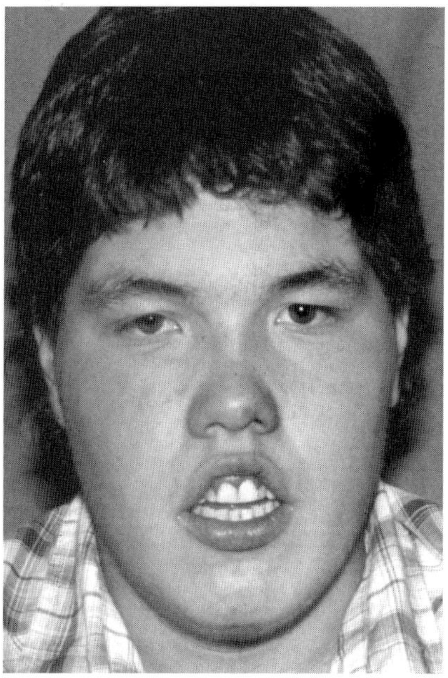
C

Chudley-Lowry Syndrome. Depressed nasal bridge, short philtrum, tented upper lip, and almond-shaped palpebral fissures in a 30-month-old male (A) and his two maternal uncles aged 19 years and 20 years (B, C). Courtesy of Dr. Albert E. Chudley, Children's Hospital, Winnipeg, Manitoba.

GROWTH AND DEVELOPMENT. Growth discordance, possibly postnatal in origin, results in head circumference and stature in the lower centiles and weight in the upper centiles. Global delay of developmental milestones is obvious from infancy.

COGNITIVE FEATURES. Moderate to severe impairment.

BEHAVIORAL MANIFESTATIONS. Short attention span, hyperactivity, and poor adaptive function were described in two cases—one of preschool age, the other adult.

NEUROLOGICAL FINDINGS. None.

HETEROZYGOTE EXPRESSION. None.

IMAGING. The CT of the brain in one case was normal.

COMMENT. Two groups of syndromes are called to mind by the clinical manifestations in Chudley-Lowry syndrome. The first group is constituted of syndromes which share hypotonia, hypogonadism, and obesity as prominent findings. Notable among these are Prader-Willi, Bardet-Biedl, Börjeson-Forssman-Lehmann, Wilson-Turner, and Vasquez syndromes. The second group of syndromes are those with hypotonic facies, minor skeletal abnormalities, and genital anomalies. The prototype syndrome of this latter group is XLMR-hypotonic facies syndrome and a number of the others with similar manifestations—XLMR arch fingerprints–hypotonia, Smith-Fineman-Myers, and XLMR-psoriasis—may, in fact, be allelic.

REFERENCE

Chudley AE, Lowry RB, Hoar DI: Mental retardation, distinct facial changes, short stature, obesity, and hypogonadism. A new X-linked mental retardation syndrome. Am J Med Genet 31:741, 1988.

Differential Matrix

Syndrome	Obesity	Hypotonia	Hypo-genitalism	Comments
Chudley-Lowry	+	+	+	Short stature, bitemporal narrowing, almond-shaped eyes, depressed nasal bridge, tented upper lip, open mouth
Börjeson-Forssman-Lehmann	+	+	+	Short stature, microcephaly, coarse face, large ears, gynecomastia, narrow sloped shoulders, visual impairment, tapered digits
Vasquez	+	+	+	Short stature, microcephaly, gynecomastia
Wilson-Turner	+	+	+	Normal growth, small hands and feet, tapered digits, gynecomastia, emotional lability
Pettigrew	0	+	+	Dandy-Walker malformation, spasticity, seizures, microcephaly or hydrocephaly, long face with macrostomia and prognathism, contractures, choreoathetosis, iron deposits in basal ganglia
Prieto	0	+	+	Ventricular enlargement, facial asymmetry, hypertelorism, prominent eyes, ptosis, long narrow nose, micrognathia, inguinal hernia, cryptorchidism
XLMR-hypotonic facies (Carpenter-Waziri) (Holmes-Gang) (Juberg-Marsidi)	0	+	+	Short stature, microcephaly, telecanthus, small triangular nose, tented upper lip, open mouth, spacing of teeth, genital anomalies, musculoskeletal anomalies, hemoglobin H inclusions in erythrocytes
Urban	+	0	+	Short stature, small hands and feet, digital contractures, osteoporosis
Young-Hughes	+	0	+	Short stature, small palpebral fissures, cupped ears, ichthyosiform scaling

CLARK-BARAITSER SYNDROME

DEFINITION. XLMR with macrocephaly, prominent forehead and large ears, broad nasal tip, thick lower lip, prominent supraorbital ridges, small lateral maxillary incisors, obesity, and macroorchidism. The gene has not been localized.
SOMATIC FEATURES. Major malformations do not occur. Overall large stature, craniofacial manifestations, and macroorchidism define the phenotype. Macrocephaly with square forehead and prominent supraorbital ridges, large ears, broad nasal tip, thick lower lips, and small lateral maxillary incisors are the dominant facial characteristics. A central maxillary diastema may also be present. Generalized obesity adds to the fullness of the face.
GROWTH AND DEVELOPMENT. Details of early growth and development are not available. As adults, affected males have macrocephaly, tall stature, and obesity.
COGNITIVE FEATURES. Moderate impairment.
HETEROZYGOTE EXPRESSION. The mother of the two affected brothers reported by Clark and Baraitser had mild mental retardation and facial features similar to her sons.
COMMENT. The phenotype is based on a single family with two affected brothers and their mildly affected mother. Initially, the authors were persuaded that the condition was the same as Atkin-Flaitz syndrome. In a subsequent publication, Baraitser et al. described another family in which two male first cousins had excessive overall growth, macrocephaly, prominence of the lower lip, obesity, and behavioral problems.

REFERENCES

Atkin JF, Flaitz K, Patil S, et al.: A new X-linked mental retardation syndrome. Am J Med Genet 21:697, 1985.

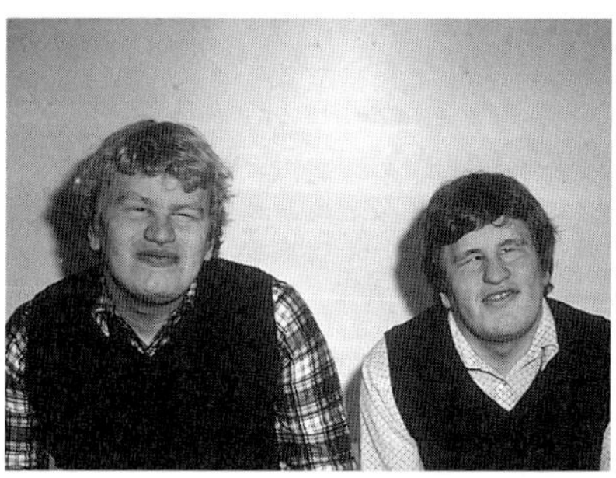

A

Clark-Baraitser Syndrome. Macrocephaly, prominent forehead, broad nasal tip, thick lower lip in brothers aged 21 and 22 years (A) and mother age 46 years (B). Courtesy of Dr. Michael Baraitser, Institute of Child Health, London.

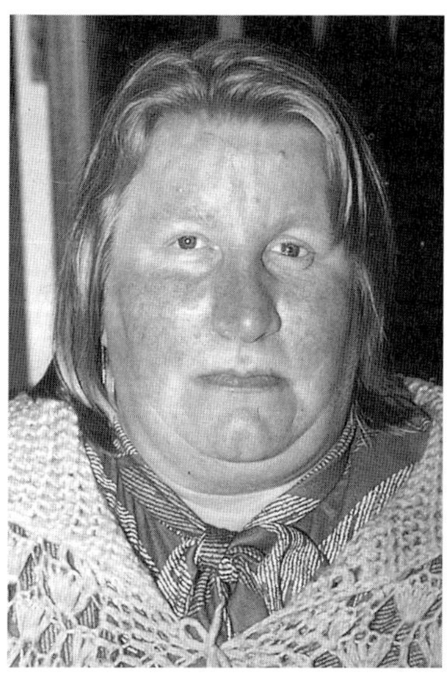

B

Baraitser M, Reardon W, Vijeratnam S: Nonspecific X-linked mental retardation with macrocephaly and obesity: a further family. Am J Med Genet 57:280, 1995.
Clark RD, Baraitser M: Letter to the Editor: a new X-linked mental retardation syndrome. Am J Med Genet 26:13, 1987.

Differential Matrix

Syndrome	Macro-cephaly	Obesity	Macro-orchidism	Comments
Clark-Baraitser	+	+	+	Large stature, dental abnormalities, broad nasal tip, thick lower lip
Atkin-Flaitz	+	+	+	Short stature, hypertelorism, downslanting palpebral fissures, broad nasal tip, thick lower lip, brachydactyly, seizures
XLMR-macrocephaly-macroorchidism	+	+	+	Elongated face, prominent mandible, clumsiness, repetitive movements
XLMR-macrocephaly	+	+	0	Downslanting palpebral fissures, elbow limitation
Fragile X	+	0	+	Normal or excessive growth, prominent forehead, long face, midface hypoplasia, large ears, prominent mandible
Lujan	+	0	+	Marfanoid habitus, asthenic build, long face, prominent forehead, high palate, micrognathia, long digits, pectus excavatum, joint hyperextensibility, seizures, hyperactivity

COFFIN-LOWRY SYNDROME

(Coffin Syndrome, Lowry Syndrome, MIM 303600)

DEFINITION. XLMR with short stature, distinctive facies, large soft hands, hypotonia, joint hyperextensibility, and skeletal changes. The gene (Rsk-2) maps to Xp22 and is a growth related serine threonine kinase.

SOMATIC FEATURES. Facial features evolve, becoming characteristic late in childhood or adolescence. In infancy, prominent forehead, hypertelorism, anteverted nares, tented upper lip, cupped ears, and hypotonia may be notable. As years pass, the head and stature grow slowly, the face elongates and coarsens, the ears become notably large, lips and nasal structures thicken, and the mouth is kept open, showing crowding of the teeth.

Musculoskeletal manifestations include large soft hands with tapering of the distal phalanges, pectus carinatum, bent knee habitus, flat feet, and generalized joint hyperextensibility. X-rays show delayed maturation, drumstick terminal phalanges with distal tufting and constriction of the adjacent shaft, short ulnas with angulation of the ulnar and radial epiphyses, short sternum with failure of

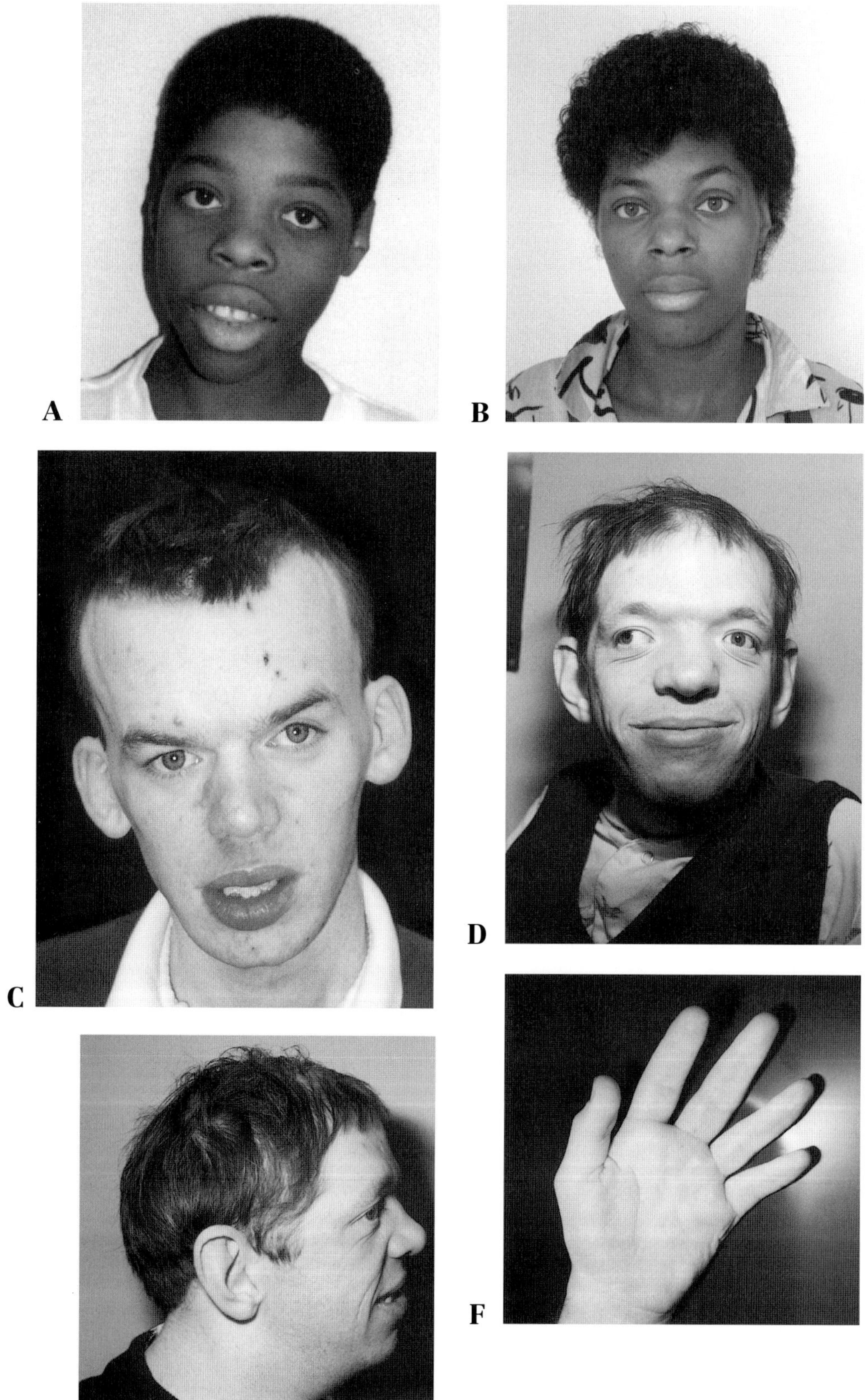
A
B
C
D
E
F

longitudinal fusion of the paired sternal segments, pectus carinatum, notches in the anterior–superior margin of the lumbar vertebrae, narrow intervertebral spaces, mild kyphosis or scoliosis, and accentuation of lumbar lordosis.

GROWTH AND DEVELOPMENT. Intrauterine growth is often slow and postnatal growth notable by continued microcephaly and short stature.

COGNITIVE FEATURES. Developmental milestones lag from the outset and ultimate cognitive function is profoundly impaired.

HETEROZYGOTE EXPRESSION. Carrier females consistently show a phenotype milder than males, consisting of short stature, coarse face with prominent brow, hypertelorism, thick nasal tissues, prominent lips, soft fleshy hands with thick fingers tapering distally, and variable radiographic findings similar to those in males. Cognitive function may be mildly impaired or normal.

COMMENT. Recognition that the entities reported by Coffin et al. in 1966 and Lowry et al. in 1971 represented one condition was reported by Temtamy et al. in 1975. The condition is represented in most large facilities for the mentally retarded. Diagnostic confusion most often results with XLMR–hypotonic facies syndrome (α-thalassemia–mental retardation) and Williams syndrome. Neither of these conditions has the large soft hands and radiographic changes found in Coffin-Lowry syndrome. Certain distinction can be achieved in cases which remain enigmatic through mutational analysis of the Rsk-2 gene (Coffin-Lowry) and XNP gene (XLMR-hypotonic facies syndrome) and through fluorescent in situ hybridization (FISH) studies of the elastin gene (Williams syndrome).

REFERENCES

Coffin GS, Siris E, Wegienka LC: Mental retardation with osteocartilaginous anomalies. Am J Dis Child 112:205, 1966.

Hanauer A, Alembik T, Gilgenkrantz S, et al.: Probable localisation of the Coffin-Lowry locus in Xp22.2-p22.1 by multipoint linkage analysis. Am J Med Genet 30:523, 1988.

Lowry B, Miller JR: A new dominant gene mental retardation syndrome. Am J Dis Child 121:496, 1971.

Temtamy SA, Miller JD, Hussels-Maumenee I: The Coffin-Lowry syndrome: an inherited faciodigital mental retardation syndrome. Pediatrics 86:724, 1975.

Trivier E, De Cesare D, Jacquot S, et al.: Mutations in the kinase Rsk-2 associated with Coffin-Lowry syndrome. Nature 384:567, 1996.

←

Coffin-Lowry Syndrome. Hypertelorism, prominent lips and open mouth at age 11 years (A); mother of patient in A showing hypertelorism and prominence of lips (B); cupped ears and prominent lips at age 29 years (C); microcephaly, hypertelorism, exotropia, large mouth, prominent lips, and thickened tapered digits at age 44 years (D–F).

Differential Matrix

Syndrome	Hypotonic Facies	Hyper-telorism	Arch Fingerprints/ Low Ridge Count	Comments
Coffin-Lowry	+	+	+	Short stature, microcephaly, anteverted nares, tented upper lip, prominent lips and large mouth, large ears, soft hands with tapered digits, pectus carinatum
Prieto	+	+	+	Ventricular enlargement, facial asymmetry, prominent eyes, ptosis, long narrow face, micrognathia, inguinal hernia, cryptorchidism
XLMR-hypotonic facies (Carpenter-Waziri) (Holmes-Gang) (Juberg-Marsidi)	+	+	0	Short stature, microcephaly, telecanthus, small triangular nose, tented upper lip, open mouth, spacing of teeth, genital anomalies, musculoskeletal anomalies, hemoglobin H inclusions in erythrocytes
Chudley-Lowry	+	0	+	Short stature, bitemporal narrowing, almond-shaped eyes, depressed nasal bridge, tented upper lip, open mouth, hypogonadism, obesity
XLMR-arch fingerprints-hypotonia	+	0	+	Tapered fingers, genu valgum, areflexia, hypotonia

Cranioorodigital Syndrome

(Otopalatodigital Syndrome Type II, OPD II Syndrome, OPD2, Faciopalatoosseous Syndrome, FPO, MIM 304120)

Definition. XLMR with facial features similar to otopalatodigital syndrome (OPD) I but more severe skeletal anomalies and with variable mental retardation. The gene for OPD II has not been mapped.

Somatic Features. Craniofacial features include prominent forehead, flat midface, flat/broad nasal bridge, hypertelorism, downslanting palpebral fissures, small mouth, marked micrognathia, cleft palate, low-set rotated ears, wide sutures, and large anterior fontanel with delayed closure. The thumbs and halluces are short and blunted. The halluces may be absent. The fingers are blunted, flexed, and overlapping. There is variable syndactyly, clinodactyly, and postaxial polydactyly of fingers and toes. The feet may be rockerbottom. The fibulae are small or absent. The other long bones are bowed and the elbows, wrists, knees, and hips may be subluxed/dislocated. The thorax is narrow with pectus excavatum.

The membranous calvarium is underossified and the base of the skull, the supraorbital ridges, and the long bones are osteosclerotic. These findings may resolve with age. Sinuses are absent or underaerated. The mandible and malar areas are hypoplastic. Phalanges (particularly distal), metacarpals, and metatarsals

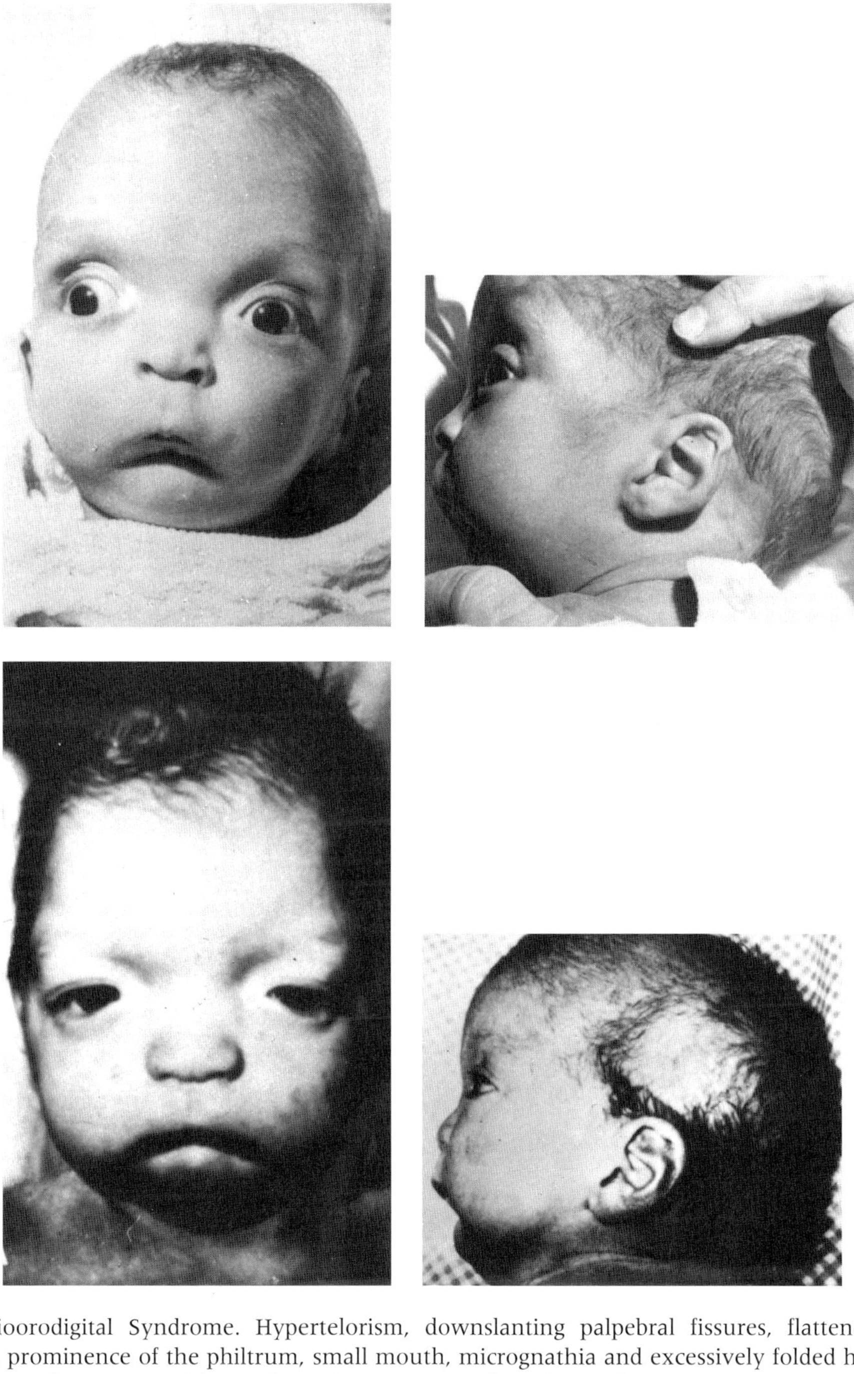

A

B

Cranioorodigital Syndrome. Hypertelorism, downslanting palpebral fissures, flattened nose, prominence of the philtrum, small mouth, micrognathia and excessively folded helices in infants reported by Fitch et al. 1983 (A) and Andre et al. 1981 (B).

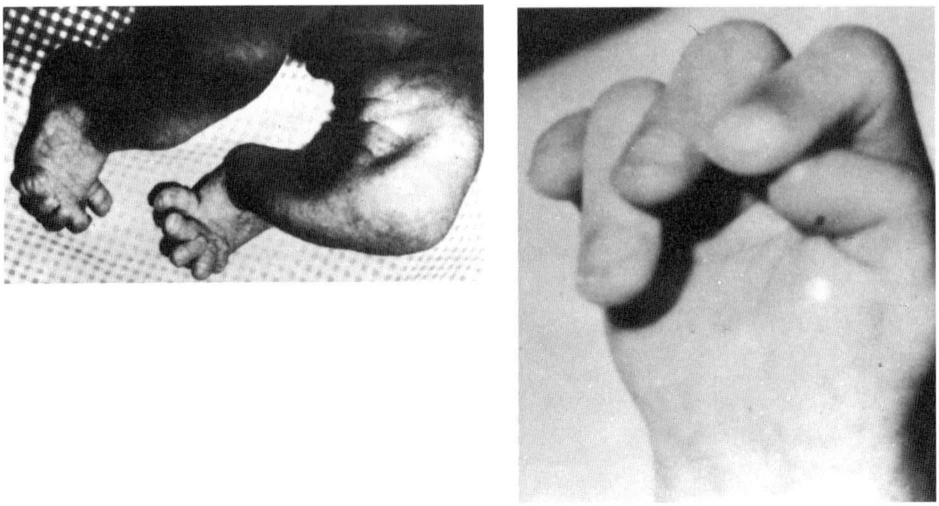

C

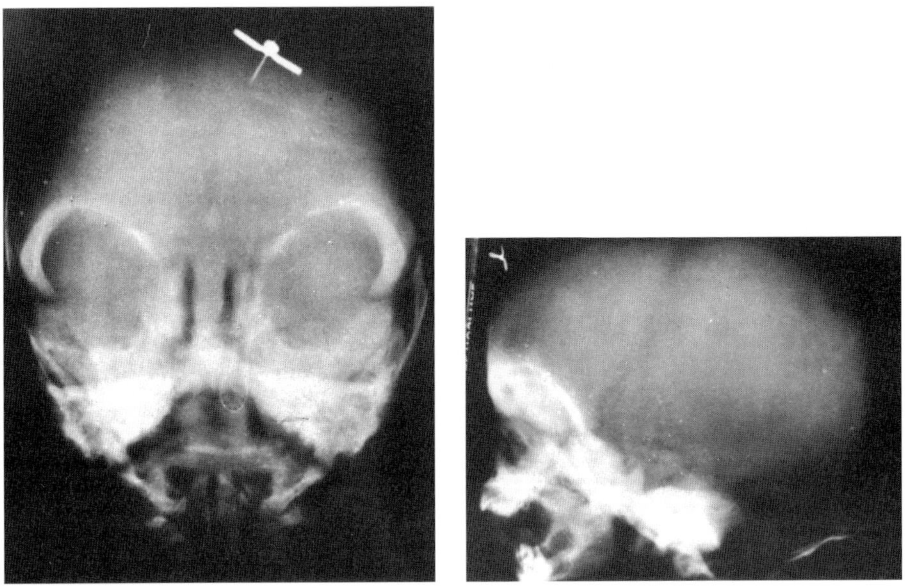

D

Cranioorodigital Syndrome. (continued) Spreading, malposition, and syndactyly of toes, and flexion and overlapping of fingers in patient reported by Andre et al. 1981 (C); skull X-rays at 1 month showing wide intraorbital distance, unusual ossification of the lateral orbital ridges, large calvarium with prominent occiput and dense base of the skull (D). Courtesy of the *American Journal of Medical Genetics,* Copyright © 1983, Alan R. Liss, Inc.

are short. Toe phalanges may not be visualized radiographically. The first metatarsals and halluces may be absent. Phalangeal bone maturation is advanced and carpal maturation delayed. The clavicles are thin and wavy. The ribs are narrow centrally and widened at the ends. Vertebral bodies may be flat.

GROWTH AND DEVELOPMENT. Survivors are undergrown.

COGNITIVE FEATURES. Most of the few survivors have some degree of mental retardation, but normal intellect has been reported. Mixed hearing impairment may affect speech development.

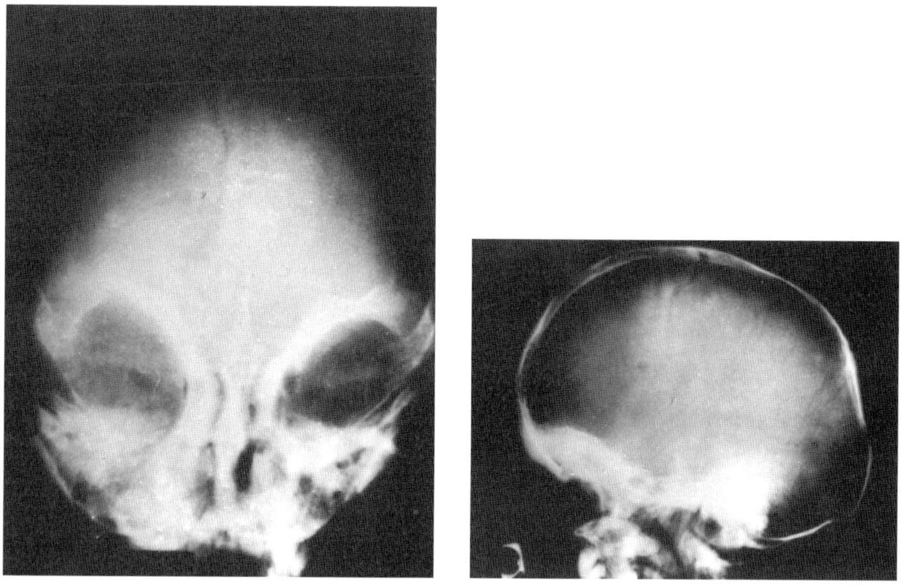

E

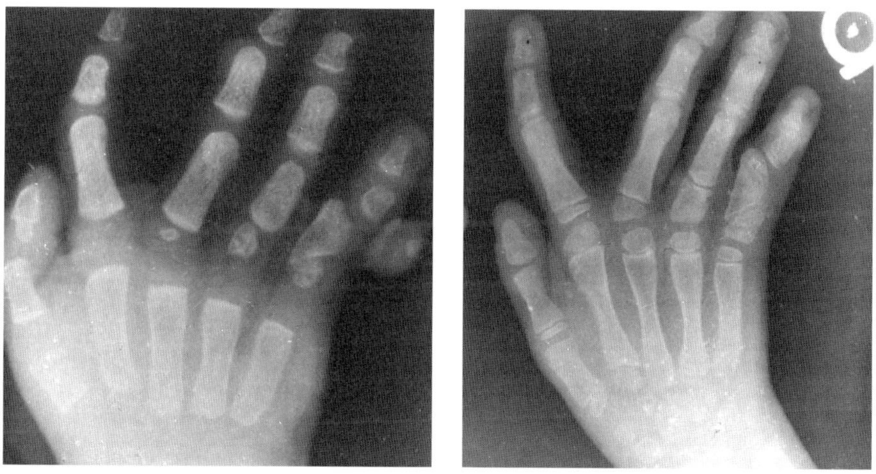

F

Cranioorodigital Syndrome. (continued) Skull X-ray at 6 years showing thickened calvarium, frontal bossing and underdevelopment of the paranasal sinuses and mastoids (E); and radiograph at ages 1 and 5 years showing shortening of the first metacarpal, peg-shaped epiphysis of the distal phalanx of the thumb, abnormal epiphyses of the proximal phalanges digits four and five, and postaxial polydactyly (F). Courtesy of *The American Journal of Medical Genetics,* copyright © 1983, Alan R. Liss, Inc.

Natural History. The majority are stillborn or die in the first year of life, usually from pulmonary infections and aspiration. Survivors are undergrown and may have orthopedic problems. Facial appearance, bone mineralization and bowing improve with age.

Heterozygote Expression. Heterozygotes may have mild facial, digital, and radiographic features. Features reported in females include frontal bossing, skull sclerosis, poorly aerated sinuses, hypertelorism, downslanting palpebral fissures, low-set ears, high arch palate, bifid uvula, micrognathia, syndactyly, and clinodactyly.

COMMENT. OPD II has not been mapped. Based on clinical similarities, it has been suggested that it is a variant of or allelic to OPD I or Melnick-Needles. It has also been suggested that it is contiguous to X-linked cerebellar hypoplasia/hydrocephalus.

REFERENCES

Fitch N, Jequier S, Papageorgiou A: A familial syndrome of cranial, facial, oral and limb anomalies. Clin Genet 10:226, 1976.

Fitch N, Jequier S, Gorlin R: The oto-palato-digital syndrome, proposed type II. Am J Med Genet 15:655, 1983.

Holder SE, Winter RM: Otopalatodigital syndrome type II. J Med Genet 30:310, 1993.

Preis S, Kemperdick H, Majewski F: Oto-palato-digital syndrome type II in two unrelated boys. Clin Genet 45:154, 1994.

Stratton RF, Bluestone DL: Oto-palato-digital syndrome type II with X-linked cerebellar hypoplasia/hydrocephalus. Am J Med Genet 41:169, 1991.

Differential Matrix

Syndrome	Cleft Palate	Hearing Impairment	Hypoplastic Fibulae	Comments
Cranioorodigital	+	+	+	Undergrowth, prominent forehead, flat/broad nasal bridge, ocular hypertelorism, downslanting palpebral fissures, flat midface, blunted, flexed, overlapping fingers, rockerbottom feet, subluxed/dislocated joints
Otopalatodigital I	+	+	+	Short stature, prominent brow, broad nasal root, apparent ocular hypertelorism, downslanting palpebral fissures, blunted distal phalanges, irregular curvature and spacing of digits, limitation of elbow movement

DUCHENNE MUSCULAR DYSTROPHY

(Pseudohypertrophic Muscular Dystrophy, MIM 310200)

DEFINITION. XLMR associated with pseudohypertrophic muscular dystrophy. Duchenne muscular dystrophy and the milder Becker muscular dystrophy are allelic disorders caused by mutations in dystrophin, a large gene occupying most of Xp21.3.

SOMATIC FEATURES. Major malformations or distinctive craniofacial manifestations do not occur. Hypertrophy of muscles, particularly those of the calf, pro-

Duchenne Muscular Dystrophy. Five-year-old male showing hypertrophy of the calf muscles.

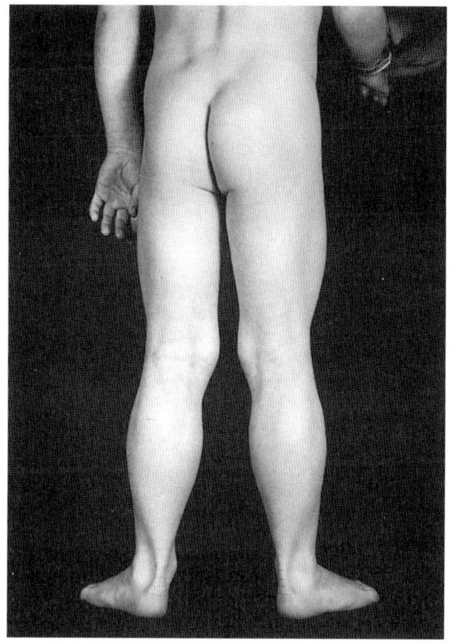

vides an early diagnostic clue, even before weakness is notable. Muscle destruction persists and progresses relentlessly leading to loss of ambulation in the teen years and death in early adult life. In the final stage, widespread muscle wasting, weakness, and contractures are evident.

Cognitive Features. A wide range of cognitive function can be found. Most cases have normal intelligence, but the average IQ measures 80–85 and about 20% will have IQ measures below 70. Three percent have severe mental retardation. Verbal abilities test lower than performance abilities. Affected brothers tend to have comparable cognitive function. An adequate explanation for the cognitive impairment has not been established but is presumed to be a pleiotropic effect of abnormal dystrophin on brain development.

Heterozygote Expression. Although carriers usually have normal muscle strength and intellectual function, 5%–10% may have slight muscle weakness and a lesser number may have cognitive impairment. Carrier manifestations have been attributed to preferential inactivation of the normal X chromosome. Carriers frequently have high normal or elevated creatine kinase levels. Muscle biopsy may show centralization of nuclei and variability in size of muscle fibers.

Neurological Findings. Neuromuscular findings generally follow a predictable and relentlessly progressive pattern. Weakness of the lower limbs and pelvic girdle initially manifests as clumsiness and inability to climb stairs. Hypertrophy of the calf muscles may give parents a false sense that the muscles are strong. Toe walking leads to pelvic tilt and compensatory hyperlordosis of the lumbar spine, both evident during the preschool years and accompanied by loss of deep tendon reflexes.

REFERENCES

Duchenne GBA: Recherches sur la paralysie musculaire pseudo-hypertrophique, ou paralysie myosclérosique. Gén Méd 11:5, 1868. Translation in Arch Neurol 19:629, 1968.

Differential Matrix

Syndrome	Muscle Hypertrophy	Weakness	Areflexia	Comments
Duchenne muscular dystrophy	+	+	+	Hypertrophy of calf muscles, elevated muscle enzymes, muscle wasting, contractures
Charcot-Marie-Tooth neuropathy, Cowchock variant	0	+	+	Peripheral motor and sensory neuropathy, deafness, pes cavus
Charcot-Marie-Tooth neuropathy, Ionasescu variant	0	+	+	Peripheral motor and sensory neuropathy, wasting of intrinsic hand muscles, enlarged ulnar nerves, pes cavus
Arts	0	+	+	Growth deficiency, hypotonia, ataxia, deafness, vision loss, seizures, childhood death
Myotubular myopathy	0	+	+	Hypotonic facies, open mouth, tented upper lip, hydrocephaly, long digits, cryptorchidism, hypotonia
Phosphoglycerate kinase deficiency	0	+	+	Expressionless face, seizures, myoglobinuria, hemolytic anemia

Dyskeratosis Congenita

(Zinsser-Engmann-Cole Syndrome, MIM 305000)

Definition. XLMR associated with dyskeratosis, hyperpigmentation, leukoplakia, alopecia, pancytopenia, predisposition to malignancy, and hypersplenomegaly. The gene is linked to DXS52 (Xq28), lod score 5.33.

Somatic Features. The major cutaneous manifestation is reticulate hyperpigmentation with predisposition for the neck, upper chest, and arms. The lesions may be telangiectatic and have interspersed areas of hypopigmented atrophic skin. The palms and soles have hyperkeratosis, and alopecia and hyperhidrosis are common. Bullae may follow minimal trauma. The nails develop longitudinal ridging or splitting, and friability, and may decrease in size or may be completely lost. Fingernail changes precede toenail changes. Leukoplakia forms on the oral mucosa but may affect other mucosal linings as well. When the epithelia of the lacrimal ducts is involved, blepharitis, conjunctivitis, and epiphora may result. Excessive cavities or tooth loss may be a part of the condition. In some cases, the

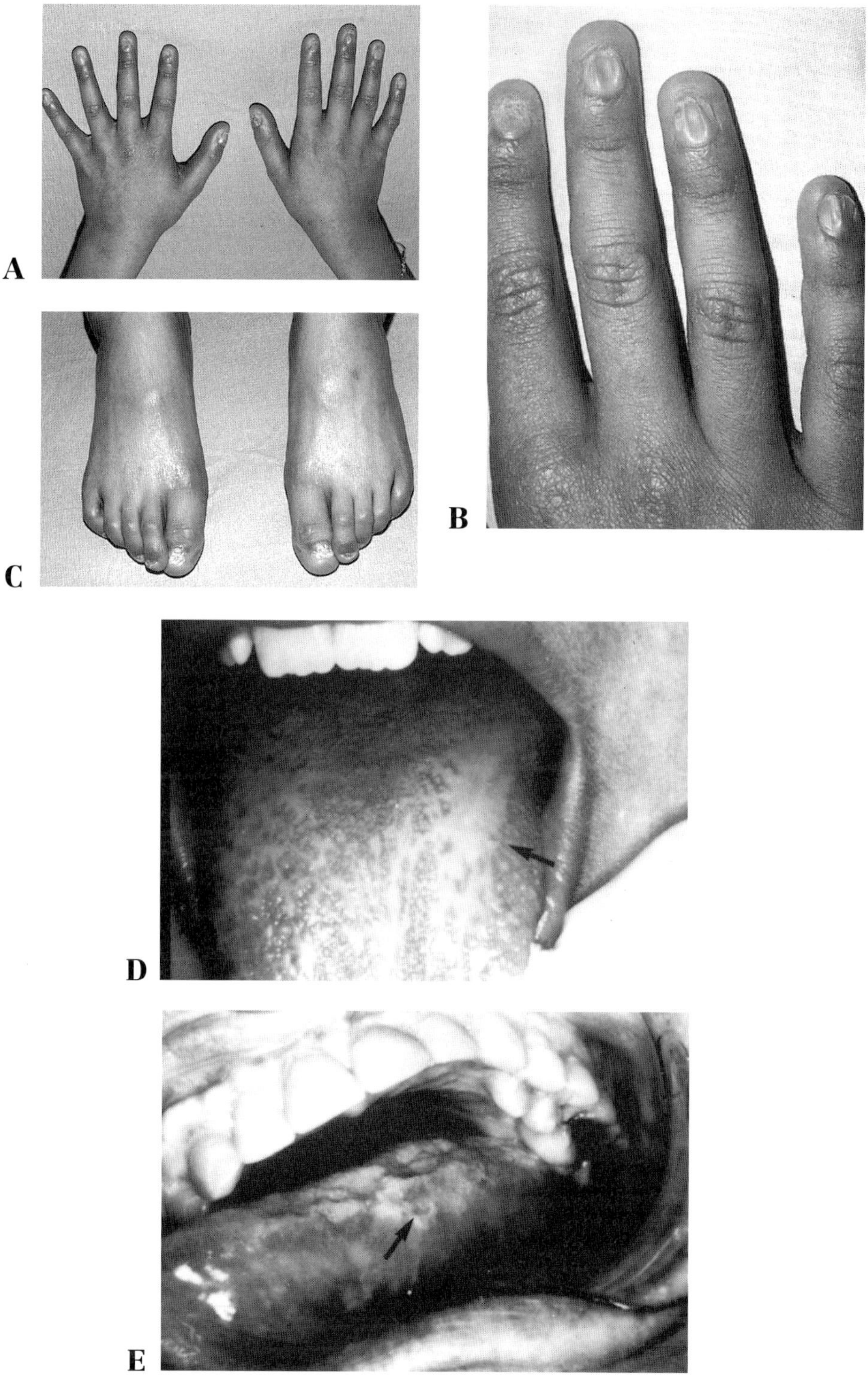

Dyskeratosis Congenita. Dystrophic nails of hands and feet (A-C); white plaques [arrows] of the tongue (D, E). Courtesy of Dr. Shashidhar Pai, Medical University of South Carolina, Charleston.

face appears pinched secondary to loss of subcutaneous tissue. Small penis and testes have been described, but hypogonadism appears quite rare.

Pancytopenia occurs in about half of cases, heralded by thrombocytopenia or anemia. Squamous cell carcinoma may occur in areas of cutaneous lesions or mucosal leukoplakia. Esophageal and pancreatic carcinomas and Hodgkin lymphoma occur in a small minority of cases.

GROWTH AND DEVELOPMENT. Usually normal with occasional cases having short stature.

COGNITIVE FEATURES. Normal cognitive function is the rule but with mild impairment in about a third of cases.

NATURAL HISTORY. Only rarely are any cutaneous manifestations present at birth. Usually they make their appearance between ages 5 and 12 years. Mucous membrane lesions appear slightly later and hematologic abnormalities occur in the midteen years with malignancy in young adult life.

HETEROZYGOTE EXPRESSION. None. The cases of female involvement likely represent autosomal inheritance.

LABORATORY. Excessive chromatid breakage, both spontaneous and radiation induced, has been reported in fibroblast cultures.

COMMENT. Cognitive impairment is not a prerequisite nor common feature of dyskeratosis congenita. Genetic heterogeneity exists with autosomal and X-linked forms.

REFERENCES

Arngrimsson R, Dokal I, Luzzatto L, et al.: Dyskeratosis congenita: three additional families show linkage to a locus in Xq28. J Med Genet 30:618, 1993.

Connor JM, Gatherer D, Gray FC, et al.: Assignment of the gene for dyskeratosis congenita to Xq28. Hum Genet 72:348, 1986.

Davidson HR, Connor JM: Dyskeratosis congenita. J Med Genet 25:843, 1988.

DeBauche DM, Pai GS, Stanley WS: Enhanced G_2 chromatid radiosensitivity in dyskeratosis congenita fibroblasts. Am J Hum Genet 46:350, 1990.

Sirinavin C, Trowbridge AA: Dyskeratosis congenita: clinical features and genetic aspects. J Med Genet 12:339, 1975.

Zinsser F: Atrophia cutis reticularis cum pigmentatione, dystrophia unguim et leukoplakia oris. Ikonographia Dermatol 5:219, 1910.

Differential Matrix

Syndrome	Cutaneous Lesions	Hair and/or Nail Abnormality	Malignancy Predisposition	Comments
Dyskeratosis congenita	+	+	+	Short stature, alopecia, hyperpigmented lesions, palmar and plantar hyperkeratosis, mucosal leukoplakia, pancytopenia
Cantu	+	+	0	Short stature, follicular keratosis, cortical atrophy, alopecia, microcephaly, seizures
Fitzsimmons	+	+	0	Pes cavus, hyperkeratosis of palms and soles, spastic paraplegia
Golabi-Ito-Hall	+	+	0	Microcephaly, short stature, telecanthus, high nasal root, cupped ears, cardiac malformation, thoracic asymmetry, sacral dimple, cutis marmorata
Goltz	+	+	0	Cataracts, ocular dysgenesis, linear areas of dermal aplasia, cutaneous adipose herniations, abnormal teeth, vertebral anomalies, limb reduction defects, genitourinary anomalies
Incontinentia pigmenti	+	0	0	Verrucous lesions, irregular hyperpigmentation, microcephaly, ocular anomalies, oligodontia, abnormally-shaped teeth, spasticity, seizures
MIDAS	+	0	0	Microphthalmia, ocular dysgenesis, corneal opacification, dermal aplasia, dysgenesis of corpus callosum, cardiac defects, cardiomyopathy
X-linked hereditary bullous dystrophy	+	+	0	Microcephaly, short stature, upslanting palpebral fissures, protruding ears, short and tapered digits, cardiac defects, small testes, early death from pulmonary infection

FITZSIMMONS SYNDROME

(XLMR–Spastic paraplegia–Palmoplantar Hyperkeratosis, MIM 309560)

DEFINITION. XLMR with lower limb spasticity, pes cavus, and hyperkeratosis of the palms and soles. The gene has not been localized.

SOMATIC FEATURES. Lower limb spasticity with pes cavus, clawing of the toes, wasting of the distal legs and ankles, and shuffling gait become apparent at about age 2 years. The upper limbs remain normal. Hyperkeratosis of the palms and soles becomes apparent later, in midchildhood. The soles are more severely af-

A

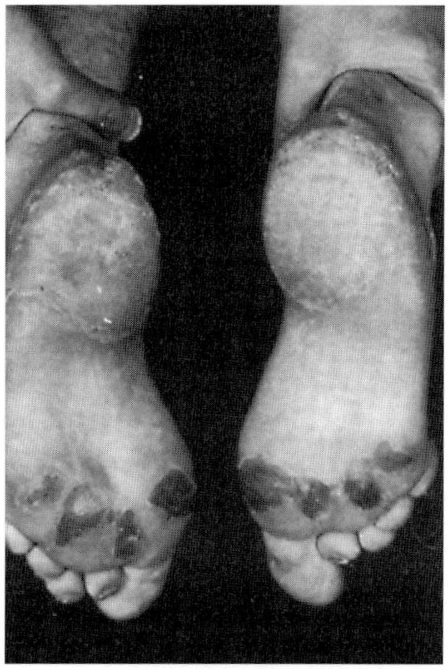

B

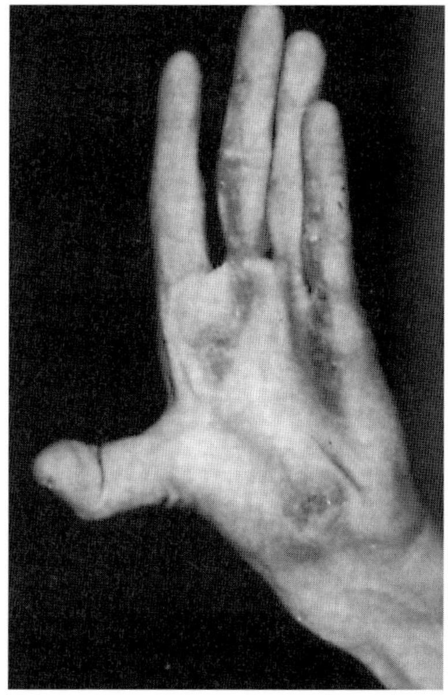

C

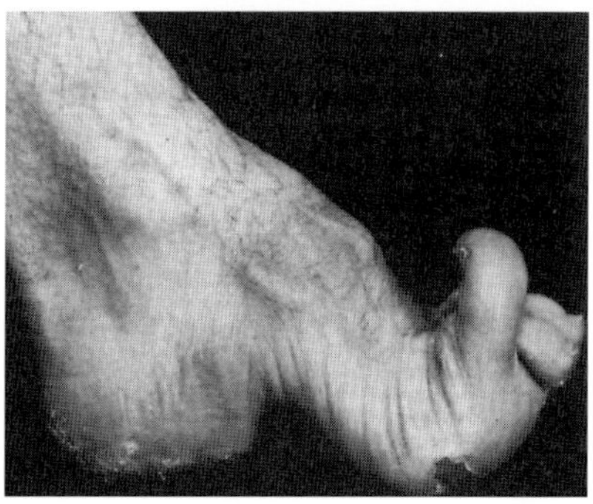

Fitzsimmons Syndrome. Hyperkeratosis of the soles (A); hyperkeratosis of the palms and dislocated thumb (B); pes cavus with dorsiflexion of the halux and clawing of the toes (C). Courtesy of *Clinical Genetics*, copyright 1983, Munksgaard, Copenhagen.

fected and erosions may occur over pressure points. The nails are thickened and fissured. Teeth and sweat production appear normal. A facial phenotype with high forehead, prominent nose, frontal balding, and sparse hair was noted in the index family. Hyperextensibility of the digits has been seen and in one case resulted in spontaneous thumb dislocation.

GROWTH AND DEVELOPMENT. Prenatal and postnatal growth appears normal. Developmental delay is obvious prior to age 1 year.

COGNITIVE FEATURES. Mild impairment.

NEUROLOGICAL FINDINGS. Hyperreflexia and spasticity begin by age 2 years and appear to become static during adulthood.

HETEROZYGOTE EXPRESSION. Females may show evidence of cutaneous and neurological involvement but have normal intelligence. While quite mild in comparison to the manifestations in males, fissuring and erythema of the palms, thickening of the soles, and thickened and fissured nails have been described in females. Deep tendon reflexes in the lower limbs are increased and the toes may show some clawing.

COMMENT. Ectodermal manifestations occur in only a few XLMR syndromes.

REFERENCE

Fitzsimmons JS, Fitzsimmons EM, McLachlan JI, et al.: Four brothers with mental retardation, spastic paraplegia and palmoplantar hyperkeratosis. A new syndrome? Clin Genet 23:329, 1983.

Differential Matrix

Syndrome	Alopecia/ Sparse Hair	Cutaneous Manifestation	Spastic Paraplegia	Comments
Fitzsimmons	+	+	+	Pes cavus, hyperkeratosis of palms and soles, dystrophic nails
Cantu	+	+	0	Short stature, microcephaly, hyperpigmented lesions, follicular keratosis, cortical atrophy, seizures, pancytopenia
Dykeratosis congenita	+	+	0	Short stature, hyperpigmented lesions, palmar and plantar hyperkeratosis, mucosal leukoplakia, nail ridging or splitting, pancytopenia, skin and mucosal lesions premalignant
X-linked hereditary bullous dystrophy	+	+	0	Microcephaly, short stature, upslanting palpebral fissures, protruding ears, digits short and tapered, cardiac defects, small testes, early death from pulmonary infection

FRAGILE X SYNDROME

(Marker X Syndrome, Fragile XA syndrome, Martin-Bell Syndrome, MIM 309550)

DEFINITION. XLMR with prominent forehead, long face, recessed midface, large ears, prominent mandible, and macroorchidism. The gene, FMR1, is located at Xq27.3. Greater than 99% of the mutations described are expansions of an unstable CGG repeat in the 5′ untranslated region of the gene.

SOMATIC FEATURES. A characteristic facial appearance—prominent forehead, elongation of the face, large ears with incompletely folded helices, hypoplasia of the midface, pale irides, and prominent mandible—evolves during the childhood and teenage years. In early childhood, the facial elongation and prominence of

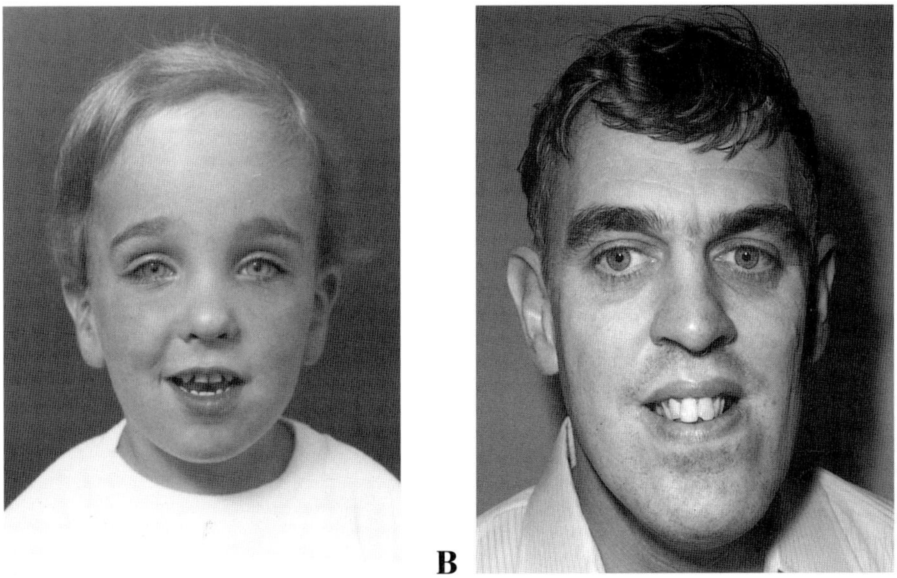

A B

Fragile X Syndrome. Microcephaly and prominent forehead at 3 years of age (A); typical adult facial appearance with long face, large ears and prominent jaw. (B).

the mandible may be less notable. The palate may be high and the teeth crowded. There is a tendency to joint laxity, manifesting as excessive hyperextensibility of digits, flat feet, and, less commonly, scoliosis and mitral valve prolapse. Testicular enlargement may be detected by measurement at any age. In adulthood, testicular volume usually exceeds 25 ml. Major malformations do not occur.

Growth and Development. Prenatal and early postnatal growth is robust with head circumference, length, and weight exceeding the average for age. Motor milestones lag from the outset, usually requiring twice the time for achievement of sitting alone, pulling up, and walking. Language development may be even further delayed.

Behavioral Manifestations. Perhaps the most formidable management issue in the fragile X syndrome is the difficult temperament. Children exhibit hyperactivity, attention deficiency, tantrums, perseverative speech, shyness, social anxiety, aggressive outbursts, autistic behaviors, tactile defensiveness, hand flapping, hand biting, and gaze avoidance. Most of these behaviors persist into adult life.

Neurological Findings. Childhood hypotonia and generalized seizures commonly resolve by adulthood.

Heterozygote Expression. About half of females with full mutations will have mental retardation, usually of less severe degree than males with full mutations. Somatic or cognitive manifestations are not to be anticipated among males or females with premutation alleles.

Imaging. Many children have had CNS imaging because of developmental delay and macrocephaly. The brain in fragile X syndrome appears overgrown with an increase in ventricular volume and a decrease in size of the cerebellar vermis.

COMMENT. Fragile X syndrome is the most commonly diagnosed XLMR syndrome. In the general population, males have a prevalence of one in 4000–6000. Fragile X syndrome accounts for about 2% of males and about 0.3% percent of females with mental retardation. Premutations with 50–230 CGG repeats in the 5′ untranslated region of the FMR1 gene do not cause mental retardation or other phenotypic abnormalities in males or females, but in females confer a risk for expansion of the CGG repeat to full mutation range (> 230 repeats) with transmission to the next generation.

REFERENCES

de Vries BBA, Halley DJJ, Oostra BA, Niermeijer MF: The fragile X syndrome. J Med Genet 35:579–589, 1998.

Lubs H: A marker X chromosome. Am J Hum Genet 21:231, 1969.

Martin JP, Bell J: A pedigree of mental defect showing sex-linkage. J Neur Psychiat 6:154, 1943.

Oberle I, Rousseau F, Heitz D, et al.: Instability of a 550-base pair DNA segment and abnormal methylation in fragile X syndrome. Science 252:1097, 1991.

Differential Matrix

Syndrome	Macro-cepahly	Macro-orchidism	Behavioral Aberrations	Comments
Fragile X	+	+	+	Normal or excessive growth, prominent forehead, long face, midface hypoplasia, large ears, prominent mandible
Atkin-Flaitz	+	+	0	Short stature, hypertelorism, downslanting palpebral fissures, broad nasal tip, thick lower lip, brachydactyly, seizures
Clark-Baraitser	+	+	0	Large stature, obesity, dental abnormalities, broad nasal tip, thick lower lip
XLMR-macrocephaly-macroorchidism	+	+	0	Elongated face, prominent mandible, clumsiness, repetitive movements
PPM-X	0	+	+	Spastic paraplegia, psychosis, parkinsonian features
Mucopolysaccharidosis IIA	+	0	+	Short stature, coarse facies, hepatosplenomegaly, hernias, joint stiffness, thick skin, hirsutism
Waisman-Laxova	+	0	+	Spasticity

GLYCEROL KINASE DEFICIENCY

(XLMR-Hyperglycerolemia, MIM 307030)

DEFINITION. XLMR and slow growth, hypogonadism, spasticity, muscular dystrophy, and osteoporosis associated with hyperglycerolemia, glyceroluria, and glycerol kinase deficiency. The full syndrome is seen only where glycerol kinase deficiency is a component of the contiguous gene syndrome involving adjacent genes for gonadotropin deficiency, adrenal hypoplasia, and Duchenne muscular dystrophy. Isolated glycerol kinase deficiency may be asymptomatic or may cause recurrent episodes of lethargy, hypothermia, vomiting, and acidemia. The gene, GKD, is located in Xp21.3.

SOMATIC FEATURES. No somatic manifestations should be anticipated in isolated glycerol kinase deficiency. Short stature, hypogonadotropic hypogonadism, osteoporosis with fractures, muscular weakness with pseudohypertrophy, spasticity, seizures, esotropia, and developmental impairment may occur when adjacent genes are deleted as part of the complex glycerol kinase deficiency contiguous gene syndrome.

GROWTH AND DEVELOPMENT. Postnatal growth deficiency and delayed development occur only when genes adjacent to glycerol kinase are deleted as part of a contiguous gene syndrome.

NEUROLOGICAL FINDINGS. Recurrences of lethargy and hypothermia and of vomiting, acidemia, and stupor have occurred in children with isolated glycerol kinase deficiency. These symptoms resolved with institution of a low-fat diet. Muscle weakness and spasticity may occur in patients with large deletions involving adjacent genes.

HETEROZYGOTE EXPRESSION. Female carriers of isolated glycerol kinase deficiency do not show clinical manifestations, nor do those females with deletions of adjacent genes as part of the complex glycerol kinase deficiency contiguous gene syndrome.

COMMENT. Most patients with glycerol kinase deficiency have had deletions of this gene which extended to involve adjacent genes. The gene order appears to be Xpter-GTD-AHC-GK-DMD-OTC-Xcen. It is not clear that glycerol kinase deficiency alone causes mental retardation. Certainly there exist adult forms of glycerol kinase deficiency which have no clinical manifestations. Grier et al. have reported a case of presumed isolated glycerol kinase deficiency in a male infant with recurrent hypothermia and lethargy. Ginns et al. and Eriksson et al. reported children with recurrent episodes of vomiting, acidemia, and stupor. A low-fat diet resulted in clinical and developmental improvement in these cases. Developmental impairment might result from these recurrent episodes. Perhaps more likely, mental retardation may result from involvement of a separate gene. There appears to be one such gene distal to the adrenal hypoplasia gene. Alternatively, mental impairment may result from deletions that extend into the 3′ end of the DMD gene.

REFERENCES

Bartley JA, Patil S, Davenport S, et al.: Duchenne muscular dystrophy, glycerol kinase deficiency, and adrenal insufficiency associated with Xp21 interstitial deletion. J Pediatr 108:189, 1986.

Eriksson A, Lindstedt S, Ransnas L, et al.: Deficiency of glycerol kinase (EC2.7.1.30). Clin Chem 29:718, 1983.

Ginns EI, Barranger JA, McClean SW, et al.: Hyperglycerolemia secondary to glycerol kinase deficiency in a child without neurological deficits. Pediatr Res 16:191A, 1982.

Grier RE, Howell RR, Wu D, et al.: Isolated glycerol kinase deficiency: nutritional and molecular genetic studies. Am J Hum Genet 45(Suppl):A6, 1989.

Matsumoto T, Kondoh T, Yoshimoto M, et al.: Complex glycerol kinase deficiency: molecular-genetic, cytogenetic, and clinical studies of five Japanese patients. Am J Med Genet 31:603, 1988.

McCabe ERB, Guggenheim MA, Fennessey PV, et al.: Glyceroluria, psychomotor retardation, spasticity, dystrophic myopathy, and osteoporosis in a sibship. Pediatr Res 11:527, 1977.

McCabe ERB, Fennessey PV, Guggenheim MA, et al.: Human glycerol kinase deficiency with hyperglycerolemia and glyceroluria. Biochem Biophys Res Commun 78:1327, 1977.

Walker AP, Muscatelli F, Monaco AP: Isolation of the human Xp21 glycerol kinase gene by positional cloning. Hum Mol Genet 2:107, 1993.

Willard HF: Cloning of the X-linked glycerol kinase gene. Hum Mol Genet 2:95, 1993.

Differential Matrix

Syndrome	Hypothermia	Lethargy	Recurrent Vomiting	Comments
Glycerol kinase deficiency	+	+	+	Short stature, hypogonadotrophic hypogonadism, osteoporosis, fractures, muscle weakness, spasticity and seizures when a part of GKD contiguous gene syndrome. Isolated GKD may be asymptomatic.
Menkes	+	+	0	Growth deficiency, sparse kinky hair, pallor, limited movement, hypertonicity, seizures, metaphyseal widening and spurs, arterial tortuosity, childhood death
Ornithine transcarbamylase deficiency	0	+	+	Chronic or intermittent hyperammonemia, microcephaly, protein-induced vomiting and lethargy, ataxia, seizures
Pyruvate dehydrogenase deficiency	0	+	+	Lactic acidosis, microcephaly, hypotonia, ataxia, dysarthria, CNS anomalies

G_{M3} GANGLIOSIDOSIS

(G_{M3} Sphingolipodystrophy, MIM 305650)

This entity is listed for historical purposes. It has been reported in only a single case and is believed by many authorities not to exist as a specific disorder.

The single male case reported showed widespread manifestations of lysosomal storage disease at birth, including coarsening of the facies, gingival hypertrophy, macroglossia, thick skin, hirsutism, broad hands and feet with digital stiffness or contractures, inguinal and umbilical hernias, and enlarged liver and spleen. Prior to death at $3^1/_2$ months, the course was complicated by lethargy or unresponsiveness, hypotonia, respiratory distress, pneumonia, and seizures.

Radiographs at birth were normal. Urine was negative for mucopolysaccharide excretion. G_{M3} gangliosides were found in the liver and a defect in ganglioside biosynthesis was proposed.

COMMENT. Clinical phenotype appeared identical to G_{M1} gangliosidosis although progression to death was faster. The suggestion of X-linkage was based on the history of a maternal uncle with similar signs who died at age $2^1/_2$ months. Other cases have not been reported and a specific defect of lysosomal metabolism was not demonstrated in the proband.

REFERENCES

Maclaren NK, Max SR, Cornblath M, et al.: GM_3 gangliosidosis: a novel human sphingolipodystrophy. Pediatrics 57:106, 1976.

Max SR, Maclaren NK, Brady RO, et al.: GM_3 (hematoside) sphingolipodystrophy. NEJM 291:929, 1974.

GOLABI-ITO-HALL SYNDROME

DEFINITION. XLMR with short stature, microcephaly, narrow or triangular face, telecanthus, epicanthus, upslanting palpebral fissures, cupped ears, and ectodermal manifestations. The gene has not been mapped.

SOMATIC FEATURES. Characteristic manifestations are found in each of the craniofacial segments. The cranium is small and the triangular facial configuration present in childhood elongates during the teen years. The upper face is perhaps most distinctive because of the narrow forehead with prominence of the glabella or metopic ridging, telecanthus, epicanthus, and upslanting palpebral fissures. A long nose with high nasal root and cupped ears are the major midfacial manifestations. The lower facial segment shows a thin upper lip, prominent maxillary central incisors, narrow palate with wide palatine ridges, and, at least in early childhood, a small mandible. A variety of ectodermal manifestations, including dry brittle scalp hair, nail hypoplasia, cutis marmorata, and large maxillary central incisors have been described. Chest asymmetry was noted in two cases and atrial septal defect in two cases.

Golabi-Ito-Hall Syndrome. Affected male at age 21 years showing short stature, microcephaly, triangular face, cupped ears, upslanted palpebral fissures, long nose, thin upper lip, and small mandible (A–C); affected cousin at age 13 years (D). Courtesy of Dr. Herbert A. Lubs, University of Miami School of Medicine, Miami.

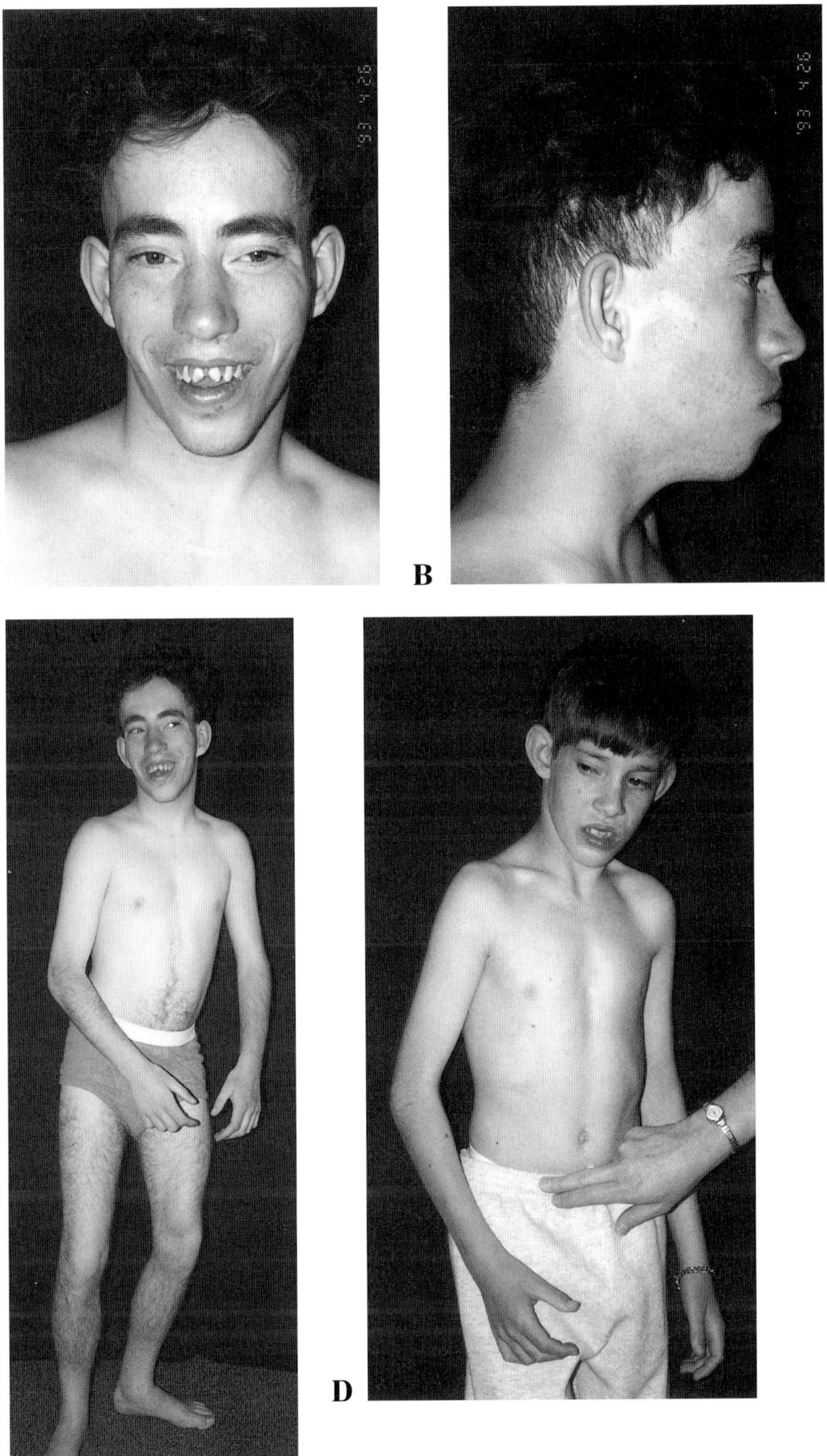

A B C D

GROWTH AND DEVELOPMENT. Birth weight and head circumference are normal but in the lower percentiles. Postnatally, all growth percentiles lag, leading to microcephaly and short stature. Global developmental delay becomes obvious during infancy and early childhood.

COGNITIVE FEATURES. The degree of cognitive impairment was not reported. An IQ of 23 was found in one affected male who also had neonatal complications.

NEUROLOGICAL FINDINGS. Abnormal neurologic findings—lower limb hyperreflexia, Babinski signs, petit mal seizures, and mild sensorineural hearing loss—were described in only one case who required resuscitation at birth.

HETEROZYGOTE EXPRESSION. None reported.

LABORATORY. Chronic hematuria of unknown cause occurred in one case.

COMMENT. Only a single family has been reported. The presence of chronic hematuria and sensorineural hearing loss in one affected male suggests Alport syndrome, an X-linked entity which does not have mental retardation.

REFERENCES

Golabi M, Ito M, Hall BD: A new X-linked multiple congenital anomalies/mental retardation syndrome. Am J Med Genet 17:367, 1984.

Differential Matrix

Syndrome	Distinctive Craniofacial Findings	Cardiac Malformation	Ectodermal Manifestation	Comments
Golabi-Ito-Hall	+	+	+	Microcephaly, short stature, telecanthus, high nasal root, cupped ears, thoracic asymmetry, sacral dimple, dry/brittle/sparse hair, cutis marmorata, nail hypoplasia
MIDAS	+	+	+	Microphthalmia, ocular dysgenesis, corneal opacification, dermal aplasia, dysgenesis of corpus callosum
X-linked hereditary bullous dystrophy	+	+	+	Microcephaly, short stature, upslanting palpebral fissures, protruding ears, short and tapered digits, bullous dystrophy, small testes, early death from pulmonary infection
Lenz microphthalmia	+	+	0	Microcephaly, microphthalmia, ocular dysgenesis, malformed ears, cleft lip/palate, cardiac and genitourinary anomalies, thumb duplication or hypoplasia, narrow shoulders
Opitz FG	+	+	0	Macrocephaly, broad forehead, down-slanted palpebral fissures, everted lower lip, dysgenesis of corpus callosum, imperforate anus, constipation, flat thumbs and great toes, hypotonia
Simpson-Golabi-Behmel	+	+	0	Somatic overgrowth, supernumerary nipples, polydactyly
Telecanthus-hypospadias	+	+	0	High broad nasal root, dysplastic ears, cleft lip/palate, abnormal cranial contour or symmetry
XLMR-hypotonic facies (Carpenter-Waziri) (Holmes-Gang) (Juberg-Marsidi)	+	+	0	Microcephaly, short stature, small testes, telecanthus, small triangular nose, tented upper lip, open mouth, spacing of teeth, genital anomalies, musculoskeletal anomalies, hemoglobin H inclusions in erythrocytes
Oral-facial-digital I	+	0	+	Sparse scalp hair, dystopia canthorum, flat midface, hypoplastic alae nasi, hypertrophic and aberrant oral frenuli, intraoral clefts and pseudoclefts, lingual hamartomas, brachydactyly, syndactyly, clinodactyly, structural brain anomalies, polycystic kidneys

GOLDBLATT SPASTIC PARAPLEGIA SYNDROME

(MIM 312920)

DEFINITION. XLMR with nystagmus, optic atrophy, muscle hypoplasia, contractures, ataxia, and spasticity. The gene is linked to marker pDP34 (DXYS1X) in Xq21.3, lod score 3.3.

SOMATIC FEATURES. Malformations or facial abnormalities do not occur. Optic atrophy, nystagmus and exotropia are present. The leg muscles are underdeveloped and signs of spasticity and ataxia are present.

GROWTH AND DEVELOPMENT. Not known.

COGNITIVE FEATURES. Mildly impaired.

NEUROLOGICAL FINDINGS. Nystagmus, exotropia, spastic paraplegia with increased deep tendon reflexes and Babinski signs are present from infancy. Ataxia, dysarthria, dysmetria, and dysdiadochokinesia may be present as well. Independent ambulation is not achieved, but muscle power of the arms and continence of bowel and bladder are normal.

HETEROZYGOTE EXPRESSION. None.

COMMENT. Although more clinically severe, the neuromuscular and ocular findings suggest that this syndrome may be a variant of Pelizaeus-Merzbacher syndrome, the gene for which has been localized to Xq21.1.

REFERENCE

Goldblatt J, Ballo R, Sachs B, et al.: X-linked spastic paraplegia: evidence for homogeneity with a variable phenotype. Clin Genet 35:116, 1989.

Differential Matrix

Syndrome	Ataxia	Spastic Paraplegia	Muscle Hypoplasia	Comments
Goldblatt spastic paraplegia	+	+	+	Optic atrophy, exotropia, nystagmus, dysarthria, contractures
Allan-Herndon-Dudley	+	+	+	Childhood hypotonia, dysarthria, athetosis, large ears with cupping or abnormal architecture, contractures
Apak ataxia-spastic diplegia	+	+	+	Short stature, clubfoot
Arena	+	+	+	Clubfoot, iron deposits in basal ganglia, rigidity, dystonia
XLMR-spastic paraplegia-athetosis	+	+	+	Nystagmus, weakness, dysarthria, contractures
Mohr-Tranebjaerg (Jensen)	+	+	0	Neurologic deterioration with childhood onset, dystonia
Pelizaeus-Merzbacher	+	+	0	Optic atrophy, nystagmus, hypotonia, dystonia, DNA dysmyelination
Pettigrew	+	+	0	Microcephaly or hydrocephaly, long face with macrostomia and prognathism, Dandy-Walker malformation, small testes, contractures, choreoathetosis, iron deposits in basal ganglia
X-linked spastic paraplegia, type 7	+	+	0	Nystagmus, reduced vision, absent speech and ambulation, bowel and bladder dysfunction

GOLTZ SYNDROME

(Focal Dermal Hypoplasia, MIM 305600)

DEFINITION. XLMR in females associated with linear areas of thin or absent skin, herniated cutaneous papules of adipose tissue, dystrophic nails, abnormal teeth and hair, cataracts, and reduction defects of the limbs. On the basis of X chromosome deletions and rearrangements, the gene appears to be located in the distal short arm at Xp22.3.

SOMATIC FEATURES. Focal areas of dermal hypoplasia or aplasia date from birth, occur on all skin surfaces except the palms and soles, vary considerably in size, and tend to be linear when on the limbs. Affected areas of skin are thin and depressed, forming irregular plaques which may be darker or lighter than adjacent normal skin. Histologically, the connective tissue of the corium is replaced completely or partially by adipose tissue. Yellowish saccular herniations of fat encased in the thinnest covering of epidermis occur, perhaps with a predilection in

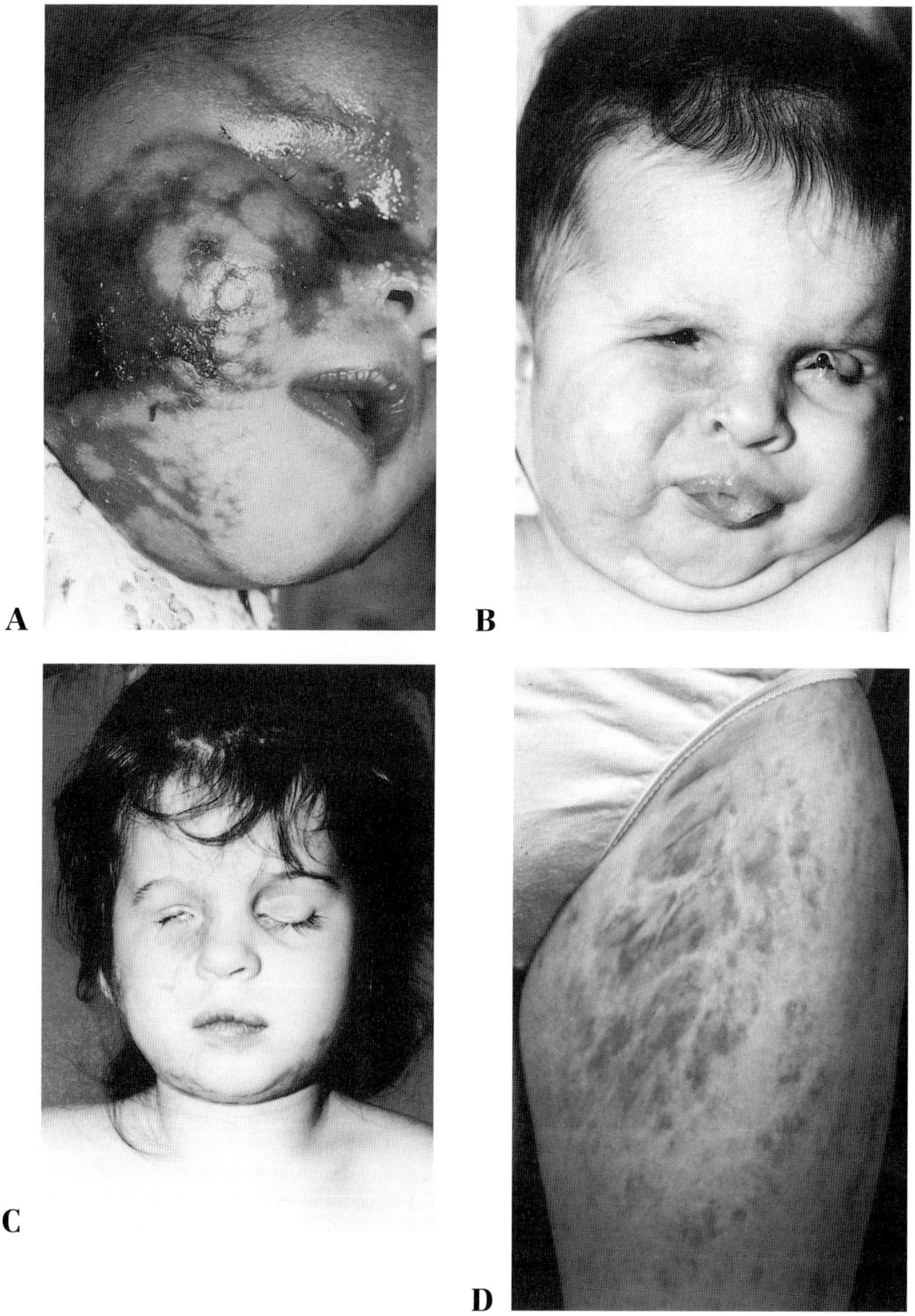

Goltz Syndrome. Oculocutaneous manifestations involving the face showing microphthalmia, small palpebral fissures, and hypoplastic or aplastic areas of skin at ages 2 weeks, 3 months, and 2 years (A–C); thinning of skin of the proximal thigh with herniations of adipose tissue (D).

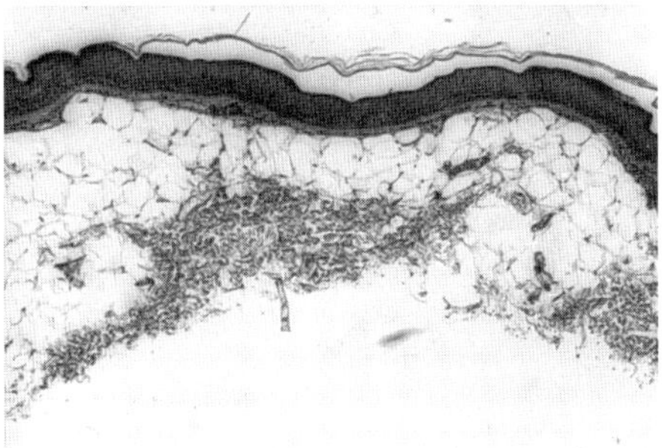
E

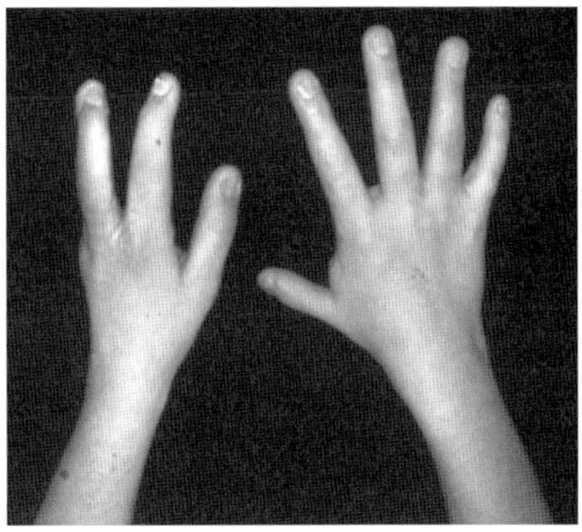
F

Goltz Syndrome. (continued) Replacement of connective tissue of the corium with adipose tissue (E); upper limb malformation with absence of the ulnar rays of the left hand and thumb hypoplasia of the right hand (F). Illustrations A–C courtesy of Dr. Arthur S. Aylsworth, University of North Carolina School of Medicine, Chapel Hill. Illustrations D–F courtesy of Dr. Robert Gorlin, University of Minnesota, Minneapolis.

body folds and in the perioral and perianal areas and are considered a pathognomonic finding.

Other ectodermal tissues have involvement as well. The hair is generally sparse and in localized areas of the scalp and pubic area may be totally absent. Dystrophic or absent nails occur, particularly when adjacent skin is involved. Oligodontia, hypoplastic teeth, notched incisors, malocclusion or irregular spacing, or delayed eruption can be found in nearly half of cases.

Ocular defects, often unilateral or asymmetric, include epiphora, strabismus, microphthalmia, iris colobomas, cataracts, optic atrophy, and retinal colobomas.

In addition to contributions from the ocular, dental, and cutaneous abnormalities, the facies may be otherwise distinctive, with facial asymmetry, simply formed and cupped ears, broad nasal tip and, in some cases, notching of the alae nasi. Cleft lip, cleft palate, cleft tongue, and notching of the alveolar ridges may also occur.

Most cases have malformations of the hands and feet, typically reduction defects with the missing rays being central, medial, or lateral. Limb asymmetry, syndactyly, hemivertebrae, and clavicular anomalies occur as well. Longitudinal striations in the metaphyses of the long bones have been demonstrated in about 20% of cases.

Other anomalies may include omphalocele, inguinal hernia, hiatal hernia, and unusually placed hernias at the sites of dermal hypoplasia. Renal dysplasia and horseshoe kidney have also been reported.

GROWTH AND DEVELOPMENT. Growth is globally impaired, beginning prior to birth and often resulting in microcephaly and short stature. Asymmetry commonly affects the face, limbs, and trunk. Most achieve developmental milestones at the normal times; others are variably delayed.

COGNITIVE FEATURES. In most cases, cognitive function is normal. The minority of cases with impaired function, perhaps 15%, are represented primarily among those with microcephaly and severe ocular malformations.

IMAGING. The CNS structures are usually normal. Rarely noted abnormalities include hydrocephalus and agenesis of the corpus callosum.

COMMENT. Most cases are sporadic, although in some instances female relatives have had mild evidence of ectodermal involvement. As with other female-limited disorders, gestational lethality in males has been proposed. Several mildly affected males have been reported, their involvement being limited to the skin and so mild as to preclude diagnosis until they fathered daughters with typical manifestations. These males likely represent mosaics with only a minority of somatic cells affected.

REFERENCES

Burgdorf WHC, Dick GF, Soderberg MD, et al.: Focal dermal hypoplasia in a father and daughter. Am Acad Dermatol 4:273, 1981.

Goltz RW, Peterson WC, Gorlin RJ, et al.: Focal dermal hypoplasia. Arch Dermatol 86:52, 1962.

Goltz RW: Focal dermal hypoplasia syndrome. An Update. Arch Dermatol 128:1108, 1992.

Temple IK, MacDowall P, Baraitser M, et al.: Focal dermal hypoplasia (Goltz syndrome). J Med Genet 27:180, 1990.

Differential Matrix

Syndrome	Ocular Abnormality	Urogenital Anomalies	Cutaneous Abnormality	Comments
Goltz	+	+	+	Linear areas of dermal aplasia, dystrophic nails, abnormal teeth and hair, vertebral anomalies, limb reduction defects
Lenz microphthalmia	+	+	+	Short stature, microcephaly, microphthalmia, cupped or dysplastic ears, thumb anomalies, cleft lip/palate, sloped shoulders, clavicular hypoplasia, barrel chest, kyphoscoliosis
Cerebrooculogenital	+	+	0	Short stature, microcephaly, hydrocephaly, agenesis of corpus callosum, microphthalmia, ptosis, hypospadias, cryptorchidism, clubfoot, spasticity
Lowe	+	+	0	Short stature, hypotonia, aminoaciduria, progressive renal disease
Wittwer	+	+	0	Growth deficiency, microcephaly, microphthalmia, hearing loss, vision loss, hypertelorism, hypotonia, seizures
MIDAS	+	0	+	Corneal opacification, dermal aplasia, dysgenesis of corpus callosum, cardiac defects, cardiomyopathy

GRAHAM ANOPHTHALMIA SYNDROME

(Graham Syndrome, X-Linked Anophthalmia, MIM 301590)

DEFINITION. XLMR with anophthalmia and ankyloblepharon. Linkage analysis suggests that the gene may be in Xq27-q28.
SOMATIC FEATURES. Clinical anophthalmia, ankyloblepharon, shallow orbits, and short eyebrows and eyelids make up the facial phenotype. Other common characteristics have not been described. One male had preauricular tags and cleft soft palate.
COGNITIVE FEATURES. Severe impairment.
GROWTH AND DEVELOPMENT. Unknown.
HETEROZYGOTE EXPRESSION. None.
COMMENT. Only a single family with seven affected males in two generations has been reported. Limitation of the clinical manifestations to the ocular and periocular region makes possible differentiation from other microphthalmia–mental retardation syndromes.

A
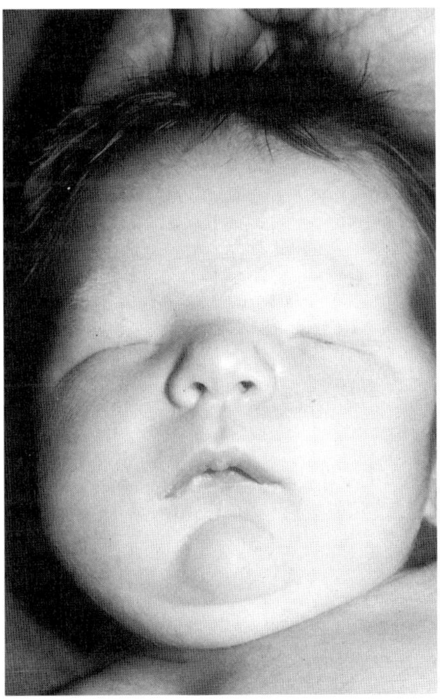

B
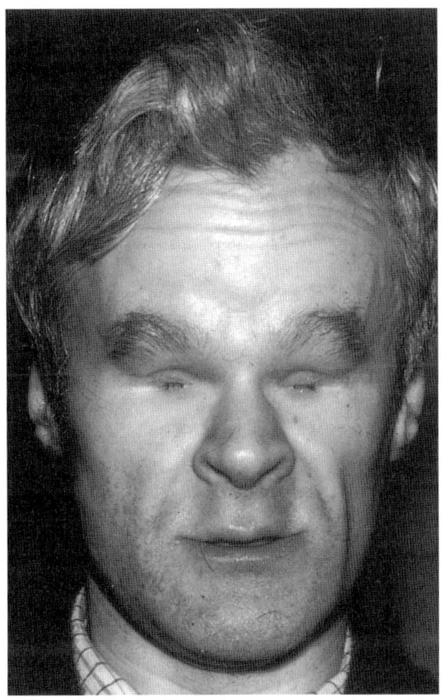

Graham Anophthalmia Syndrome. Affected males in infancy and adulthood showing bilateral anophthalmia and ankyloblepharon. Courtesy of Dr. Norman Nevin, Northern Ireland Regional Genetic Center, Belfast.

REFERENCE

Graham CA, Redmond RM, Nevin NC: X-linked clinical anophthalmos: localization of the gene to Xq27-Xq28. Ophthalmic Pediatr Genet 12:43, 1990.

Differential Matrix

Syndrome	Ocular Dysgenesis	Short or Fused Palpebral Fissures	Comments
Graham anophthalmia	+	+	Microphthalmia, shallow orbits, short eyebrows
Aicardi	+	+	Lacunar retinopathy, costovertebral anomalies, agenesis of corpus callosum, seizures
Goltz	+	+	Cataracts, linear areas of dermal aplasia, cutaneous adipose herniations, dystrophic nails, abnormal teeth and hair, vertebral anomalies, limb reduction defects, genitourinary anomalies
MIDAS	+	+	Microphthalmia, corneal opacification, dermal aplasia, dysgenesis of corpus callosum, cardiac defects, cardiomyopathy
Lenz microphthalmia	+	0	Short stature, microcephaly, cupped or dyplastic ears, thumb anomalies, urogenital anomalies, cleft lip/palate, sloped shoulders, clavicular hypoplasia, barrel chest, kyphoscoliosis
Cerebrooculogenital	+	0	Short stature, microcephaly, hydrocephaly, agenesis of corpus callosum, microphthalmia, ptosis, hypospadias, cryptorchidism, clubfoot, spasticity
Wittwer	+	0	Growth deficiency, microcephaly, hearing loss, vision loss, hypertelorism, genitourinary anomalies, hypotonia, seizures

Gustavson Syndrome

(XLMR–Optic Atrophy–Deafness–Seizures, MIM 309555)

Definition. XLMR with microcephaly, short stature, blindness, deafness, seizures, spasticity, and early death. The gene has been localized to the region flanked by DXS424 (Xq23) and DXS297 (Xq27.3), lod score 3.35.

Somatic Features. Microcephaly, optic atrophy, large ears, marked short stature, and contractures of the large joints give a distinctive, if not specific, presentation. The fontanels are quite small if palpable at all. Vertical talus gives the foot a rockerbottom or calcaneovalgus configuration. Ultrasound and CT imaging have demonstrated marked undergrowth of the brain, enlarged cerebral ventricles, cerebellar hypoplasia, and, in one case, Dandy-Walker malformation.

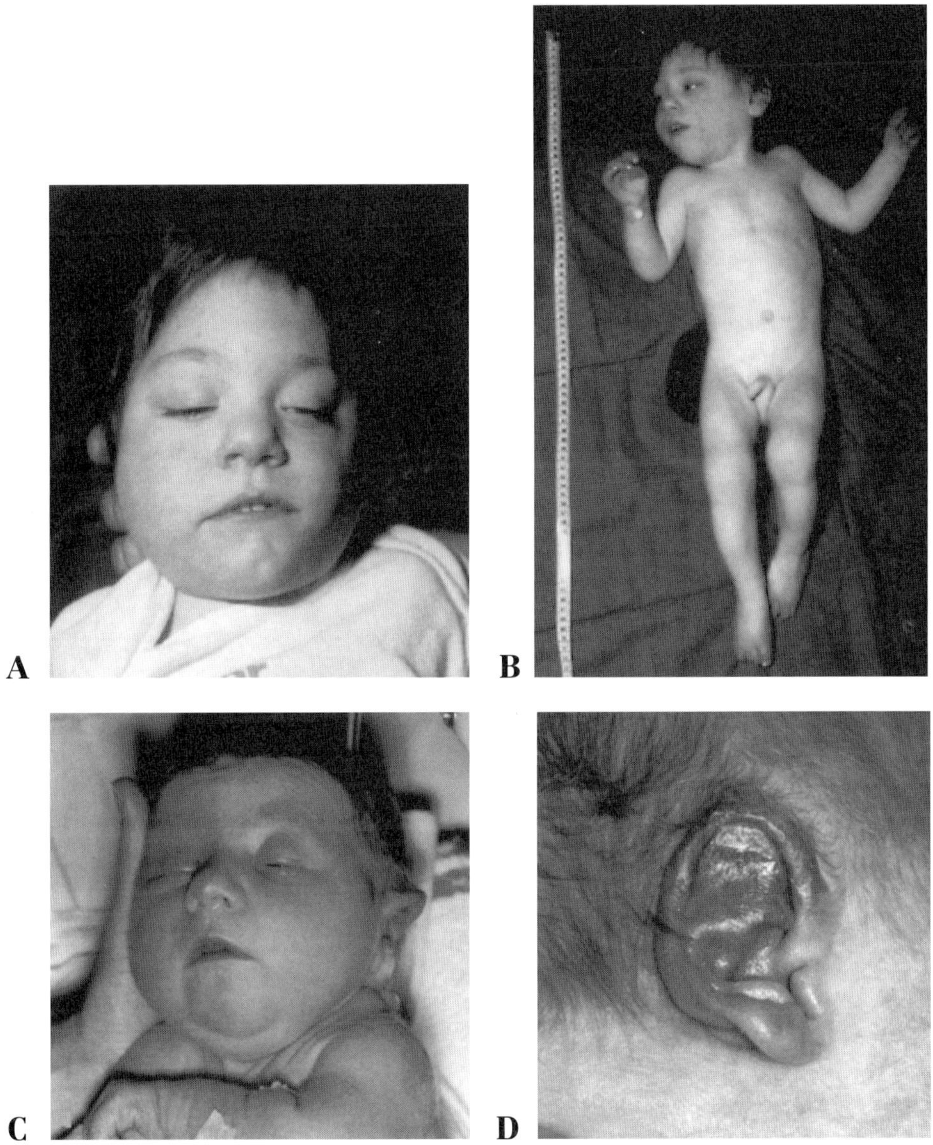

Gustavson Syndrome. Affected male at age 14 months showing short broad nose, large ears, and spastic positioning (A, B); 3-day-old male cousin with receding chin and large dysplastic ears (C, D). Courtesy of Dr. Karl-Henrik Gustavson, University of Uppsala, Sweden and *The American Journal of Medical Genetics,* Copyright © 1993 Wiley-Liss, Inc.

GROWTH AND DEVELOPMENT. Marked intrauterine growth impairment occurs with decreased head circumference, length, and weight. Length appears to be more severely reduced than other growth parameters. Growth impairment continues postnatally. No meaningful developmental progress is made and death occurs in infancy or early childhood.

COGNITIVE FEATURES. No apparent cognitive skills develop prior to death.

NEUROLOGICAL FINDINGS. From birth, these infants are severely impaired with increased muscle tone and hyperreflexia. They do not respond to visual or auditory stimulation. Seizures and apneic episodes occur. Contractures of the large joints and equinovarus, calcaneovalgus, or rockerbottom feet are present at birth.
HETEROZYGOTE EXPRESSION. Carrier females typically show no manifestations. One infant girl, however, was severely and typically affected, a circumstance possibly explained by preferential inactivation of her normal X chromosome.
IMAGING. Brain undergrowth, especially affecting the cerebellum, enlarged cerebral ventricles, and Dandy-Walker malformation (one case), have been demonstrated by ultrasound and cranial tomography.
COMMENT. A similar phenotype (microcephaly, short stature, impaired vision and hearing, spasticity and contractures) and course (profound developmental failure, seizures, and early death) are shared by a number of conditions in which severe intrauterine brain injury has been sustained. Prenatal infections with herpes virus, cytomegalovirus, rubella, and toxoplasma gondii constitute environmental causes which may be distinguished by serological testing, intracranial calcifications, and evidence of continuing postnatal infection of various tissues. Reardon et al. have reviewed a number of genocopies, some possibly X-linked, which may in some cases be distinguished by the presence of intracranial calcifications and thrombocytopenia. Two entities with cerebellar hypoplasia, Arena and Christianson syndromes, map to Xq21-q27 and may be due to mutations of the same gene.

REFERENCES

Arena JF, Schwartz C, Stevenson R, et al.: Spastic paraplegia with iron deposits in the basal ganglia: a new X-linked mental retardation syndrome. Am J Med Genet 43:479, 1992.

Christianson AL, Stevenson RE, van der Meyden CH, et al.: X-linked mental retardation, mild craniofacial dysmorphology, epilepsy, ophthalmoplegia, and cerebellar atrophy in a large South African kindred. J Med Genet, in press, 1999.

Gustavson K-H, Annerén G, Malmgren H, et al.: New X-linked syndrome with severe mental retardation, severely impaired vision, severe hearing defect, epileptic seizures, spasticity, restricted joint mobility, and early death. Am J Med Genet 45:654, 1993.

Malmgren H, Sundvall M, Dahl N, et al.: Linkage mapping of a severe X-linked mental retardation syndrome. Am J Hum Genet 52:1046, 1993.

Reardon W, Hockey A, Silberstein P, et al.: Autosomal recessive congenital intrauterine infection-like syndrome of microcephaly, intracranial calcification, and CNS disease. Am J Med Genet 52:58, 1994.

Differential Matrix

Syndrome	Cerebellar Hypoplasia	Seizures	Spasticity	Comments
Gustavson	+	+	+	Microcephaly, short stature, optic atrophy with blindness, large ears, deafness, joint contractures, rockerbottom feet, brain undergrowth, hydrocephaly
Arena	+	+	+	Muscle hypoplasia, clubfoot, iron deposits in basal ganglia, rigidity, dystonia
Paine	+	+	+	Microcephaly, optic atrophy, short stature, vision and hearing loss
Pettigrew	+	+	+	Dandy-Walker malformation, microcephaly or hydrocephaly, long face with macrostomia and prognathism, small testes, contractures, myoglobinuria, hemolytic anemia
Schimke	+	+	+	Microcephaly, sunken eyes, downslanting palpebral fissures, narrow nose, spacing of teeth, cupped ears, hypotonia, abducens palsy, hearing loss, vision loss, choreoathetosis, contractures
Christianson	+	+	0	Short stature, microcephaly, general asthenia, contractures, ophthalmoplegia
Bertini	+	+	0	Macular degeneration, hypotonia, childhood death, developmental delays and regression, postnatal growth impairment

HOLMES-GANG SYNDROME

DEFINITION. XLMR with microcephaly, large fontanel, hypotonic facies with short nose and anteverted nares, and clubfoot. A mutation has been found in XNP, confirming allelism with XLMR–hypotonic facies syndrome.

SOMATIC FEATURES. Microcephaly, large anterior fontanelle, apparent hypertelorism, epicanthus, short nose with flat nasal bridge and anteverted nares, and tented upper lip with short philtrum make up the craniofacial phenotype. The feet are clubbed. In one case, renal hypoplasia/dysplasia, thyroglossal duct cyst and incomplete lung lobation were found at autopsy.

GROWTH AND DEVELOPMENT. Intrauterine growth is slow and postnatally growth delay persists. Developmental progress is severely delayed with death in infancy or early childhood.

HETEROZYGOTE EXPRESSION. None.

NEUROPATHOLOGY. Markedly small brain with hypoplasia of cerebral white matter and indistinct temporal gyri.

COMMENT. This syndrome is based on observations in a single family. Similarity of the craniofacial findings, largely due to hypotonia, with those in the XLMR–hypotonic facies syndrome (α-thalassemia mental retardation), has led to the identification of a mutation in the XNP gene in Xq13.

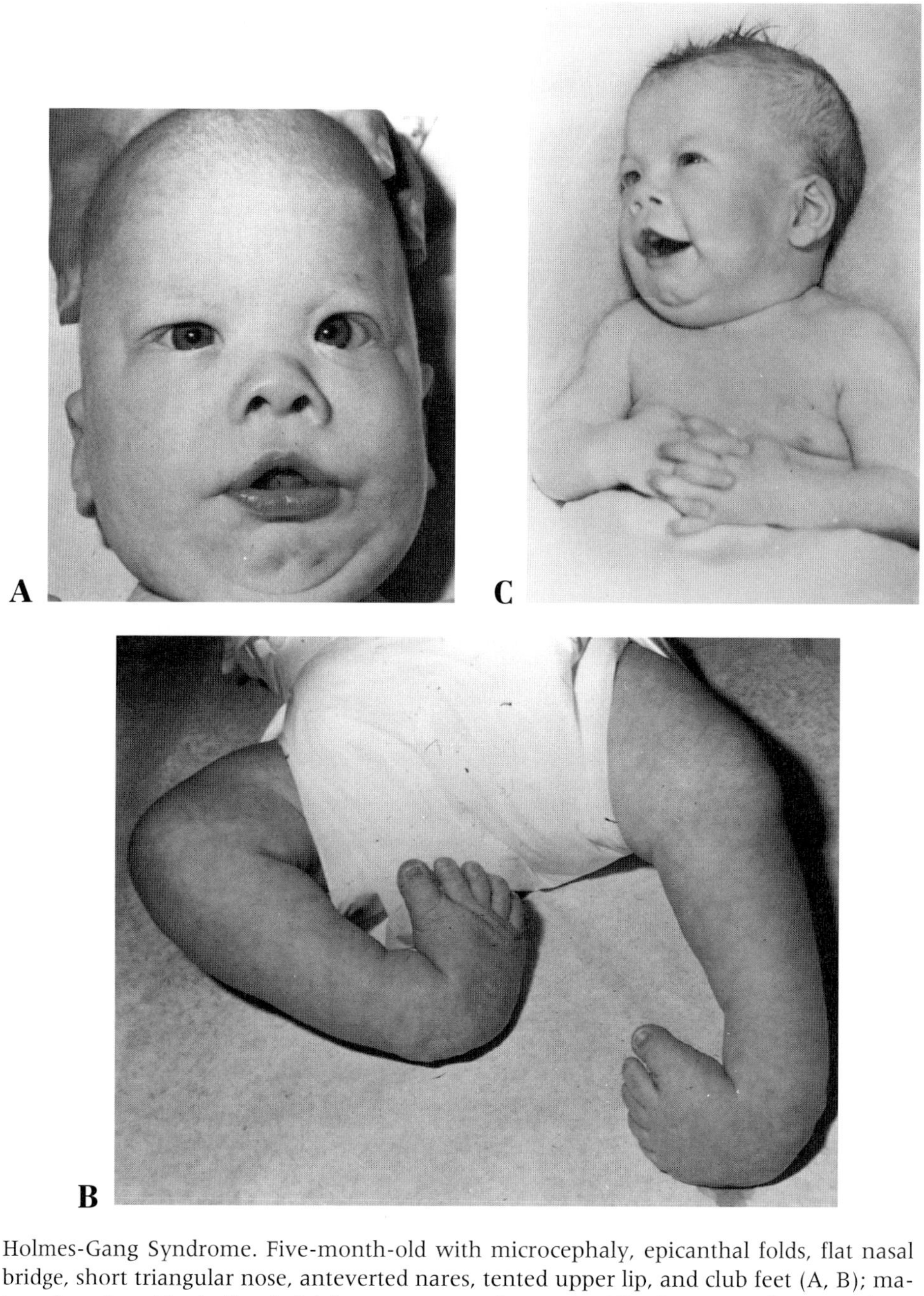

Holmes-Gang Syndrome. Five-month-old with microcephaly, epicanthal folds, flat nasal bridge, short triangular nose, anteverted nares, tented upper lip, and club feet (A, B); maternal uncle with similar facial features at age 5 months (C). Courtesy of Dr. Lewis B. Holmes, Massachusetts General Hospital, Boston

REFERENCE

Holmes LB, Gang DL: Brief clinical report: An X-linked mental retardation syndrome with craniofacial abnormalities, microcephaly and club foot. Am J Med Genet 17:375, 1984.

Differential Matrix

Syndrome	Micro-cephaly	Hypotonic Facies	Short Nose	Comments
Holmes-Gang (Carpenter-Waziri) (Juberg-Marsidi) (XLMR-hypotonic facies)	+	+	+	Short stature, small testes, telecanthus, small triangular nose, tented upper lip, open mouth, spacing of teeth, genital anomalies, musculoskeletal anomalies, hemoglobin H inclusions in erythrocytes
Coffin-Lowry	+	+	0	Short stature, hypertelorism, anteverted nares, tented upper lip, prominent lips and large mouth, large ears, soft hands with tapered digits, pectus carinatum
Miles-Carpenter	+	+	0	Short stature, ptosis, small palpebral fissures, open mouth, pectus excavatum, scoliosis, long hands, camptodactyly, rockerbottom feet, arch fingerprints, spasticity, unsteady gait
Proud	+	+	0	Hearing loss, vision loss, agenesis of corpus callosum, cryptorchidism, inguinal hernias, ataxia, spasticity, seizures
Smith-Fineman-Myers	+	+	0	Ptosis, flat philtrum, scoliosis, midfoot varus, narrow feet, seizures
Chudley-Lowry	0	+	+	Short stature, bitemporal narrowing, almond-shaped eyes, depressed nasal bridge, tented upper lip, open mouth, hypogonadism, hypotonia, obesity
XLMR-psoriasis	0	+	+	Hypertelorism, open mouth, large ears, seizures, psoriasis

HYDE-FORSTER SYNDROME

Hyde-Forster reported two brothers with brachycephaly, flat occiput, plagiocephaly, "coarse features," and severe developmental delay. One brother had microcephaly, seizures, and mild cerebral atrophy on CT imaging. The younger brother had prominence of the forehead. Two maternal aunts had learning problems but no craniofacial manifestations. In the absence of additional details or other similar cases, designation of these cases as a unique XLMR syndrome should be deferred.

REFERENCE

Hyde-Forster I, McCarthy G, Berry AC: A new X linked syndrome with mental retardation and craniofacial dysmorphism? J Med Genet 29:736, 1992.

HYDROCEPHALY-CEREBELLAR AGENESIS SYNDROME

(XLMR–Hydrocephalus–Cerebellar Agenesis Syndrome, MIM 307010)

DEFINITION. XLMR with hydrocephaly, cerebellar agenesis, hypotonia, seizures, and early death. The gene has not been localized.

SOMATIC FEATURES. No craniofacial manifestation aside from enlarged head circumference secondary to hydrocephaly has been described. In one case, rudimentary scrotum was present. Focal glomerulosclerosis and mild hemosiderin deposits in multiple organs were noted.

GROWTH AND DEVELOPMENT. Prenatal growth was impaired in one case. Delivery by caesarian section is required because of hydrocephalus.

NEUROLOGICAL FINDINGS. Hypotonia, areflexia, hyporeflexia, and seizures manifest almost immediately and the infants die shortly after birth.

NEUROPATHOLOGY. Absent cerebellar hemispheres, thinning and gliosis of the cerebral cortex, absence of the foramina of Magendie and Luschka, and dilation of the lateral ventricles, aqueduct of Sylvius, foramen of Monro, and third and fourth ventricles were found at postmortem examination.

COMMENT. This entry is based on one family with three affected males, one of whom had postmortem examination. A hydrocephalic female second cousin related through males was presumed to have a coincidental unrelated hydrocephalus. The early demise of the affected males makes comparison with other X-linked conditions with cerebellar anomalies and hydrocephalus problematic. Based on a case of oral-facial-digital (OFD) II with cerebellar hypoplasia and hydrocephalus it has been suggested that these two X-linked conditions may be allelic.

REFERENCES

Riccardi VM, Marcus ES: Congenital hydrocephalus and cerebellar agenesis. Clin Genet 13:443, 1978.

Stratton RF, Bluestone DL: Oto-palato-digital syndrome type II with X-linked cerebellar hypoplasia/hydrocephalus. Am J Med Genet 41:169, 1991.

Differential Matrix

Syndrome	Hydro-cephaly	Cerebellar Anomalies	Seizures	Comments
Hydrocephaly-cerebellar agenesis	+	+	+	Absent cerebellar hemispheres, hypotonia
Gustavson	+	+	+	Microcephaly, short stature, optic atrophy with blindness, large ears, deafness, joint contractures, rockerbottom feet, brain undergrowth, cerebellar hypoplasia, spasticity
Pettigrew	+	+	+	Dandy-Walker malformation, spasticity, microcephaly or hydrocephaly, long face with macrostomia, small testes, contractures, choreoathetosis, iron deposits in basal ganglia
Bertini	0	+	+	Macular degeneration, hypotonia, ataxia, childhood death, hypoplasia of cerebellar vermis and corpus callosum, developmental delays and regression, postnatal growth impairment
Christianson	0	+	+	Short stature, microcephaly, general asthenia, contractures, ophthalmoplegia
Paine	0	+	+	Microcephaly, short stature, optic atrophy, vision and hearing loss, spasticity
Armfield	+	0	+	Short stature, cataracts or glaucoma, dental anomalies, small hands and feet, joint stiffness

INCONTINENTIA PIGMENTI

(Bloch-Sulzberger Syndrome, IP-1, IP-2, MIM 308310)

DEFINITION. XLMR associated with incontinentia pigmenti. Gene loci in Xp11 and Xq28 have been found on the X chromosome. The Xp11 locus was identified by chromosome rearrangements in sporadic cases (IP-1); the Xq28 locus was established by linkage analysis in familial cases (IP-2), placing the gene distal to factor 8.

SOMATIC FEATURES. Pigmentary changes are required for the diagnosis. Typically, these changes are triphasic, beginning at birth or within the first 6 weeks of life as irregular crops of erythematous vesicular lesions. Within 6–8 weeks, these lesions become verrucous in nature and persist for several months. Irregular hyperpigmentation replaces the verrucous lesions and persists for years. The hyperpigmented skin follows the lines of Blaschko and histologically shows incontinence of pigment in the basal layer of the epidermis and phagocytosis of

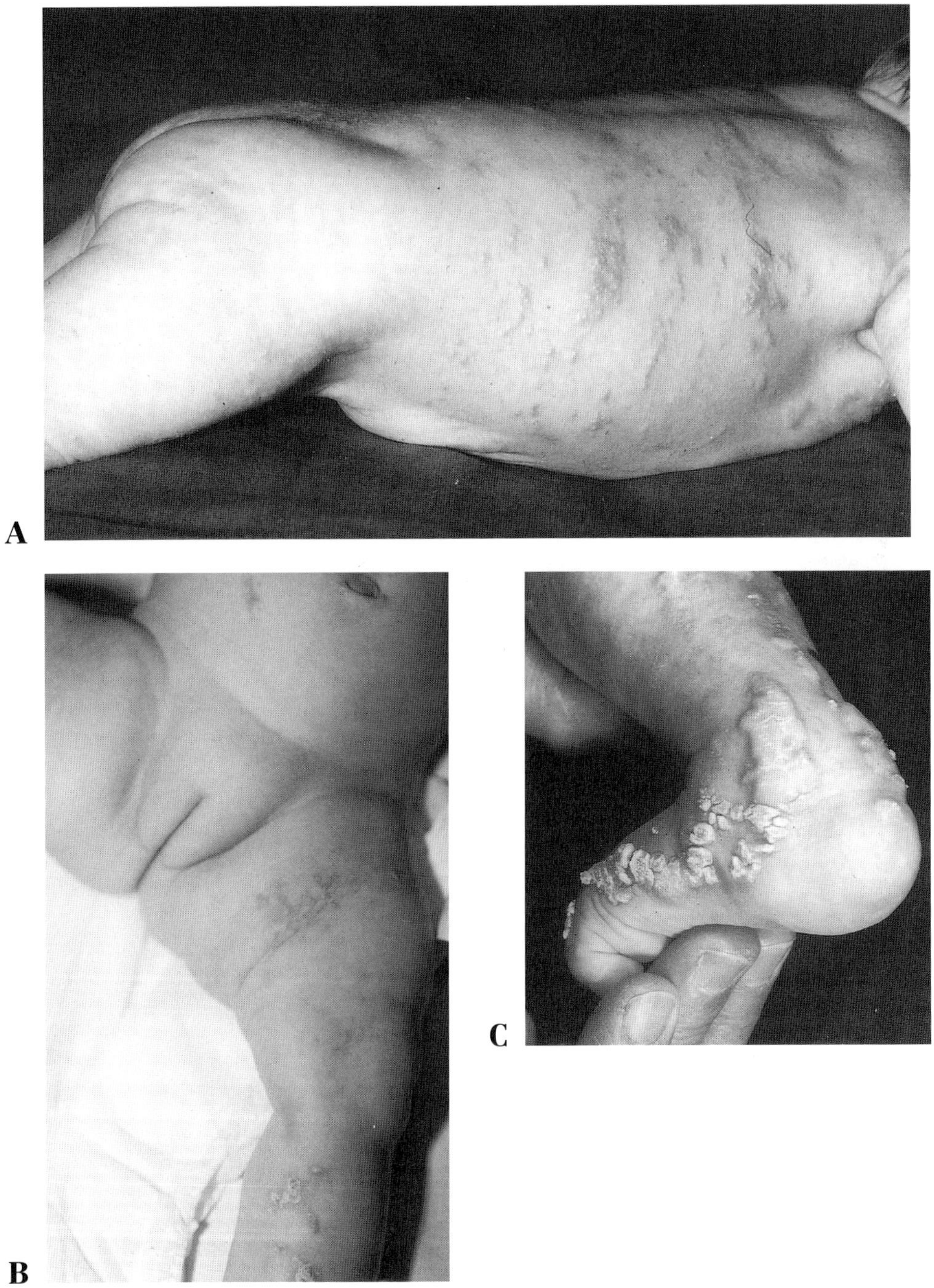

Incontinentia Pigmenti. Vesicular lesions (A), and verrucous lesions (B, C) during infancy.

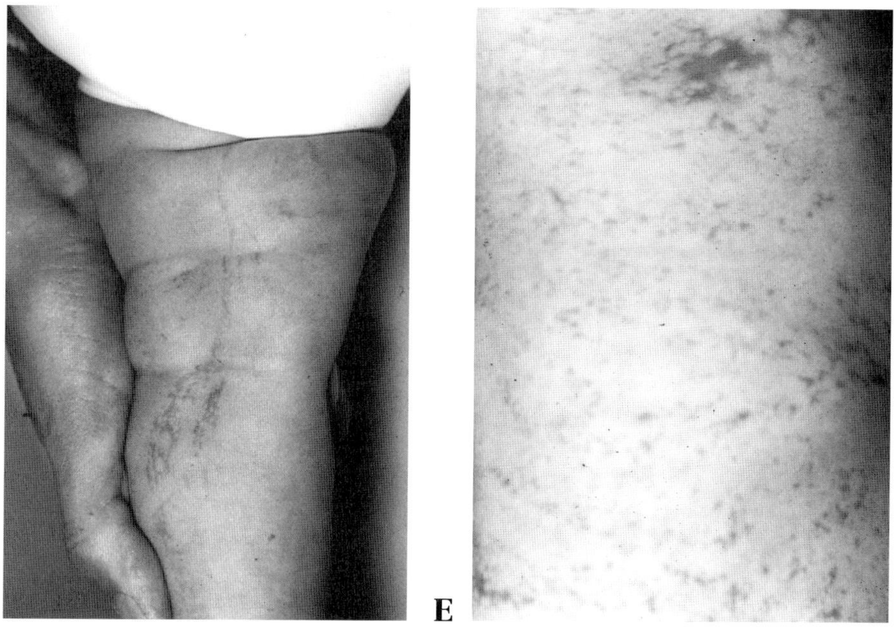

D E

Incontinentia Pigmenti. (continued) Residual hyperpigmented lesions during childhood (D, E). A, C, and E courtesy of Dr. Robert G. Carney, Jr., Decatur, Illinois.

the dendritic processes of melanocytes. By adult life, the hyperpigmentation fades, leaving atrophic depigmented scarring.

A variety of neurological, ocular, and dental abnormalities have been reported. Over half of patients have microcephaly, mental retardation, spasticity, or seizures. Microphthalmia, strabismus, nystagmus, cataracts, optic atrophy, and blindness may occur. Oligodontia, abnormally shaped teeth, and delayed dental eruption are particularly common.

GROWTH AND DEVELOPMENT. Intrauterine and postnatal growth appear normal. Delay of developmental milestones occurs predominantly among cases with neurological manifestations.

COGNITIVE FEATURES. The variable cognitive function appears dependent upon involvement of the central nervous system. Those cases with seizures and/or spasticity are most likely to have cognitive impairment.

COMMENT. At least two gene loci for incontinentia pigmenti exist on the X chromosome: IP-1 has been mapped tentatively to Xp11 on the basis of X chromosome rearrangements in sporadic cases; IP-2 has been mapped to Xq28 by linkage analysis in familial cases. Sporadic (IP-1) and familial types (IP-2) are similar in all respects except that the vesicular phase of cutaneous eruption may not occur in IP-1. Incontinentia pigmenti usually occurs in females. Pedigrees showing a paucity of males and an increased number of spontaneous abortions lend support to the concept that it represents a dominant X-linked disorder with gestational lethality in males.

REFERENCES

Bloch B: Krankendemonstrationen aus der dermatologischen klinik Zürich. Schweiz Med Wochenschr 57:404–405, 1926.

Carney RG: Incontinentia pigmenti. A world statistical analysis. Arch Dermatol 112:535–542, 1976.

Gilgenkrantz S, Tridon P, Pinel-Briquel N, et al.: Translocation X;9 (p11;q34) in a girl with incontinentia pigmenti. Ann Genet (Paris) 28:90–92, 1985.

Hodgson SV, Neville B, Jones RWA, et al.: Two cases of X autosome translocation in females with incontinentia pigmenti. Hum Genet 75:98–99, 1985.

Landy SJ, Donnai D: Incontinentia pigmenti (Block-Sulzberger syndrome). J Med Genet 30:53–59, 1993.

Lenz W: Half chromatid mutations may explain incontinentia pigmenti in males. Am J Hum Genet 27:690–691, 1975.

Sefiani A, Abel L, Heuertz S, et al.: The gene for incontinentia pigmenti is assigned to Xq28. Genomics 4:427–429, 1989.

Sulzberger MB: Über eine bisher nicht beschriebene congenitale Pigmentanomalie (Incontinentia pigmenti). Arch Dermatol Syph 154:19–32, 1927.

Differential Matrix

Syndrome	Cutaneous Changes	Ocular Anomalies	Dental Anomalies	Comments
Incontinentia pigmenti	+	+	+	Cutaneous vesicles, verrucous lesions, and irregular hyperpigmentation, microcephaly, ocular anomalies, oligodontia, abnormally-shaped teeth, spasticity, seizures
Goltz	+	+	+	Cataracts, ocular dysgenesis, linear areas of dermal aplasia, cutaneous adipose herniations, dystrophic nails, abnormal teeth and hair, vertebral anomalies, limb reduction defects, genitourinary anomalies
MIDAS	+	+	0	Microphthalmia, ocular dysgenesis, corneal opacification, dermal aplasia, dysgenesis of corpus callosum, cardiac defects, cardiomyopathy
Dyskeratosis congenita	+	0	+	Short stature, alopecia, hyperpigmented lesions, palmar and plantar hyperkeratosis, mucosal leukoplakia, nail ridging or splitting, pancytopenia, skin and mucosal lesions premalignant

JENSEN SYNDROME

(Nerve Deafness–Optic Atrophy–Dementia Syndrome, Mohr-Mageroy Syndrome, Mohr-Tranebjaerg Syndrome, MIM 304700, Formerly 311150)

Jensen reported a single family with infancy-onset sensorineural hearing loss, mutism, progressive optic atrophy, loss of vision, and adult-onset dementia. The dementia was accompanied by behavioral disturbances manifest by confusion, unsociable behavior, and aggressiveness. A mutation in the deafness-dystonia protein (DDP) gene has been demonstrated in this family and hence Jensen syndrome is allelic to the Mohr-Tranebjaerg syndrome.

REFERENCES

Jensen PKA: Nerve deafness, optic nerve atrophy, and dementia: a new X-linked recessive syndrome? Am J Med Genet 9:55, 1981.

Jin H, May M, Tranebjaerg L, et al: A novel X-linked gene, DDP, shows mutations in families with deafness (DFN-1), dystonia, mental deficiency and blindness. Nat Genet 14: 177, 1996.

Mohr J, Magerøy K: Sex-linked deafness of a possibly new type. Acta Genet Stat Med 10:54, 1960.

Tranebjaerg L, Schwartz C, Eriksen H, et al.: A new X linked recessive deafness syndrome with blindness, dystonia, fractures, and mental deficiency is linked to Xq22. J Med Genet 32:257, 1995.

Juberg-Marsidi Syndrome

Juberg and Marsidi reported three males with severe mental retardation and growth impairment, cupped ears, deafness, epicanthus, strabismus, flat nasal bridge, arched upper lip, and hypogenitalism. Two of the three cases died in childhood. Mattei et al. reported a second family with similar growth failure, craniofacial findings, and genital anomalies. A mutation has been found in the helicase V domain of the XNP gene in the second family, indicating that Juberg-Marsidi syndrome is a variant form of the XLMR–hypotonic facies syndrome (α-thalassemia mental retardation). Mutational analysis has not been reported in the original family.

REFERENCES

Juberg RC, Marsidi I: A new form of X-linked mental retardation with growth retardation, deafness, and microgenitalism. Am J Hum Genet 32:714, 1980.

Mattéi JF, Collignon P, Ayme S, et al.: X-linked mental retardation, growth retardation, deafness and microgenitalism. A second familial report. Clin Genet 23:70, 1983.

Villard L, Gecz J, Mattéi JF, et al.: XNP mutation in a large family with Juberg-Marsidi syndrome. Nat Genet 12:359, 1996.

Kang Syndrome

(X-Linked Agenesis of Corpus Callosum)

Definition. XLMR with microcephaly, frontal prominence, telecanthus, downturned mouth, short broad hands with brachydactyly, agenesis of corpus callosum, and spastic diplegia. The gene has not been localized.

A

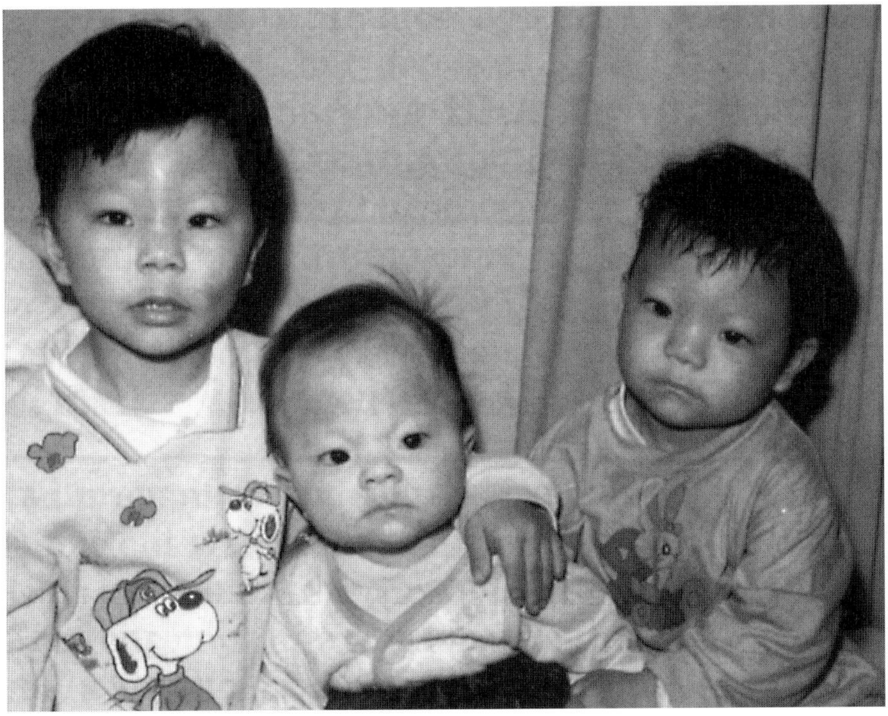

B

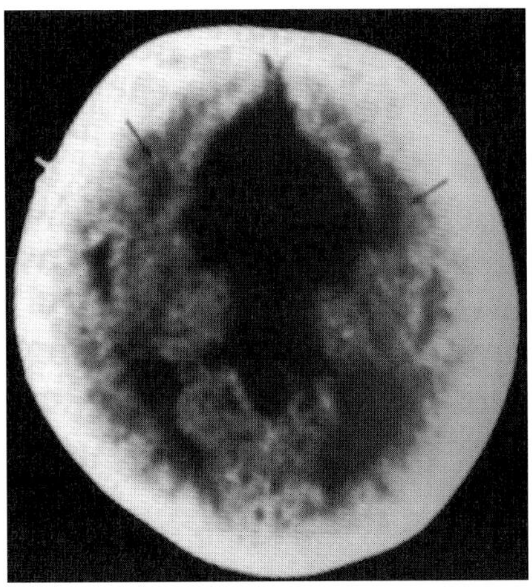

Kang Syndrome. Affected brothers at ages 8 years (left) and 3 years (right) and maternal cousin at age 8 months (center), showing frontal prominence, telecanthus, broad nasal root, and downturned mouth (A); cranial tomography of infant at age 8 months showing a large interhemispheric cyst and displacement of lateral ventricles [arrows] (B). Courtesy of Dr. Shio-Jean Lin, National Cheng Kung University Hospital, Taiwan.

SOMATIC FEATURES. The face appears broad with frontal prominence, telecanthus, small nose with anteverted nares, and downturned mouth. Microcephaly or hydrocephaly occurs with malformations of the brain (agenesis of corpus callosum, interhemispheric cysts, gyral dysplasia, and lateral displacement of the ventricles). One case had unilateral cataract. The hands are short and broad with short fingers and single flexion creases on the fifth fingers. The genitalia appear normal. Spastic diplegia ensues.

GROWTH AND DEVELOPMENT. Details of postnatal growth and development have not been reported. Birth weights are normal.

COGNITIVE FEATURES. Mild impairment.
NEUROLOGICAL FINDINGS. Spastic diplegia becomes evident during infancy.
HETEROZYGOTE EXPRESSION. None.
IMAGING. Ultrasound and CT show dysgenesis of the corpus callosum, interhemispheric cysts, dilation of the lateral and third ventricles, and cortical gyral dysplasia.
COMMENT. Although dysgenesis of the corpus callosum may be found in apparently asymptomatic individuals in the general population, this developmental anomaly occurs more commonly among individuals with mental retardation and especially among the subgroup with metabolic errors. Other anomalies of the central nervous system often accompany dysgenesis of the corpus callosum and may be responsible for neurological symptoms. Complete or partial agenesis of the corpus callosum occurs consistently in a number of XLMR syndromes: Aicardi, cerebrooculogential, Goltz, Lujan, MIDAS, Opitz FG, oral-facial-digital, Proud, pyruvate dehydrogenase deficiency, and X-linked hydrocephaly-MASA syndromes. As such, it seems a helpful but nonmandatory clue to diagnosis.

REFERENCES

Bamforth F, Bamforth S, Poskitt K, et al.: Abnormalities of corpus callosum in patients with inherited metabolic diseases. Lancet 2:451, 1988.

Grogono JL: Children with agenesis of the corpus callosum. Dev Med Child Neurol 10:613, 1968.

Kang W-M, Huang C-C, Lin S-J: X-linked recessive inheritance of dysgenesis of corpus callosum in a Chinese Family. Am J Med Genet 44:619, 1992.

Differential Matrix

Syndrome	Micro-cephaly	Dysgenesis of Corpus Callosum	Spastic Paraplegia	Comments
Kang	+	+	+	Frontal prominence, telecanthus, small nose, short hands, seizures, downslanted mouth, brachydactyly
Proud	+	+	+	Hearing loss, vision loss, agenesis of corpus callosum, cryptorchidism, inguinal hernias, ataxia, seizures
Pyruvate dehydrogenase deficiency	+	+	+	Lactic acidosis, hypotonia, ataxia, dysarthria, CNS anomalies
Goltz	+	+	0	Cataracts, ocular dysgenesis, linear areas of dermal aplasia, cutaneous adipose herniations, dystrophic nails, abnormal teeth and hair, vertebral anomalies, limb reduction defects, genitourinary anomalies
X-linked hydrocephaly-MASA spectrum	0	+	+	Hydrocephaly, adducted thumbs
Paine	+	0	+	Short stature, optic atrophy, vision and hearing loss, seizures
Pettigrew	+	0	+	Dandy-Walker malformation, seizures, microcephaly or hydrocephaly, long face with macrostomia and prognathism, small testes, contractures, choreoathetosis, iron deposits in basal ganglia
Schimke	+	0	+	Sunken eyes, downslanting palpebral fissures, narrow nose, spacing of teeth, cupped ears, hypotonia, abducens palsy, hearing loss, vision loss, spasticity, choreoathetosis, contractures

LENZ MICROPHTHALMIA SYNDROME

(Lenz Syndrome, MIM 309800)

DEFINITION. XLMR with microcephaly, microphthalmia, malformed or cupped ears, cleft lip and cleft palate, dental anomalies, urogenital anomalies, narrow shoulders, duplication of the thumbs or other digital malformations, and spinal curvature. The gene has not been localized.

SOMATIC FEATURES. The facies appear normal except for asymmetric and often colobomatous microphthalmia, blepharoptosis, and dysplastic ears. The colobomas may extend to the optic discs and retinal detachment, lens dislocation, and cataract may be present. The ears may be simply formed and cupped or be small

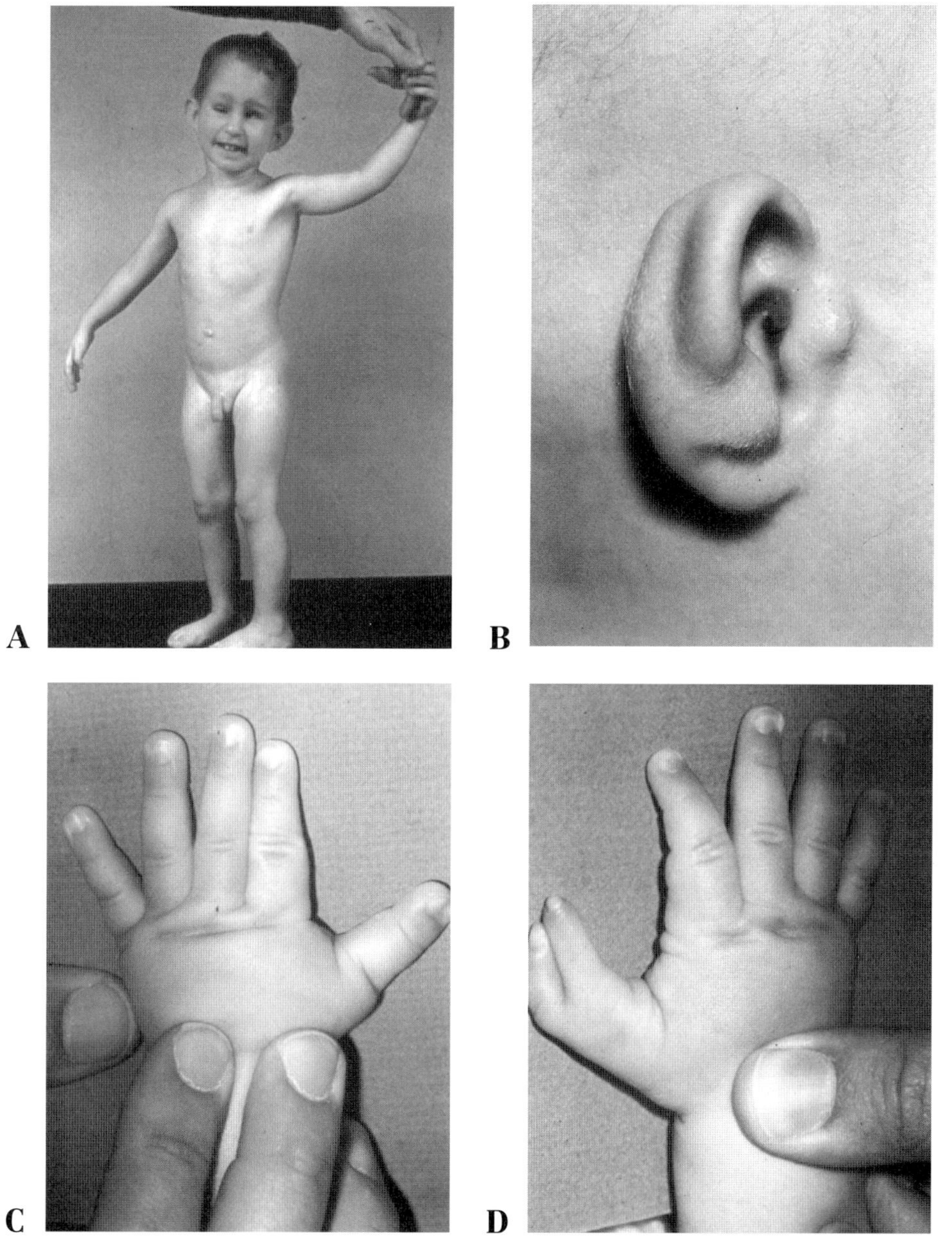

Lenz Microphthalmia Syndrome. Three-year-old male with bilateral microphthalmia, more severe on the right, short palpebral fissure on right, cupped ears, and hypoplastic thumbs (A); manifestations in a second patient showing dysplastic ears, preaxial polydactyly, syndactyly, choreoretinal coloboma involving the nerve head and iris coloboma with subluxed lens (B–H). Courtesy of Dr. Elias Traboulsi, Cleveland Clinic, Cleveland.

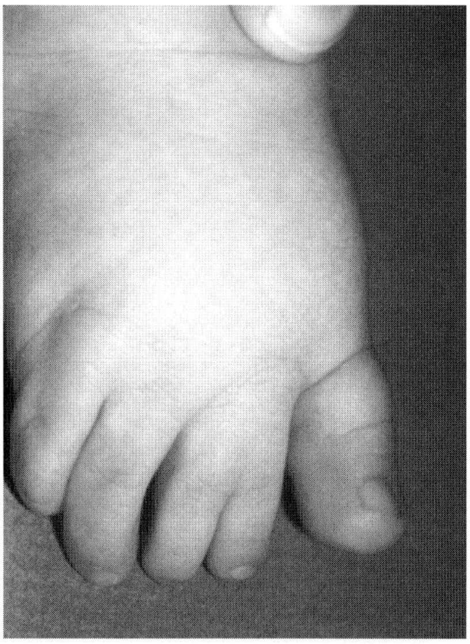

E

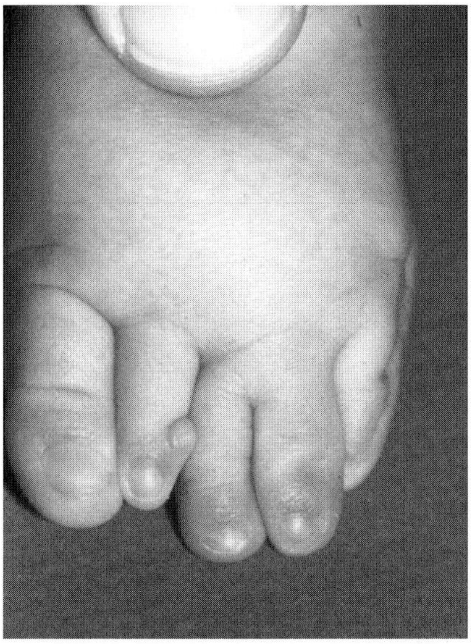

F

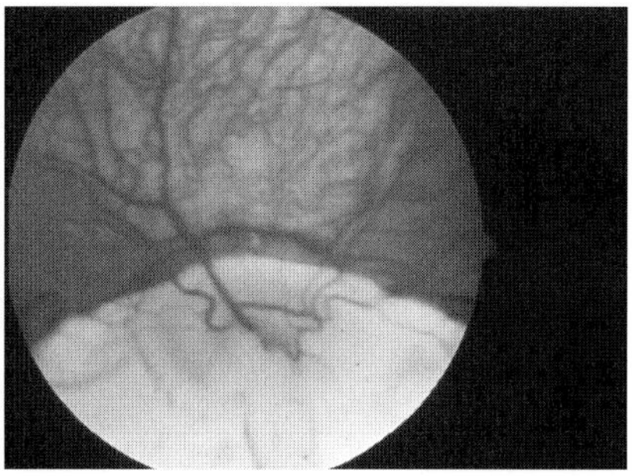

G

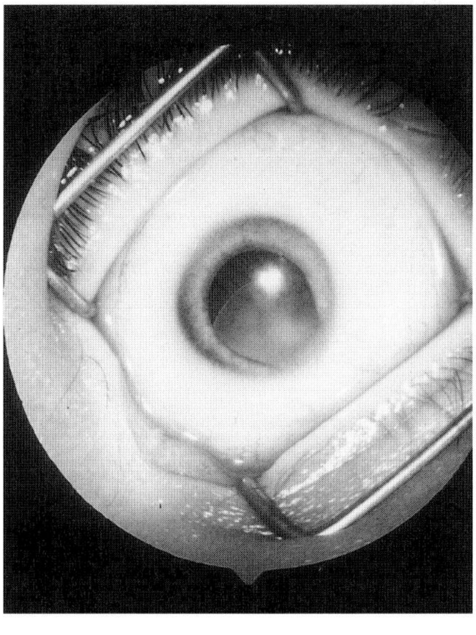

H

Lenz Microphthalmia Syndrome. (continued)

and dysplastic. Thumb duplication or hypoplasia is the usual hand malformation. Syndactyly, camptodactyly, and clinodactyly may affect hands and feet. A variety of urogenital anomalies include renal agenesis, hydronephrosis, hypospadias, and cryptorchidism. Cleft lip and palate, crowding or wide spacing of the teeth, and cardiac malformations are seen in a minority of cases. Sloping shoulders, thinning of the lateral third of the clavicles, barrel chest, kyphoscoliosis, and gibbus anomaly are common.

Growth and Development. Detailed information on growth is not available. Some affected males have intrauterine growth impairment. All parameters of postnatal growth appear slow with measurements ultimately falling below the third centiles. Developmental milestones are globally but variably delayed.

COGNITIVE FEATURES. Some degree of cognitive impairment occurs in all cases, but considerable variation in severity has been reported.
IMAGING. No intracranial malformations have been described.
HETEROZYGOTE EXPRESSION. Carrier females may have short stature, microcephaly, and digital anomalies.
COMMENT. Lenz microphthalmia syndrome may be distinguished from other X-linked microphthalmia syndromes on the basis of associated manifestations. Norrie disease has congenital bilateral blindness and retinal dysplasia, progressing to collapse of the ocular globe and hearing loss. Goltz syndrome has dermal aplasia, cutaneous herniations of fat, and dysplasia of other ectodermal tissues and is expressed in females only. The MIDAS syndrome, another disorder with female limited expression, has linear areas of dermal aplasia, CNS and cardiac malformations, and cardiomyopathy.

REFERENCES

Glanz A, Forse A, Polomeno RC, et al.: Lenz microphthalmia: a malformation syndrome with variable expression of multiple congenital anomalies. Can J Ophthalmol 18:41, 1983.

Lenz W: Recessiv-geschlechtsgebundene mikrophthalmie mit multiplen missbildungen. Zeit Kinderheil 77:384, 1955. Translation in Proc Greenwood Genet Ctr 17:5, 1998.

Traboulsi EI, Lenz W, Gonzales-Ramos M, et al.: The Lenz microphthalmia syndrome. Am J Ophthalmol 105:40, 1988.

Differential Matrix

Syndrome	Ocular Anomaly	Limb Anomaly	Urogenital Anomaly	Comments
Lenz microphthalmia	+	+	+	Microcephaly, malformed ears, cleft lip/palate, cardiac anomalies, thumb duplication or hypoplasia, narrow shoulders
Goltz	+	+	+	Linear areas of dermal aplasia, cutaneous adipose herniations, dystrophic nails, abnormal teeth and hair, vertebral anomalies
Cerebrooculogenital	+	0	+	Short stature, microcephaly, hydrocephaly, agenesis of corpus callosum, microphthalmia, ptosis, hypospadias, cryptorchidism, clubfoot, spasticity
Lowe	+	0	+	Short stature, hypotonia, aminoaciduria, progressive renal disease
Wittwer	+	0	+	Growth deficiency, microcephaly, hearing loss, hypertelorism, hypotonia, seizures

LESCH-NYHAN SYNDROME

(XLMR-Hyperuricemia, Hypoxanthine Guanine Pyrophosphate Ribosyl Transferase Deficiency, MIM 308000)

DEFINITION. XLMR with uric acid urinary stones, spasticity, choreoathetosis, seizures, and self-mutilation, associated with hyperuricemia. The gene, HPRT, is located in Xq26.

SOMATIC FEATURES. Malformations and developmental abnormalities of the craniofacial structures do not occur. The lips and tongue may be irregular, avulsed, or scarred secondary to biting. The digits may be similarly mutilated. Hematuria, crystalluria, and stones result from hyperuricemia.

GROWTH AND DEVELOPMENT. Intrauterine growth is normal. There is a tendency toward poor weight gain and general asthenia, but the head circumference and length are usually normal. Profound developmental failure accompanied by choreoatheotoid and dystonic movement becomes obvious by 6 months of age. In most cases, speech and independent sitting or ambulation are never achieved.

COGNITIVE FEATURES. Variable cognitive impairments have been documented with IQ measurements between 40 and 65.

A

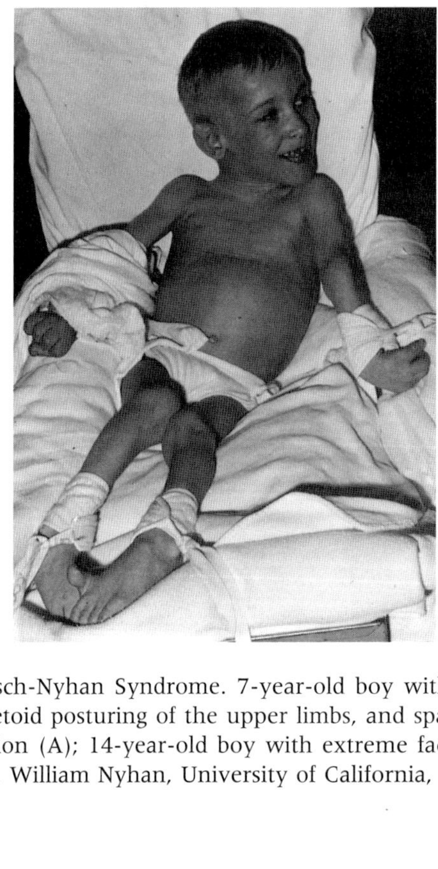

B

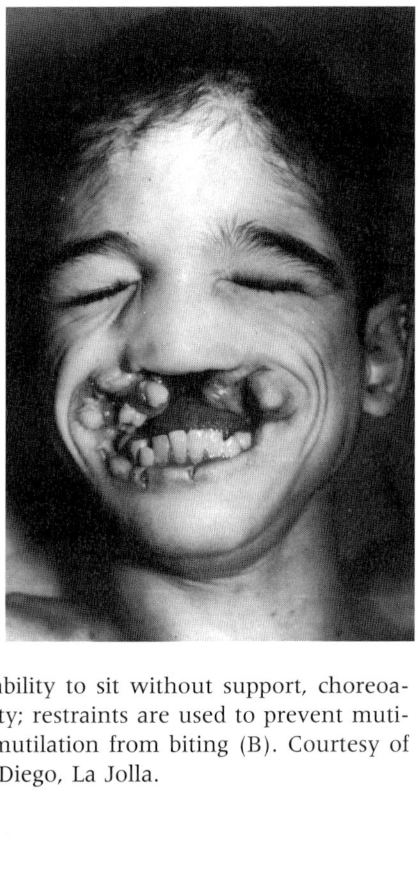

Lesch-Nyhan Syndrome. 7-year-old boy with inability to sit without support, choreoathetoid posturing of the upper limbs, and spasticity; restraints are used to prevent mutilation (A); 14-year-old boy with extreme facial mutilation from biting (B). Courtesy of Dr. William Nyhan, University of California, San Diego, La Jolla.

Behavioral Manifestations. Uncontrollable urge to self-mutilation by biting constitutes the most dramatic behavioral abnormality. Patients may attempt injury to their heads or limbs and appear unusually aggressive toward others in their environment.

Neurological Findings. Constant involuntary movements dominate the neurological phenotype. Choreoathetoid movement of the fingers, flailing movement of the limbs, excessive startle reactions and opisthotonic posturing are interrupted only by sleep. Spasticity with hypertonicity, increased deep tendon reflexes, clonus, and Babinski signs dates from infancy but usually becomes notable after choreoathetosis is well established. Most distressing is the self-mutilation of the lips and digits from biting, a clearly painful phenomenon which usually begins after age 2 years. Seizures occur in about half of cases.

Imaging. Brain malformations do not occur but the overall brain size may be small and the ventricles mildly dilated.

Laboratory. Excessive production of uric acid leads to hyperuricemia, excessive urinary excretion of uric acid, elevated urinary uric acid:creatine ratios, crystalluria, and uric acid stones. A megaloblastic anemia occurs in a minority of cases.

Comment. Although self-injury is a common phenomenon among persons with severe mental retardation, self-mutilation by biting appears unique to individuals with Lesch-Nyhan syndrome. They do not appear to have any reduction in sensation to pain. No therapy, other than protection against self-mutilation by tooth extraction and wrapping of the hands, has been successful.

REFERENCES

Hoefnagel D, Andrew ED, Mireault NG, et al.: Hereditary choreoathetosis, self-mutilation and hyperuricemia in young males. N Engl J Med 273:130, 1965.

Lesch M, Nyhan WL: A familial disorder of uric acid metabolism and central nervous system function. Am J Med 36:561, 1964.

Differential Matrix

Syndrome	Spasticity	Choreo-athetosis	Seizures	Comments
Lesch-Nyhan	+	+	+	Self-mutilation, hyperuricemia
Pettigrew	+	+	+	Dandy-Walker malformation, microcephaly or hydrocephaly, long face with macrostomia and prognathism, small testes, contractures, iron deposits in basal ganglia
Proud	+	+	+	Microcephaly, hearing loss, vision loss, agenesis of corpus callosum, cryptorchidism, inguinal hernias, ataxia
XLMR-spastic paraplegia-athetosis	+	+	+	Nystagmus, weakness, dysarthria, muscle wasting, contractures
Allan-Herndon-Dudley	+	+	0	Large ears with cupping or abnormal architecture, muscle hypoplasia, childhood hypotonia, contractures, dysarthria, athetosis, ataxia
Schimke	+	+	0	Microcephaly, sunken eyes, downslanting palpebral fissures, narrow nose, spacing of teeth, cupped ears, hypotonia, abducens palsy, hearing loss, vision loss, contractures
Goldblatt spastic paraplegia	+	0	+	Optic atrophy, exotropia, nystagmus, ataxia, dysarthria, muscle hypoplasia, contractures
Gustavson	+	0	+	Microcephaly, short stature, optic atrophy with blindness, large ears, deafness, joint contractures, rockerbottom feet, brain undergrowth, hydrocephaly, cerebellar hypoplasia
Paine	+	0	+	Microcephaly, short stature, optic atrophy, vision and hearing loss
Pelizaeus-Merzbacher	+	0	+	Optic atrophy, nystagmus, hypotonia, ataxia, dystonia, CNS dysmyelination
X-linked ataxia-deafness-dementia	+	0	+	Optic atrophy, vision loss, hearing loss, ataxia, hypotonia, childhood death

LOWE SYNDROME

(Oculocerebrorenal Syndrome, MIM 309000)

DEFINITION. XLMR with short stature, cataracts, renal tubular dysfunction, and hypotonia. The gene, OCRL1, codes for phosphotidylinositol 4,5-bisphospate 5-phosphatase and is located in Xq26.1.

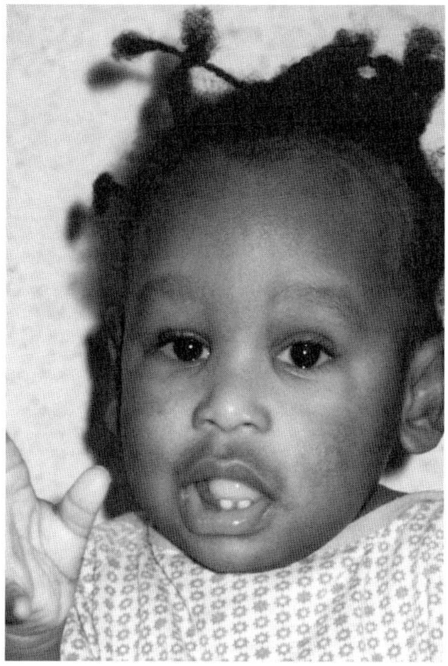

Lowe Syndrome. Fifteen-month-old male with cataracts, epicanthus, and hypotonia.

SOMATIC FEATURES. Congenital cataracts provide the initial diagnostic lead in almost all cases. The eyes may appear deep-set and in time may develop glaucoma and corneal keloids. These ocular features, frontal prominence with normal head circumference, marked hypotonia, and areflexia round out the phenotype in infancy and early childhood. Progressive renal disease ultimately leads to death. During childhood, tubular dysfunction is manifest by urinary loss of protein, amino acids, carnitine, bicarbonate, and phosphate. Glomerular function is little affected during childhood but steadily declines during the adult years. Metabolic disturbances from the renal dysfunction may result in undermineralization, fractures, and rickets. Renal failure occurs during the fourth decade.
GROWTH AND DEVELOPMENT. Intrauterine growth appears normal but linear growth falls below the third centile by age 1–3 years. Weight follows a similar pattern although normal weight may persist for the first few years. Head circumference may remain in the midcentiles in the preschool years, fall to or below the lower centiles in late childhood, but thereafter gain toward the mean.
COGNITIVE FEATURES. Moderate to severe impairment generally occurs although one-fourth of cases will score 70 or higher on IQ tests.
BEHAVIORAL MANIFESTATIONS. Maladaptive behavior consisting of stubbornness, temper tantrums, and repetitive shaking of the limbs occurs in many cases.
HETEROZYGOTE EXPRESSION. Carrier females can be identified by fine opacities in the lenses. Slit lamp examination may be required.
LABORATORY. Proteinuria, aminoaciduria, and low urine osmolality are the first evidence of tubular dysfunction. There are subsequent excess renal losses of bicarbonate, phosphate, potassium, and carnitine. Metabolic acidosis, hypophosphatemia, hypokalemia, and low serum carnitine result. With glomerular involvement, there is progressive evidence of renal insufficiency.

COMMENT. Manifestations are present from birth and follow a predictable course. Because of the cataracts and renal tubular dysfunction, Lowe syndrome may be readily differentiated from other hypotonia syndromes.

REFERENCES

Attree O, Olivos IM, Okabe I, et al.: The Lowe's oculocerebrorenal syndrome gene encodes a protein highly homologous to inositol polyphosphate-5-phosphatase. Nature 358:239, 1992.

Charnas LR, Bernardini I, Rader D, et al.: Clinical and laboratory findings in the oculocerebrorenal syndrome of Lowe, with special reference to growth and renal function. N Eng J Med 324:1318, 1991.

Lowe CU, Terrey M, MacLachlan EA: Organic-aciduria, decreased renal ammonia production, hydrophthalmos, and mental retardation: a clinical entity. Am J Dis Child 83:164, 1952.

Mueller OT, Hartsfield JK Jr, Gallardo LA, et al.: Lowe oculocerebrorenal syndrome in a female with a balanced X;20 translocation: mapping of the X chromosome breakpoint. Am J Hum Genet 49:804, 1991.

Differential Matrix

Syndrome	Ocular Anomaly	Renal Dysfunction or Anomalies	Hypotonia	Comments
Lowe	+	+	+	Short stature, cataracts, aminoaciduria, progressive renal failure
Wittwer	+	+	+	Growth deficiency, microcephaly, microphthalmia, hearing loss, vision loss, hypertelorism, genitourinary anomalies, seizures
Cerebrooculogenital	+	+	0	Short stature, microcephaly, hydrocephaly, agenesis of corpus callosum, microphthalmia, ptosis, hypospadias, cryptorchidism, clubfoot, spasticity
Goltz	+	+	0	Cataracts, ocular dysgenesis, linear areas of dermal aplasia, cutaneous adipose herniations, dystrophic nails, abnormal teeth and hair, vertebral anomalies, limb reduction defects, genitourinary anomalies
Lenz microphthalmia	+	+	0	Microcephaly, microphthalmia, ocular dysgenesis, malformed ears, cleft lip/palate, cardiac and genitourinary anomalies, thumb duplication or hypoplasia, narrow shoulders
Arts	+	0	+	Growth deficiency, paucity of muscles, areflexia, ataxia, deafness, vision loss, seizures, childhood death
Bertini	+	0	+	Macular degeneration, ataxia, seizures, childhood death, hypoplasia of cerebellar vermis and corpus callosum, developmental delays and regression, postnatal growth impairment

LUJAN SYNDROME

(Lujan-Fryns Syndrome, XLMR–Marfanoid Habitus, MIM 309520)

DEFINITION. XLMR with marfanoid skeletal habitus and behavioral aberrations. The gene has not been mapped.

SOMATIC FEATURES. Patients are generally tall and thin with stature and head circumference in the upper centiles. The face is long with prominent forehead, high nasal bridge, high palate, low-set retroverted but normal length ears, and micrognathia. Hands and feet are long and thin with long digits. Pectus excavatum and joint hyperextensibility may be present. One patient had an extra row of upper teeth at 17 years and another had an atrial septal defect. Speech is high-pitched and hypernasal but velopharyngeal incompetence or submucous cleft palate has not been reported. Seizures, hyperactivity, and aggressiveness have been significant management issues. Testicular enlargement has been noted in several cases.

GROWTH AND DEVELOPMENT. From early childhood, height and head circumference measure in the upper growth centiles. Weight is usually below the 50th centile. Speech and motor milestones are delayed, but the severity varies considerably.

COGNITIVE FEATURES. A wide range of cognitive function accompanies the prominent behavioral manifestations. In most cases, mild to moderate cognitive impairment occurs.

BEHAVIORAL MANIFESTATIONS. Various males have exhibited hyperactive, aggressive, autistic and psychotic behaviors, as well as shyness and jovialness.

NEUROLOGICAL FINDINGS. None.

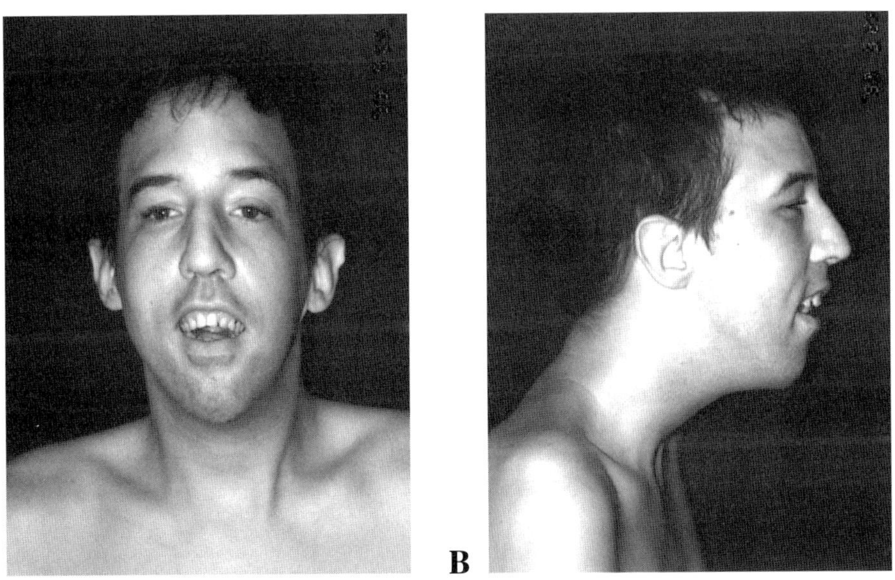

A B

Lujan Syndrome. Twenty-eight-year-old with prominent forehead and long face, high nasal bridge, receding chin, and low-set simply formed ears (A, B).

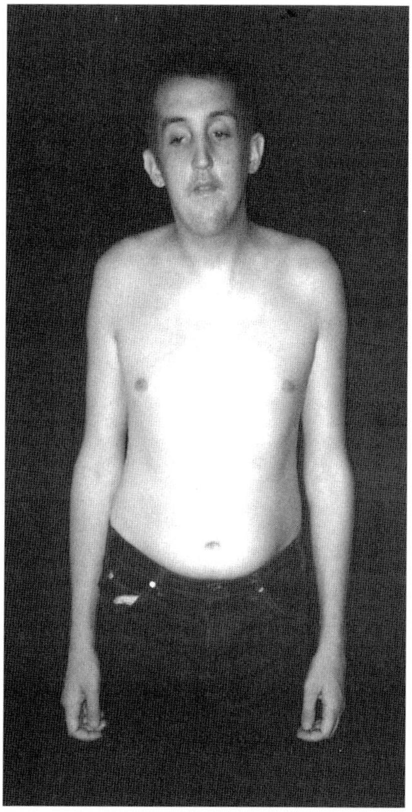

C

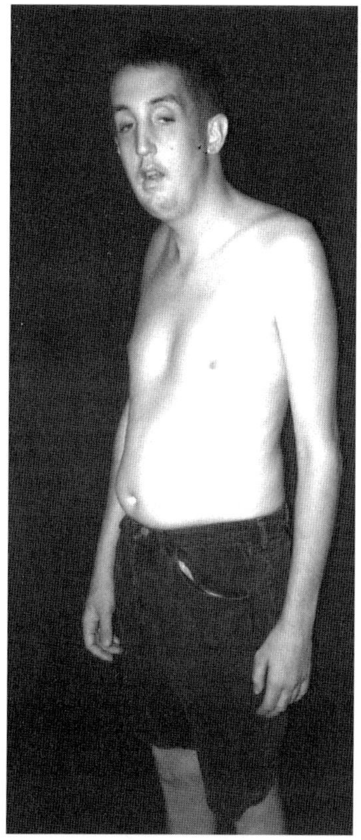

D

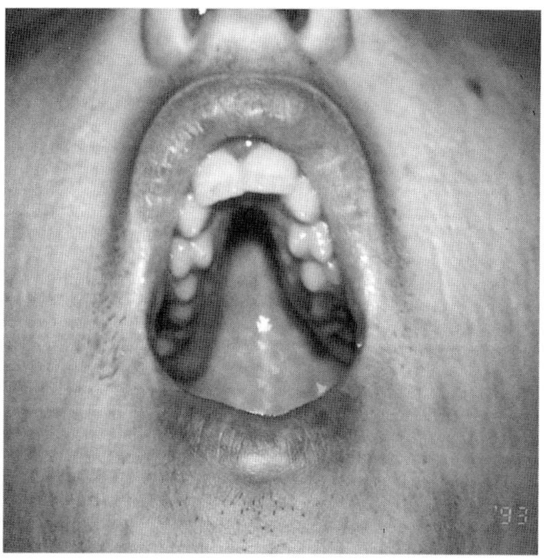

E

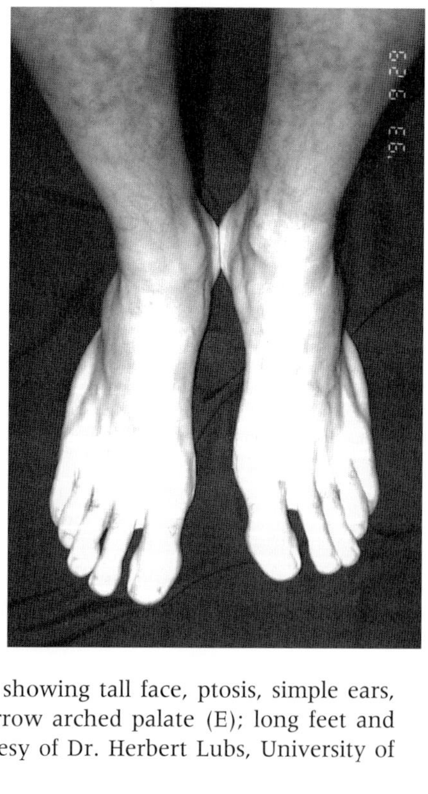

F

Lujan Syndrome. (continued) 33-year-old brother showing tall face, ptosis, simple ears, large mandible, and pectus excavatum (C, D); narrow arched palate (E); long feet and toes with spacing between toes 1 and 2 (F). Courtesy of Dr. Herbert Lubs, University of Miami School of Medicine, Miami.

HETEROZYGOTE EXPRESSION. One carrier female with normal intellect has marfanoid habitus and high-pitched nasal speech.

IMAGING. One case with agenesis of corpus callosum and one with suspected partial absence of corpus callosum were present in the original Lujan syndrome family.

COMMENT. A number of cases and a few families have been reported since the Lujan et al. report of 1984. It is not clear that genetic heterogeneity is not represented in those reports.

REFERENCES

Fryns J-P, Buttiens M: X-linked mental retardation with Marfanoid habitus. Am J Med Genet 28:267, 1987.

Lacombe D, Bonneau D, Verloes A, et al.: Lujan-Fryns syndrome (X-linked mental retardation with Marfanoid habitus): report of three cases and review. Genet Couns 4:193, 1993.

Lalatta F, Livini E, Selicorni A, et al.: X-linked mental retardation with Marfanoid habitus: first report of four Italian patients. Am J Med Genet 38:228, 1991.

Lujan JE, Carlin ME, Lubs HA: A form of X-linked mental retardation with Marfanoid habitus. Am J Med Genet 17:311, 1984.

Differential Matrix

Syndrome	Marfanoid Habitus	Behavioral Disturbance	Seizures	Comments
Lujan	+	+	+	Asthenic build, long face, prominent forehead, high palate, micrognathia, long digits, pectus excavatum, joint hyperextensibility, hyperactivity
Ornithine transcarbamylase deficiency	0	+	+	Chronic or intermittent hyperammonemia, microcephaly, protein-induced vomiting and lethargy, ataxia
Rett	0	+	+	Acquired microcephaly, developmental regression, truncal ataxia, repetitive hand movements, autistic features
Monoamine oxidase-A deficiency	0	+	0	Aggressive behavior, repetitive hand movements

MEHMO SYNDROME

(Mental Retardation–Epileptic Seizures–Hypogonadism and Hypogenitalism–Microcephaly–Obesity Syndrome, XLMR-Microcephaly-Obesity-Hypogonadism-Seizures)

DEFINITION. XLMR with short stature, microcephaly, hypogonadism, obesity, seizures, and early childhood death. The gene maps between CYBB (Xp21.1) and DXS365 (Xp22.13), lod score 2.3.

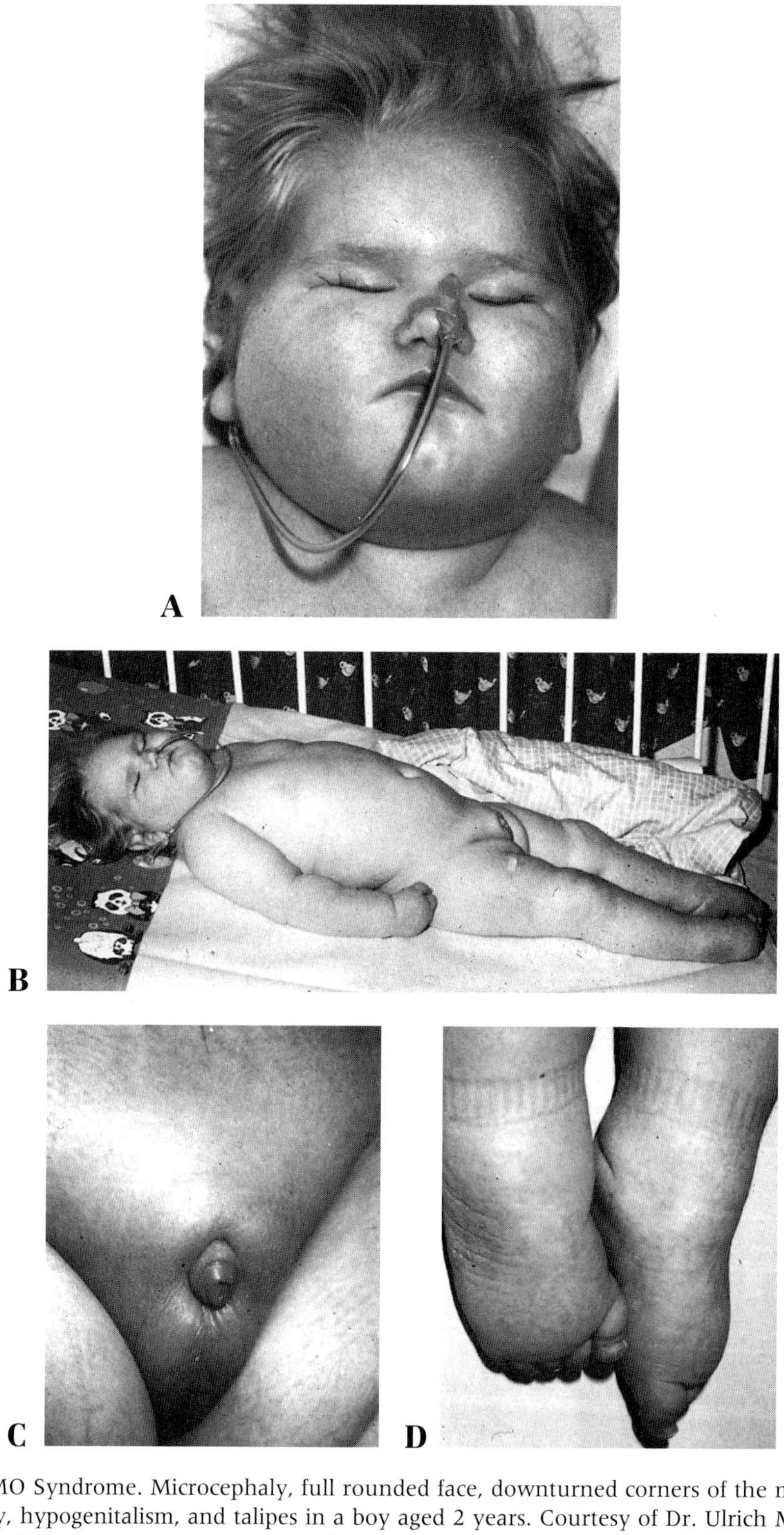

MEHMO Syndrome. Microcephaly, full rounded face, downturned corners of the mouth, obesity, hypogenitalism, and talipes in a boy aged 2 years. Courtesy of Dr. Ulrich Müller, Institut für Humangenetik, Universität Giessen, Giessen, Germany.

SOMATIC FEATURES. Major malformations do not occur. Microcephaly and facial features suggestive of hypotonia (thick helices with upturned earlobes, thick alae nasi, tented upper lip with downturned angles of the mouth, and puffy cheeks) were present in the child described most completely. The penis was small and the testes undescended. Hands and feet were edematous; fingers were tapered and the feet had equinovarus deformations. Generalized obesity was present. Death occurs during infancy or early childhood.

GROWTH AND DEVELOPMENT. At birth, growth parameters measure in the lower centiles. Thereafter, head growth and stature are further slowed but weight gain is excessive. No significant developmental milestones are achieved.

COGNITIVE FEATURES. Severe impairment.

NEUROLOGICAL FINDINGS. Details of the neurological examination are not available.

HETEROZYGOTE EXPRESSION. None.

COMMENT. This XLMR syndrome suffers profound developmental failure, seizures, and death in infancy or early childhood and in this regard differs from other XLMR syndromes with hypotonia, hypogonadism, and obesity.

REFERENCE

Steinmüller R, Steinberger D, Müller U: MEHMO (mental retardation, epileptic seizures, hypogonadism and -genitalism, microcephaly, obesity), a novel syndrome: assignment of disease locus to Xp21.1-p22.13. Eur J Hum Genet 6:201, 1998.

Differential Matrix

Syndrome	Obesity	Hypotonia	Hypo-gonadism	Comments
MEHMO	+	+	+	Short stature, microcephaly, edematous hands and feet, equinovarus deformity, seizures, early childhood death
Vasquez	+	+	+	Short stature, microcephaly, gynecomastia
Börjeson-Forssman-Lehmann	+	+	+	Short stature, microcephaly, coarse face, large ears, gynecomastia, narrow sloped shoulders, visual impairment, tapered digits
Chudley-Lowry	+	+	+	Short stature, bitemporal narrowing, almond-shaped eyes, depressed nasal bridge, tented upper lip, open mouth
Wilson-Turner	+	+	+	Normal growth, small hands and feet, tapered digits, gynecomastia, emotional lability
XLMR-hypotonic facies (Carpenter-Waziri) (Holmes-Gang) (Juberg-Marsidi)	0	+	+	Short stature, microcephaly, telecanthus, small triangular nose, tented upper lip, open mouth, spacing of teeth, genital anomalies, musculoskeletal anomalies, hemoglobin H inclusions in erythrocytes
Pettigrew	0	+	+	Dandy-Walker malformation, spasticity, seizures, microcephaly or hydrocephaly, long face with macrostomia and prognathism, small testes, contractures, choreoathetosis, iron deposits in basal ganglia
Urban	+	0	+	Short stature, small hands and feet, digital contractures, osteoporosis
XLMR-panhypopituitarism	+	0	+	Short stature, hypogenitalism, small sella turcica, deficiency of pituitary, thyroid, adrenal, and gonadal hormones
Young-Hughes	+	0	+	Short stature, small palpebral fissures, cupped ears, ichthyosiform scaling

MENKES SYNDROME

(XLMR–Kinky Hair, XLMR–Copper Transport Defect, MIM 309400)

DEFINITION. XLMR with growth deficiency, full cheeks, sparse kinky hair, metaphyseal changes, limited spontaneous movement, hypertonicity, seizures, hypothermia, lethargy, arterial tortuosity, and death in early childhood, associated with low serum copper and ceruloplasmin and deficient cellular transport of cop-

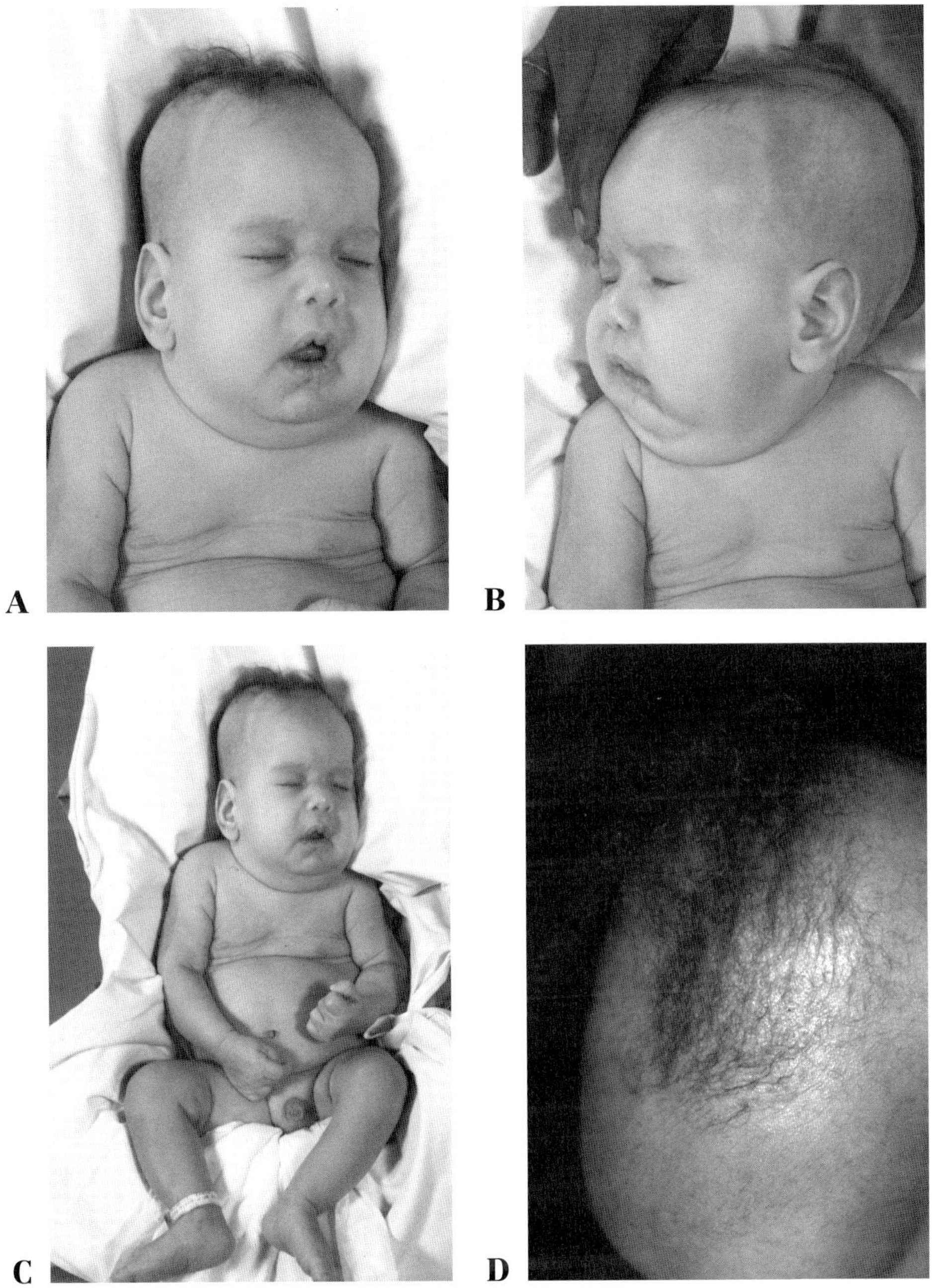

Menkes Syndrome. Four-month-old infant with generalized hypotonia, puffiness and sagging of the cheeks, and sparse hair. Courtesy of Dr. Arthur S. Aylsworth, University of North Carolina School of Medicine, Chapel Hill.

per. The gene, ATP7A, has properties of a copper transporting protein and is located in Xp13.3.

SOMATIC FEATURES. Although the face may be pale, expressionless, and have full cheeks, it is the hair that is most distinctive. Scalp hair is sparse and hypopigmented, often with the shafts broken near the skin. Eyebrows are similarly sparse, horizontal, and twisted in appearance. The characteristic twisting of pili torti is the only structurally visible change in the hair shafts. The skin is also hypopigmented and tends to be lax. Seborrheic dermatitis, predominantly affecting the face and scalp, may persist throughout life. Major malformations do not occur. The arteries are tortuous with irregularly narrowed lumens. Wormian bones may be found in the sagittal and lambdoid sutures. Metaphyses of the ribs and long bones are widened and spurs may occur at the metaphyses of the long bones.

Growth and Development. Although premature delivery occurs commonly, intrauterine growth is normal or nearly so. Postnatal growth appears variable with some infants maintaining normal growth velocity while others lag behind and eventually fall below −2 SD in head circumference and stature. Development is profoundly delayed, with most infants never progressing beyond smiling and control of the head position, skills which are quickly lost.

Cognitive Features. In the usual case, no significant cognitive skills are attained. Milder variants with less severe impairments have been described.

Neurological Findings. From the early days or weeks of life, these infants appear lethargic with little spontaneous movement and very little progress in development. They become mildly hypertonic, often exhibit hypothermia, and develop seizures of generalized or myoclonic types. Death occurs within the first few years.

Natural History. The classic presentation is early and lethal. The hair is fine but normal microscopically at birth. Hypothermia, hyperbilirubinemia, frequent infections, poor feeding, and hypotonia may complicate the first days and weeks of life. After several months of limited development, relentless developmental and neurologic deterioration ensues, manifest in the form of myoclonic seizures, spasticity, limited movement, and minimal responsiveness. The facial, cutaneous, hair, and joint findings become apparent in the first months. Death occurs in the first 3 years of life. The few survivors beyond early childhood have profound mental and neurologic impairments.

Several milder variants with ATP7A mutations have been described. In some cases, developmental delay and milder mental retardation, ataxia, dysarthria, seizures, pili torti, and facial and connective tissue features are described. In the occipital horn syndrome, connective tissue (lax skin, loose joints, diverticulae of bladder, hernias) and skeletal changes (occipital exostoses, expansion of the lateral clavicles, wavy long bone cortices) predominate, but intelligence is low normal, borderline, or in the mild-MR range.

Heterozygote Expression. Carrier females may have pili torti but this is not an obligate finding. Neurologic or cognitive abnormalities do not occur.

Neuropathology. The brain is moderately undergrown, has diffuse neuronal loss, gliosis, and areas of microcystic degeneration. There appears to be a predisposition to subdural hematomas. Cerebral arteries may be thin walled, tortuous, and dilated.

Laboratory. Low levels of copper and ceruloplasmin may be demonstrated in the serum. Defective intracellular trafficking of copper leads to deficient movement of copper transplacentally, decreased intestinal absorption of copper, and excessive accumulation of copper in the tissues.

COMMENT. Various clinical manifestations appear due to deficient activities of enzymes requiring copper (lysyl oxidase, cytochrome *c* oxidase, dopamine β-hydroxylase, and superoxide mutase). The hope that parenteral administration of copper would be therapeutic has not been completely fulfilled. Parenteral copper administration can normalize serum copper and ceruloplasmin. Success in modifying the clinical course appears to be due in part to the time when therapy begins. When initiated prior to the onset of neurological signs, subcutaneous copper-histidine treatment may prevent altogether the neurological manifestations and mental retardation in some patients. Other cases do not respond so beneficially. Long-term treatment, however, does not prevent development, progression, and complications of occipital horn syndrome. The success of treatment may depend, in part, on the type of ATP7A mutation.

REFERENCES

Chelly J, Türner Z, Tønnesen T, et al.: Isolation of a candidate gene for Menkes disease that encodes a potential heavy metal binding protein. Nat Genet 3:14, 1993.

Christodoulou J, Danks DM, Bibidhendra S, et al.: Early treatment of Menkes disease with parenteral copper-histidine: Long-term follow-up of four treated patients. Am J Med Genet 76:154, 1998.

Danks DM, Campbell PE, Stevens BJ, et al.: Menkes's kinky hair syndrome. An inherited defect in copper absorption with widespread effects. Pediatrics 50:188, 1972.

Menkes JH, Alter M, Steigleder GK, et al.: A sex-linked recessive disorder with retardation of growth, peculiar hair and focal cerebral and cerebellar degeneration. Pediatrics 29:764, 1962.

Mercer JFB, Livingston J, Hall B, et al.: Isolation of a partial candidate gene for Menkes disease by positional cloning. Nat Genet 3:20, 1993.

Proud VK, Mussell HG, Kaler SG, et al.: Distinctive Menkes disease variant with occipital horns: delineation of natural history and clinical phenotype. Am J Med Genet 65:44, 1996.

Vulpe C, Levinson B, Whitney S, et al.: Isolation of a candidate gene for Menkes disease and evidence that it encodes a copper transporting ATPase. Nat Genet 3:7, 1993.

Differential Matrix

Syndrome	Hair Abnormality	Skeletal Changes	Seizures	Comments
Menkes	+	+	+	Growth deficiency, hypothermia, pallor, limited movement, hypertonicity, metaphyseal widening and spurs, arterial tortuosity, childhood death
Oral-facial-digital I	+	+	+	Sparse scalp hair, dystopia canthorum, flat midface, hypoplastic alae nasi, hypertrophic and aberrant oral frenuli, intraoral clefts and pseudoclefts, lingual hamartomas, brachydactyly, syndactyly, clinodactyly, structural brain anomalies, polycystic kidneys
Fitzsimmons	+	+	0	Pes cavus, hyperkeratosis of palms and soles, dystrophic nails, spastic paraplegia
Goltz	+	+	0	Cataracts, ocular dysgenesis, linear areas of dermal aplasia, cutaneous adipose herniations, dystrophic nails, abnormal teeth and hair, vertebral anomalies, limb reduction defects, genitourinary anomalies
X-linked hereditary bullous dystrophy	+	+	0	Microcephaly, short stature, upslanting palpebral fissures, protruding ears, short and tapered digits, cardiac defects, bullous dystrophy, small testes, early death from pulmonary infection
Cantu	+	0	+	Short stature, microcephaly, alopecia, hyperpigmented lesions, follicular keratosis, cortical atrophy, pancytopenia

MIDAS SYNDROME

(Microphthalmia–Dermal Aplasia–Sclerocornea Syndrome, Microphthalmia–Linear Skin Defects Syndrome, MIM 309801)

DEFINITION. XLMR in females with microphthalmia, corneal opacification, and linear areas of dermal aplasia on the face, neck, and upper torso. On the basis of chromosome deletions and translocations, the gene has been located in Xp22.1-p22.3

SOMATIC FEATURES. At birth, infants have irregular linear skin defects of the face and upper torso, generalized facial erythema, microphthalmia, and corneal opacification. Additional ocular findings may include glaucoma, iris coloboma, embryotoxin, cataracts, retinopathy, retinal detachment, and orbital cysts. Vision is limited to light perception. The skin defects heal over the initial months of life, leaving linear atrophic scars.

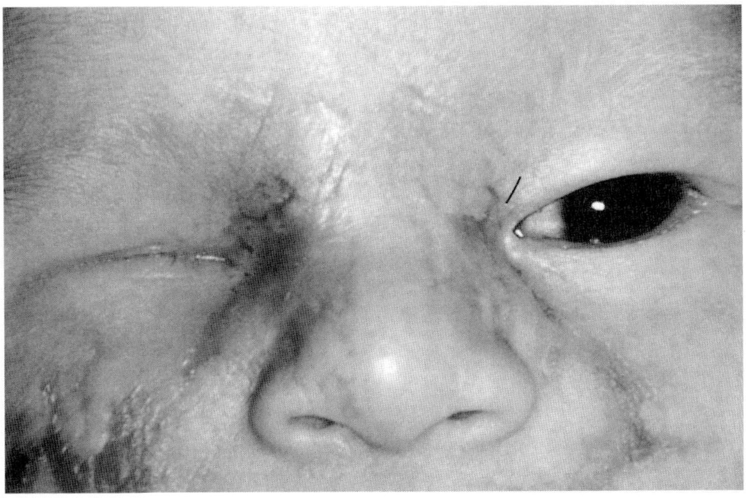

MIDAS Syndrome. Female infant with a de novo X;Y translocation with irregular areas of erythematous skin hypoplasia in the periocular area, microophthalmia, and corneal opacity. Courtesy of Dr. Robert Mueller, Leeds General Infirmary, England.

Aside from the ocular and cutaneous manifestations, the facial appearance is usually normal. Hypertelorism, abnormally formed ears, and micrognathia have been described. A wide variety of other structural anomalies have been described. Central nervous system and cardiac malformations are most notable. Dysgenesis of the corpus callosum, absent septum pellucidum, cystic lesions of the cerebrum, and enlarged ventricles number among the CNS anomalies. Structural cardiac anomalies include atrial septal defects (ASD), ventricular septal defects (VSD), and overriding aorta. Arrhythmias have also been described. Bird et al. have pointed out the particular association with oncocytic cardiomyopathy. Diaphragmatic hernia and anterior placement of the anus have been seen in one or more cases.

GROWTH AND DEVELOPMENT. Short stature becomes obvious within a few months after birth. Microcephaly has been noted in only one case.

COGNITIVE FEATURES. Cognitive impairment seems to be restricted to those who have associated CNS anomalies.

COMMENT. Translocations, deletions, or other rearrangements involving the X chromosome have been documented in most cases. As all cases reported have been females, MIDAS syndrome may be lethal in males. Among cases not associated with X chromosome rearrangements, an alternative explanation may be the emergence in females of paternal germline mutations.

REFERENCES

Al-Gazali LI, Mueller RF, Caine A, et al.: Two 46,XX,t(X;Y) females with linear skin defects and congenital microphthalmia: a new syndrome at Xp22.3. J Med Genet 27:59, 1990.

Bird LM, Krous HF, Eichenfield LF, et al.: Female infant with oncocytic cardiomyopathy and microphthalmia with linear skin defects (MLS): a clue to the pathogenesis of oncocytic cardiomyopathy? Am J Med Genet 53:141, 1994.

Differential Matrix

Syndrome	Ectodermal Dysplasia	Ocular Anomaly	CNS Anomaly	Comments
MIDAS	+	+	+	Microphthalmia, ocular dysgenesis, corneal opacification, dermal aplasia, dysgenesis of corpus callosum, cardiac defects, cardiomyopathy
Goltz	+	+	+	Cataracts, ocular dysgenesis, linear areas of dermal aplasia, cutaneous adipose herniations, dystrophic nails, abnormal teeth and hair, vertebral anomalies, limb reduction defects, genitourinary anomalies
Incontinentia pigmenti	+	+	0	Cutaneous vesicles, verrucous lesions, irregular hyperpigmentation, microcephaly, ocular anomalies, oligodontia, abnormally-shaped teeth, spasticity, seizures
Aicardi	0	+	+	Ocular dysgenesis, lacunar retinopathy, costovertebral anomalies, agenesis of corpus callosum, seizures
Cerebrooculogenital	0	+	+	Short stature, microcephaly, hydrocephaly, agenesis of corpus callosum, microphthalmia, ptosis, hypospadias, cryptorchidism, clubfoot, spasticity
Wittwer	0	+	+	Growth deficiency, microcephaly, microphthalmia, hearing loss, vision loss, hypertelorism, genitourinary anomalies, hypotonia, seizures

MILES-CARPENTER SYNDROME

(Miles Syndrome, MRXS4, XLMR with contractures and arch fingerprints, MIM 309605)

DEFINITION. XLMR with short stature, microcephaly, exotropia, long hands, digit contractures, rockerbottom feet, arch fingerprints, and spasticity. Gene location is between OTC (Xp11.4) and DXS94 (Xq22.2), lod score 2.7.

SOMATIC FEATURES. Craniofacial, skeletal, and cutaneous features distinguish the Miles-Carpenter syndrome. Microcephaly is present but not so marked as to cause craniofacial disproportion. Facial characteristics include medial flair of the eyebrows, exotropia, ptosis, small palpebral fissures, maxillary hypoplasia, thick alae nasi, open mouth with arched palate and thick alveolar ridges, and obtuse mandibular angle. Facial asymmetry, bitemporal narrowing, and small teeth with

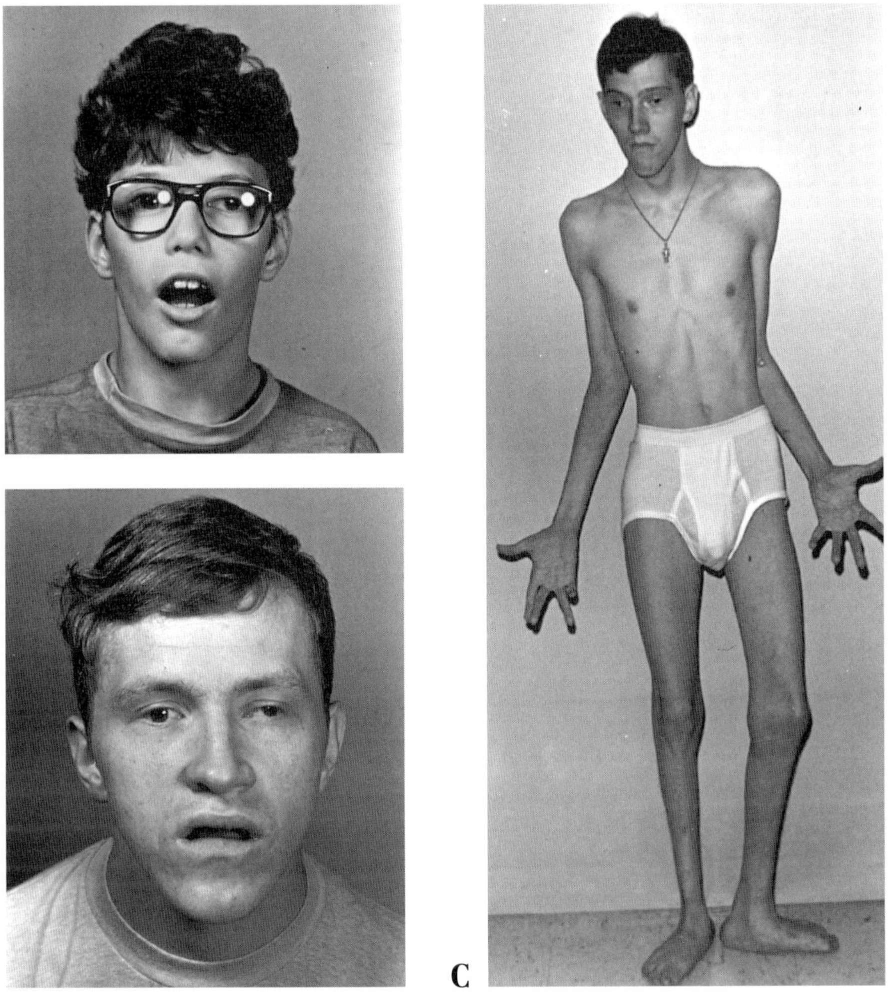

A B C

Miles-Carpenter Syndrome. Twenty-two-year-old male with exotropia, smooth philtrum, and tented upper lip (A); 31-year-old male cousin with facial asymmetry, left exotropia, and ptosis (B); 32-year-old male with slender build, pectus excavatum, scoliosis, high nasal bridge, long palms, accessory hypothenar crease, camptodactyly of fifth fingers, proximally placed thumbs, and pes planus with prominent heel (C–E).

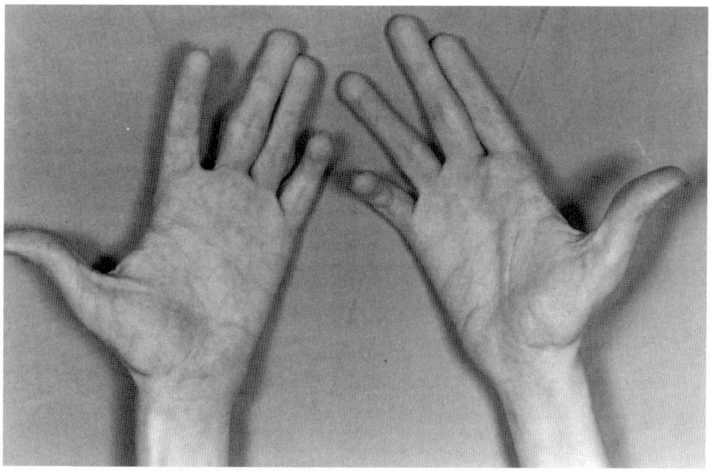

D

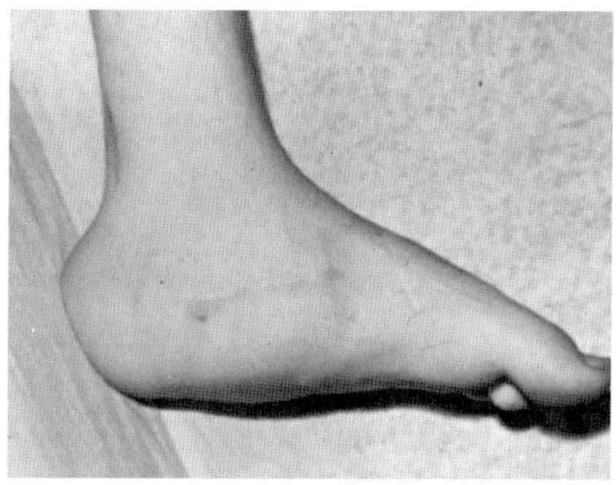

E

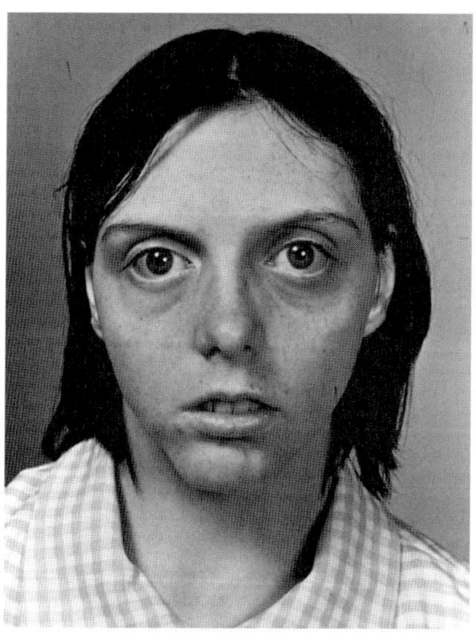

F

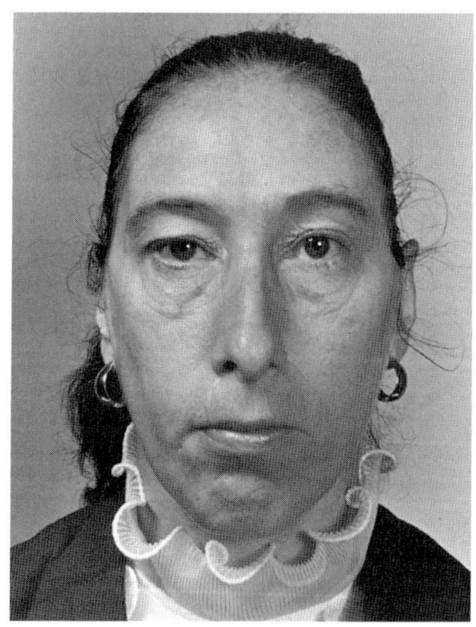

G

Miles-Carpenter Syndrome. (continued) Long palms, accessory hypothenar crease, camptodactyly of fifth fingers, proximally placed thumbs, and pes planus with prominent heel in 32-year-old male (D, E); 25-year-old carrier female with microcephaly, facial asymmetry, proptosis, and small mandible (F); 36-year-old carrier female with long face and high nasal bridge (G). Courtesy of Dr. Judith Miles, University of Missouri Health Sciences Center, Columbia.

irregular placement may be present. Ear size and architecture are not remarkable. The axial skeleton shows pectus excavatum and thoracic scoliosis. Hands are long, especially the palms, hyperextensible at the metacarpophalangeal joints, and have proximal thumb placement, finger 5 camptodactyly, abnormal palmar creases, cupping of the palms, and hyperconvex nails. Mild cutaneous syndactyly may be present. Feet are equally distinctive, with rockerbottom configuration due to vertical talus, and they show valgus positioning of the great toes and contractures of toes 4 and 5. The legs taper distally, the elbows and knees hyperextend, and stature may be shortened by flexed knee posture and scoliosis. The constant presence of 10 low fingerprint arches adds a distinctive and diagnostically helpful manifestation. Radiographs of one male demonstrated thickened calvaria, hyperostosis frontalis interna, bifid sternum, coxa valga, narrow diaphyses of the long bones, and epiphyseal delay.

GROWTH AND DEVELOPMENT. Birth weights range from 2.4 to 3.2 kg. Postnatal growth shows short stature and microcephaly. Genitalia appear normal although secondary sexual characteristics may be underdeveloped.

COGNITIVE FEATURES. Affected males have severe mental retardation; carrier females may be mildly impaired.

NEUROLOGICAL FINDINGS. Mild spasticity, toe walking, and unsteady gait.

HETEROZYGOTE EXPRESSION. Carrier females may have both somatic features and cognitive impairment although milder than in males. Microcephaly and craniofacial features may be present. The long cupped hands with digital contractures, hyperextensible MCP joints, and proximally placed thumbs typically occur in carrier females, but rockerbottom feet do not, although toe contractures and lateral deviation of the great toes may be present. Arches predominate in the fingerprint patterns.

COMMENT. The phenotype is based on observation in a single family with four affected males and six carrier females. Hoefnagel reported a brother and sister with similar findings. Four other XLMR syndromes have an excess of arch fingerprints or a low total ridge count: Chudley-Lowry, Coffin-Lowry, Prieto, and XLMR-arch fingerprints–hypotonia syndromes.

REFERENCES

Hoefnagel D: Malformation syndromes with mental deficiency. Birth Defects Orig Art Ser V(2): 11, 1969.

Miles JH, Carpenter NJ: Unique X-linked mental retardation syndrome with fingertip arches and contractures linked to Xq21.31. Am J Med Genet 38:215, 1991.

Tackels D, Thibodeau SN, Michaels V, et al.: Gene localization for the Miles-Carpenter syndrome (MCS). Am J Med Genet, in press, 1999.

Differential Matrix

Syndrome	Micro-cephaly	Skeletal Abnormality	Spasticity	Comments
Miles-Carpenter	+	+	+	Short stature, ptosis, small palpebral fissures, open mouth, pectus excavatum, scoliosis, long hands, camptodactyly, rockerbottom feet, arch fingerprints, unsteady gait
Cerebrooculogenital	+	+	+	Short stature, hydrocephaly, agenesis of corpus callosum, microphthalmia, ptosis, hypospadias, cryptorchidism, clubfoot
Gustavson	+	+	+	Short stature, optic atrophy with blindness, large ears, deafness, joint contractures, rockerbottom feet, brain undergrowth, hydrocephaly, cerebellar hypoplasia, seizures
Kang	+	+	+	Frontal prominence, telecanthus, small nose, short hands, dysgenesis of corpus callosum, seizures, downslanted mouth, brachydactyly
Pettigrew	+	+	+	Dandy-Walker malformation, seizures, microcephaly or hydrocephaly, long face with macrostomia and prognathism, small testes, contractures, choreoathetosis, iron deposits in basal ganglia
Proud	+	+	+	Hearing loss, vision loss, agenesis of corpus callosum, cryptorchidism, inguinal hernias, ataxia, seizures
Schimke	+	+	+	Sunken eyes, downslanting palpebral fissures, narrow nose, spacing of teeth, cupped ears, hypotonia, abducens palsy, hearing loss, vision loss, choreoathetosis, contractures

MOHR-TRANEBJAERG SYNDROME

(Mohr Syndrome, Mohr-Mageroy Syndrome, Deafness-Blindness-Dementia Syndrome, MIM 304700)

DEFINITION. XLMR with progressive deafness, blindness, and neurologic deterioration with onset in early childhood. The gene maps to Xq22 and has been identified as the deafness dystonia polypeptide (DDP).

SOMATIC FEATURES. Normal growth and craniofacial appearance. Fractures are common and perhaps are related to injury because of unsteady gait.

GROWTH AND DEVELOPMENT. Intrauterine and postnatal growth are normal. Early developmental milestones are normal, but verbal abilities may be impaired because of hearing loss.

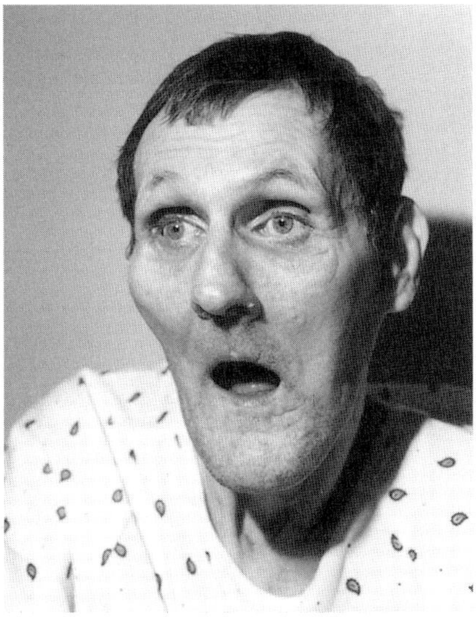
A
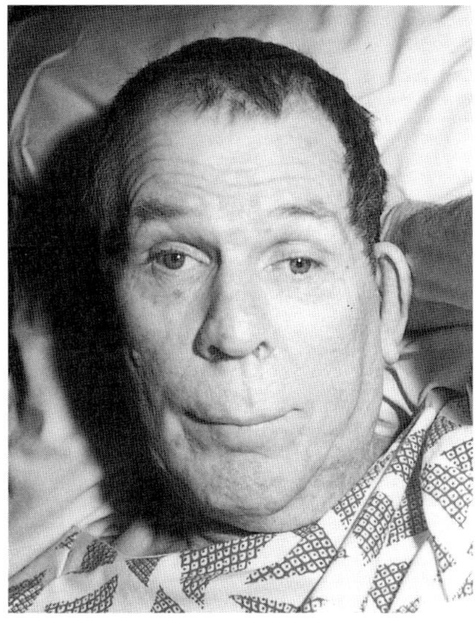
B

Mohr-Tranebjaerg Syndrome. Fifty-five-year-old male with wasting of facial muscles and sunken eyes (A); 62-year-old with facial asymmetry, upslanting palpebral fissures, and blindness (B).

Cognitive Features. Progressive loss of cognitive skills eventually leads to severe impairment. The onset coincides with other neurologic findings, usually by late childhood or early adult life.

Behavioral Manifestations. Restlessness, irritability, and aggressiveness may occur in childhood. Following the onset of dementia, there may be confusion, unsociable behavior, and paranoid ideation.

Neurological Findings. Hearing loss develops after birth and rapidly worsens. Speech develops among those in whom hearing loss is delayed beyond the first few years. Vision becomes impaired and is lost at a later age, generally becoming symptomatic in the 30s and progressively worsening. Photophobia and scotomas may precede vision loss by a number of years. Retinal changes are compatible with central choroidal areolar dystrophy with central scotomas. Retinal dysfunction is usually not seen on electroretinogram (ERG). Motor skills become impaired early in life, in some cases before age 10 years. Ataxia, dystonia, and spasticity interfere with speech, feeding, and ambulation. Some cases become opisthotonic. Mental deterioration coincides with the other neurological impairments. Irritability, aggressiveness, and paranoia occur in some cases. Mild neurogenic muscle atrophy has been verified by EMG and muscle biopsy.

Heterozygote Expression. Mild hearing loss, pallor of the optic discs and possible signs of motor-sensory neuropathy have been noted in several obligate carriers.

Neuropathology. Generalized brain atrophy is the typical postmortem finding.

Imaging. Cerebral atrophy occurs as early as age 7 years.

Laboratory. Long chain fatty acids, phytanic acid, plasmalogens, and muscle staining for amyloid are normal.

COMMENT. The initial family was reported as isolated X-linked deafness (DFN-1). The neurodegenerative manifestations were recognized on later follow-up. Progressive sensorineural hearing loss has onset between 1 and 5 years, usually after acquisition of some speech. Loss of vision and onset of neurological abnormalities and dementia are often delayed until adult life, but may begin in late childhood. Neurodegeneration appears relentless with eventual loss of motor skills, lack of contact with the environment, dysphagia, spasticity, and psychosis. Although rapid progression to death occurred in one teenage patient, life expectancy does not appear shortened in most cases.

REFERENCES

Jensen PKA: Nerve deafness, optic nerve atrophy and dementia: a new X-linked recessive syndrome? Am J Med Genet 9:55, 1981.

Jin H, May M, Tranebjaerg L, et al.: A novel X-linked gene, DDP, shows mutations in families with deafness (DFN-1), dystonia, mental deficiency and blindness. Nat Genet 14:177, 1996.

Mohr J, Magerøy K: Sex-linked deafness of a possibly new type. Acta Genet Stat Med 10:54, 1960.

Ponjavic V, Andreasson S, Tranebjaerg L, et al.: Full-field electroretinograms in a family with Mohr-Tranebjaerg syndrome. Acta Ophthalmol Scand 74:632, 1996.

Tranebjaerg L, Schwartz C, Eriksen H, et al.: A new X linked recessive deafness syndrome with blindness, dystonia, fractures, and mental deficiency is linked to Xq22. J Med Genet 32:257, 1995.

Differential Matrix

Syndrome	Hearing Loss	Vision Loss	Spasticity, Dystonia, or Ataxia	Comments
Mohr-Tranebjaerg (Jensen)	+	+	+	Neurologic deterioration with childhood onset
Gustavson	+	+	+	Microcephaly, short stature, optic atrophy, large ears, joint contractures, rockerbottom feet, brain undergrowth, hydrocephaly, cerebellar hypoplasia, seizures
Paine	+	+	+	Microcephaly, short stature, optic atrophy, seizures
Proud	+	+	+	Microcephaly, agenesis of corpus callosum, cryptorchidism, inguinal hernias, seizures
Schimke	+	+	+	Microcephaly, sunken eyes, downslanting palpebral fissures, narrow nose, spacing of teeth, cupped ears, hypotonia, abducens palsy, choreoathetosis, contractures
X-linked ataxia-deafness-dementia	+	+	+	Optic atrophy, spastic paraplegia, hypotonia, seizures, childhood death
Norrie	+	+	0	Ocular dysplasia and degeneration, adult-onset hearing loss
Wittwer	+	+	0	Growth deficiency, microcephaly, microphthalmia, hypertelorism, genitourinary anomalies, hypotonia, seizures
Arts	0	+	+	Growth deficiency, paucity of muscles, hypotonia, areflexia, seizures, childhood death
Bertini	0	+	+	Macular degeneration, hypotonia, seizures, childhood death, hypoplasia of cerebellar vermis and corpus callosum, developmental delays and regression, postnatal growth impairment
X-linked spastic paraplegia, type 7	0	+	+	Nystagmus, reduced vision, absent speech and ambulation, bowel and bladder dysfunction, spastic quadriplegia

Monoamine Oxidase-A Deficiency

(Brunner syndrome, MIM 309850)

Definition. X-linked behavioral disorder and borderline intelligence secondary to monoamine oxidase (MAO)-A deficiency. A mutation in the MAO-A gene in Xp11.3-p11.4 has been documented.

SOMATIC FEATURES. Growth appears normal and major malformations or distinctive facial features have not been reported.

GROWTH AND DEVELOPMENT. Normal growth. Early developmental progress is not notably abnormal.

COGNITIVE FEATURES. Normal to borderline low cognitive function.

BEHAVIORAL MANIFESTATIONS. A withdrawn and shy demeanor punctuated by disordered behavior, particularly aggressive and violent behavior out of proportion to provocation, is typical. Recurrent clusters of aggressive behavior, insomnia, and night terrors last several days. Additional behaviors include setting fires, exhibitionism, voyeurism, rape, and unwelcome embracing.

NEUROLOGICAL FINDINGS. Repetitive hand wringing, plucking, and fiddling occur commonly but neurological examination is grossly normal.

HETEROZYGOTE EXPRESSION. None described.

LABORATORY. Urine analysis shows elevated monamine substrates (normetanephrine, 3-methoxytyramine, and tyramine) and reduced monamine products (vanilacetic acid, vanilglycolic acid, 5-hydroxyindole-3-acetic acid, and 3-methoxy-4-hydroxyphenylglycol). Activity of MAO-B is normal in platelets.

COMMENT. MAO-A and MAO-B are closely linked genes in Xp11.3-11.4. Deletion of both genes has been associated with severe mental retardation, but deletion of the MAO-B gene alone does not appear to cause any disability.

REFERENCES

Brunner HG, Nelen MR, van Zandvoort P, et al.: X-linked borderline mental retardation with prominent behavioral disturbance: phenotype, genetic localization, and evidence for disturbed monoamine metabolism. Am J Hum Genet 52:1032, 1993.

Brunner HG, Nelen M, Breakefield XO, et al.: Abnormal behavior associated with a point mutation in the structural gene for monoamine oxidase A. Science 262:578, 1993.

Differential Matrix

Syndrome	Aggressive or Violent Behavior	Repetitive Movements	Metabolic Disturbances	Comments
Monoamine oxidase-A deficiency	+	+	+	-
Lowe	0	+	+	Short stature, cataracts, hypotonia, aminoaciduria, progressive renal failure
Mucopolysaccharidosis IIA	+	0	+	Macrocephaly, short stature, coarse facies, hepatosplenomegaly, hernias, joint stiffness, thick skin, hirsutism

MUCOPOLYSACCHARIDOSIS IIA

(Hunter Syndrome, MPS IIA, MIM 309900)

DEFINITION. XLMR with generalized mucopolysaccharide storage due to sulfoiduronate sulfatase deficiency. The gene is located in the proximal portion of Xq28.

SOMATIC FEATURES. Two more or less distinctive types of mucopolysaccharidosis II are recognized clinically. In the "severe form" (MPS IIA) profound mental

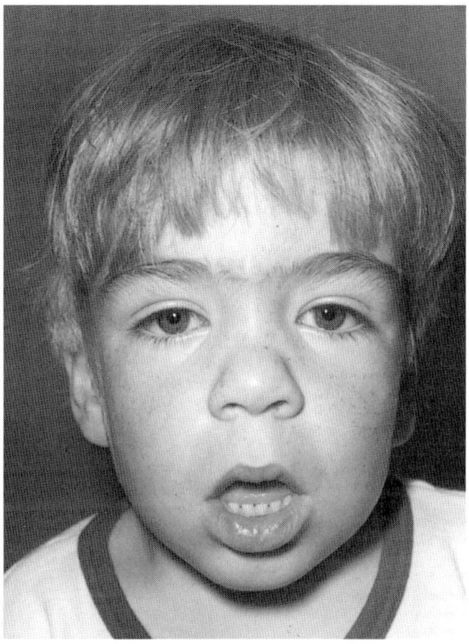

A

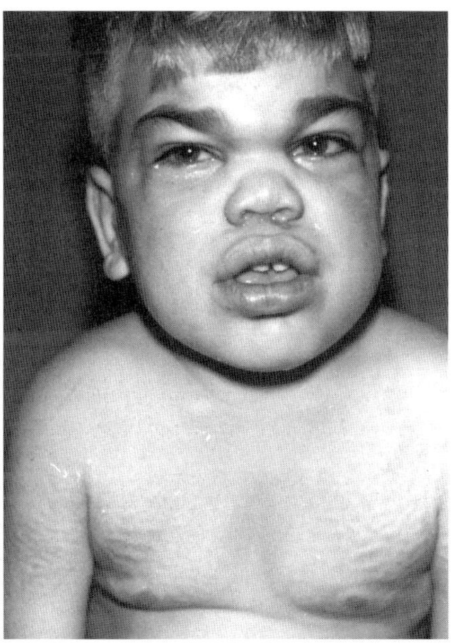

B

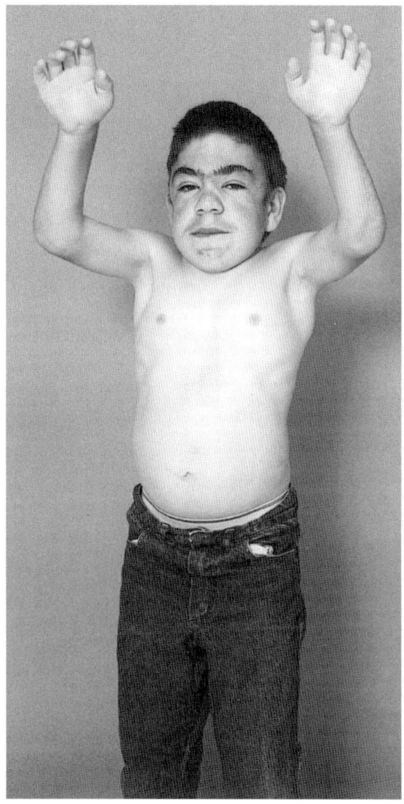

C

Mucopolysaccharidosis IIA. Coarse facies, depressed nasal bridge, full lower face, thickened lips, facial acne, and joint contractures at ages 4 and 16 years (A, C); 14-year-old with prominent lower face, depressed nasal bridge, full lips, and nodular skin lesions over the chest and arms (B).

retardation becomes obvious by late childhood. In the "mild form" (MPS IIB) mentation may be normal and deterioration of mental function only slowly progressive. At birth, infants usually appear normal. They experience normal or excessive growth during the first 1 to 2 years. There is a paucity of clinical signs except respiratory symptoms (noisy breathing from upper airway obstruction, recurrent rhinorrhea), large scaphoid head, and herniae (inguinal and umbilical) during infancy. Coarsening of facial features with thickening of the nostrils, lips, and tongue; joint stiffness; growth failure; excessive growth of fine body hair; and hepatosplenomegaly become obvious at about 2 years and progress in severity. Thick skin, short neck, widely spaced teeth, hearing loss of some degree, and papilledema are commonly present. Nodular skin lesions on the arms or posterior chest wall, retinal pigmentation, mild pectus excavatum, pes cavus, mucoid diarrhea, and seizures occur less commonly. Valvular and coronary heart disease develop during childhood and mental function, hearing, and joint mobility deteriorate steadily. The spine is straight and corneas clear grossly.

COGNITIVE FEATURES. Function is severely impaired prior to the end of the first decade and disruptive, destructive behavior is the rule.

NEUROLOGICAL FINDINGS. Progressive hearing loss.

LABORATORY. Roentgenologic findings include scaphoid skull, enlarged sella with anterior excavation, skeletal findings of dysostosis multiplex, minimal vertebral changes, and precocious osteoarthritis of the femoral heads. Laboratory findings include excessive urinary excretion of dermatan sulfate and heparan sulfate; leukocytes, fibroblasts, and serum are deficient in the enzyme sulfoiduronate sulfatase; leukocytes and fibroblasts show metachromatic staining; cultured fibroblasts accumulate sulfated mucopolysaccharides at an enhanced rate and can be "corrected" with purified Hunter factor or with fibroblast secretions from non-Hunter individuals.

COMMENT. Hunter syndrome is the only X-linked mucopolysaccharidosis. The two types (MPS IIA and MPS IIB) are examples of allelic variation which result in remarkably different neurobehavioral phenotypes but the same somatic phenotype. Severe mental deterioration and disruptive, destructive behavior, typical of MPS IIA is also seen in Sanfilippo syndrome (MPS III).

REFERENCES

Hunter C: A rare disease in two brothers. Proc R Soc Med 10:104, 1917.

Wilson PJ, Morris CP, Anson DS, et al.: Hunter syndrome: isolation of an iduronate-2-sulfatase cDNA clone and analysis of patient DNA. Proc Natl Acad Sci USA 87:8531, 1990.

Differential Matrix

Syndrome	Short Stature	Coarse Facies	Macro-cephaly	Comments
Mucopoly-saccharidosis IIA	+	+	+	Hepatosplenomegaly, hernias, joint stiffness, thick skin, hirsutism, behavioral disturbance
Atkin-Flaitz	+	+	+	Hypertelorism, downslanting palpebral fissures, broad nasal tip, thick lower lip, brachydactyly, seizures
XLMR-hypotonic facies (Carpenter-Waziri) (Holmes-Gang) (Juberg-Marsidi)	+	+	0	Small testes, telecanthus, small triangular nose, tented upper lip, open mouth, spacing of teeth, genital anomalies, musculoskeletal anomalies, hemoglobin H inclusions in erythrocytes
Börjeson-Forssman-Lehmann	+	+	0	Obesity, hypotonia, hypogonadism, microcephaly, large ears, gynecomastia, narrow shoulders, visual impairment, tapered digits
Coffin-Lowry	+	+	0	Hypertelorism, anteverted nares, tented upper lip, prominent lips and large mouth, large ears, soft hands with tapered digits, pectus carinatum, hypotonia

Myotubular Myopathy

(Centronuclear Myopathy, MIM 310400)

Definition. XLMR associated with hypotonia, weakness, and absent deep tendon reflexes secondary to myotubular myopathy. A locus (MTM1) in Xq28 has been identified by linkage analysis; genetic heterogeneity is likely since at least one three-generation family does not show linkage to Xq28.

Somatic Features. A craniofacial phenotype, due in large measure to hypotonia, may be recognized. Ptosis, arched upper lip, high palate, open mouth, thick alae nasi, and thick auricular helices accent an elongated and immobile face. The head tends to be large and elongated in its anteroposterior diameter. Hydrocephalus has been demonstrated in patients with intracranial hemorrhage in the perinatal period and in patients without this complication. Long slender digits are typical, contractures may be present, and cryptorchidism is commonly noted.

Growth and Development. Birth length and head circumference, but not birth weight, tend to be large. Hydrocephaly contributes to the increased head circumference in some cases. The hydrocephaly is communicating and may arrest spontaneously or progressively worsen. The tendency toward increased body length persists among those who survive the early months of life. Pervasive delay of developmental milestones is typical in these usually ventilator-dependent children.

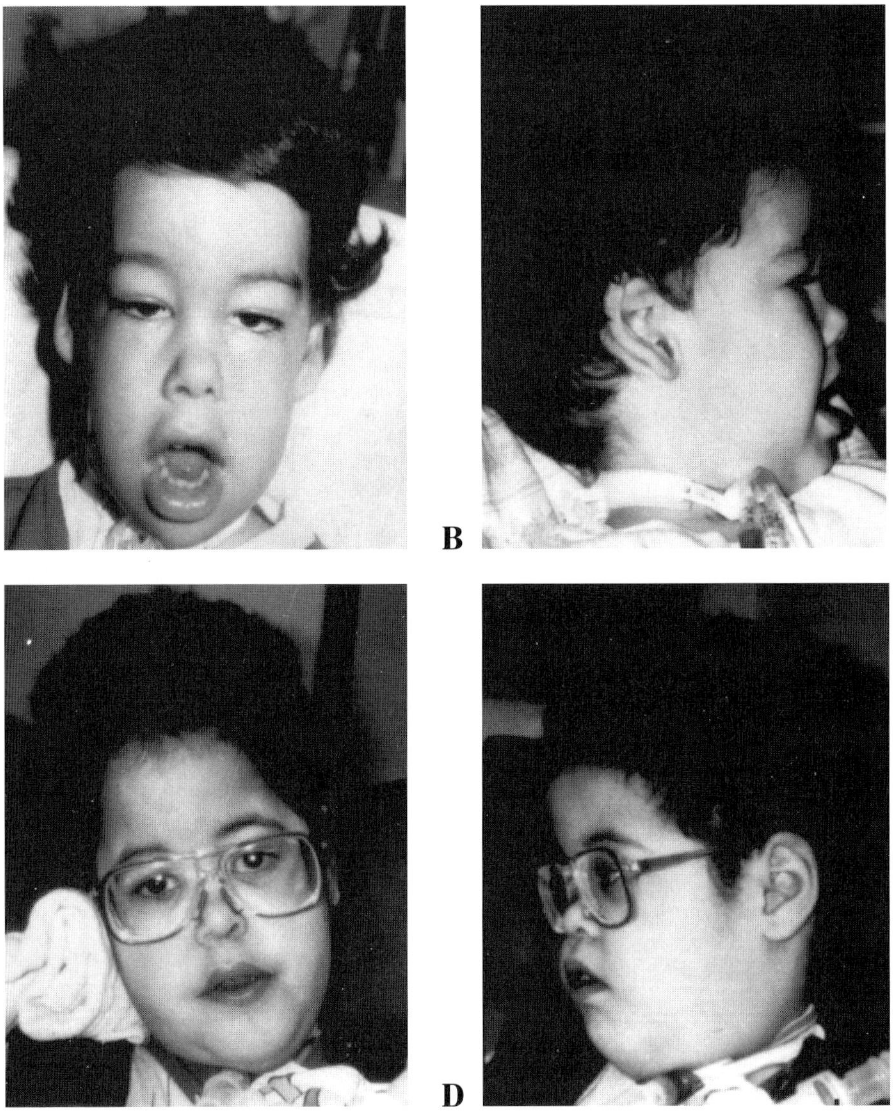

A B C D

Myotubular Myopathy. Four-year-old with macrocephaly and myopathic facies including ptosis, thickening of the alae nasi, and tenting of the upper lip (A, B); 6-year-old with macrocephaly, narrow bifrontal area, long facies, and tented upper lip (C, D). Courtesy of Dr. Shashidhar Pai, Medical University of South Carolina, Charleston.

COGNITIVE FEATURES. Severe motor impairment, ventilator dependency, and early death prevent adequate assessment of cognitive function.

NEUROLOGICAL FINDINGS. Profound hypotonia, weakness, and areflexia exist from birth and presumably from early in fetal life. Respiratory efforts are insufficient, generally requiring ventilator support.

HETEROZYGOTE EXPRESSION. Although not clinically weak, carriers may show myopathic changes on muscle histology. This finding is inconsistent, however.

LABORATORY. Small muscle fibers with centralization of nuclei and absence of central myofibrils can be demonstrated by light and electron microscopy.
IMAGING. Hydrocephaly is present in some cases. Intracranial hemorrhage and evidence of ischemia may also be present.
COMMENT. Myotubular myopathy has been suspected in at-risk pregnancies by the paucity of fetal movement and the appearance, often only in the third trimester, of polyhydramnios. Most patients die in the first few months of life. Survival has been possible with early and continued ventilator support.

REFERENCES

Darnfors C, Larsson HE, Oldfors A, et al.: X-linked myotubular myopathy: a linkage study. Clin Genet 37:335, 1990.
DeAngelis MS, Palmucci L, Leone M, et al.: Centronuclear myopathy: clinical morphologic and genetic characters. A review of 288 cases. J Neurol Sci 103:2, 1991.
Joseph M, Pai GS, Holden KR, et al.: X-linked myotubular myopathy: clinical observations in ten additional cases. Am J Med Genet 59:168, 1995.
Samson F, Mesnard L, Heimburger M, et al.: Genetic linkage heterogeneity in myotubular myopathy. Am J Hum Genet 57:120, 1995.
Van Wijngaarden GK, Fleury P, Bethlem J, et al.: Familial myotubular myopathy. Neurology 19:901, 1969.

Differential Matrix

Syndrome	Muscle Wasting	Hypotonia	Areflexia, Hypo-reflexia	Comments
Myotubular myopathy	+	+	+	Open mouth, tented upper lip, hydrocephaly, long digits, cryptorchidism, weakness
Arts	+	+	+	Growth deficiency, paucity of muscles, ataxia, deafness, vision loss, seizures, childhood death
Charcot-Marie-Tooth neuropathy, Cowchock variant	+	0	+	Peripheral motor and sensory neuropathy, deafness, pes cavus, weakness
Charcot-Marie-Tooth neuropathy, Ionasescu variant	+	0	+	Peripheral motor and sensory neuropathy, weakness, wasting of intrinsic hand muscles, enlarged ulnar nerves, pes cavus
Duchenne muscular dystrophy	+	0	+	Hypertrophy of calf muscles, elevated muscle enzymes, progressive weakness, contractures
Phosphoglycerate kinase deficiency	+	0	+	Expressionless face, weakness, seizures, myoglobinuria, hemolytic anemia

NANCE-HORAN SYNDROME

(XLMR-Cataract-Dental Syndrome, MIM 302350)

DEFINITION. XLMR with congenital cataracts, microcorneas, dental anomalies, and brachydactyly. The gene has been linked to markers in Xp22, lod score 3.23.
SOMATIC FEATURES. Congenital cataracts almost invariably bring this condition to attention at birth or in early infancy. The dense bilateral nuclear cataracts may be detected on routine examination or in the course of evaluating the accompanying nystagmus. Microcornea and, less frequently, microphthalmia and glaucoma may be present. Vision is severely impaired. Dental anomalies include supernumerary maxillary medial incisors (mesiodens), peg-shaped teeth, notching of the incisors, and spacing of the central incisors (diastema). The ears are frequently cupped, prominent, and simply formed. Other facial features include long facies, prominent nasal bridge and nose, prominent mandible, retracted midface, and high arched palate. Short fourth metacarpals and short broad fingers complete the phenotype.
GROWTH AND DEVELOPMENT. Growth appears to be normal. Development is delayed and cognition is impaired in about 20% of males. The visual impairment is contributory but does not appear to be the sole cause.
COGNITIVE FEATURES. Mild to moderate cognitive impairment has been suspected in a minority of cases.
HETEROZYGOTE EXPRESSION. Young females may have posterior sutural cataracts that are only detected by slit lamp and do not limit vision. Increasing lens opac-

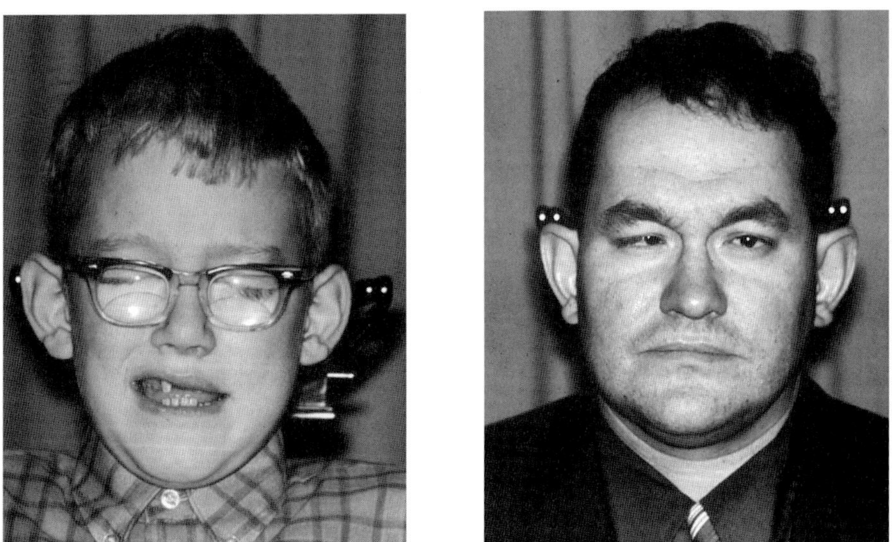

A B

Nance-Horan Syndrome. Nine-year-old male with cupped ears, microcornea, and congenital cataracts (A); 38-year-old with cupped ears, microcornea, and congenital cataracts (B).

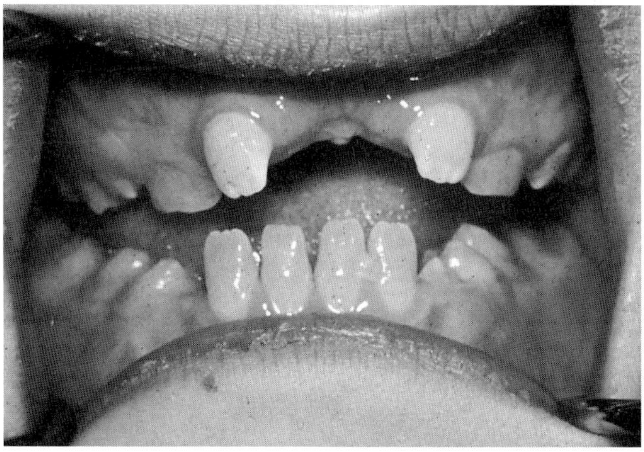

C

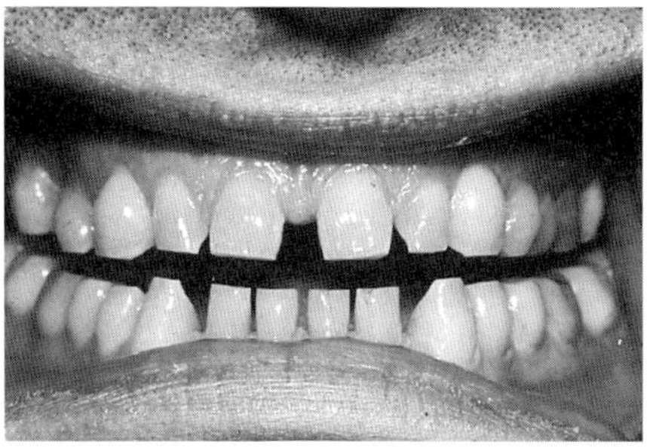

D

Nance-Horan Syndrome. (continued) Teeth of patient shown in A showing spacing of incisors and narrow incisal edges (C); teeth of patient shown in B showing spacing of incisors and tapering of incisal edges (D). Courtesy of Dr. Walter Nance, Medical College of Virginia, Richmond.

ity with age has been reported. Tapering, notching, and spacing of the incisors have been observed.

COMMENT. Cataracts, apparently X-linked, have been reported in families without other features of Nance-Horan. It is possible that the manifestations of Nance-Horan may be pleiotrophic effects of a single gene or components of a contiguous gene deletion.

REFERENCES

Bergen AAB, ten Brink J, Schuurman EJM, et al.: Nance-Horan syndrome: linkage analysis in a family from the Netherlands. Genomics 21:238, 1994.

Horan MB, Billson FA: X-linked cataract and Hutchinsonian teeth. Aust Paediat J 10:98, 1974.

Nance WE, Warburg M, Bixler D, et al.: Congenital X-linked cataract, dental anomalies and brachymetacarpalia. Birth Defects Orig Art Ser X(4):285, 1974.

Walpole IR, Hockey A, Nicoll A: The Nance-Horan syndrome. J Med Genet 27:632, 1990.

Differential Matrix

Syndrome	Cataracts	Dental Anomalies	Digital Anomalies	Comments
Nance-Horan	+	+	+	Microcornea, nystagmus, cupped ears, short fourth metacarpals
Armfield	+	+	+	Short stature, cataracts or glaucoma, small hands and feet, hydrocephaly, joint stiffness, seizures
Goltz	+	+	+	Ocular dysgenesis, linear areas of dermal aplasia, cutaneous adipose herniations, dystrophic nails, vertebral anomalies, limb reduction defects, genitourinary anomalies
Lenz microphthalmia	+	+	+	Microcephaly, microphthalmia, ocular dysgenesis, malformed ears, cleft lip/palate, cardiac and genitourinary anomalies, thumb duplication or hypoplasia, narrow shoulders
Incontinentia pigmenti	+	+	0	Cutaneous vesicles, verrucous lesions, irregular hyperpigmentation, microcephaly, ocular anomalies, oligodontia, spasticity, seizures
Albright hereditary osteodystrophy	+	0	+	Short stature, obesity, brachydactyly, short metacarpals and metatarsals, ectopic calcifications

NORRIE DISEASE

(Norrie Retinal Dysplasia, MIM 310600)

DEFINITION. XLMR with a progressive ophthalmopathy (iris atrophy, uveal ectropion, anterior and posterior synechiae, cataract, hyperplastic vitreous, and retrolental mass) and adult-onset hearing loss. The gene, norrin, codes for a cysteine knot-containing growth factor and is located in Xp11.3.

SOMATIC FEATURES. Ocular dysplasia and degeneration dominate the physical phenotype. Apart from the ocular findings, major malformations and facial manifestations do not occur. Binocular blindness is present from birth. The corneas vary in size and in clarity. The anterior chamber is likewise variable in depth. Iris atrophy occurs in most and is associated with anterior and posterior synechiae. Cataracts will develop in many but not all cases. Retinal dysplasia manifesting as impaired vascularization, aplasia of sensory cells, and hyperplasia of pigment cells combines with hyperplasia of the vitreous to form a yellowish gray retrolental mass constituting an obligatory finding. The degeneration may ultimately progress to collapse of the ocular globe. Moderate to severe sensorineural hearing loss appears in the second or third decade.

GROWTH AND DEVELOPMENT. Intrauterine and postnatal growth is normal. Developmental delay in childhood identifies those who will be mentally retarded.
COGNITIVE FEATURES. Cognitive impairment of varying severity affects the majority but not all cases.
NEUROLOGICAL FINDINGS. Aside from blindness and deafness, neurological abnormalities do not occur.
HETEROZYGOTE EXPRESSION. None.
IMAGING. Abnormalities of brain structure have not been described.
COMMENT. The X chromosome hosts a disproportionate share of genes that disturb formation and function of the eye. Mutations in these genes also produce CNS malformations or functional impairments but do so quite inconsistently. As yet, reasons for the variable expression have not been found. Missense mutations in the Norrie disease gene have also been found in X-linked familial exudative vitreoretinopathy and in X-linked recessive primary retinal dysplasia, entities in which mental retardation and hearing loss do not occur. Vision loss appears later and may be unilateral and less severe.

REFERENCES

Chen Z-Y, Battinelli EM, Fielder A, et al.: A mutation in the Norrie disease gene (NDP) associated with X-linked familial exudative vitreoretinopathy. Nat Genet 5:180, 1993.

Chen Z-Y, Battinelli EM, Kendriks RW, et al.: Norrie disease gene: characterization of deletions and possible function. Genomics 16:533, 1993.

Norrie G: Causes of blindness in children. Acta Ophthalmol 5:7, 1927.

Shastry BS, Hejtmancik JF, Trese MT: Identification of novel missense mutations in the Norrie disease gene associated with one X-linked and four sporadic cases of familial exudative vitreoretinopathy. Hum Mutat 9:396, 1997.

Strasberg P, Liede HA, Stein T, et al.: A novel mutation in the Norrie disease gene predicted to disrupt the cystine knot growth factor motif. Hum Mol Genet 4:2179, 1995.

Warburg M: Norrie's disease. A new hereditary bilateral pseudotumour of the retina. Acta Ophthalmol 39:757, 1961.

Differential Matrix

Syndrome	Ocular Dysgenesis	Vision Loss	Hearing Loss	Comments
Norrie	+	+	+	Adult-onset hearing loss
Wittwer	+	+	+	Growth deficiency, microcephaly, microphthalmia, hypertelorism, genitourinary anomalies, hypotonia, seizures
Cerebrooculogenital	+	+	0	Short stature, microcephaly, hydrocephaly, agenesis of corpus callosum, microphthalmia, ptosis, hypospadias, cryptorchidism, clubfoot, spasticity
Goltz	+	+	0	Cataracts, linear areas of dermal aplasia, cutaneous adipose herniations, dystrophic nails, abnormal teeth and hair, vertebral anomalies, limb reduction defects, genitourinary anomalies
Lenz microphthalmia	+	+	0	Microcephaly, microphthalmia, malformed ears, cleft lip/palate, cardiac and genitourinary anomalies, thumb duplication or hypoplasia, narrow shoulders
Lowe	+	+	0	Short stature, cataracts, hypotonia, aminoaciduria, progressive renal failure
MIDAS	+	+	0	Microphthalmia, corneal opacification, dermal aplasia, dysgenesis of corpus callosum, cardiac defects, cardiomyopathy

OPITZ FG SYNDROME

(FG Syndrome, Opitz-Kaveggia Syndrome, MIM 305450)

DEFINITION. XLMR with macrocephaly, broad flat thumbs, imperforate anus or constipation, and hypotonia. One gene has been localized to Xq12-q21.3 but all families do not show linkage to this region. Another gene locus may be in Xq28.
SOMATIC FEATURES. The facial characteristics include absolute or relative macrocephaly, broad forehead, frontal hair upsweep, hypertelorism, epicanthus, downslanted palpebral fissures, thick alae nasi, small cupped simply formed ears,

→

Opitz FG Syndrome. Turricephaly, hypertelorism, downslanting palpebral fissures, small and low-set simply formed ears, and tented and thin upper lip at age 5 years (A); macrocephaly, dolichocephaly, hypertelorism, downslanting palpebral fissures, tented upper lip, maxillary overbite, notching of the upper central incisors, broad thumbs, and great toes in an 8-year-old boy (B–D). Figure A courtesy of Dr. John Graham, Cedars-Sinai Medical Center, Los Angeles; Figures B–D courtesy of Dr. Curtis Rogers, Greenwood Genetic Center, Greenwood, SC.

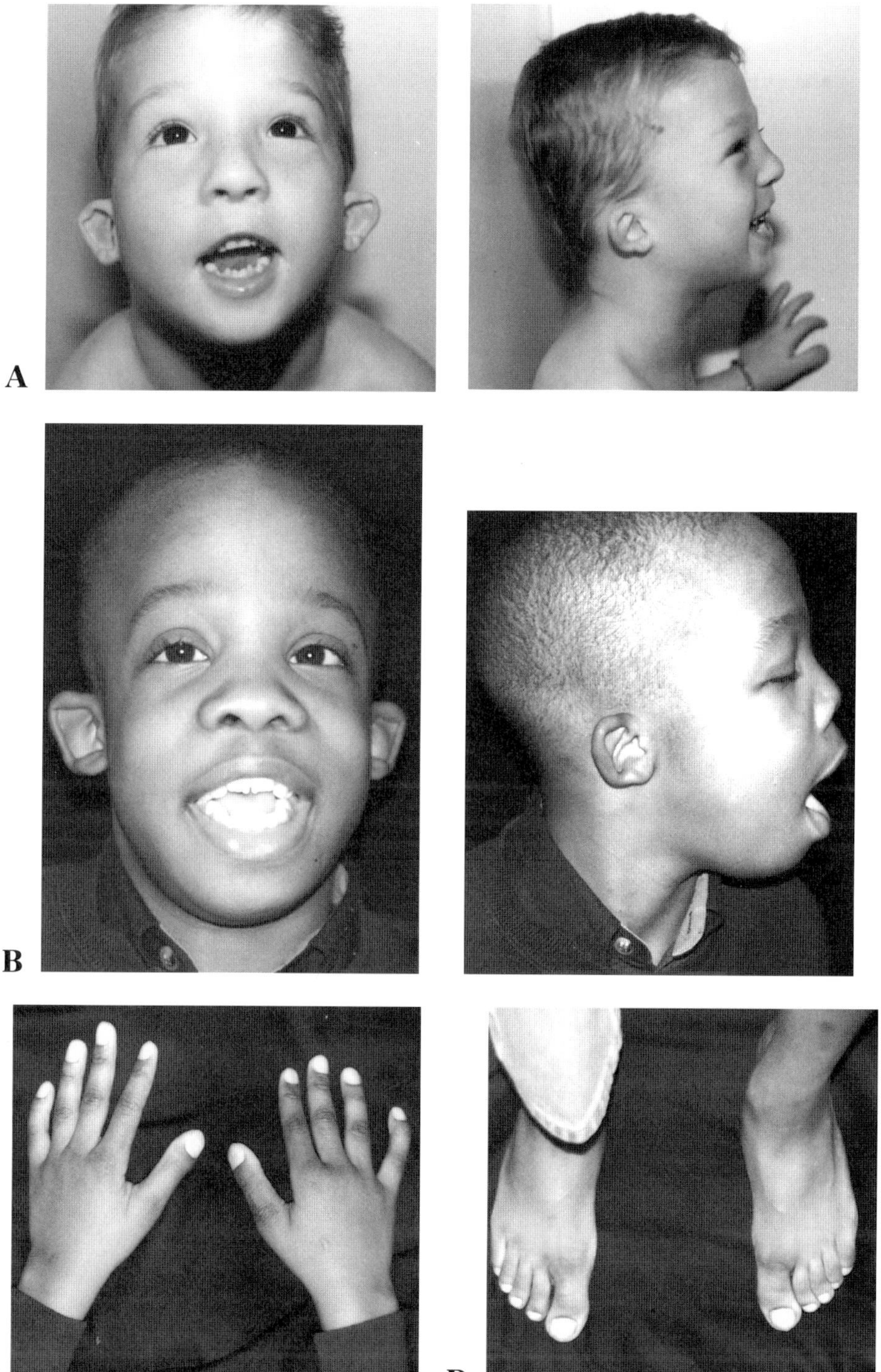

A B C D

open mouth, high arched palate, and everted lower lip. Hypotonia is notable and may be responsible for some of the facial features. A wide variety of structural anomalies of the central nervous system, heart, and genitourinary tract have been described. Complete or partial agenesis of the corpus callosum is the most common CNS anomaly but dilated ventricles, pachygyria, and cerebral heterotopias have been noted. Cardiac defects, present in one-third of cases, include ventricular septal defect and hypoplastic left heart. Dilation of the urinary system, cryptorchidism, and hypospadias are the most common genitourinary tract abnormalities. Pyloric stenosis and hernias have been reported. Imperforate anus or severe childhood constipation without imperforate anus appears to be a distinguishing feature found in most cases. Musculoskeletal manifestations include broad flat thumbs and great toes, cutaneous syndactyly of fingers 2 and 3, horizontal palmar creases, camptodactyly, pectus excavatum, kyphoscoliosis, and large joint contractures. Joint hyperextensibility is typical. Split hand has been noted in a single case.

GROWTH AND DEVELOPMENT. Intrauterine growth is usually normal or only mildly impaired. Stature usually remains in lower centiles, but in some cases it falls below the third centile. The head grows disproportionately, becoming macrocephalic or relatively macrocephalic in comparison to stature. The anterior fontanel may be large and delayed in closure. Motor and language development lags from the outset.

COGNITIVE FEATURES. Severe impairment is the rule although milder impairment has been seen occasionally.

BEHAVIORAL MANIFESTATIONS. An affable personality with excessive talkativeness and hyperactivity has been described in some.

NEUROLOGICAL FINDINGS. Hypotonia dominates the neurological examination but in some cases gives way to spasticity, contractures, and unsteadiness during adult life. Seizures and sensorineural hearing loss occur in a minority.

HETEROZYGOTE EXPRESSION. No consistent manifestations are present in carrier females, although broad forehead, hypertelorism, and anterior upsweep of the scalp hair have been noted.

IMAGING. Partial or complete agenesis of the corpus callosum occurs most commonly. In some cases, the ventricles may be dilated. Pachygyria and cerebral heterotopias have been described in a few cases.

COMMENT. Genetic heterogeneity exists in this entity and perhaps explains in part the clinical difficulty in diagnosis. The diagnosis is most compelling in the presence of macrocephaly, hypotonia, and imperforate anus. Diagnosis on the basis of the rather subtle and variable craniofacial manifestations requires an experienced eye. Localization and isolation of the causative genes may help.

REFERENCES

Briault S, Hill R, Shrimpton A, et al.: A gene for FG syndrome maps in the Xq12-21.31 region. Am J Med Genet 73:87, 1997.

Graham JM, Tackels D, Dibbern K, et al.: FG syndrome: report of three new families with linkage to Xq12-q21.31. Am J Med Genet 80:145, 1998.

Opitz JM, Kaveggia EG: Studies of malformation syndromes of man XXXIII: the FG syndrome. An X-linked recessive syndrome of multiple congenital anomalies and mental retardation. Z Kinderheilk 117:1, 1974.
Opitz JM, Richieri-da Costa A, Aase JM, et al.: FG syndrome update 1988: note of 5 new patients and bibliography. Am J Med Genet 30:309, 1988.
Sorge G, Polizzi A, Ruggieri M, et al.: Early fatal course in three brothers with FG syndrome. Clin Pediatr 35:365, 1996.

Differential Matrix

Syndrome	Macro-cephaly	Digital Anomalies	Hypotonia	Comments
Opitz FG	+	+	+	Broad forehead, downslanted palpebral fissures, everted lower lip, dysgenesis of corpus callosum, cardiac defects, imperforate anus, constipation, broad flat thumbs and great toes
Simpson-Golabi-Behmel	+	+	+	Somatic overgrowth, supernumerary nipples, polydactyly
Atkin-Flaitz	+	+	0	Short stature, hypertelorism, downslanting palpebral fissures, broad nasal tip, thick lower lip, brachydactyly, seizures
Mucopoly-saccharidosis IIA	+	+	0	Short stature, coarse facies, hepato-splenomegaly, hernias, joint stiffness, thick skin, hirsutism, behavioral disturbance
XLMR-hypotonic facies (Carpenter-Waziri) (Holmes-Gang) (Juberg-Marsidi)	0	+	+	Microcephaly, short stature, small testes, telecanthus, small triangular nose, tented upper lip, open mouth, spacing of teeth, genital anomalies, musculoskeletal anomalies, hemoglobin H inclusions in erythrocytes
Coffin-Lowry	0	+	+	Short stature, microcephaly, hypertelorism, anteverted nares, tented upper lip, prominent lips and large mouth, large ears, soft hands with tapered digits, pectus carinatum
Miles-Carpenter	0	+	+	Microcephaly, short stature, ptosis, small palpebral fissures, open mouth, pectus excavatum, scoliosis, long hands, camptodactyly, rockerbottom feet, arch fingerprints, spasticity, unsteady gait

ORAL-FACIAL-DIGITAL SYNDROME I

(Orofaciodigital Syndrome I, OFD1, MIM 311200)

DEFINITION. XLMR associated with dystopia canthorum, midface anomalies, intraoral clefts and pseudoclefts, lingual hamartomas, hypertrophied oral frenuli, structural anomalies of the brain, polycystic kidneys, brachydactyly, and syndactyly manifest predominantly in females. The gene has been localized between DXS996 and DXS7105 in Xp22.2-Xp22.3.

SOMATIC FEATURES. Craniofacial manifestations, especially those involving the oral structures, predominate. Externally obvious facial features are transient facial milia, dystopia canthorum, flattening of the midface, hypoplasia of alar cartilages, and midline pseudocleft of the lip. Intraoral anomalies include high arch or cleft (often irregular) of the palate, pseudocleft or lobation of the tongue, hamartomas on the tongue, hypertrophied and aberrant frenuli, malocclusion, and hypodontia. The fingers are asymmetrically short with proximal cutaneous syndactyly and clinodactyly, especially of fingers 2 and 5. Polydactyly rarely occurs. Other anomalies include dry, sparse scalp hair, alopecia, agenesis of corpus callosum, hydrocephaly, porencephaly, and adult-type polycystic kidneys.

GROWTH AND DEVELOPMENT. Growth is usually normal, but developmental milestones may be delayed.

COGNITIVE FEATURES. About half of cases have cognitive impairment.

NEUROLOGICAL FINDINGS. The presence and type of neurologic symptoms and signs presumably depend on cerebral involvement, which is variable. Findings include seizures, ataxia, dysarthria, dysmetria, and trembling of the hands.

IMAGING. Structural anomalies of the brain include agenesis of corpus callosum, neuronal heterotopias, hydrocephaly, porencephaly, cerebral infarcts, cerebral cysts, brain atrophy, cerebellar hypoplasia/dysplasia, and hypothalamic hamartomas.

COMMENT. OFD-1 is one of the X-linked conditions that has been found almost exclusively in females. Most cases, up to 75%, are sporadic, perhaps arising from mutations in the paternal germline. Available pedigrees are also consistent with X-linked dominant inheritance with lethality in hemizygous males. Affected males have been reported. Some have had the karyotype 47,XXY. Others may have an orofaciodigital syndrome other than OFD I. Edwards et al. reported a family with an OFD II–like syndrome having an X-linked recessive pattern of transmission. Vallaud et al. described a family in which females with OFD I were related through unaffected transmitting males.

REFERENCES

Edwards M, Mulcahy D, Turner G: X-linked recessive inheritance of an orofaciodigital syndrome with partial expression in females and survival of affected males. Clin Genet 34:325, 1988.

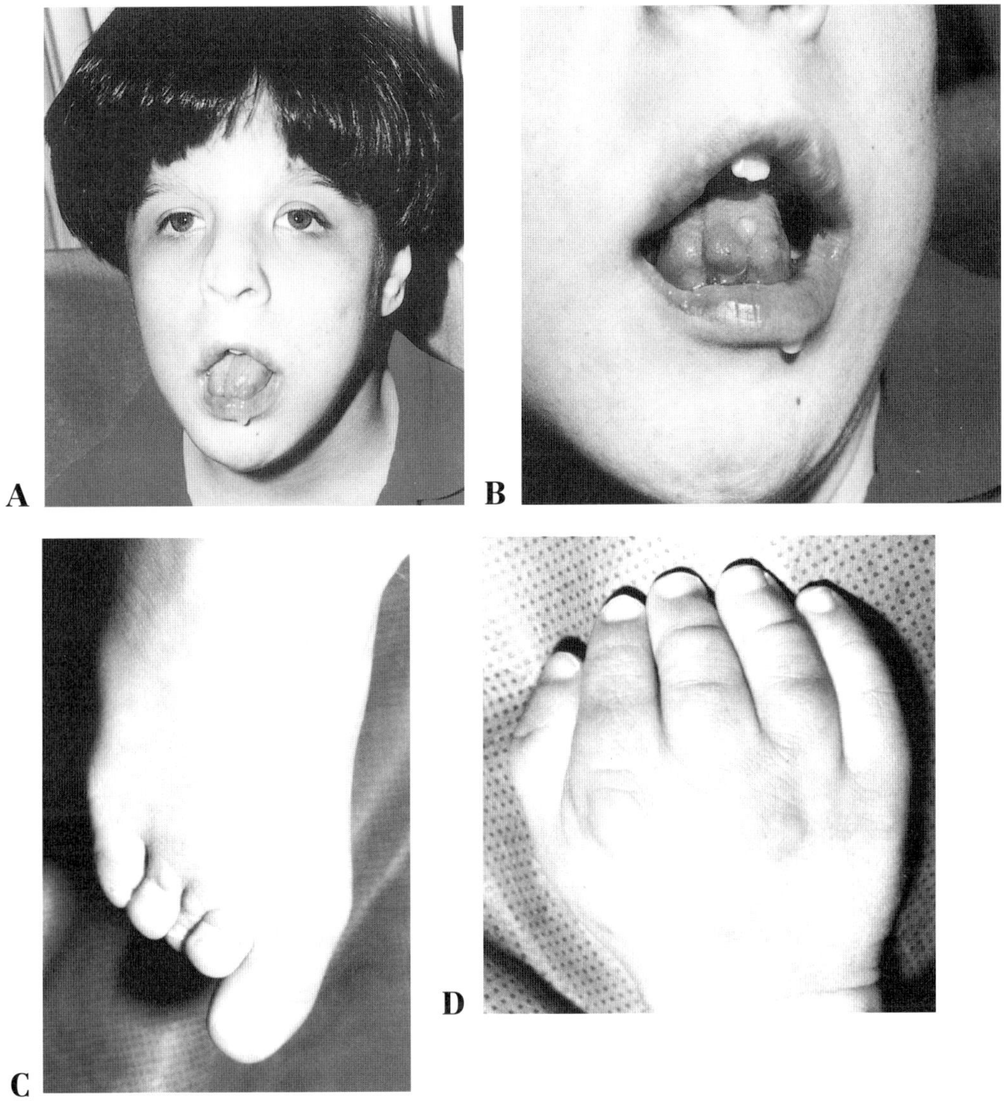

Oral-Facial-Digital 1 Syndrome. (continued) Seventeen-year-old girl with epicanthus, downslanting palpebral fissures, nasal deformation, gaping mouth, tongue nodule, and brachydactyly. Courtesy of Dr. Arthur S. Aylsworth, University of North Carolina School of Medicine, Chapel Hill.

Feather SA, Woolf AS, Donnai D, et al.: The oral-facial-digital syndrome type I (OFDI), a cause of polycystic kidney disease and associated malformations, maps to Xp22.2-Xp22.3. Hum Mol Genet 6:1163, 1997.

Gorlin RJ, Anderson VE, Scott CR: Hypertrophied frenuli, oligophrenia, familial trembling and anomalies of the hand. N Engl J Med 264:486, 1961.

Leão MJ, Ribeiro-Silva ML: Orofaciodigital syndrome type I in a patient with severe CNS defects. Pediatr Neurol 13:247, 1995.

Papillon-Léage Mme, Psaume J: Une malformation héréditaire de la muqueuse buccale brides et freins anormaux. Rev Stomatol (Paris) 55:209, 1954.
Vaillaud JC, Martin J, Szepetowski G, et al.: Le syndrome oro-facial-digital. Etude clinique et génétique à propos de 10 cas observés dans une même famille. Rev Pédiat 5:383, 1968.
Wettke-Schäfer R, Kantner G: X-linked dominant inherited diseases with lethality in hemizygous males. Hum Genet 64:1, 1983.

Differential Matrix

Syndrome	Orofacial Clefting	Oral Frenula/ Tongue Hamartomas	Brachy-dactyly	Comments
Oral-facial-digital I	+	+	+	Sparse scalp hair, dystopia canthorum, flat midface, hypoplastic alae nasi, syndactyly, clinodactyly, structural brain anomalies, polycystic kidneys
Armfield	+	0	+	Short stature, cataracts or glaucoma, dental anomalies, small hands and feet, hydrocephaly, joint stiffness, seizures
Cranioorodigital	+	0	+	Undergrowth, hearing impairment, prominent forehead, flat/broad nasal bridge, ocular hypertelorism, downslanting palpebral fissures, flat midface, blunted flexed overlapping fingers, rockerbottom feet, hypoplastic fibulas, subluxed/ dislocated joints
Otopalatodigital I	+	0	+	Short stature, conductive hearing impairment, prominent brow, broad nasal root, apparent ocular hypertelorism, downslanting palpebral fissures, cleft palate, blunted distal phalanges, irregular curvature and spacing of digits, limitation of elbow movement

Ornithine Transcarbamylase Deficiency

(Ornithine Carbamyltransferase Deficiency, OTC Deficiency, MIM 311250)

Definition. XLMR condition caused by chronic or intermittent hyperammonemia due to deficiency of ornithine transcarbamylase. The gene for ornithine transcarbamylase is about 12 cm proximal to the Duchenne muscular dystrophy locus in Xp21.

Somatic Features. Malformations and other distinctive somatic manifestations do not occur.

Growth and Development. Intrauterine growth is normal. Those who experience hyperammonemic encephalopathy early in infancy have subsequent growth failure including microcephaly. Delay of developmental milestones may likewise be related to early hyperammonemia.

Cognitive Features. Neonatal hyperammonemia causes mental retardation. Later onset hyperammonemic encephalopathy results in some cognitive impairment. Even those with intermittent, self-limited episodes and apparently asymptomatic females may have lower IQs than unaffected family members.

Behavioral Manifestations. Agitation or irritability followed by disorientation and lethargy may be associated with hyperammonemia.

Neurological Findings. Cerebral edema and subsequent compromise of cerebral perfusion lead to a variety of neurological findings including changes in sensorium, ataxia, hemiparesis, slurred speech, seizures, amblyopia, and coma.

Natural History. Presentation is variable depending on the residual enzyme activity and, in heterozygotes, on lyonization in hepatocytes. With negligible enzyme activity, presentation occurs early, in the second or third day of life, with poor feeding, vomiting, lethargy, and hyperventilation, progressing to coma, respiratory arrest, and death. Survivors have mental retardation and often cerebral palsy.

Presentation is more variable in the later onset group. Symptoms may present in infancy with advancement to a higher protein diet, in children and adults with a high-protein meal, and at any age with an infection or with no apparent precipitating event. Symptoms include vomiting, headache, hyperventilation, and changes in sensorium or behavior in the form of irritability, agitation, lethargy, or disorientation. Slurred speech, hemiparesis, seizures, ataxia, and amblyopia may appear. Untreated, coma, respiratory arrest, and death may ensue. All survivors of hyperammonemic encephalopathy have some cognitive impairment.

Heterozygote Expression. Expression in females depends on residual enzyme activity and on lyonization of enzyme activity in hepatocytes. Females have been reported with early presentation, but this is unusual. Usually expressing females have later onset and episodic symptoms. Two-thirds of asymptomatic women have elevated plasma ammonia and glutamine compared to controls.

Neuropathology. Neurologic symptoms and signs stem from cerebral edema and compromise of cerebral blood flow. This appears to be primarily due to high glutamine concentrations in glial cells with subsequent osmotic swelling of the cells.

IMAGING. Cerebral imaging reveals edema acutely and atrophy with prolonged or repeated episodes.

LABORATORY. Chronically in the early onset and intermittently in the late onset, there is respiratory alkalosis, hyperammonemia, and oroticaciduria. Plasma glutamine and alanine may be elevated. In neonatal presentation, plasma citrulline is absent or very low. Allopurinol challenge test may detect mildly affected patients between episodes and asymptomatic heterozygotes. Direct mutational analysis of the OTC gene is possible.

TREATMENT. Prevention of encephalopathic episodes offers the best prognosis. Hyperammonemic encephalopathy causes brain damage. Even asymptomatic hyperammonemia may cause mild but permanent cerebral dysfunction. Elevated plasma glutamine may predict an impending encephalopathy. Those infants diagnosed prenatally should be started on treatment at birth. Treatment for all ages consists of a low-protein diet, citrulline or arginine as a source of arginine, and sodium phenylbutyrate for alternative nitrogen excretion. Hemodialysis is the best form of ammonia/glutamine removal in encephalopathic coma.

REFERENCES

Bachmann C: Ornithine carbamoyl transferase deficiency: findings, models and problems. J Inherit Metab Dis 15:578, 1992.

Brusilow SW: Urea cycle disorders: diagnosis, pathophysiology, and therapy. Adv Pediatr 43:127, 1996.

Lindgren V, De Martinville B, Horwich AL, et al.: Human ornithine transcarbamylase locus mapped to band Xp21.1 near the Duchenne muscular dystrophy locus. Science 226:698, 1984.

Tuchman M: The clinical, biochemical, and molecular spectrum of ornithine transcarbamylase deficiency. J Lab Clin Med 120:836, 1992.

Differential Matrix

Syndrome	Metabolic Disturbance	Sensorium Change	Ataxia	Comments
Ornithine transcarbamylase deficiency	+	+	+	Chronic or intermittent hyperammonemia, microcephaly, protein-induced vomiting and lethargy, seizures
Pyruvate dehydrogenase deficiency	+	+	+	Lactic acidosis, microcephaly, hypotonia, dysarthria, CNS anomalies

Otopalatodigital Syndrome I

(Otopalatodigital Syndrome, OPD Syndrome, OPD I, MIM 311300)

Definition. XLMR with distinctive facial appearance, cleft palate, conductive hearing impairment, short stature, skeletal dysplasia, and, in some cases, mild cognitive impairment. The OPD I gene has been localized distal to DXS52 in Xq28, lod score 3.19.

Somatic Features. A "pugilistic" facial appearance and digital anomalies suggest OPD I. Craniofacial features include occipital prominence, frontal bossing, overhanging brow, broad depressed nasal bridge, apparent ocular hypertelorism,

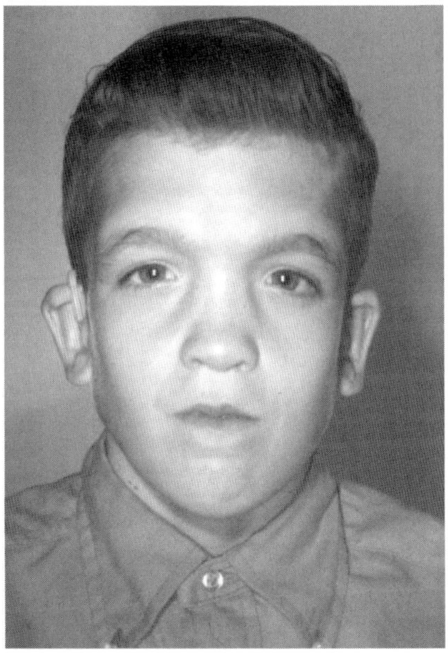

A

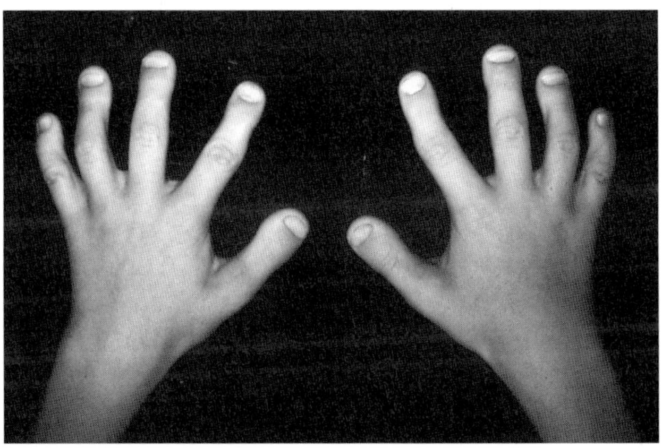

B

Otopalatodigital 1 Syndrome. Facies of boy (A); hands with brachydactyly and expansion of the distal phalanges (B).

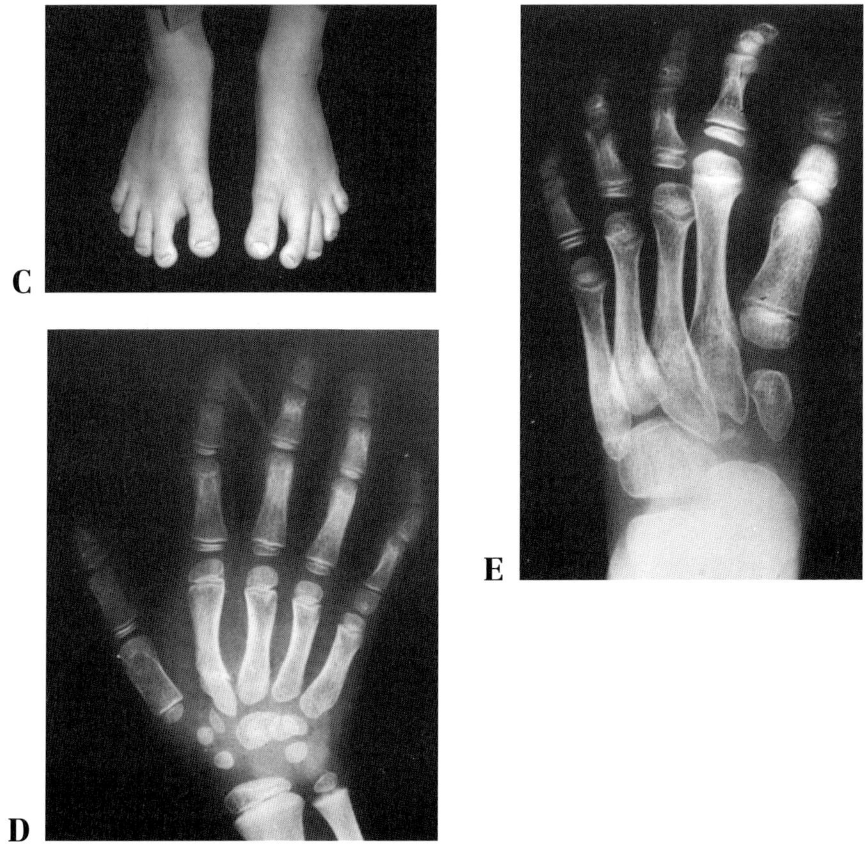

Otopalatodigital 1 Syndrome. (continued) Foot with expansion of the distal phalanges and increased spacing between toes 1 and 2 (C); radiograph of the hand showing changes (D); foot (E). Courtesy of Dr. Robert J. Gorlin, University of Minnesota School of Dentistry, Minneapolis.

downslanting palpebral fissures, small mouth, micrognathia, and cleft palate. The trunk is short with pectus excavatum. The thumbs and halluces are short and broad. The terminal fingers and toes are blunted and bulbous with short nails. The digits are also irregular in curvature and the toes widely spaced. The long bones of the limbs may be involved, with limitation of elbow movement, bowing, and abnormal modeling. Some of the facial and skeletal findings are mirrored in the radiographs—thick skull base, prominent supraorbital ridges, hypoplastic facial bones, small mandible with obtuse angle, hypoplastic/aplastic paranasal sinuses, short broad distal phalanges of digits, accessory ossification centers at bases of metacarpals and metatarsals, and abnormal configurations and coalitions of carpals and tarsals.

GROWTH AND DEVELOPMENT. Stature is generally less than the 10th centile. Development may be delayed. Delay in speech development may be a manifestation of the general cognitive impairment or secondary to conductive hearing impairment due to malformed middle ear ossicles and chronic middle ear effusions.

COGNITIVE FEATURES. IQs are usually 75–90.

HETEROZYGOTE EXPRESSION. Females may have prominent supraorbital ridges, apparent hypertelorism, flat maxillary and malar areas, depressed broad nasal bridge, fifth finger clinodactyly, short nails, toe spacing, and radiographic findings.

COMMENT. Diagnosis is based on clinical and radiographic features; OPD I has craniofacial and digital manifestations similar to those in cranioorodigital syndrome (OPD II) and Pallister W syndrome.

REFERENCES

Biancalana V, LeMarec B, Odent S, et al.: Oto-palato-digital syndrome type I: further evidence for assignment of the locus to Xq28. Hum Genet 88:228, 1991.

Dudding BA, Gorlin RJ, Langer LO: The oto-palato-digital syndrome, a new symptom-complex consisting of deafness, dwarfism, cleft palate, characteristic facies, and generalized bone dysplasia. Am J Dis Child 113:214, 1967.

Gall JC, Stern AM, Poznanski AK, et al.: Oto-palato-digital syndrome: comparison of clinical and radiographic manifestations in males and females. Am J Hum Genet 24:24, 1972.

Langer LO: The roentgenographic features of the oto-palato-digital (OPD) syndrome. Am J Roentgenol 100:63, 1967.

Poznanski AK, MacPherson RI, Dijkman DJ, et al.: Otopalatodigital syndrome: radiologic findings in the hand and foot. Birth Defects Orig Art Ser X(5):125, 1974.

Taybi H: Generalized skeletal dysplasia with multiple anomalies. Am J Roentgenol 88:450, 1962.

Differential Matrix

Syndrome	Cleft Palate	Hearing Impairment	Digital Anomalies	Comments
Otopalatodigital I	+	+	+	Short stature, prominent brow, broad nasal root, apparent ocular hypertelorism, downslanting palpebral fissures, blunted distal phalanges, irregular curvature and spacing of digits, limitation of elbow movement
Cranioorodigital	+	+	+	Undergrowth, prominent forehead, flat/broad nasal bridge, ocular hypertelorism, downslanting palpebral fissures, flat midface, blunted flexed overlapping fingers, rockerbottom feet, hypoplastic fibulae, subluxed/dislocated joints
Oral-facial-digital I	+	0	+	Sparse scalp hair, dystopia canthorum, flat midface, hypoplastic alae nasi, hypertrophic and aberrant oral frenuli, intraoral clefts and pseudoclefts, lingual hamartomas, brachydactyly, syndactyly, clinodactyly, structural brain anomalies, polycystic kidneys
Pallister W	+	0	+	Short stature, prominent forehead, wide nasal tip, incomplete cleft lip/palate, spasticity, contractures

Paine Syndrome

(Paine-Seemanová Syndrome, MIM 311400)

Definition. XLMR with microcephaly, optic atrophy, spastic diplegia, and seizures. Genetic heterogeneity is likely; no gene has been localized.

Somatic Features. Microcephaly and short stature, possibly of postnatal onset, in the company of optic atrophy and spastic diplegia dominate the clinical phe-

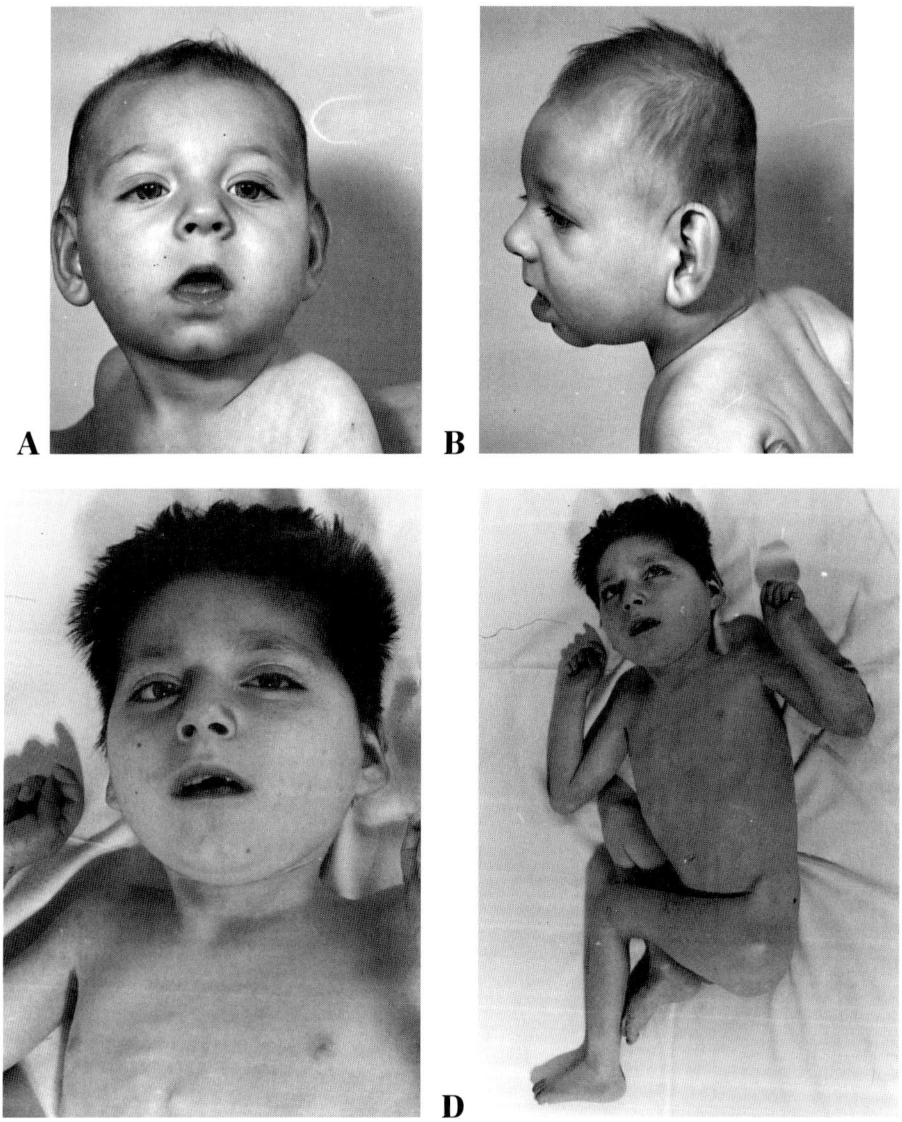

Paine Syndrome. Ten-month-old with microcephaly (A,B); $7^1/_2$-year-old with microcephaly and spasticity (C,D). Courtesy of Dr. E. Seemanová, University Children's Hospital of Charles University, Prague, Czech Republic.

notype. Impaired vision and hearing are probable. Major malformations do not occur. Dermatoglyphics in one family showed an excess of arches or low loops and distal displacement of the palmar triradius. Death in infancy or early childhood is the rule.

GROWTH AND DEVELOPMENT. Intrauterine growth may be normal but all parameters of postnatal growth are impaired. Microcephaly and short stature become obvious early in infancy if not at birth. No significant developmental milestones are achieved.

COGNITIVE FUNCTION. Severe impairment obvious from early infancy.

NEUROLOGICAL FINDINGS. Generalized spasticity with increased muscle tone, hyperreflexia, grimacing, opisthotonic body positioning, and myoclonic/opisthotonic seizures.

NEUROPATHOLOGY. Autopsy on a 15-month-old child showed generalized undergrowth of the brain with decreased cerebral neurons but without gliosis.

IMAGING. The brain shows global undergrowth or atrophy. The ventricles and extracerebral spaces may be enlarged. Radiographs show no calcifications.

LABORATORY. A mild aminoaciduria and elevated α-amino nitrogen level in the cerebrospinal fluid originally reported by Paine could not be confirmed in later studies or in the patients reported by Seemanová et al.

COMMENT. Genetic heterogeneity is almost certain. Although similar in many respects to the cases reviewed by Reardon et al., CNS calcifications and neonatal thrombocytopenia have not been reported in Paine syndrome. Other XLMR syndromes with death during childhood include Arts, Bertini, Gustavson, Holmes-Gang, hydrocephaly-cerebellar agenesis, hereditary bullous dystrophy, VACTERL-hydrocephalus, XLMR-ataxia-deafness-dementia, and X-linked lissencephaly.

REFERENCES

Paine RS: Evaluation of familial biochemically determined mental retardation in children, with special reference to aminoaciduria. N Engl J Med 262:658, 1960.

Reardon W, Hockey A, Silberstein, et al.: Autosomal recessive congenital intrauterine infection-like syndrome of microcephaly, intracranial calcifications, and CNS disease. Am J Med Genet 52:58, 1994.

Seemanová E, Lesný I, Hyánek J, et al.: X-chromosomal recessive microcephaly with epilepsy, spastic tetraplegia and absent abdominal reflexes. New variety of "Paine Syndrome"? Humangenetik 20:113, 1973.

Differential Matrix

Syndrome	Blindness and/or Deafness	Spasticity	Seizures	Comments
Paine	+	+	+	Microcephaly, short stature, optic atrophy
Proud	+	+	+	Microcephaly, agenesis of corpus callosum, cryptorchidism, inguinal hernias, ataxia
Schimke	+	+	+	Microcephaly, sunken eyes, downslanting palpebral fissures, narrow nose, spacing of teeth, cupped ears, abducens palsy, choreoathetosis, contractures
Mohr-Tranebjaerg (Jensen)	+	+	0	Neurologic deterioration with childhood onset, dystonia
Bertini	+	0	+	Macular degeneration, hypotonia, childhood death, hypoplasia of cerebellar vermis and corpus callosum, developmental delays and regression, postnatal growth impairment
Wittwer	+	0	+	Growth deficiency, microcephaly, microphthalmia, hypertelorism, genitourinary anomalies, hypotonia

PALLISTER W SYNDROME

(W Syndrome, MIM 311450)

DEFINITION. XLMR with short stature, characteristic facies (high forehead, frontal upsweep, prominent brow, hypertelorism, downslanting palpebral fissures, depressed and broad nasal bridge, wide nasal tip, incomplete cleft lip and palate, short high mandible), absent central maxillary incisors, limitation of elbow movement, and spasticity. A gene locus has not been determined.

SOMATIC FEATURES. All components of the face share in the distinctive characteristics. Head circumference is normal, but the forehead is tall and the brow prominent. Midfacial manifestations include hypertelorism, small and downslanting palpebral fissures, depression or broadness of the nasal bridge, and wide nasal tip with thick alae nasi and columella. The lower face is defined by simple short philtrum with thin upper lip, partial cleft or notching of the upper lip with extension to the alveolar ridge or anterior palate, absent central maxillary incisors, and vertically tall mandible but not prognathism. Facial asymmetry is typical. Skeletal manifestations include general asthenia with cubitus valgus, limited movement or dislocation of the elbows, pectus excavatum, camptodactyly of fingers 4 and 5, limited movement of MCP joint of finger 1, and pes cavus or pes planus with midfoot varus. Muscle tone may be decreased during early child-

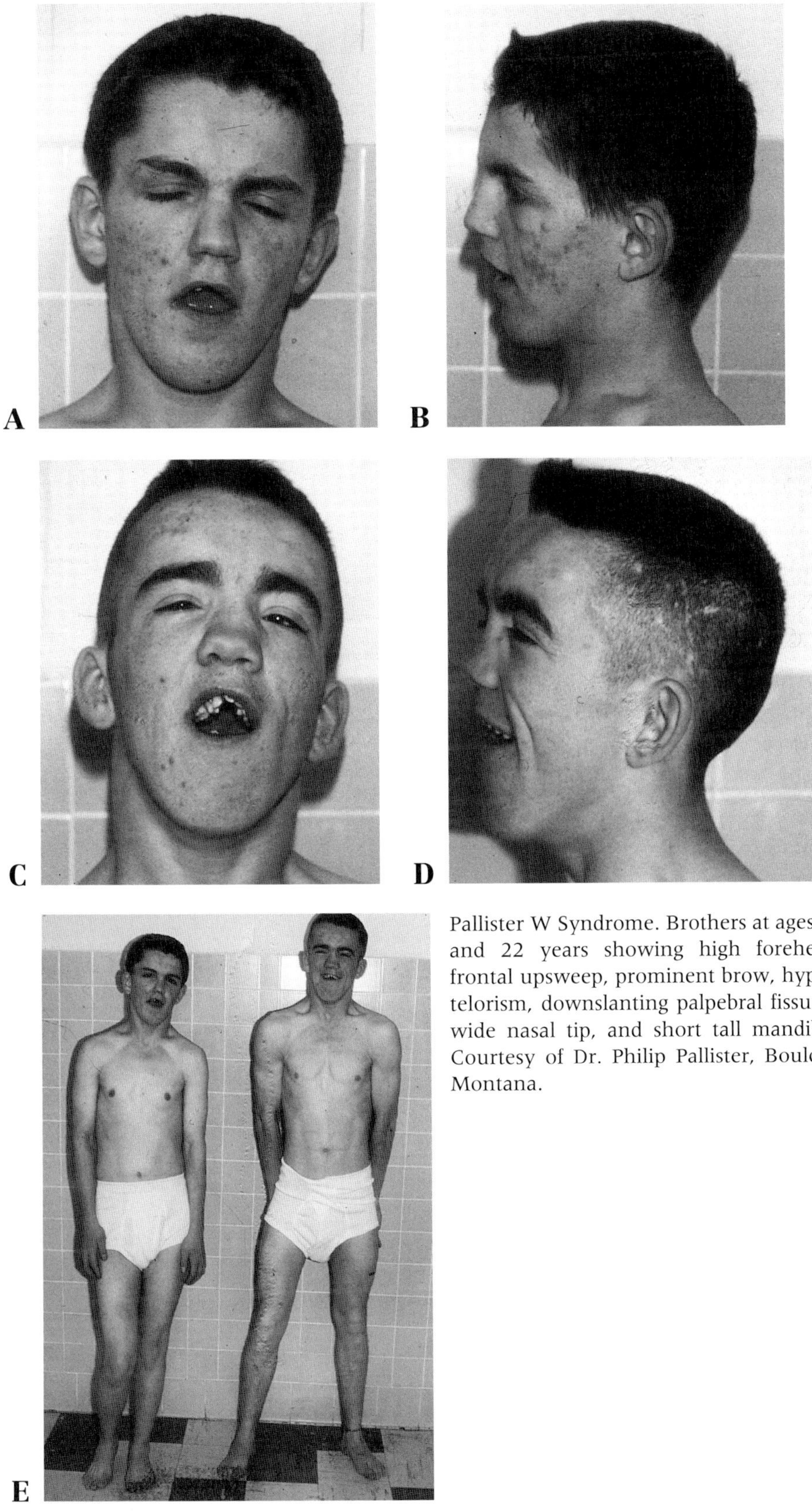

Pallister W Syndrome. Brothers at ages 20 and 22 years showing high forehead, frontal upsweep, prominent brow, hypertelorism, downslanting palpebral fissures, wide nasal tip, and short tall mandible. Courtesy of Dr. Philip Pallister, Boulder, Montana.

hood but generalized spasticity with hyperactive deep tendon reflexes develops eventually. A coarse tremor of the upper limbs was noted in two brothers.

GROWTH AND DEVELOPMENT. Intrauterine growth is variable. The head circumference remains normal, but stature falls below −2 SD during childhood. Delay of developmental milestones is obvious from early infancy.

COGNITIVE FEATURES. Severe impairment.

IMAGING. Pneumoencephalography has shown ventricular enlargement and agenesis of the corpus callosum in one case.

NEUROLOGICAL FINDINGS. Hypotonia was present in the one case in which the early childhood history was known. Spasticity with increased deep tendon reflexes and seizures of various types become the dominant neurological manifestations.

HETEROZYGOTE EXPRESSION. In the original family, carrier females had high forehead, hypertelorism, downslanting palpebral fissures, strabismus, short philtrum, and vertically tall mandible and possibly showed cognitive or neurobehavioral abnormality.

COMMENT. Only four affected males in two families have been reported. Confirmation that the responsible gene is located on the X chromosome has not been possible. Resemblance of the facial manifestations to those of otopalatodigital syndrome, another X-linked disorder, was pointed out by Pallister et al.

REFERENCE

Bottani A, Schinzel A: A third patient with median cleft upper lip, mental retardation and pugilistic facies (W syndrome): corroboration of a hitherto private syndrome. Clin Dysmorphol 2:225, 1993.

Pallister PD, Herrmann J, Spranger JW, et al.: The W syndrome. Studies of malformation syndromes of man XXVIII. Birth Defects Orig Art Ser X(7):51, 1974.

Pallister PD, Herrmann J: Pallister-W syndrome. In: Birth Defects Encyclopedia. ML Buyse, ed. Center for Birth Defects Information Services, Dover, 1990, p. 1354.

Differential Matrix

Syndrome	Short Stature	Facial Clefting	Seizures	Comments
Pallister W	+	+	+	Prominent forehead, wide nasal tip, incomplete cleft lip/palate, spasticity
Armfield	+	+	+	Cataracts or glaucoma, dental anomalies, small hands and feet, hydrocephaly, joint stiffness
Otopalatodigital	+	+	0	Conductive hearing impairment, skeletal dysplasia, mild cognitive impairment
Telecanthus-hypospadias	0	+	0	High broad nasal root, dysplastic ears, abnormal cranial contour or symmetry

PARTINGTON SYNDROME

(XLMR-Dystonia Syndrome, MRXS1, MIM 309510)

DEFINITION. XLMR with dysarthria, dystonia, hyperreflexia, and seizures. The gene is located distal to DXS28 in Xp21.3, lod score is 2.11.

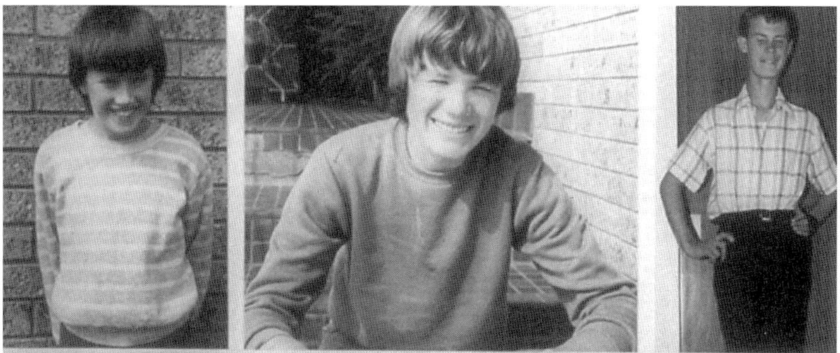

A

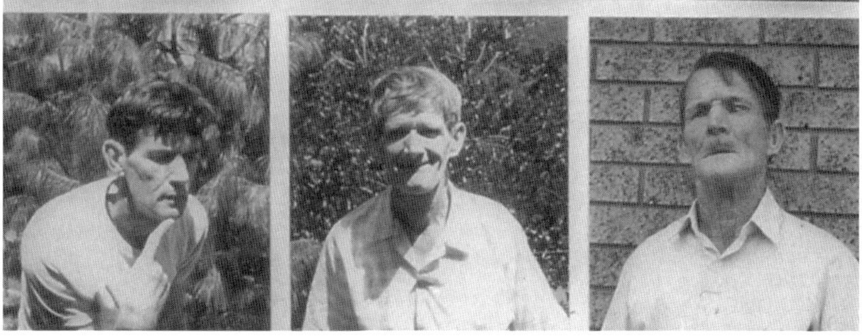

B

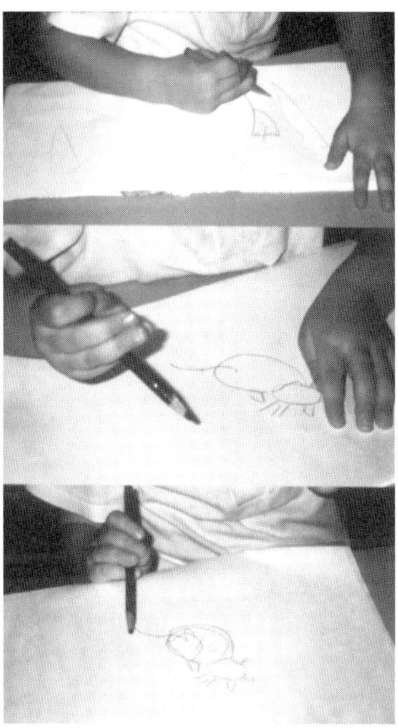

C

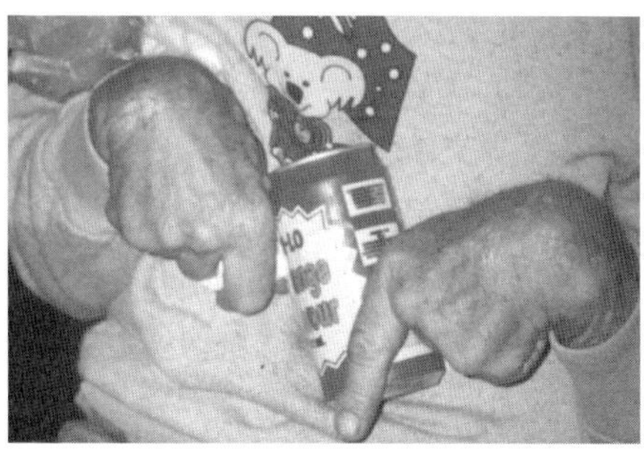

D

Partington Syndrome. Affected males at ages 12, 16, and 15 years showing normal facies (A); adult males at ages 37, 47, and 57 years (B); dystonic hand positions at ages 12 years (C) and 67 years (D). Courtesy of Dr. Michael Partington, Hunter Genetics, New South Wales, Australia.

SOMATIC FEATURES. Major malformations do not occur and craniofacial findings are not consistent. The face tends to be elongated, especially after childhood. Flexed posture and scoliosis may be present.

GROWTH AND DEVELOPMENT. Cranial and statural growth follow a normal course. Early childhood milestones lag behind but are quite variable. Difficulty in articulation is the major speech disability. The most severely affected individuals do not speak or seldom do so.

COGNITIVE FEATURES. Variable from borderline to moderate impairment.

NEUROLOGICAL FINDINGS. Recurrent dystonic spasms involving the hands and dysarthria become obvious prior to school age and progress slowly if at all. The gait appears awkward and the deep tendon reflexes are brisk. Seizures occur in a minority of cases.

HETEROZYGOTE EXPRESSION. None.

LABORATORY. Normal nerve conduction velocity and electomyography.

COMMENT. Dystonia limited to the hands and nonprogressive or only slowly progressive appears unique to the Partington syndrome. Other XLMR-dystonia syndromes have been mapped to Xq, which distinguishes them from Partington syndrome.

REFERENCE

Gedeon A, Partington M, Mulley J: X-linked mental retardation with dystonic movements of the hands (PRTS): revisited. Am J Med Genet 51:565, 1994.

Partington MW, Mulley JC, Sutherland GR, et al.: X-linked mental retardation with dystonic movements of the hands. Am J Med Genet 30:251, 1988.

Differential Matrix

Syndrome	Dystonia or Choreo-athetosis	Hyper-reflexia	Seizures	Comments
Partington	+	+	+	Scoliosis, flexed posture, dysarthria
Lesch-Nyhan	+	+	+	Spasticity, self-mutilation, hyperuricemia
Pettigrew	+	+	+	Dandy-Walker malformation, spasticity, microcephaly or hydrocephaly, long face with macrostomia and prognathism, small testes, contractures, iron deposits in basal ganglia
Proud	+	+	+	Microcephaly, hearing loss, vision loss, agenesis of corpus callosum, cryptorchidism, inguinal hernias, ataxia, spasticity
XLMR-spastic paraplegia-athetosis	+	+	+	Nystagmus, weakness, dysarthria, spastic paraplegia, muscle wasting
Allan-Herndon-Dudley	+	+	0	Large ears with cupping or abnormal architecture, muscle hypoplasia, childhood hypotonia, contractures, dysarthria, athetosis, ataxia, spastic paraplegia
Mohr-Tranebjaerg (Jensen)	+	+	0	Hearing loss, vision loss, neurologic deterioration with childhood onset, spasticity
Goldblatt spastic paraplegia	0	+	+	Optic atrophy, exotropia, nystagmus, ataxia, spastic paraplegia, dysarthria, muscle hypoplasia, contractures
Gustavson	0	+	+	Microcephaly, short stature, optic atrophy with blindness, large ears, deafness, joint contractures, rockerbottom feet, brain undergrowth, hydrocephaly, cerebellar hypoplasia, spasticity
Paine	0	+	+	Microcephaly, short stature, optic atrophy, vision loss, hearing loss, spasticity
X-linked ataxia-deafness-dementia	0	+	+	Optic atrophy, vision loss, hearing loss, spastic paraplegia, ataxia, hypotonia, childhood death

PELIZAEUS-MERZBACHER SYNDROME

(X-Linked Spastic Paraplegia, Pelizaeus-Merzbacher Type, Complicated X-Linked Spastic Paraplegia 2, SPG2, PMD, MIM 312080)

DEFINITION. XLMR with nystagmus, truncal hypotonia and progressive spastic paraplegia, ataxia, and dystonia associated with CNS dysmyelination. The responsible gene, proteolipid protein gene (PLD), has been mapped to Xq21.1.

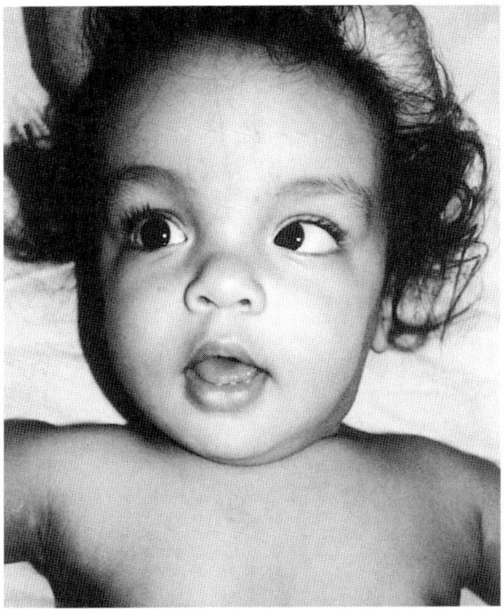

A

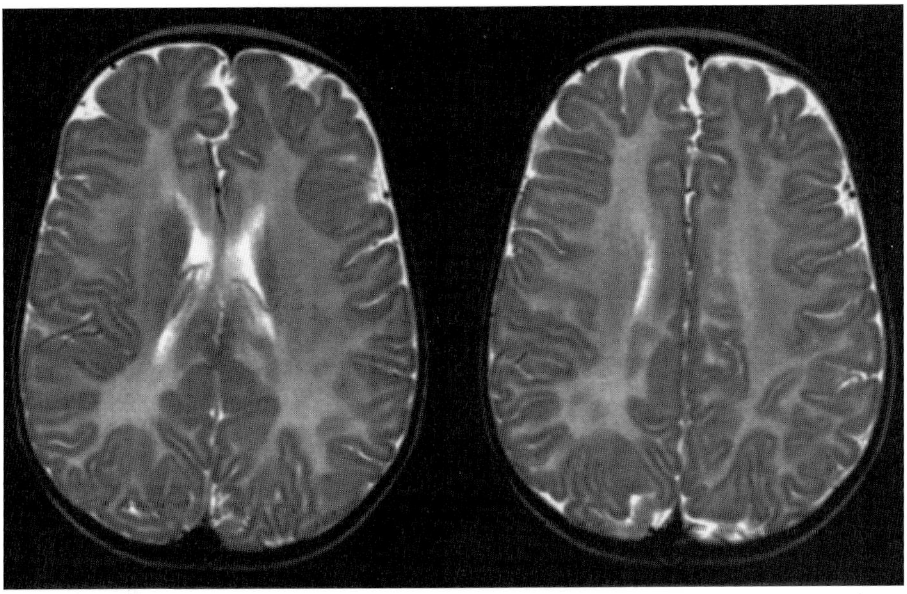

B

Pelizaeus-Merzbacher. Seven-month-old male with nystagmus, developmental delay, and normal facies (A); Axial MRI at age 44 months showing increased signal of white matter indicating deficient myelination. (B). Courtesy Dr. Arthur S. Aylsworth, University of North Carolina School of Medicine, Chapel Hill.

SOMATIC FEATURES. Neurological manifestations dominate the phenotype. Malformations and distinctive craniofacial features do not occur. Optic atrophy is found in most cases by school age. Contractures may result from the neurologic impairment.

GROWTH AND DEVELOPMENT. Intrauterine and postnatal growth appear normal in most cases. Short stature of mild degree has been reported in a minority of cases. Developmental milestones may be globally delayed with motor skills lagging further behind than language development.

COGNITIVE FEATURES. Considerable variability in cognitive function ranging from normal to moderate impairment has been noted, even among affected males of the same family.

NEUROLOGICAL FINDINGS. Nystagmus generally precedes other neurologic findings, appearing in the early months of life; it is multidirectional in nature and often becomes less pronounced in childhood. Respiratory stridor has also been noted during infancy in many cases. Truncal hypotonia and pyramidal signs appear during early childhood, manifest variably by increased tone in the lower limbs, hyperreflexia, awkward gait, and Babinski sign. The spastic paraplegia is progressive and may be accompanied by ataxia, upper limb tremors, dystonic movements, dysarthria, and dysmetria. Seizures occur in a minority. Ambulation may be sufficiently impaired in the teen or early adult years to require wheelchair or other support.

HETEROZYGOTE EXPRESSION. Although two of the cases reported by Pelizaeus were females, there is no convincing evidence of carrier manifestation.

IMAGING. Global or spotty decrease in density of the white matter appears during childhood. Overall brain atrophy and ventricular dilation are mild.

LABORATORY. Visual evoked responses and brain stem auditory evoked responses are often abnormal. Histological examination of the brain has documented a deficiency of oligodendrocytes, the myelin producing cells of the CNS. As a consequence, axons lack myelin sheaths.

COMMENT. Pelizaeus-Merzbacher syndrome was the first of the X-linked spastic paraplegias to be described (1885 and 1910), the first to be regionally mapped (1985), and the first to be attributed to mutations in a specific gene (1987). Complicated spastic paraplegia (SPG2) was shown to be allelic in 1994.

REFERENCES

Boulloche J, Aicardi J: Pelizaeus-Merzbacher disease: clinical and nosological study. J Child Neurol 1:233, 1986.

Gencic S, Abuelo D, Ambler M, et al.: Pelizaeus-Merzbacher disease: an X-linked neurologic disorder of myelin metabolism with a novel mutation in the gene encoding proteolipid protein. Am J Hum Genet 45:435, 1989.

Merzbacher L: Eine eigenartige framiliäre Erkrankungsform (aplasia axialis extracorticalis congenita)-Z Gesamte. Neurol Psychiatr 3:1, 1910.

Pelizaeus F: Über eine eigenthümliche Form spastischer Lähmung mit Cerebralerscheinungen auf hereditärer Grundlage (multiple Sklerose). Arch Psychiatr Nervenkr 16:698, 1885.

Saugier-Veber P, Munnich A, Bonneau D, et al.: X-linked spastic paraplegia and Pelizaeus-

Merzbacher disease are allelic disorders at the proteolipid protein locus. Nat Genet 6:257, 1994.

Trofatter JA, Dlouhy SR, De Meyer W, et al.: Pelizaeus-Merzbacher diseases: tight linkage to proteolipid protein gene exon variant. Proc Natl Acad Sci USA 86:9427, 1989.

Differential Matrix

Syndrome	Ataxia	Spastic Paraplegia	Nystagmus	Comments
Pelizaeus-Merzbacher	+	+	+	Optic atrophy, hypotonia, dystonia, CNS dysmyelination
Apak ataxia-spastic diplegia	+	+	+	Short stature, muscle hypoplasia, contractures
Goldblatt spastic paraplegia	+	+	+	Optic atrophy, exotropia, dysarthria, contractures, muscle hypoplasia
XLMR-spastic paraplegia-athetosis	+	+	+	Weakness, dysarthria, muscle wasting, contractures
Adrenoleukodystrophy	+	+	0	Adrenal insufficiency, diffuse skin pigmentation, progressive neurologic deterioration and dementia, elevated very long chain fatty acids in plasma
Allan-Herndon-Dudley	+	+	0	Childhood hypotonia, dysarthria, athetosis, large ears with cupping or abnormal architecture, contractures
Arena	+	+	0	Clubfoot, rigidity, dystonia, iron deposits in basal ganglia, muscle hypoplasia
Pettigrew	+	+	0	Microcephaly or hydrocephaly, long face with macrostomia and prognathism, Dandy-Walker malformation, small testes, contractures, choreoathetosis, iron deposits in basal ganglia
X-linked ataxia-deafness-dementia	+	+	0	Optic atrophy, vision loss, hearing loss, hypotonia, seizures, childhood death
X-linked ataxia-dementia	+	+	0	Adult-onset dementia
X-linked hydrocephaly-MASA spectrum	+	+	0	Hydrocephaly, adducted thumbs, dysgenesis of corpus callosum
Cerebrooculogenital	0	+	+	Short stature, microcephaly, hydrocephaly, agenesis of corpus callosum, microphthalmia, ptosis, hypospadias, cryptorchidism, clubfoot
X-linked spastic paraplegia, type 7	0	+	+	Reduced vision, absent speech and ambulation, bowel and bladder dysfunction, spastic quadriplegia

PERIVENTRICAL NODULAR HETEROTOPIA

(Hereditary Nodular Heterotopia, MIM 300049)

DEFINITION. XLMR with seizures and bilateral periventricular nodular heterotopias in female gene carriers. The gene is linked to markers distal to DXS1113 in Xq28, lod score 4.77.

SOMATIC FEATURES. Multiple subependymal nodules of heterotopic gray matter, usually bilateral, are the major somatic abnormality. Enlargement of the cisterna magna has been described in several cases. The findings are limited to females. At least one pedigree suggests gestational lethality of males.

GROWTH AND DEVELOPMENT. Normal.

COGNITIVE FEATURES. If cognitive impairment occurs, it is mild. Normal intelligence is usual.

NEUROLOGICAL FINDINGS. Seizures of multiple clinical types occur with the usual onset during the teen years, but in some cases they begin in early childhood or in adult life. Complex partial and tonic-clonic seizures are particularly common.

IMAGING. Periventricular nodular heterotopias are best demonstrated by magnetic resonance imaging. They appear isointense with gray matter.

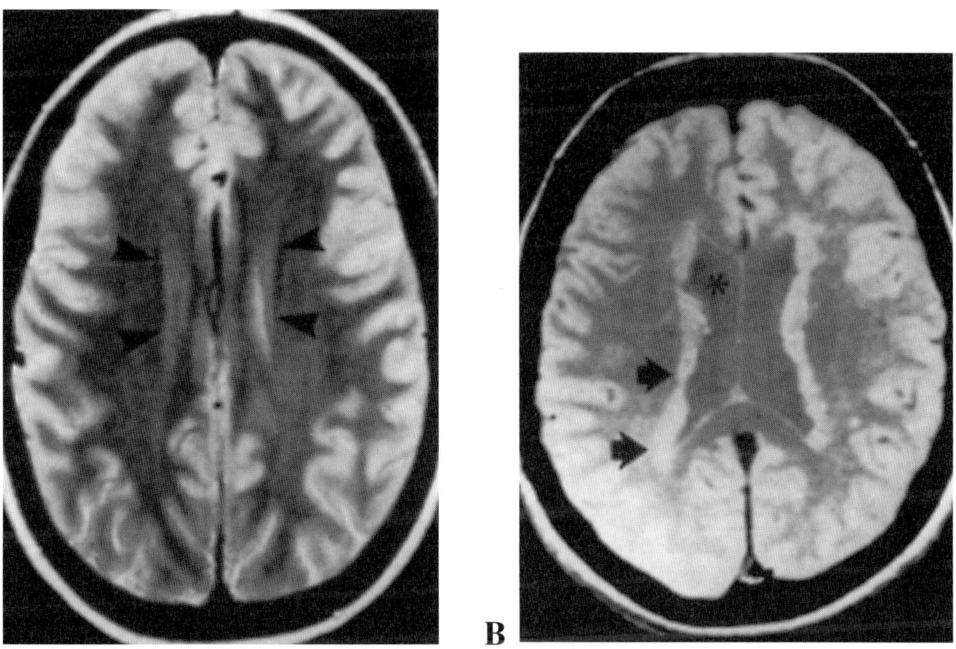

A B

Periventricular Nodular Heterotopia. T_1-weighted MRI from normal individual showing good definition of white matter and the periventricular zone [arrowheads] is extremely thin and indistinct (A); T_1-weighted MRI from a female showing heterotopias with signal characteristics identical to that of gray matter in the periventricular zone [arrows] and distortion of the lateral ventricles [asterisk] (B).

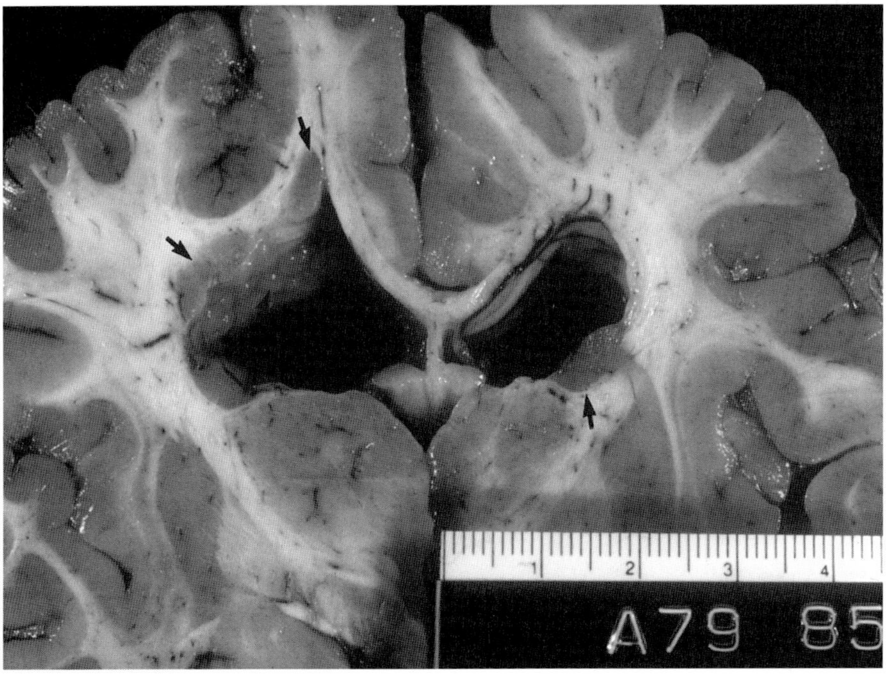

C

Periventricular Nodular Heterotopia. (continued) Coronal section of brain showing bilateral periventricular heterotopias [arrows] (C). Illustrations A and B courtesy of Dr. Peter Huttenlocher, Department of Pediatrics and Neurology, University of Chicago, and *Neuron*, Copyright 1996, Cell Press; illustration C courtesy of Dr. Alasdair G.W. Hunter and the Department of Pathology, Children's Hospital of Eastern Ontario, Ottawa.

COMMENT. The finding of periventricular nodules in a child with seizures usually leads to the diagnosis of tuberous sclerosis. Bilateral periventricular nodular heterotopias can be differentiated from tuberous sclerosis by the absence of skin lesions, cortical lesions, and hamartomas in other organs. Further, the lesions do not calcify, have the density of gray matter, and are found only in female gene carriers. Mental retardation, if it occurs at all, is mild.

REFERENCES:

Eksioglu YZ, Scheffer IE, Cardenas P, et al.: Periventricular heterotopia: an X-linked dominant epilepsy locus causing aberrant cerebral cortical development. Neuron 16:77, 1996.

Huttenlocher PR, Taravath S, Mojtahedi S: Periventricular heterotopia and epilepsy. Neurology 44:51, 1994.

Jardine PE, Clarke MA, Super M: Familial bilateral periventricular nodular heterotopia mimics tuberous sclerosis. Arch Dis Child 74:244, 1996.

Oda T, Nagai Y, Fujimoto S, et al.: Hereditary nodular heterotopia accompanied by mega cisterna magna. Am J Med Genet 47:268, 1993.

Walsh CA, Cardenas P, Ji B, et al.: Linkage of cerebral cortical periventricular heterotopia and epilepsy to markers in Xq28. Neurology 45 (Suppl 4):A440, 1995.

Differential Matrix

Syndrome	Neuronal Migration Defect	Seizures	Female-Limited Expression	Comments
Periventricular nodular heterotopia	+	+	+	Bilateral subependymal nodular heterotopias
Aicardi	+	+	+	Ocular dysgenesis, lacunar retinopathy, costovertebral anomalies, agenesis of corpus callosum
X-linked lissencephaly	+	+	0	Dysgenesis of corpus callosum, hypotonia, spasticity, genital hypoplasia
Rett	0	+	+	Acquired microcephaly, developmental regression, truncal ataxia, repetitive hand movements, autistic features
XLMR-epilepsy	0	+	+	Developmental regression, repetitive stereotypic hand movements

PETTIGREW SYNDROME

(XLMR–Dandy-Walker Malformation–Basal Ganglia Disease–Seizures, MIM 304340)

DEFINITION. XLMR with long narrow face, microcephaly or hydrocephaly, Dandy-Walker malformation, seizures, spasticity, choreoathetosis, and iron deposition in the basal ganglia. The location of the gene is not known, the originally reported localization based on linkage analysis having been withdrawn.

SOMATIC FEATURES. Although variable, the face tends to be long and narrow with high forehead, large bulbous nose, variable coarsening of facial features, macrostomia, and large lips. Strabismus may be present. Lacking hydrocephaly, patients are microcephalic. Tower skull was present in several cases. Contractures and kyphoscoliosis appear with progressive spasticity. Other skeletal findings include long thin digits, pectus deformation, pes planus, and pes equinovarus. Cystic dilation of the fourth ventricle or Dandy-Walker malformation is present in half of patients. Hypotonia, present from infancy, becomes overlaid with choreoathetosis, ataxia, spasticity, and seizures in early childhood. Testicular volume appears small.

GROWTH AND DEVELOPMENT. Head growth is slow unless complicated by hydrocephaly. Growth parameters are otherwise normal.

COGNITIVE FEATURES. Severe impairment.

NEUROLOGICAL FINDINGS. Hypotonia is present in early infancy. Within the first few years, choreoathetosis and spasticity of progressive nature become superimposed. Increased deep tendon reflexes are demonstrable in all limbs and contractures occur by young adult life. Seizures may begin at any age.

HETEROZYGOTE EXPRESSION. Some carrier females have dull mentation. One carrier experienced early dementia and at autopsy had a small brain with iron deposition in basal ganglia and cerebellum.

NEUROPATHOLOGY. Postmortem examination has documented hydrocephaly with Dandy-Walker malformations or cystic dilation of the forth ventricle and

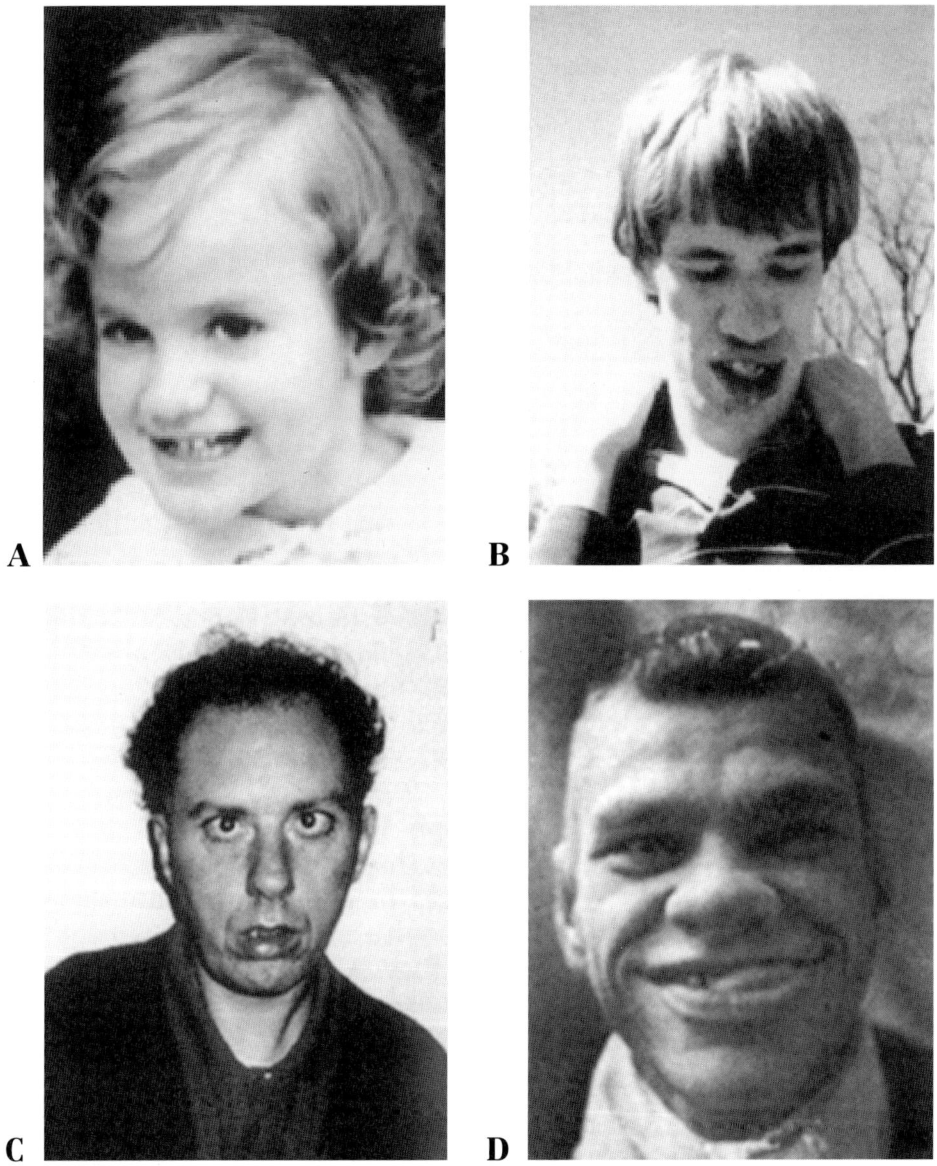

Pettigrew Syndrome. Prominent forehead and bulbous nose in childhood (A); long face with broad nose, and thick lips at age 25 years (B); tall forehead, narrow face, broadening of the nasal tip and small jaw at age 39 years (C); coarse facies with broad nose, large mouth and thick lower lip at age 25 years (D). Courtesy of Dr. David Ledbetter, University of Chicago and the *American Journal of Medical Genetics*, Copyright 1991, Wiley-Liss, Inc.

cerebellar hypoplasia (vermis and hemispheres). Iron deposition was found in scattered areas of the midbrain but most prominently in the basal ganglia. In the absence of hydrocephaly, the brain was small with iron deposition.

IMAGING. Hydrocephaly, posterior fossa cyst or Dandy-Walker malformation, hypoplasia of the cerebellum, underdeveloped frontal cortex, and iron deposits in the basal ganglia have been demonstrated.

LABORATORY. Hemosiderin deposits can be found in liver and spleen.

COMMENT. Various forms of underdevelopment of the cerebellum include total absence of the cerebellum except for a small remnant, aplasia or hypoplasia of the vermis, aplasia or hypoplasia of one or both cerebellar hemispheres, and generalized hypoplasia of the entire cerebellum. Dandy-Walker malformation may occur, particularly among those cases with aplasia or hypoplasia of the vermis. Mutations in one or more X-linked genes may lead to underdevelopment of the cerebellum and, especially among those cases with other central nervous system anomalies, may have associated mental retardation.

REFERENCES

Huang TH-M, Hejtmancik JF, Edwards A, et al.: Linkage of the gene for an X-linked mental retardation disorder to a hypervariable $(AGAT)_n$ repeat motif within the human hypoxanthine phosphoribosyltransferase (HPRT) locus (Xq26). Am J Hum Genet 49:1312, 1991.

Pettigrew AL, Jackson LG, Ledbetter DH: New X-linked mental retardation disorder with Dandy-Walker malformation, basal ganglia disease, and seizures. Am J Med Genet 38:200, 1991.

Differential Matrix

Syndrome	Cerebellar Hypoplasia	Spastic Paraplegia	Iron Deposits or Calcification of Basal Ganglia	Comments
Pettigrew	+	+	+	Dandy-Walker malformation, seizures, microcephaly or hydrocephaly, long face with macrostomia, small testes, contractures, choreoathetosis
Arena	+	+	+	Muscle hypoplasia, clubfoot, ataxia, rigidity, dystonia
Christianson	+	+	+	Short stature, microcephaly, general asthenia, contractures, seizures, ophthalmoplegia
Gustavson	+	+	+	Microcephaly, short stature, optic atrophy with blindness, large ears, deafness, joint contractures, rockerbottom feet, brain undergrowth, hydrocephaly, seizures
Schimke	+	+	+	Microcephaly, sunken eyes, downslanting palpebral fissures, narrow nose, spacing of teeth, cupped ears, hypotonia, abducens palsy, hearing loss, vision loss, choreoathetosis, contractures
Paine	+	+	0	Microcephaly, short stature, optic atrophy, vision and hearing loss, seizures
XLMR-hydrocephaly-basal ganglia calcifications	0	+	+	Hydrocephaly, muscle hypoplasia, sensory impairment

PHOSPHOGLYCERATE KINASE DEFICIENCY

(PGK Deficiency, MIM 311800)

DEFINITION. XLMR with muscle weakness, diminished deep tendon reflexes, seizures, and recurrent myoglobinuria due to phosphoglycerate kinase deficiency. The gene, PGK1, has been localized to Xq13.3

SOMATIC FEATURES. Major malformations do not occur. The face may be relatively expressionless. Muscle bulk and distribution are not unusual.

GROWTH AND DEVELOPMENT. Intrauterine and postnatal growth progresses normally, but mild to moderate delay of motor and speech development occurs.

COGNITIVE FEATURES. Moderate impairment.

NEUROLOGICAL FINDINGS. Seizures may precipitate episodes of generalized muscle pain, weakness, hemolytic anemia, and myoglobinuria. Deep tendon reflexes are depressed.

IMAGING. Normal.

LABORATORY. Phosphoglycerate kinase activity in muscle measures below 10% of normal levels. Nonetheless, glycogen accumulation is not demonstrably increased. During episodes of myoglobinuria, creatine kinase and lactate dehydrogenase (LDH) are elevated.

COMMENT. Phosphoglycerate kinase, phosphoglycerate mutase, and lactic dehydrogenase M-subunit deficiencies constitute a group of muscle glycogenoses which may be associated with recurrent episodes of myoglobinuria. PGK alone is X-linked.

REFERENCE

Sugie H, Sugie Y, Nishida M, et al.: Recurrent myoglobinuria in a child with mental retardation: phosphoglycerate kinase deficiency. J Child Neurol 4:95, 1989.

Differential Matrix

Syndrome	Muscle Weakness	Areflexia, Hypo-reflexia	Seizures	Comments
Phosphoglycerate kinase deficiency	+	+	+	Expressionless face, decreased deep tendon reflexes, myoglobinuria, hemolytic anemia
Arts	+	+	+	Growth deficiency, paucity of muscles, hypotonia, ataxia, deafness, vision loss, childhood death
Charcot-Marie-Tooth neuropathy, Cowchock variant	+	+	0	Peripheral motor and sensory neuropathy, deafness, pes cavus
Charcot-Marie-Tooth neuropathy, Ionasescu variant	+	+	0	Peripheral motor and sensory neuropathy, weakness, wasting of intrinsic hand muscles, enlarged ulnar nerves, pes cavus
Duchenne muscular dystrophy	+	+	0	Hypertrophy of calf muscles, elevated muscle enzymes, progressive weakness, muscle wasting, contractures
Myotubular myopathy	+	+	0	Hypotonic facies, open mouth, tented upper lip, hydrocephaly, long digits, cryptorchidism, hypotonia

PLOTT SYNDROME

(XLMR With Laryngeal Abductor Palsy, MIM 308850)

DEFINITION. XLMR with laryngeal abductor palsy. The gene has not been localized.

SOMATIC FEATURES. Expressionless facies result from a paucity of spontaneous movement of the facial muscles. Volitional movement, however, appears normal and electromyography of facial muscles is normal. No malformations occur. Respiratory stridor is present from the first breath and does not resolve. It may become less symptomatic or may worsen leading to tracheotomy or death. Stridor is due to paralysis of the posterior cricoarytenoid muscle, which leaves the vo-

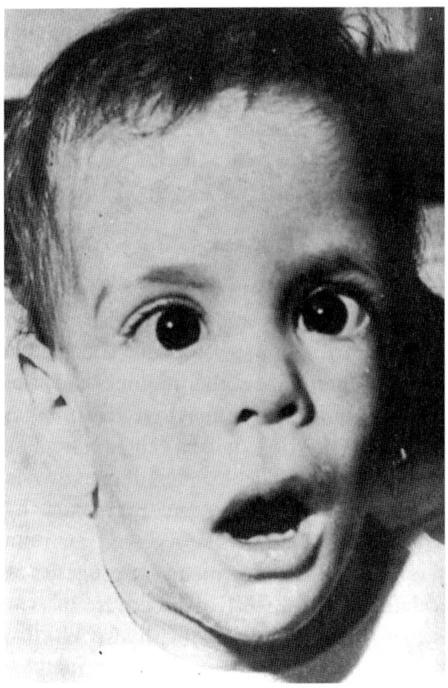

Plott Syndrome. Seventeen-month-old male with expressionless and staring facies with open mouth, opisthotonus, and tonic posturing of hands and feet. Courtesy of Dr. Gordon Watters, Montreal Children's Hospital, Montreal.

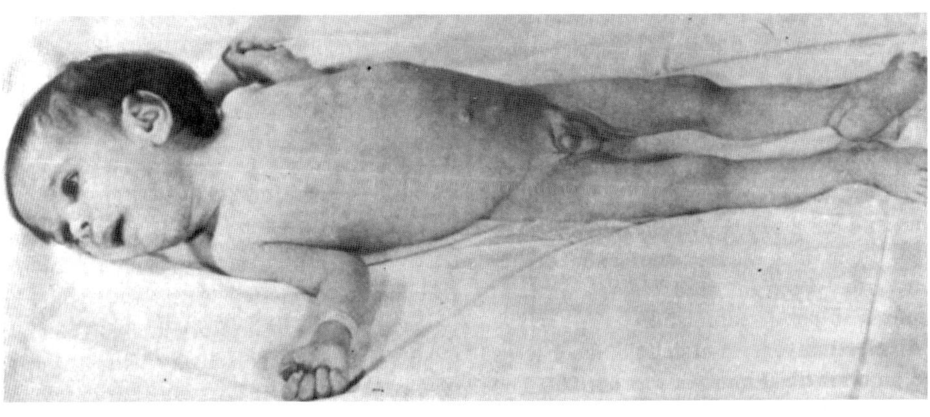

cal cords in the adducted position. During crying, the vocal cords close completely; during quiet respiration, the vocal cords are relaxed, yielding a slit-like opening. Abductor palsy has been attributed to dysgenesis of the nucleus ambiguus. One case had unilateral abducens palsy and unilateral deafness.

GROWTH AND DEVELOPMENT. Although birth weights in some cases register in the lower centiles, in other cases intrauterine growth is normal. Postnatal growth proceeds at a normal rate. Early motor development is characterized by clumsiness, awkward gait, and poor hand–eye coordination. Muscle strength and tone are normal.

COGNITIVE FUNCTION. Mild cognitive impairment occurred in three cases in the original report (IQ 56–73).

COMMENT. Three males in a second family reported by Watters and Fitch (1973) had more severe laryngeal stridor associated with sucking and swallowing difficulties, poor weight gain, apneic episodes, floppiness, stiffening, nystagmus, blindness, optic atrophy, and either early death or survival with profound psychomotor and neurologic impairments.

Perinatal hypoxia may be a significant factor in the mental impairment. Alternatively, the dysgenetic process, presumed to cause faulty development of the medulla, may also affect other areas of the brain.

REFERENCE

Plott D: Congenital laryngeal-abductor paralysis due to nucleus ambiguus dysgenesis in three brothers. N Engl J Med 271:593, 1964.

Watters GV, Fitch N: Familial laryngeal abductor paralysis and psychomotor retardation. Clin Genet 4:429, 1973.

Differential Matrix

Syndrome	Respiratory Difficulty From Birth	Expres-sionless Face	Normal Muscle Strength	Comments
Plott	+	+	+	Laryngeal abductor paralysis
Myotubular myopathy	+	+	0	Hypotonic facies, open mouth, tented upper lip, hydrocephaly, long digits, cryptorchidism, hypotonia, weakness, areflexia

PORTEOUS SYNDROME

The phenotype of Porteous syndrome is based on a single report. Affected males have short stature, normal head circumference, high forehead, receding hairline, high-pitched voice, and mild to moderate cognitive impairment. Testicular volume is normal. Carrier females have no somatic or cognitive manifestations. The gene links to markers between DXS991 (Xp11.21) and AR (Xq12), lod score of 3.15.

A
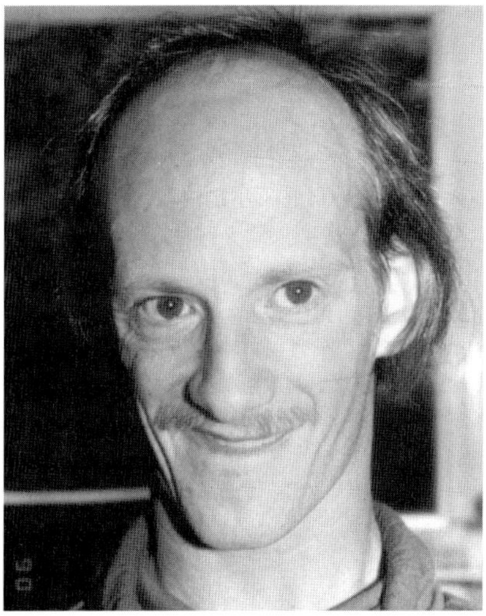

B
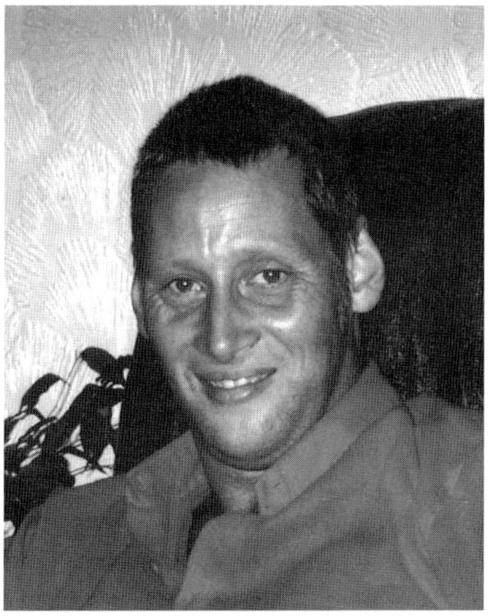

Porteous Syndrome. Cousins showing long facies, prominent forehead, receding hairline, and prominent mandible. Courtesy of Dr. Mary Porteous, South East of Scotland Clinical Genetic Service, Edinburgh.

REFERENCE

Porteous MEM, Johnson H, Burn J, et al.: A new mental retardation syndrome mapping to the pericentromeric region of the X-chromosome. Am J Hum Genet 51: A106, 1992.

PPM-X SYNDROME

(Psychosis–Pyramidal Signs–Macroorchidism Syndrome, MIM 300055)

DEFINITION. XLMR with macroorchidism, pyramidal signs, and manic-depressive psychosis. The gene maps distal to DXS1691 in Xq28, lod score 3.3.

SOMATIC FEATURES. The craniofacies appear normal and head size is normal. Several males have had short stature. Macroorchidism is consistently present. Neuropsychiatric features predominate with onset in childhood. Manic and de-

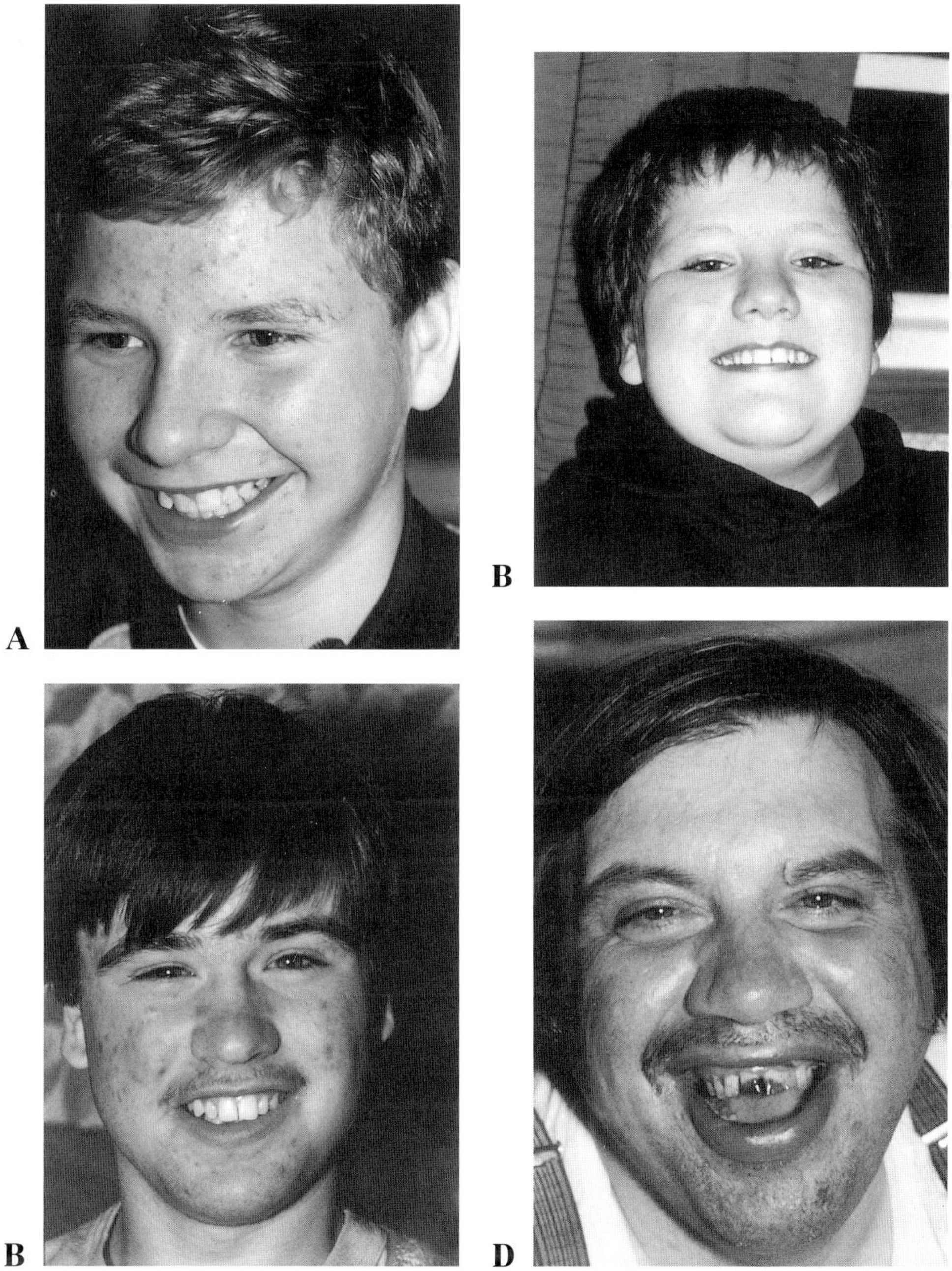

PPM-X Syndrome. Normal facial appearance in affected males at ages 11, 12, 25, 38, 39, and 41 years (A–F). Courtesy of Dr. Susan Lindsay, University of Newcastle upon Tyne, Newcastle upon Tyne, UK.

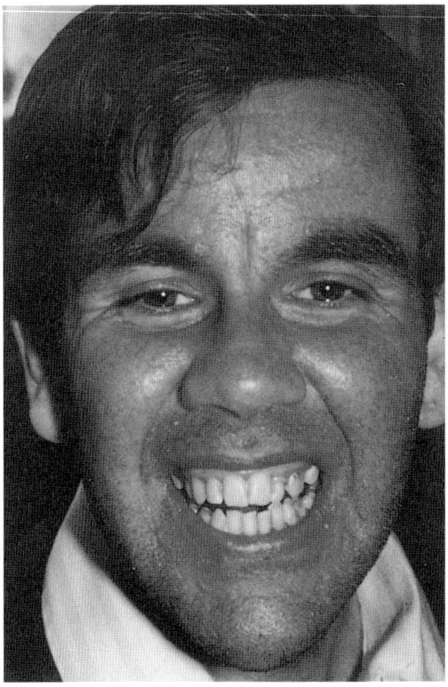

E

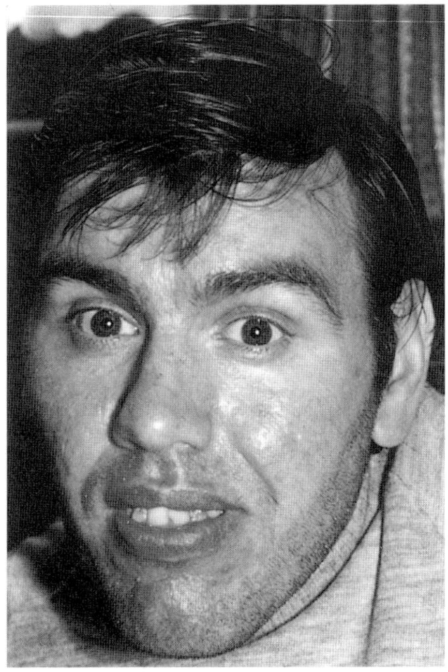

F

PPM-X Syndrome. (continued)

pressive episodes are periodically imposed on a background of hyperreflexia or spastic paraplegia, tremors, and parkinsonian features.

Growth and Development. Prenatal growth normal but adult stature is short in some individuals. Cephalic growth is normal.

Cognitive Features. Moderate impairment.

Neurological Findings. Increased muscle tone, hyperreflexia, Babinski signs, stiffness, stooped posture, shuffling gait and resting tremors may be noted as early as age 10 years. Episodes of depression (despondency, weepiness, fearfulness, poor appetite, sleep disturbances) and episodes of irritability, overactivity, aggressiveness, insomnia, and talkativeness punctuate late childhood and adult life. A contribution of antipsychosis medications to the neurologic findings was possible in some cases.

Heterozygote Expression. Female carriers have below average intelligence.

Imaging. Not known.

Comment. Macroorchidism occurs in a limited number of XLMR syndromes, specifically Atkin-Flaitz, XLMR-macroorchidism, fragile X, and PPM-X syndromes. In the family reported by Atkin-Flaitz, macroorchidism occurred in affected and nonaffected males. Spasticity, parkinsonian signs, and psychosis do not typically occur in any of the XLMR-macroorchidism syndromes other than PPM-X syndrome.

REFERENCE

Lindsay S, Splitt M, Edney S, et al.: PPM-X: A new X-linked mental retardation syndrome with psychosis, pyramidal signs, and macroorchidism maps to Xq28. Am J Hum Genet 58:1120, 1996.

Differential Matrix

Syndrome	Macro-orchidism	Spasticity	Tremors or Rigidity	Comments
PPM-X	+	+	+	Psychosis, parkinsonian features
Arena	0	+	+	Muscle hypoplasia, clubfoot, iron deposits in basal ganglia, ataxia, dystonia
Gustavson	0	+	+	Microcephaly, short stature, optic atrophy with blindness, large ears, deafness, joint contractures, rockerbottom feet, brain undergrowth, hydrocephaly, cerebellar hypoplasia, seizures
Lesch-Nyhan	0	+	+	Choreoathetosis, self-mutilation, hyperuricemia
Pelizaeus-Merzbacher	0	+	+	Optic atrophy, nystagmus, hypotonia, ataxia, dystonia, CNS dysmyelination
Pettigrew	0	+	+	Dandy-Walker malformation, seizures, microcephaly or hydrocephaly, long face with macrostomia and prognathism, small testes, contractures, choreoathetosis, iron deposits in basal ganglia
Waisman-Laxova	0	+	+	-
XLMR-spastic paraplegia-athetosis	0	+	+	Nystagmus, weakness, dysarthria, muscle wasting, contractures

PRIETO SYNDROME

DEFINITION. XLMR with distinctive facies, optic atrophy, ventriculomegaly, hypotonia, and skeletal anomalies. The syndrome location is between the genes for ornithine transcarbamylase (OTC) and monoamine oxidase–A deficiency (MAO-A) in Xp11, lod score 3.58.

SOMATIC FEATURES. The cranium measures within the normal range (2–70 centiles) but may be asymmetric. The face may be asymmetric as well with triangular configuration, hypertelorism, prominent eyes, epicanthus, strabismus, ptosis, long narrow nose with the tip overhanging the columella, dysplastic low set ears with small lobes, and micrognathia or retrognathia. A double row of lower incisors was present in one case. The optic discs are pale. There is generalized decrease in tone with persistent drooling, depressed reflexes, coxa valgum, dis-

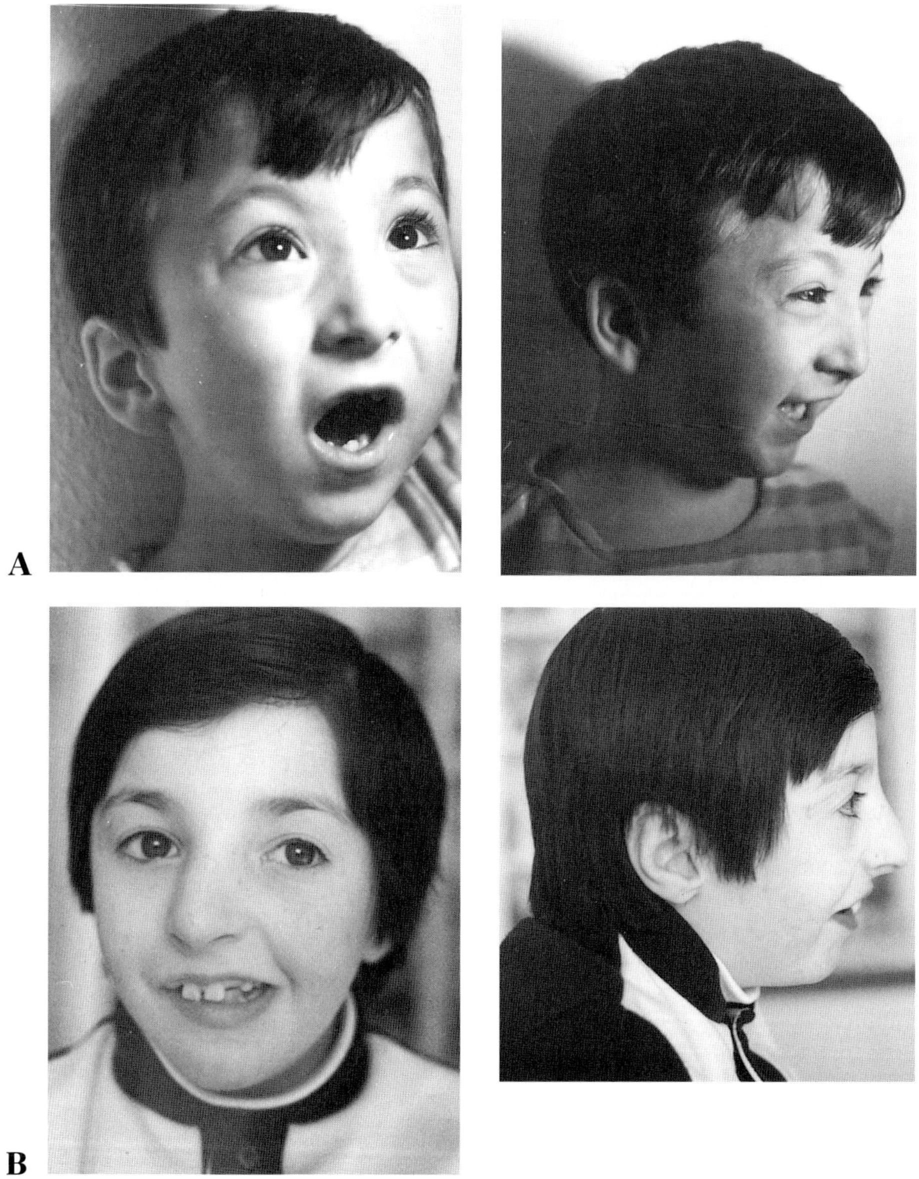

Prieto Syndrome. Triangular facies with prominent nose, absent earlobe, and retrognathia in affected males at ages 5 years (A) and 10 years (B).

located patellas, pes planus, and clubfoot. Inguinal hernia and cryptorchidism may occur. Clinodactyly of finger 5 is present. A skin dimple is found over the lower spine. The ventricles are enlarged, secondary to cerebral atrophy. Seizures occur with fever during childhood.

GROWTH AND DEVELOPMENT. Intrauterine growth appears normal with birth weight 2.9–3.8 kg. Postnatal statural and head growth is likewise normal. Global developmental delay is obvious from early infancy.

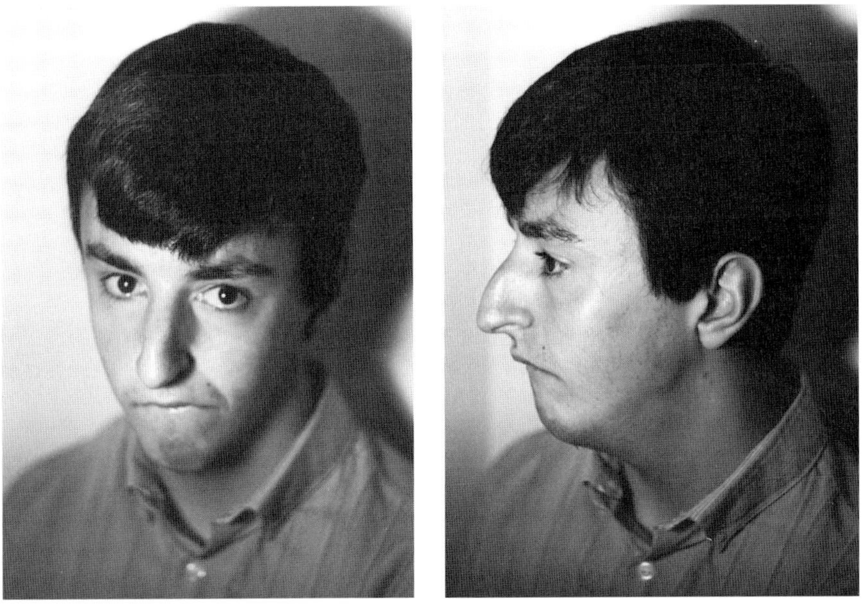

C

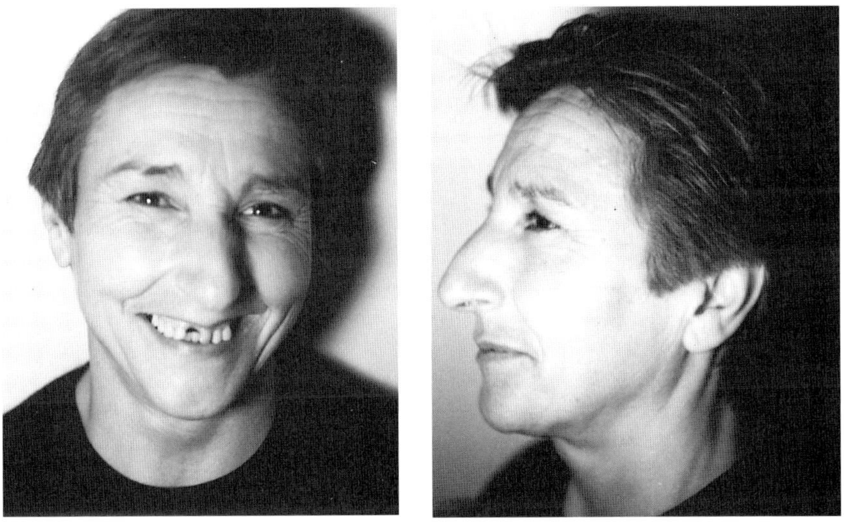

D

Prieto Syndrome. (continued) Triangular faces, prominent nose and retrognathia in an affected male at age 17 years (C), and in a carrier mother (D). Courtesy of Dr. Félix Prieto, La Fe University Hospital, Valencia, Spain.

COGNITIVE FUNCTION. Formal testing was not reported but delay of developmental milestones suggests severe mental retardation.

NEUROLOGIC FINDINGS. Decreased muscle tone and deep tendon reflexes are typical. Independent ambulation may be achieved but lost in adult life. Generalized seizures, usually with fever, occur during childhood.

HETEROZYGOTE EXPRESSION. Carrier females show no cognitive impairment.

IMAGING. Pneumoencephalography and CT demonstrated enlarged ventricles with subcortical central atrophy.

COMMENT. The description is based on a single family with eight males affected in two generations.

REFERENCES

Martínez F, Prieto F, Gal A: Refined localization of the Prieto-Syndrome locus. Am J Med Genet 64:82, 1996.

Prieto F, Badia L, Mulas F, et al.: X-linked dysmorphic syndrome with mental retardation. Clin Genet 32:326, 1987.

Watty A, Prieto F, Beneyto M, et al.: Gene localization in a family with X-linked syndromal mental retardation (Prieto Syndrome). Am J Med Genet 38:234, 1991.

Differential Matrix

Syndrome	Optic Atrophy	Hydro-cephaly	Hypotonia	Comments
Prieto	+	+	+	Ventricular enlargement, facial asymmetry, hypertelorism, prominent eyes, ptosis, long narrow nose, micrognathia, inguinal hernia, cryptorchidism
Brooks	+	+	+	Microcephaly, short stature, deep-set eyes, blepharophimosis, cupped ears, bulbous nose, small mouth, thin upper lip, pectus excavatum, flexion contractures, dysgenesis of corpus callosum
VACTERL-hydrocephaly	+	+	+	Vertebral anomalies, radial limb defects, tracheal and esophageal anomalies, renal malformations, anal anomalies
Gustavson	+	+	0	Microcephaly, short stature, blindness, large ears, deafness, joint contractures, rockerbottom feet, brain undergrowth, cerebellar hypoplasia, spasticity, seizures
Pettigrew	0	+	+	Dandy-Walker malformation, spasticity, seizures, microcephaly or hydrocephaly, long face with macrostomia and prognathism, small testes, contractures, choreoathetosis, iron deposits in basal ganglia
Arts	+	0	+	Growth deficiency, paucity of muscles, areflexia, ataxia, deafness, vision loss, seizures, childhood death
Pelizaeus-Merzbacher	+	0	+	Nystagmus, spasticity, ataxia, dystonia, CNS dysmyelination
XLMR-ataxia-deafness-dementia	+	0	+	Vision loss, hearing loss, spastic paraplegia, ataxia, seizures, childhood death

PROUD SYNDROME

DEFINITION. XLMR with short stature, microcephaly, agenesis of corpus callosum, skeletal anomalies, tapered digits, spasticity, seizures, and impairments of vision and hearing. The gene has not been localized.

SOMATIC FEATURES. Although normal at birth, growth of the head falls below the third centile in early childhood. The facies are mildly coarse, perhaps related in part to anticonvulsant therapy. Other facial features include prominent supraorbital ridges, apparent hypertelorism, prominent ears with thick lobes, and high palate. Nystagmus, wandering eye movements, and strabismus occur. Kyphoscoliosis, hip dislocation, limb contractures, and spasticity develop. Vision and hearing are impaired.

Malformations include agenesis of the corpus callosum, cryptorchidism, hypospadias, and inguinal hernia.

COGNITIVE FEATURES. Males are severely and globally impaired from birth. None learn to walk or talk. Females have had variable cognitive impairment and somatic manifestations.

NEUROLOGICAL FINDINGS. Intractable myoclonic and generalized seizures, nystagmus, impaired vision and hearing, spasticity, clonus, and athetosis appear in infancy or early childhood.

NATURAL HISTORY. Males are severely impaired from birth. Several males who were probably affected died in infancy or early childhood; others have survived to early adult life. One female carrier appeared affected to the same degree as the males; other carrier females have less severe cognitive and physical manifestations.

HETEROZYGOTE EXPRESSION. Carrier females are cognitively impaired and may have agenesis of corpus callosum, strabismus, contractures, visual defects, and seizures.

IMAGING. Agenesis of corpus callosum and ventricular dilation have been documented by CT and MRI. One case had porencephaly. Carriers were variably affected with cerebral atrophy, ventricular dilation, and partial absence of corpus callosum.

COMMENT. A single family with three affected males and three affected females has been described. Three other males died early, one at 6 months as a "blue baby" and two others in early childhood with growth failure, seizures, and other features of the condition. Linkage analysis was attempted but the gene location could not be established.

REFERENCE

Proud VK, Levine C, Carpenter NJ: New X-linked syndrome with seizures, acquired micrencephaly, and agenesis of the corpus callosum. Am J Med Genet 43:458, 1992.

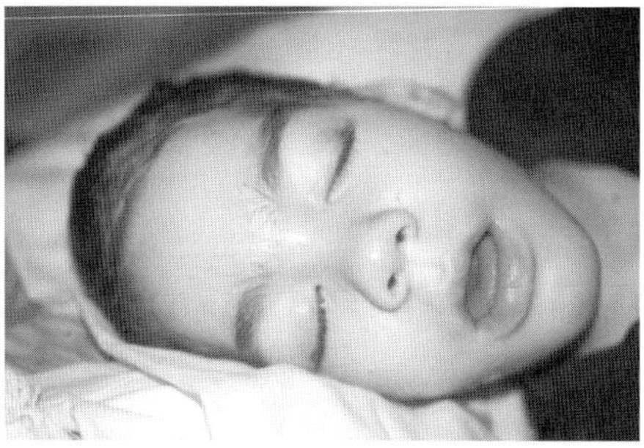
A

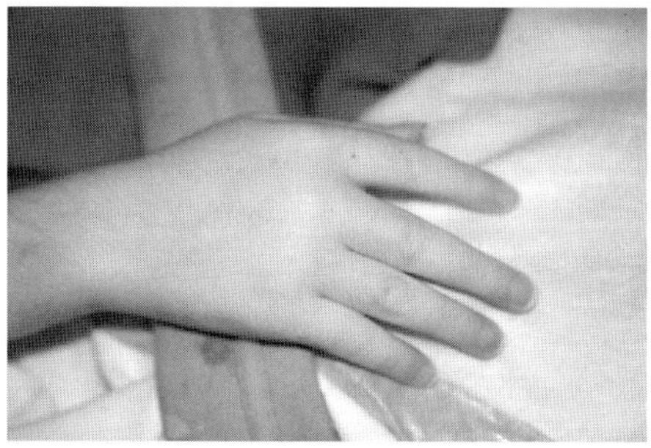
B

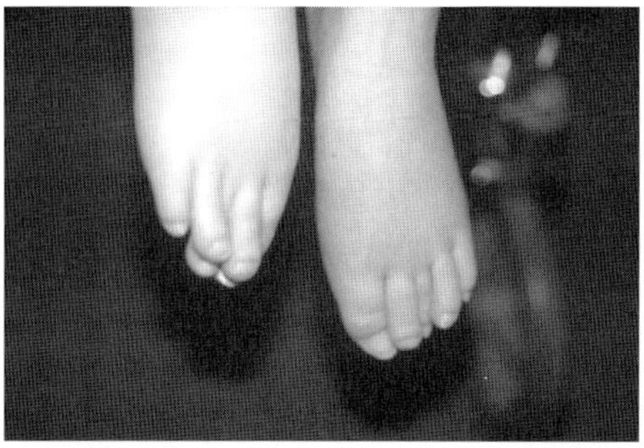
C

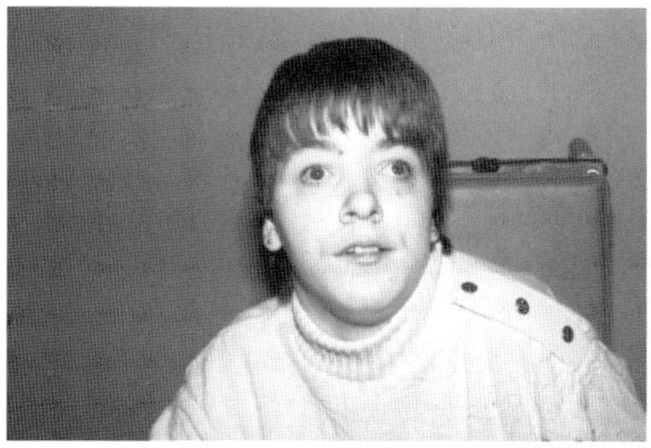
E

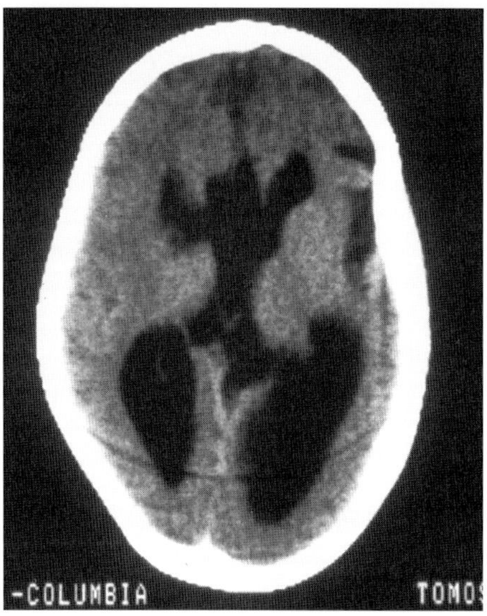

D

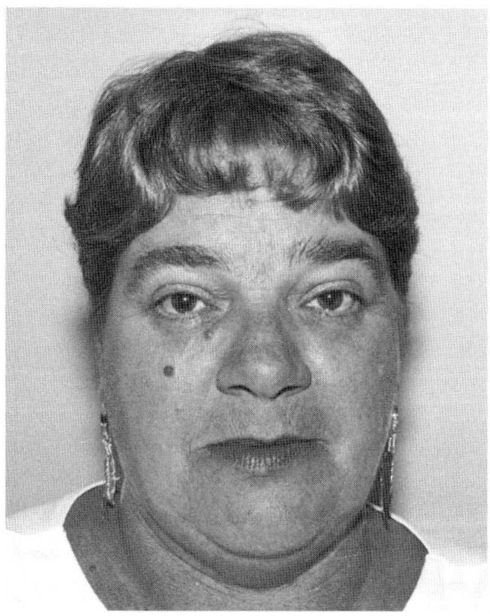
F

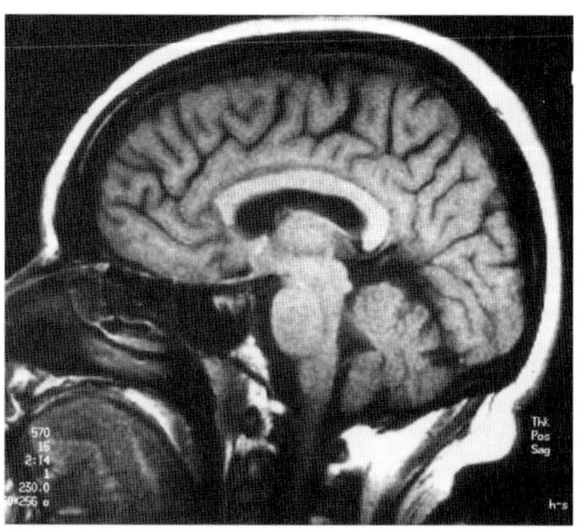
G

Differential Matrix

Syndrome	Dysgenesis of Corpus Callosum	Impaired Vision and/or Hearing	Spasticity	Comments
Proud	+	+	+	Microcephaly, cryptorchidism, inguinal hernias, ataxia, seizures
Cerebrooculogenital	+	+	+	Short stature, microcephaly, hydrocephaly, agenesis of corpus callosum, microphthalmia, ptosis, hypospadias, cryptorchidism, clubfoot
Aicardi	+	+	0	Ocular dysgenesis, lacunar retinopathy, costovertebral anomalies, seizures
Gustavson	0	+	+	Microcephaly, short stature, large ears, joint contractures, rockerbottom feet, brain undergrowth, hydrocephaly, cerebellar hypoplasia, seizures
Mohr-Tranebjaerg (Jensen)	0	+	+	Neurologic deterioration with childhood onset, dystonia
Pettigrew	0	+	+	Dandy-Walker malformation, seizures, microcephaly or hydrocephaly, long face with macrostomia and prognathism, small testes, contractures, choreoathetosis, iron deposits in basal ganglia
Schimke	0	+	+	Microcephaly, sunken eyes, downslanting palpebral fissures, narrow nose, spacing of teeth, cupped ears, hypotonia, abducens palsy, choreoathetosis, contractures
XLMR-ataxia-deafness-dementia	0	+	+	Optic atrophy, ataxia, hypotonia, seizures, childhood death
X-linked spastic paraplegia, type 7	0	+	+	Nystagmus, absent speech and ambulation, bowel and bladder dysfunction
Kang	+	0	+	Microcephaly, frontal prominence, telecanthus, small nose, short hands, seizures, downturned mouth, brachydactyly
X-linked hydrocephaly-MASA spectrum	+	0	+	Hydrocephaly, adducted thumbs

◄———

Proud Syndrome. 8-year-old male with long face, thickened alae nasi, prominent lips, tapered fingers, crowded and overlapping toes (A–C); cranial tomography in a 23-year-old male showing dilated ventricles and porencephaly (D); carrier female with strabismus and spasticity (E); carrier mother with upslanted palpebral fissures, strabismus, broad nasal tip, and hypoplasia of the rostrum of the corpus callosum (F, G). Courtesy of Dr. Virginia Proud, Norfolk, Virginia.

PYRUVATE DEHYDROGENASE DEFICIENCY

(Pyruvate Dehydrogenase E1-α Deficiency, Leigh Syndrome With Pyruvate Dehydrogenase Deficiency, Intermittent Ataxia With Pyruvate Dehydrogenase Deficiency, MIM 312170)

DEFINITION. XLMR with variable clinical manifestations ranging from profound neuromuscular failure, developmental arrest, and early death associated with overwhelming lactic acidosis to chronic or intermittent ataxia, dysarthria, and developmental impairment with or without demonstrable lactic acidosis. Deficient enzyme activity of the pyruvate dehydrogenase (PDH) complex is responsible as a result of a mutation in the E1α subunit of pyruvate decarboxylase. The E1α gene is in Xp22.22-p22.1 between DXS999 and DXS365.

SOMATIC FEATURES. A minority of patients will have craniofacial abnormalities including microcephaly, bossed forehead, wide nasal bridge, upturned nose, and long philtrum, manifestations not unlike those of fetal alcohol syndrome. Dysgenesis of the corpus callosum, cerebral atrophy, and cysts of the brain stem, basal ganglia, and cerebrum have been described.

GROWTH AND DEVELOPMENT. Survivors usually have variable developmental delay. Growth impairment and microcephaly may result from the lactic acidosis and cerebral damage.

COGNITIVE FEATURES. Survivors usually have variable degrees of mental retardation.

NEUROLOGICAL FINDINGS. Presentation may be the neurologic features of Leigh disease. Males may present with intermittent ataxia and dysarthria. Hypotonia is common and may progress to hypertonia. Seizures occur.

NATURAL HISTORY. In males, the severity may correlate with enzyme activity. Absent or negligible enzyme activity presumably is not compatible with prenatal survival. Low activity results in persistent severe lactic acidosis and death in the first 6 months. Survivors may have more residual enzyme activity. Their mild to moderate lactic acidosis may only be symptomatic with infections or may be detected in evaluation of psychomotor delay/mental retardation. There may be a neurodegenerative course with seizures, spasticity, cortical blindness, and risk of death from apnea. An even milder form presents with intermittent or chronic ataxia/dysarthria with or without mental retardation. The neurologic symptoms and mild lactic acidosis may be precipitated by carbohydrate intake.

HETEROZYGOTE EXPRESSION. The male to female ratio of documented cases is about 1:1. Females predominate in the survivors and may have any presentation except possibly carbohydrate-induced episodic ataxia.

NEUROPATHOLOGY. The brain is dependent on glucose as an energy (ATP) source. Pyruvate dehydrogenase is the rate limiting step in the entry of glucose through pyruvate into the Krebs cycle and subsequently into the respiratory chain for production of ATP. Neuronal cell death results from lactic acidosis or ATP deficit and may be generalized or localized to regions of high-energy utilization. The fetal brain is dependent on glucose oxidation and cerebral disruption may occur in utero.

IMAGING. Agenesis or hypogenesis of corpus callosum, cerebral atrophy, and cysts of the cerebral cortex, basal ganglia, and brain stem have been described. In those with ataxic episodes, neuroimaging is initially normal but may later reveal cystic lesions in the brain stem. On proton magnetic resonance spectroscopy of the brain, signals for lactate are increased and those for N-acetylaspartate decreased.
LABORATORY. Blood lactate and pyruvate are chronically or intermittently increased, but the lactate:pyruvate ratio is normal. Elevations in lactate are greater in and may be limited to the cerebral spinal fluid. Decreased PDH activity is found in skin fibroblasts and other tissues. In heterozygotes, the decreased PDH activity varies in different tissues. Most mutations are unique.
TREATMENT. Those with episodic ataxia may benefit from a low-carbohydrate ketogenic diet. A trial of thiamine and a low-carbohydrate ketogenic diet rarely are of benefit to others.
COMMENT. The clinical variability in males is presumably related to the level of enzyme activity, but the correlation is not always apparent in *in vitro* studies. In addition, in females, the capacity of normal cells to eliminate lactate but not to supply ATP for abnormal cells, as well as lyonization, contribute to the variability.

REFERENCES

Børglum AD, Flint T, Hansen LL, et al.: Refined localization of the pyruvate dehydrogenase E1α gene (PDHA1) by linkage analysis. Hum Genet 99:80, 1997.

Brown GK, Otero LJ, LeGris M, et al.: Pyruvate dehydrogenase deficiency. Med Genet 31:875, 1994.

Robinson BH, MacMillan H, Petrova-Benedict R, et al.: Variable clinical presentation in patients with defective E1 component of pyruvate dehydrogenase complex. J Pediatr 111:525, 1987.

Shevell MI, Matthews PM, Scriver CR, et al.: Cerebral dysgenesis and lactic acidemia: An MRI/MRS phenotype associated with pyruvate dehydrogenase deficiency. Pediatr Neurol 11:224, 1994.

Differential Matrix

Syndrome	Microcephaly	Structural Brain Anomalies	Lactic Acidosis	Comments
Pyruvate dehydrogenase deficiency	+	+	+	Hypotonia, ataxia, dysarthria
Ornithine transcarbamylase deficiency	+	+	+	Chronic or intermittent hyperammonemia, protein-induced vomiting and lethargy, ataxia, seizures

RENPENNING SYNDROME

DEFINITION. XLMR with short stature, microcephaly, and small testes. The gene locus maps between DXS1039 (Xp11.4) and DXS1003 (Xp11.2), with lod score of 3.13.

SOMATIC FEATURES. Alterations in growth contribute the major components of the phenotype. The craniofacial structure is distinctive only in having microcephaly or head circumference in the lower centiles. Palpebral fissures slant up-

A
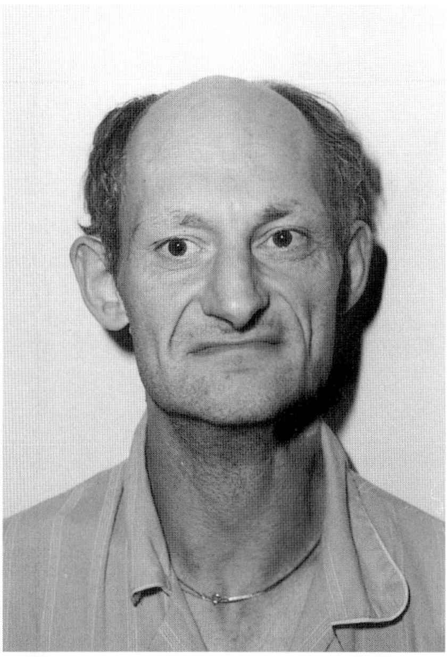

B
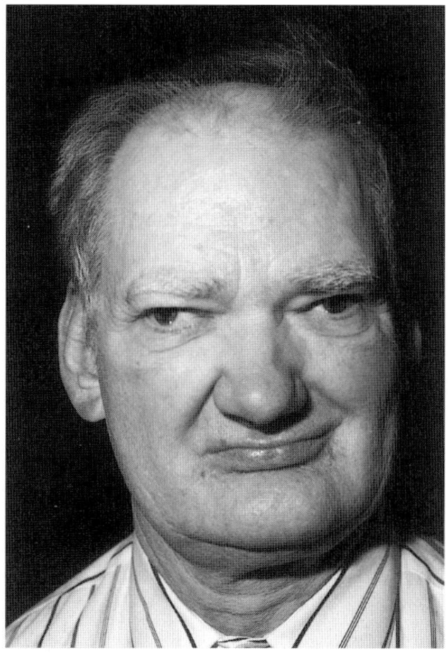

C
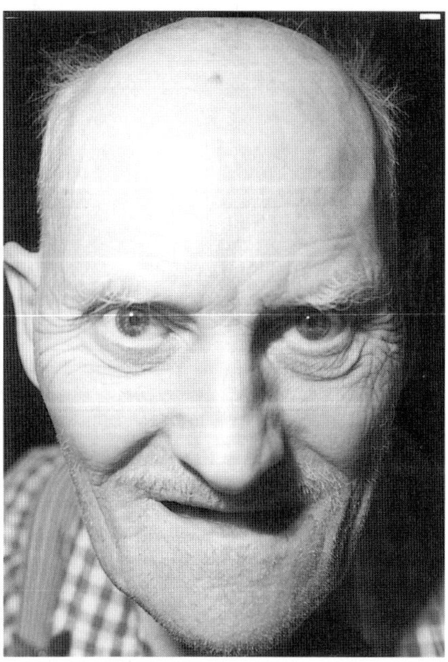

Renpenning Syndrome. Adults at ages 40, 55, and 65 years showing balding, upslanting palpebral fissures, and short philtrum. The head circumference in each measures near or below the third centile.

ward. Statural growth likewise is near or below the lower centiles. Testicular volumes are similarly small. Major malformations do not occur and the musculoskeletal system appears normal. Two males have been blind, one in association with an ocular coloboma.

COGNITIVE FEATURES. Early childhood development is severely and globally delayed. Ultimate cognitive impairment is severe.

HETEROZYGOTE EXPRESSION. Carrier females do not show growth or cognitive impairments.

NEUROPATHOLOGY. Examination of the brain in two cases has confirmed small size (780 g and 984 g) and in one case the neurons of the left cortex were arranged in columns suggesting a defect in neuronal migration or maturation.

COMMENT. In the 1970s, the term *Renpenning syndrome* came to be used as a generic reference to X-linked mental retardation (Steele and Chorazy 1974; Howard-Peebles et al. 1979; Jennings et al. 1980; Proops and Webb 1981). This broad usage was applied to syndromic XLMR, including the fragile X syndrome, and nonsyndromic XLMR. Turner et al. (1970, 1971, 1972) argued that this designation be used only for nonsyndromic XLMR—specifically, for cases lacking macrocephaly or microcephaly, epilepsy, major malformations or more than one minor malformation, and neurological signs. We propose that these practices be abandoned and that Renpenning syndrome be reserved for that condition which maps to Xp11.2-11.4 and is characterized by severe mental impairment, microcephaly, and a tendency toward short stature and small testes. Those males with XLMR who lack physical, behavioral, or neurological findings should be designated nonsyndromic (or nonspecific) XLMR, at least in the short term until the responsible genes are isolated.

REFERENCES

Archidiacono N, Rocchi M, Rinaldi A, et al.: X-linked mental retardation. II. Renpenning syndrome and other types (report of 14 families). J Génét Hum 35:381, 1987.

Filippi G, Rinaldi A, Archidiacono N, et al.: Brief report: linkage between G6PD and fragile-X syndrome. Am J Med Genet 15:113, 1983.

Fox P, Fox D, Gerrard JW: X-linked mental retardation: Renpenning revisited. Am J Med Genet 7:491, 1980.

Gerrard JW, Renpenning HJ: Sex-linked mental retardation. Lancet 1:1346, 1974

Howard-Peebles PN, Stoddard GR, Mims MG: Familial X-linked mental retardation, verbal disability, and marker X chromosomes. Am J Hum Genet 31:214, 1979.

Jennings M, Hall JG, Hoehn H: Significance of phenotypic and chromosomal abnormalities in X-linked mental retardation (Martin-Bell or Renpenning Syndrome). Am J Med Genet 7:417, 1980.

McLaughlin JF, Kriegsmann E: Developmental dyspraxias in a family with X-linked mental retardation (Renpenning syndrome). Dev Med Child Neurol 22: 1980.

Proops R, Webb T: The 'fragile' X chromosome in the Martin-Bell-Renpenning syndrome and in males with other forms of familial mental retardation. J Med Genet 18:366, 1981.

Renpenning H, Gerrard JW, Zaleski WA, et al.: Familial sex-linked mental retardation. Can Med Assoc J 87:954, 1962.

Richards BW: "Renpenning" syndrome. Lancet 2:520, 1970

Steele MW, Chorazy AL: Renpenning's syndrome. Lancet 2:752, 1974.

Stevenson RE, Arena JF, Ouzts E, et al.: Renpenning syndrome maps to Xp11. Am J Hum Genet 62:1092, 1998.

Turner G, Turner B, Collins E: Renpenning's syndrome—X-linked mental retardation. Lancet 2:365, 1970.

Turner G, Turner B, Collins E: X-linked mental retardation without physical abnormality: Renpenning's syndrome. Dev Med Child Neurol 13:71, 1971.

Turner G, Engisch B, Lindsay DG, et al.: X-linked mental retardation without physical abnormality (Renpenning's syndrome) in sibs in an institution. J Med Genet 9:324, 1972.

Differential Matrix

Syndrome	Micro-cephaly	Short Stature	Small Testes	Comments
Renpenning	+	+	+	Upslanting palpebral fissures
Sutherland-Haan	+	+	+	Upslanting palpebral fissures, asthenic habitus, pectus excavatum, scoliosis, stiff joints, pes cavus, spasticity
Börjeson-Forssman-Lehmann	+	+	+	Obesity, hypotonia, hypogonadism, coarse facies, large ears, gynecomastia, narrow sloped shoulders, visual impairment, tapered digits
Chudley-Lowry	+	+	+	Bitemporal narrowing, almond-shaped eyes, depressed nasal bridge, tented upper lip, open mouth, hypogonadism, hypotonia, obesity
X-linked hereditary bullous dystrophy	+	+	+	Upslanting palpebral fissures, protruding ears, digits short and tapered, cardiac defects, bullous dystrophy, early death from pulmonary infection
XLMR-hypotonic facies (Carpenter-Waziri) (Holmes-Gang) (Juberg-Marsidi)	+	+	+	Telecanthus, small triangular nose, tented upper lip, open mouth, spacing of teeth, genital anomalies, musculoskeletal anomalies, hemoglobin H inclusions in erythrocytes
Miles-Carpenter	+	+	0	Ptosis, small palpebral fissures, open mouth, pectus excavatum, scoliosis, long hands, camptodactyly, rockerbottom feet, arch fingerprints, spasticity, unsteady gait
Pettigrew	+	0	+	Microcephaly or hydrocephaly, long face with macrostomia and prognathism, Dandy-Walker malformation, spasticity, seizures, contractures, choreoathetosis, iron deposits in basal ganglia

RETT SYNDROME

(Ataxia-Dementia-Autism Syndrome, Autism–Dementia–Ataxia–Loss of Purposeful Hand Use Syndrome, MIM 312750)

DEFINITION. XLMR in females associated with cessation and regression of development in early childhood, truncal ataxia, autistic features, and acquired microcephaly. Haplotype analysis in multiplex families including an affected mother and daughter indicates that the Xq telomere is a candidate region for Rett syndrome. X:autosome translocations suggest the possibility of a locus on Xp.

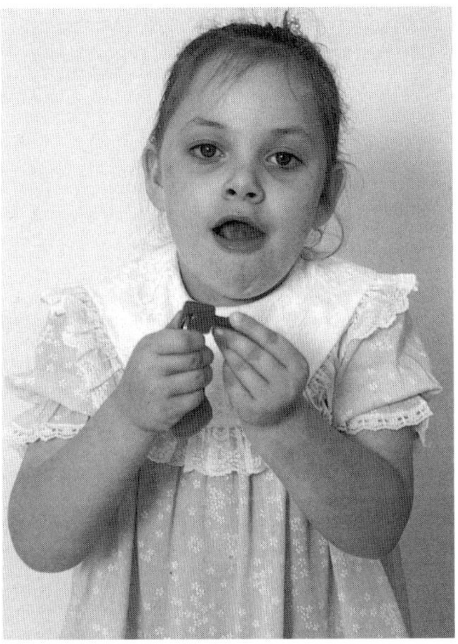

A

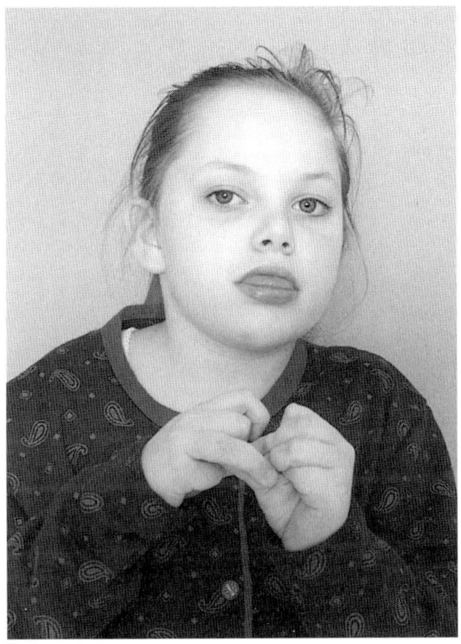

B

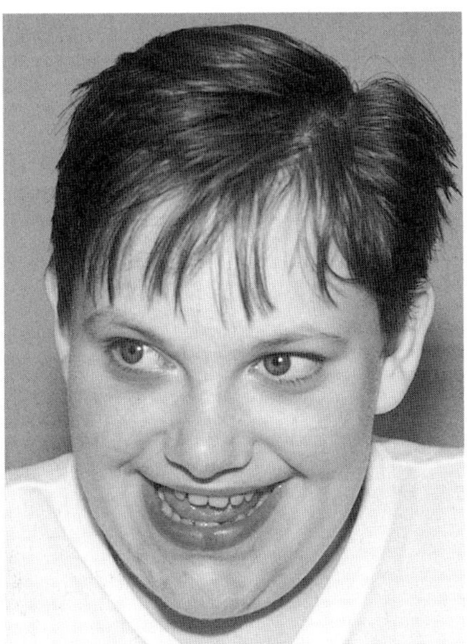

C

Rett Syndrome. Microcephaly and hand wringing activity in a girl at ages 5, 7, and 14 years.

SOMATIC FEATURES. Major malformations do not occur. Microcephaly is evident by age 3 years although the birth head circumference is normal. The facial appearance in childhood, while not distinctive, tends to be delicate and is thereby distinguished from the facial coarseness that accompanies other developmental regression syndromes, notably the lysosomal storage disorders. A pattern of neurologic deterioration dominates and defines the phenotype.

GROWTH AND DEVELOPMENT. Intrauterine growth appears normal; postnatal growth slows during the first year leading to microcephaly and short stature in early childhood. A variable period of normal development follows birth but gives way first to a slowing of development and then to a loss of skills.

COGNITIVE FEATURES. Progression to severe impairment occurs during the preschool years, usually with accompanying characteristics of autism.

NEUROLOGICAL FINDINGS. A series of neurological stages define the natural history of Rett syndrome. Following a period of normal developmental progress, acquisition of new skills slows and stops, hypotonia appears, interaction with the environment wanes, and the growth rates of the head and body decrease. By age 1–3 years, this stage merges into one of relatively rapid deterioration in which hand use, cognitive, speech, and social skills are lost and stereotypic hand movements, jerky/apraxic limb and truncal movements, autistic mannerisms, disorganized breathing with hyperventilation and apneic episodes, and seizures appear. Thereafter, unsteadiness and seizures become more notable while cognitive impairment, autistic features, and loss of motor skills plateau. In the early school years, motor function begins to deteriorate further, eventually leading to muscle wasting, loss of mobility, hypertonicity, hyperreflexia, clonus, extensor plantar reflexes, vasomotor disturbances, and cachexia.

IMAGING. Mild and nonspecific atrophy is noted on brain imaging.

ELECTROENCEPHALOGRAPHY. In all cases, the EEG is abnormal. Although a specific pattern should not be anticipated, single or multiple epileptic foci, generalized background slowing and disorganization, and loss of normal sleep patterns occur and progressively worsen.

COMMENT. Although perhaps one of the more common of the X-linked disorders with mental retardation, Rett syndrome has been enigmatic. A variety of serum and CSF biochemical changes have been observed, but none has proved to be specific, primary, or consistent. Rett syndrome occurs only in females and in this regard is similar to XLMR-epilepsy, the only other X-linked condition to be considered in the differential. Since most affected females do not reproduce, the majority of cases likely represent new mutations, possibly arising in the father's germline.

REFERENCES

Hagberg B, Aicardi J, Dias K, et al.: A progressive syndrome of autism, dementia, ataxia, and loss of purposeful hand use in girls: Rett's syndrome: report of 35 cases. Ann Neurol 14:471, 1983.

Moeschler JB, Charman CE, Berg SZ, et al.: Rett syndrome: natural history and management. Pediatrics 82:1, 1988.

Naidu S, Murphy M, Moser HW: Rett syndrome—natural history in 70 cases. Am J Med Genet 24 (Suppl 1):61, 1983.
Rett A: Uber ein eigenartiges hirnatrophisches syndrom bei hyperammonämie im kindesalter. Wien Med Wochenschr 116:723, 1966.
Xiang F, Zhang Z, Clarke A, et al.: Chromosome mapping of Rett syndrome: a likely candidate region on the telomere of Xq. J Med Genet 35:297, 1998.

Differential Matrix

Syndrome	Developmental Regression	Repetitive Stereotypic Hand Movements	Seizures	Comments
Rett	+	+	+	Acquired microcephaly, truncal ataxia, autistic features
XLMR-epilepsy	+	+	+	-

SAY-MEYER SYNDROME

(MIM 314320)

DEFINITION. XLMR with short stature, microcephaly, hypotelorism, and craniosynostosis. The gene has not been mapped.

SOMATIC FEATURES. Microcephaly with metopic ridging due to synostosis of the metopic suture, synostosis affecting other cranial sutures, narrow frontal diameter, hypotelorism, and small fontanels are the major features. Low-set or retroverted ears and high palate may be present.

GROWTH AND DEVELOPMENT. Global growth retardation dates from the intrauterine period. Although long-term developmental outcome is not known, early childhood development is moderately delayed.

NEUROLOGICAL FINDINGS. Seizures.

HETEROZYGOTE EXPRESSION. None.

COMMENT. The phenotype is based on a single family with three affected males in two generations. Craniosynostosis is rare among the XLMR syndromes and, when present, it usually affects the metopic suture.

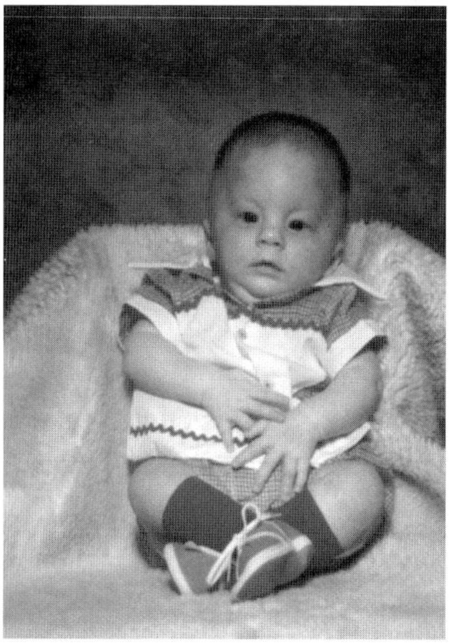

A

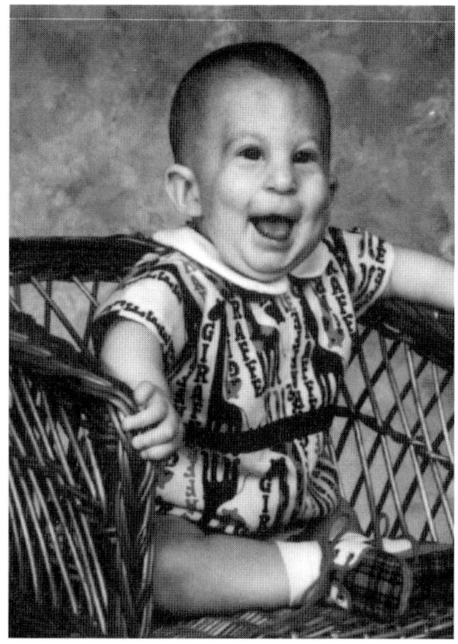

B

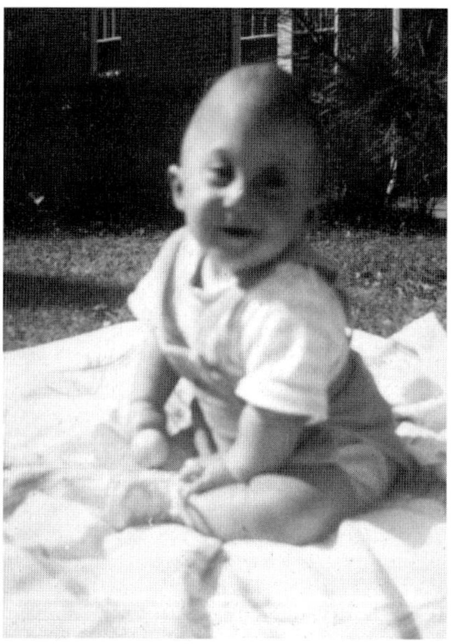

C

Say-Meyer Syndrome. Infant with microcephaly, bifrontal narrowing, prominent metopic ridging, and hypotelorism (A); cousin with microcephaly, trigonencephaly, prominent metopic ridging, epicanthal folds, and hypotelorism (B); maternal uncle with microcephaly trigonencephaly, narrow forehead with metopic ridge, and hypotelorism (C). Courtesy of Dr. Burhan Say, Tulsa Medical College, Tulsa, Oklahoma.

REFERENCE

Say B, Meyer J: Familial trigonocephaly associated with short stature and developmental delay. Am J Dis Child 135:711, 1981.

Differential Matrix

Syndrome	Micro-cephaly	Metopic Ridging or Synostosis	Hypo-telorism	Comments
Say-Meyer	+	+	+	Short stature, craniosynostosis
Golabi-Ito-Hall	+	+	0	Short stature, telecanthus, high nasal root, cupped ears, cardiac malformations, thoracic asymmetry, sacral dimple, dry/brittle/sparse hair, cutis marmorata, nail hypoplasia
XLMR-hypospadias	+	+	0	Trigonocephaly, synophrys, beaked-nose, hypospadias
Christian	0	+	+	Vertebral anomalies, abducens palsy
Brooks	+	0	+	Short stature, deep-set eyes, blepharophimosis, cupped ears, bulbous nose, small mouth, thin upper lip, pectus excavatum, flexion contractures, dysgenesis of corpus callosum
Schimke	+	0	+	Sunken eyes, downslanting palpebral fissures, narrow nose, spacing of teeth, cupped ears, hypotonia, abducens palsy, hearing loss, vision loss, spasticity, choreoathetosis, contractures

SCHIMKE SYNDROME

(Schimke XLMR Syndrome, XLMR-Choreoathetosis, MIM 312840)

DEFINITION. XLMR with short stature, microcephaly, strabismus, sunken eyes, thin nose, impaired vision and hearing, abducens palsy, choreoathetosis, and spasticity. The gene has not been localized.

SOMATIC FEATURES. Sunken eyes, downslanting palpebral fissures, apparent hypotelorism, narrow nose and alae nasi, strabismus, spacing of the teeth, and cupped ears give the distinctive facial appearance. Major malformations do not occur. In infancy males are hypotonic and feed poorly. This gives way to spasticity with increased deep tendon reflexes and Babinski signs. Microcephaly, spasticity, and involuntary limb movements become obvious during the first year. Hearing and vision are impaired and esotropia occurs secondary to abducens palsy. The spasticity progressively worsens with age, eventually leading to rigidity and joint contractures, muscle atrophy, and loss of spontaneous movement.

GROWTH AND DEVELOPMENT. Prenatal growth is impaired although the head circumference may be normal at birth. Microcephaly and short stature become obvious during the first year.

COGNITIVE FEATURES. Not available.

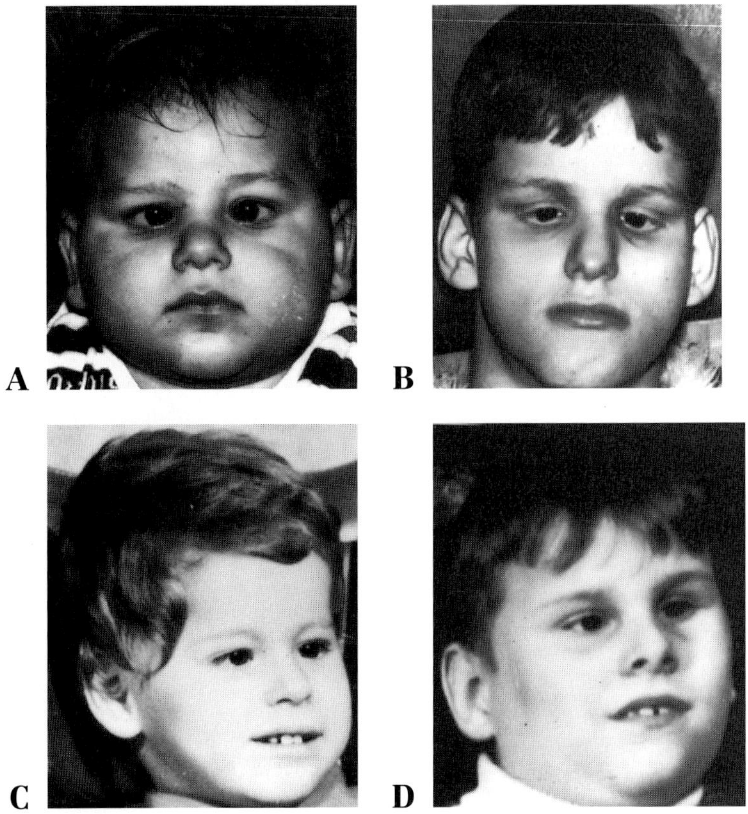

Schimke Syndrome. Cousins (A, C), maternal uncle (B), and sporadic case (D) showing microcephaly, hypotelorism, deep-set eyes, downslanting palpebral fissures, strabismus, narrow nose and alae nasi, cupped ears, and spacing of the teeth. Courtesy of Dr. Neil Schimke, Kansas University College of Health Sciences, Kansas City.

NEUROLOGICAL FINDINGS. By early childhood, spasticity and choreoathetosis replace hypotonia. The spasticity is reflected in increased deep tendon reflexes and Babinski signs and leads to widespread muscle wasting and joint contractures.
HETEROZYGOTE EXPRESSION. Mild congenital hearing loss was described in one carrier female and facial characteristics similar to affected males in another carrier female. No cognitive deficit has been reported.
NEUROPATHOLOGY. One patient, who died at age 4 years of pneumonia, had postmortem examination. The brain was small with hypoplastic cerebellum, cystic changes in the globus pallidus, calcification of the basal ganglia, gliosis of the thalamus, and loss of Purkinje cells.
COMMENT. Schimke et al. reported this syndrome in three males in one family and one male in a second family. Linkage analysis was not possible. Abducens palsy has been described in only two other XLMR syndromes (Christian and Christianson syndromes). In other clinical aspects, Schimke syndrome is also similar to Mohr-Tranebjaerg and Goldblatt Spastic Paraplegia syndromes.

REFERENCE

Schimke RN, Horton WA, Collins DL, et al.: A new X-linked syndrome comprising progressive basal ganglion dysfunction, mental and growth retardation, external ophthalmoplegia, postnatal microcephaly and deafness. Am J Med Genet 17:323, 1984.

Differential Matrix

Syndrome	Impaired Vision and/or Hearing	Abducens Palsy	Spasticity or Ataxia	Comments
Schimke	+	+	+	Microcephaly, sunken eyes, downslanting palpebral fissures, narrow nose, spacing of teeth, cupped ears, hypotonia, choreoathetosis, contractures
Christianson	0	+	+	Short stature, microcephaly, general asthenia, contractures, seizures, ophthalmoplegia
Christian	0	+	0	Vertebral anomalies, metopic ridge
Cerebrooculogenital	+	0	+	Short stature, microcephaly, hydrocephaly, agenesis of corpus callosum, microphthalmia, ptosis, hypospadias, cryptorchidism, clubfoot
Goldblatt spastic paraplegia	+	0	+	Nystagmus, optic atrophy, exotropia, muscle hypoplasia, spastic paraplegia, contractures
Mohr-Tranebjaerg (Jensen)	+	0	+	Neurologic deterioration with childhood onset, dystonia
Proud	+	0	+	Seizures, short stature, microcephaly, agenesis of corpus callosum, cryptorchidism, inguinal hernias

SIMPSON-GOLABI-BEHMEL SYNDROME

(Simpson Dysmorphia Syndrome, MIM 312870)

DEFINITION. XLMR with generalized overgrowth, prominent glabella, full midface, large mouth, prominent mandible, supernumerary nipples, cardiac defects, short hands and feet, and postaxial polydactyly. The responsible gene, GPC3, codes for an extracellular proteoglycan and maps to Xq26.

SOMATIC FEATURES. Structural features are quite variable but more consistent than cognitive impairment. Generalized overgrowth is typical although the head may be large and stature normal. The facies appear coarse and often are misinterpreted in early childhood as representing Hurler syndrome or another storage disorder. The glabella is full, metopic ridging may occur, the eyes are widely set, the palpebral fissures often slant downward, the nasal bridge may be broad and

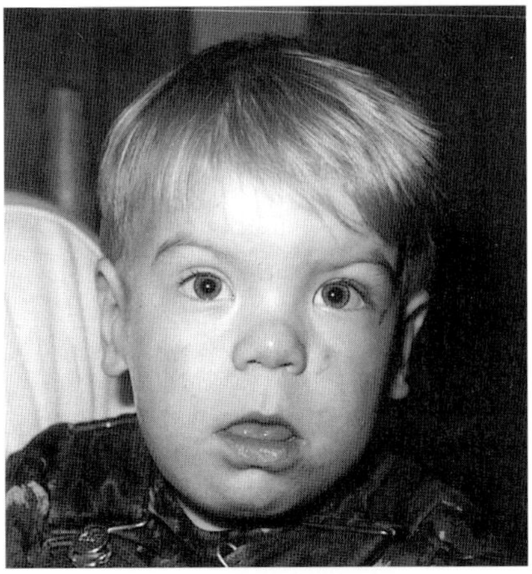
A

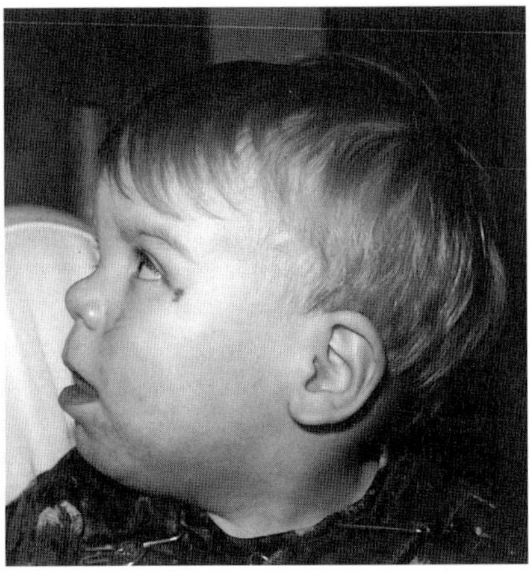
B

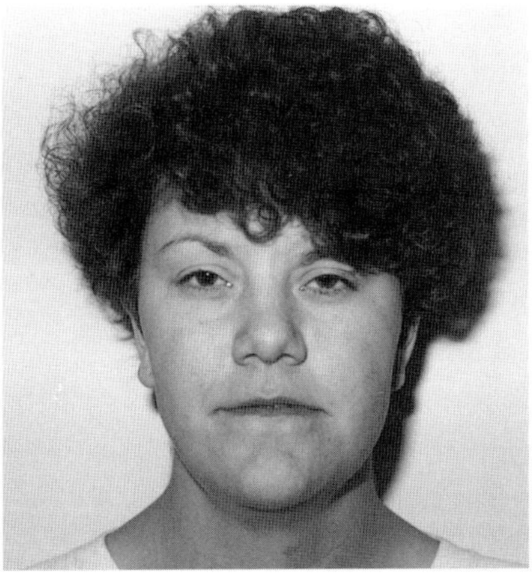
C

Simpson-Golabi-Behmel Syndrome. Male, age 20 months, with prominent forehead and depressed nasal bridge, short nose, long philtrum, and full lower lip (A, B); mother with macrocephaly, prominent forehead, flat midface and prominent mandible (C).

flat with the nasal tip broad and upturned, the maxilla and mandible are prominent, and the mouth and tongue are large. The palate may be tall but only uncommonly is cleft. The lips are thick and there may be a midline indentation of the lower lip. The neck may appear broad but not webbed. The ears usually have normal architecture. Supernumerary nipples are common. Perioral and palatal pigmentation have been reported. Heart defects in the form of structural anomalies and conduction defects have been present in some affected individuals.

The hands are broad and short with blunting of the distal phalanges. Postaxial polydactyly of the hands is typical, but broad thumbs and halluces and preaxial polysyndactyly of the halluces may occur as well. Hypoplasia and ridging of the index fingernails have been seen. Feet are likewise short. Inguinal hernias often occur in infancy. Large lobated or cystic kidneys with duplication of the collecting system and mild hydronephrosis have been seen. Crytoorchidism is common. Radiographs show advanced bone age, furrow of C2–3, cervical ribs, six lumbar vertebrae, and variable sacrococcygeal defects. A variety of other malformations have been occasionally noted.

GROWTH AND DEVELOPMENT. Prenatal and postnatal overgrowth occurs. Large head circumference is more consistent than excessive statural growth. Mild obesity may occur and the liver and spleen may be enlarged.

COGNITIVE FEATURES. While most patients will have normal cognitive function, the IQ is less than in nonaffected individuals in the family. Less commonly, mild to moderate cognitive impairment is present; severe impairment is uncommon. The unusual facial appearance and clumsy motor function may contribute to the appearance of mental retardation.

NEUROLOGICAL FINDINGS. Hypotonia of variable degree commonly occurs in early life. Winging of the scapulae, midchest depression, and wasting of the calf muscles may be manifestations of the hypotonia. There is a tendency to appear clumsy with stiff and wide-based gait. Seizures occur in a minority.

HETEROZYGOTE EXPRESSION. Carrier females are usually larger than noncarrier sisters and tend to have large facies, large mouth, and supernumerary nipples. Cognitive function is usually normal but some carrier females have had mild impairment.

COMMENT. Simpson-Golabi-Behmel syndrome shares with other overgrowth syndromes a predisposition to development of malignant tumors. Only intraabdominal tumors, including hepatocellular carcinoma, Wilms tumor, and neuroblastoma, have been described.

REFERENCES

Behmel A, Plöchl E, Rosenkranz W: A new X-linked dysplasia gigantism syndrome: Identical with the Simpson dysplasia syndrome? Hum Genet 67:409, 1984.

Garganta CL, Bodurtha JN: Report of another family with Simpson-Golabi-Behmel syndrome and a review of the literature. Am J Med Genet 44:129, 1992.

Golabi M, Rosen L: A new X-linked mental retardation-overgrowth syndrome. Am J Med Genet 17:345, 1984.

Gurrieri F, Cappa M, Neri G: Further delineation of the Simpson-Golabi-Behmel (SGB) Syndrome. Am J Med Genet 44:136, 1992.

Pilia G, Hughes-Benzie RM, MacKenzie A, et al.: Mutations in GPC3, a glypican gene, cause the Simpson-Golabi-Behmel overgrowth syndrome. Nat Genet 12:241, 1996.

Simpson JL, Landey S, New M, et al.: A previously unrecognized X-linked syndrome of dysmorphia. Birth Defects Orig Art Ser XI(2):18, 1975.

Xuan JY, Besner A, Ireland M, et al.: Mapping of Simpson-Golabi-Behmel syndrome to Xq25-q27. Hum Mol Genet 3:133, 1994.

Differential Matrix

Syndrome	Macro-cephaly	Digital Anomalies	Hypotonia	Comments
Simpson-Golabi-Behmel	+	+	+	Somatic overgrowth, supernumerary nipples, polydactyly
Opitz FG	+	+	+	Broad forehead, downslanted palpebral fissures, everted lower lip, dysgenesis of corpus callosum, cardiac defects, imperforate anus, constipation, broad flat thumbs and great toes
Atkin-Flaitz	+	+	0	Short stature, hypertelorism, downslanting palpebral fissures, broad nasal tip, thick lower lip, brachydactyly, seizures
Mucopoly-saccharidosis IIA	+	+	0	Short stature, coarse facies, hepato-splenomegaly, hernias, joint stiffness, thick skin, hirsutism, behavioral disturbance
XLMR-hypotonic facies (Carpenter-Waziri) (Holmes-Gang) (Juberg-Marsidi)	0	+	+	Microcephaly, short stature, small testes, telecanthus, small triangular nose, tented upper lip, open mouth, spacing of teeth, genital anomalies, musculoskeletal anomalies, hemoglobin H inclusions in erythrocytes
Coffin-Lowry	0	+	+	Short stature, microcephaly, hypertelorism, anteverted nares, tented upper lip, prominent lips and large mouth, large ears, soft hands with tapered digits, pectus carinatum
Miles-Carpenter	0	+	+	Microcephaly, short stature, ptosis, small palpebral fissures, open mouth, pectus excavatum, scoliosis, long hands, camptodactyly, rockerbottom feet, arch fingerprints, spasticity, unsteady gait

SMITH-FINEMAN-MYERS SYNDROME (MIM 309580)

Three reports have detailed the phenotypic manifestations of Smith-Fineman-Myers syndrome. Brothers were described in two reports and an isolated case in the third report. Phenotypic differences in the two sets of brothers introduce doubt that they have the same syndrome.

Smith, Fineman, and Myers reported two brothers with microdolichocephaly, upslanting palpebral fissures, ptosis, strabismus, cupped ears, flat philtrum, maxillary overbite, thin upper lip, scoliosis, bridged palmar creases, and long narrow feet with midfoot varus. There was diffuse hypotonia and severe developmental

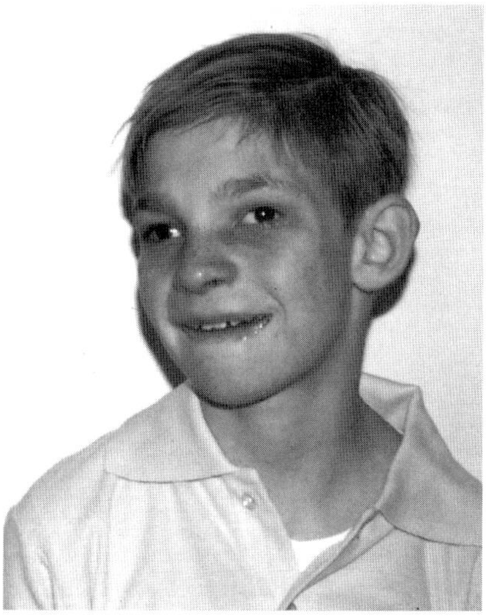

A

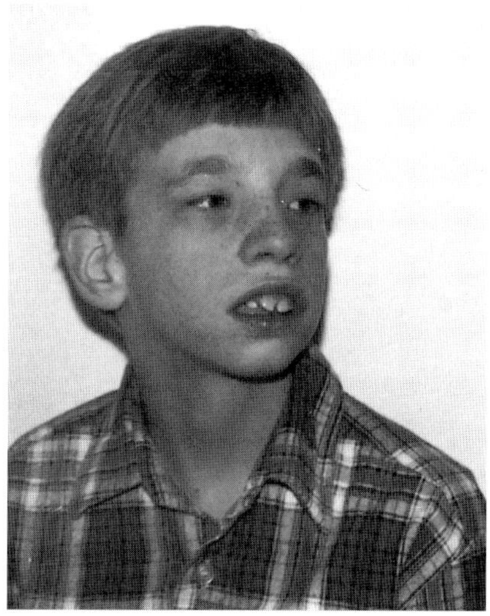

B

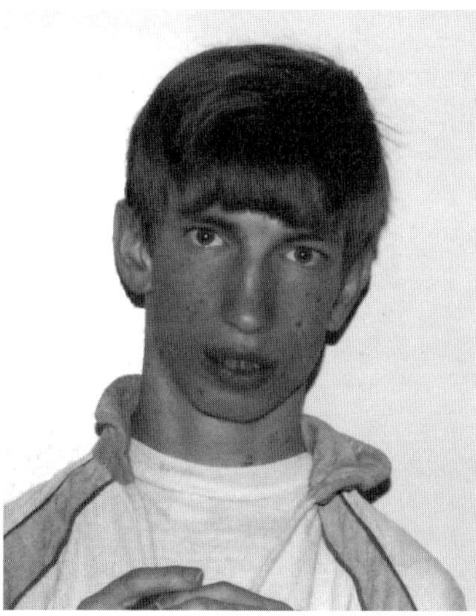

C

Smith-Fineman-Myers Syndrome. Microdolichocephaly, upslanting palpebral fissures, ptosis, strabismus, cupped ears, flat philtrum, maxillary overbite, and thin upper lip in two brothers, ages 13 years and 15 years (A, B); microdolichocephaly, narrow face, decreased nasolabial folds, smooth philtrum, maxillary overbite, patulous lower lip, and micrognathia in a sporadic case at age 22 years (C). Courtesy of Dr. John Johnson, Shodair Hospital, Helena, Montana.

impairment. Both boys had low birth weight and short stature: the older brother had generalized seizures, and the younger had minor motor seizures. Findings found in one brother but not the other included short sternum with flaring of the ribcage, femoral anteversion, hyperconvex and short fingernails, and double hair whorl. Both exhibited poor social skills and repetitive movements of the upper limbs. Pneumoencephalogram showed cortical atrophy.

Stephenson and Johnson reported a third unrelated case and follow-up of the original cases. They considered the boys to have similar craniofacial findings with microdolichocephaly, narrow face, decreased frontonasal angle, decreased nasolabial folds, smooth philtrum, prominent maxilla with overbite, prominent upper central incisors, patulous lower lip, and micrognathia. They also had short stature, thin habitus, pectus excavatum, bridged palmar creases, foot deformities, light pigmentation with freckles, and seizures. Although initially the brothers had hypotonia, they became mildly spastic with hypertonia and hyperreflexia during childhood. The isolated case lacked midfoot varus and upslanted palpebral fissures and had optic nerve hypoplasia and bifid uvula.

Adès and colleagues reported two brothers that they considered had the same syndrome. Their patients had frontal hair upsweep, hypertelorism, downslanting palpebral fissures, short nose, short philtrum with tented upper lip, prominent lower lip, open mouth, small hands with short tapered fingers, and cryptorchidism. Hall has pointed out the resemblance of these brothers to XLMR-hypotonic facies (α-thalassemia mental retardation) syndrome. They lacked hemoglobin H inclusions seen in some cases with XLMR-hypotonic facies syndrome, but mutational analysis of the XNP gene has not been reported.

REFERENCES

Adès LC, Kerr B, Turner G, et al.: Smith-Fineman-Myers syndrome in two brothers. Am J Med Genet 40:467, 1991.

Hall BD: Alpha thalassemia/mental retardation syndrome often confused with other disorders. Am J Med Genet 44:250, 1992. (Also see response by Adès: Am J Med Genet 44:251, 1992.)

Smith RD, Fineman RM, Myers GG: Short stature, psychomotor retardation, and unusual facial appearance in two brothers. Am J Med Genet 7:5, 1980.

Stephenson LD, Johnson JP: Smith-Fineman-Myers syndrome: report of a third case. Am J Med Genet 22:301, 1985.

SNYDER-ROBINSON SYNDROME

(MIM 309583)

DEFINITION. XLMR with prominent lower lip, high/cleft palate, asthenic build, kyphoscoliosis, long great toes, and nasal speech. The gene maps between DMD (Xp21.2) and DXS43 (Xp22.2), lod score is 4.21.

SOMATIC FEATURES. Facial characteristics include asymmetry, high or cleft palate, and prominent lower lip. Midface flatness or retraction may occur. General asthenic build may be accompanied by narrow thorax, pectus excavatum, kyphoscoliosis, long thin hands with hyperextensible digits, long great toes, and osteoporosis.

GROWTH AND DEVELOPMENT. Birth weight is low but adult height is above average. Motor and language milestones are moderately delayed.

COGNITIVE FEATURES. Mild cognitive impairment is the rule.

NEUROLOGICAL FINDINGS. Hypotonia occurs especially during early childhood. Asymmetric facial movement, spasticity, seizures have been noted in one or more males.

→

Snyder-Robinson Syndrome. Facial appearance in childhood and adult life (A–E).

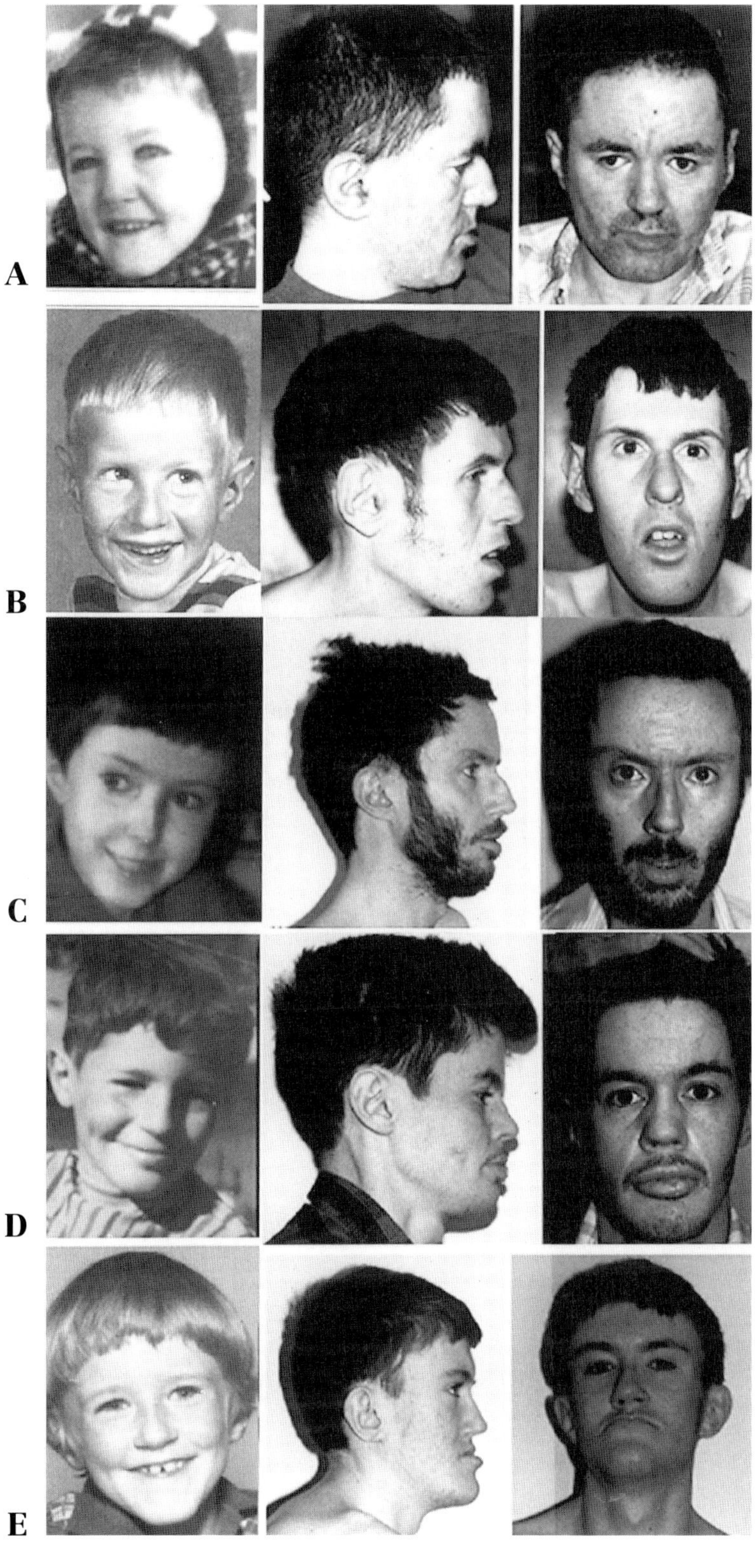
A
B
C
D
E

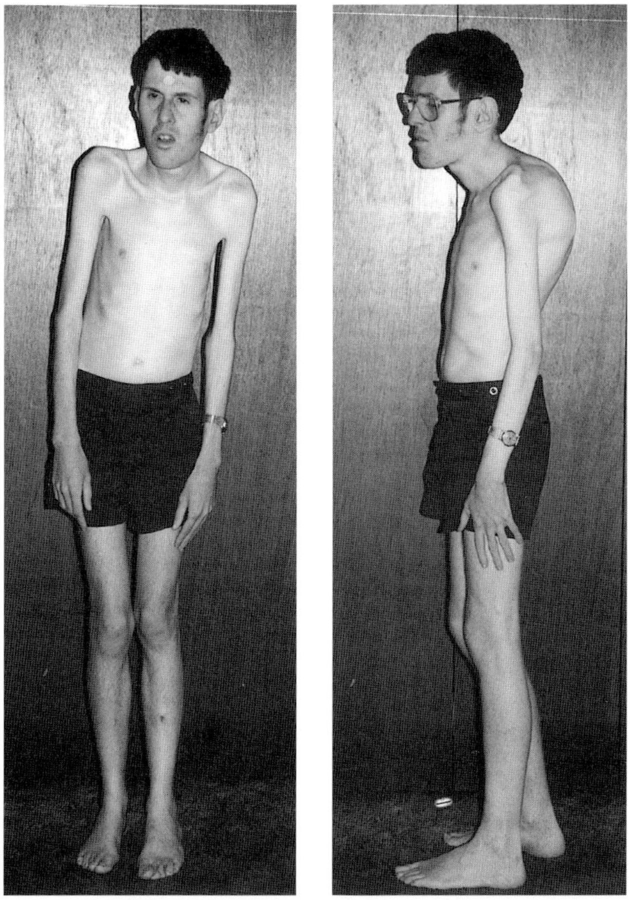

F

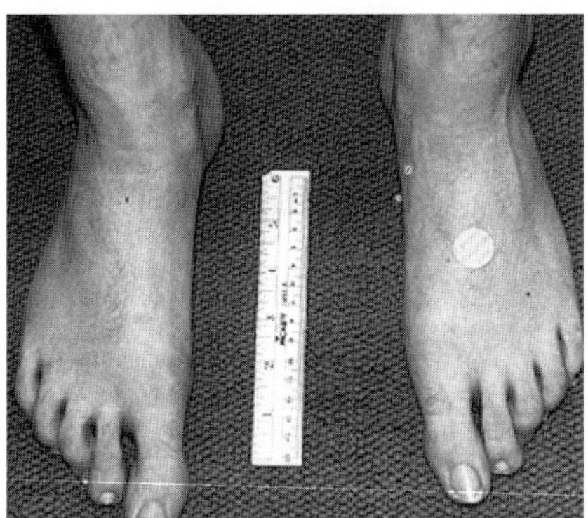

G

Snyder-Robinson Syndrome. (continued). Facial asymmetry and prominent lower lip become apparent with age. Asthenic build with decreased musculature and kyphoscoliosis in adult (F); long halluces in adult (G).

HETEROZYGOTE EXPRESSION. Carrier females have no cognitive impairment or somatic manifestation.

COMMENT. Initially reported as nonsyndromal XLMR with hypotonia, the Snyder-Robinson syndrome is now defined primarily by facial and skeletal manifestations. Muscular hypoplasia is also seen in Allan-Herndon-Dudley syndrome and Lujan syndrome.

REFERENCE

Arena JF, Schwartz C, Ouzts L, et al.: X-linked mental retardation with thin habitus, osteoporosis, and kyphoscoliosis: linkage to Xp21.3-p22.12. Am J Med Genet 64:50, 1996.

Snyder RD, Robinson A: Recessive sex-linked mental retardation in the absence of other recognizable abnormalities: report of a family. Clin Pediatr 8:669, 1969.

Differential Matrix

Syndrome	Tall Stature	Asthenic Build	Hypotonia	Comments
Snyder-Robinson	+	+	+	High or cleft palate, prominent lower lip, kyphoscoliosis, long great toes, nasal speech, hypotonia in childhood
Lujan	+	+	0	Marfanoid habitus, long face, prominent forehead, high palate, micrognathia, long digits, pectus excavatum, joint hyperextensibility, seizures, hyperactivity
Allan-Herndon-Dudley	0	+	+	Large ears with cupping or abnormal architecture, muscle hypoplasia, contractures, dysarthria, athetosis, ataxia, spastic paraplegia
Arts	0	+	+	Growth deficiency, paucity of muscles, areflexia, ataxia, deafness, vision loss, seizures, childhood death
Simpson-Golabi-Behmel	+	0	+	Somatic overgrowth, supernumerary nipples, polydactyly

STOCCO DOS SANTOS SYNDROME

DEFINITION. XLMR with low birth weight, short stature, hypertelorism, epicanthus, strabismus, hip dislocation, hirsutism, recurrent infections, and precocious puberty. The gene has been localized between DXS1003 (Xp11) and DXS8077 (Xq21), lod score 3.14.

SOMATIC FEATURES. A clear facial phenotype has not been described although photographs and clinical reports describe hypertelorism, heavy eyebrows, epicanthus, strabismus, short palpebral fissures, short philtrum, thin upper lip, and prominent nasal tip. All affected males have congenital hip dislocation, kypho-

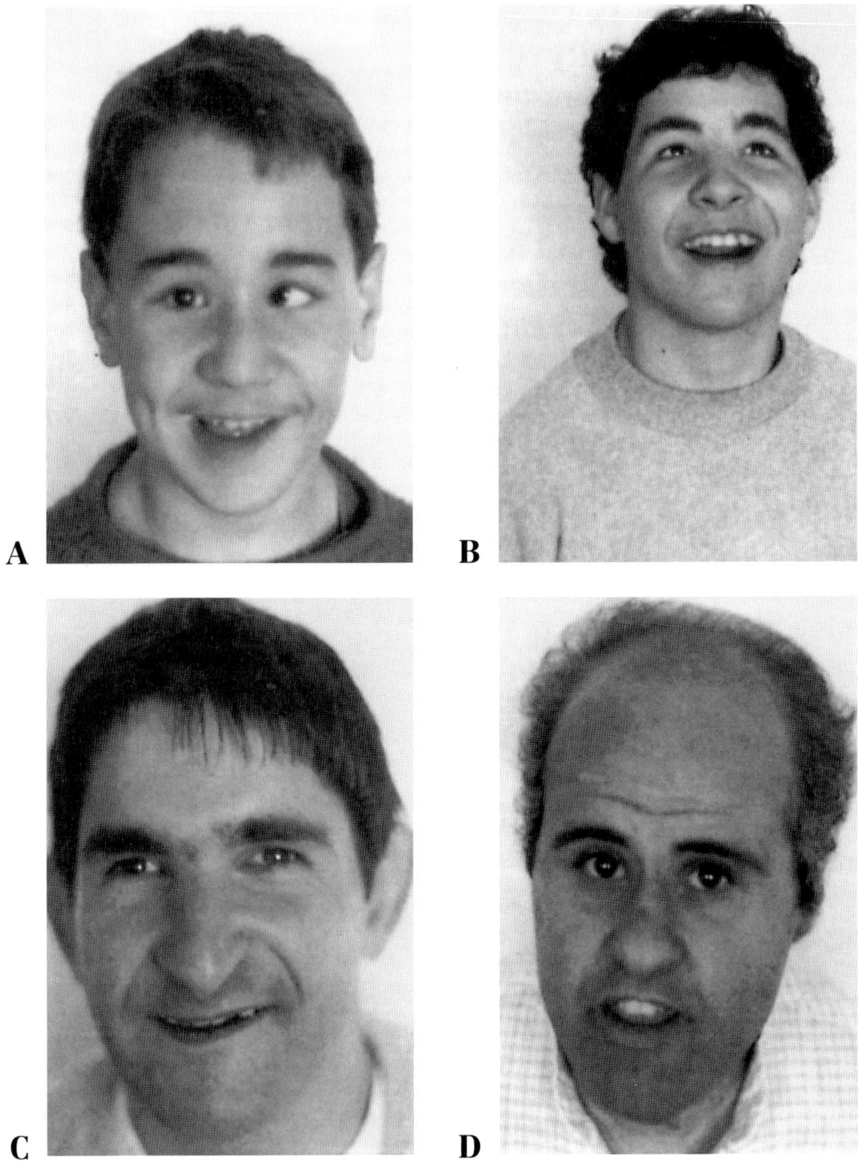

Stocco dos Santos Syndrome. Ten-year-old male with strabismus, epicanthus, hypertelorism, cataract of the right eye, long straight nose with overhanging tip, and flared alae nasi (A); cousins with similar facial manifestations but without cataract at ages 16 years (B); 28 years (C); and 30 years (D). Courtesy of Dr. Rita Stocco dos Santos, Instituto Butantan, São Paulo, Brasil.

sis, hirsutism, and precocious puberty and experience recurrent respiratory infections in childhood. Clubfoot has occurred in some cases.

GROWTH AND DEVELOPMENT. Low birth weight is described. Postnatally, short stature continues but head growth is normal. Precocious puberty has occurred at ages 7–8 years. Details of developmental progress in early childhood have not been described. Speech has been absent in some cases.

Cognitive Features. Severe impairment.
Heterozygote Expression. None.
Laboratory. A new G6PD (glucose-6-phosphate-dehydrogenase) variant was found in the family but it does not segregate with mental retardation.
Comment. Although precocious puberty occurs with increased frequency among individuals with mental retardation, its occurrence in Stocco dos Santos syndrome appears unique among the XLMR syndromes.

REFERENCE

Stocco dos Santos RC, Barretto OCO, Nonoyama K, et al.: X-linked syndrome: Mental retardation, hip luxation, and G6PD variant [Gd(+) Butantan]. Am J Med Genet 39:133, 1991.

Differential Matrix

Syndrome	Short Stature	Congenital Hip Dislocation	Recurrent Infections	Comments
Stocco dos Santos	+	+	+	Heavy eyebrows, strabismus, short palpebral fissures, short philtrum, thin upper lip, prominent nasal tip, hirsutism, kyphosis, precocious puberty
X-linked hereditary bullous dystrophy	+	0	+	Microcephaly, upslanting palpebral fissures, protruding ears, digits short and tapered, cardiac defects, bullous dystrophy, small testes, early death from pulmonary infection

Stoll Syndrome

(XLMR–Short Stature–Hypertelorism–Hypotonia)

Definition. XLMR with short stature, prominent forehead, broad nasal tip with anteverted nares, hypertension, and hypotonia. The gene has not been mapped.
Somatic Features. Short stature and craniofacial features are most notable. In addition to frontal prominence or bossing, facial characteristics include ocular hypertelorism, depressed bridge of nose, anteverted nares, and flattening of the malar area. Published photographs suggest some tenting of the upper lip. Hypotonia was evident, but only during early childhood.
Growth and Development. Although prenatal growth is normal, postnatal growth slows with short stature dating from childhood. Affected males are said to have large foreheads, but head circumference measurements have not been reported. Details of early childhood development are not available.
Cognitive Features. Mild impairment.
Neurological Findings. Hypotonia, present in infancy and early childhood, resolves within a few years.

A

B

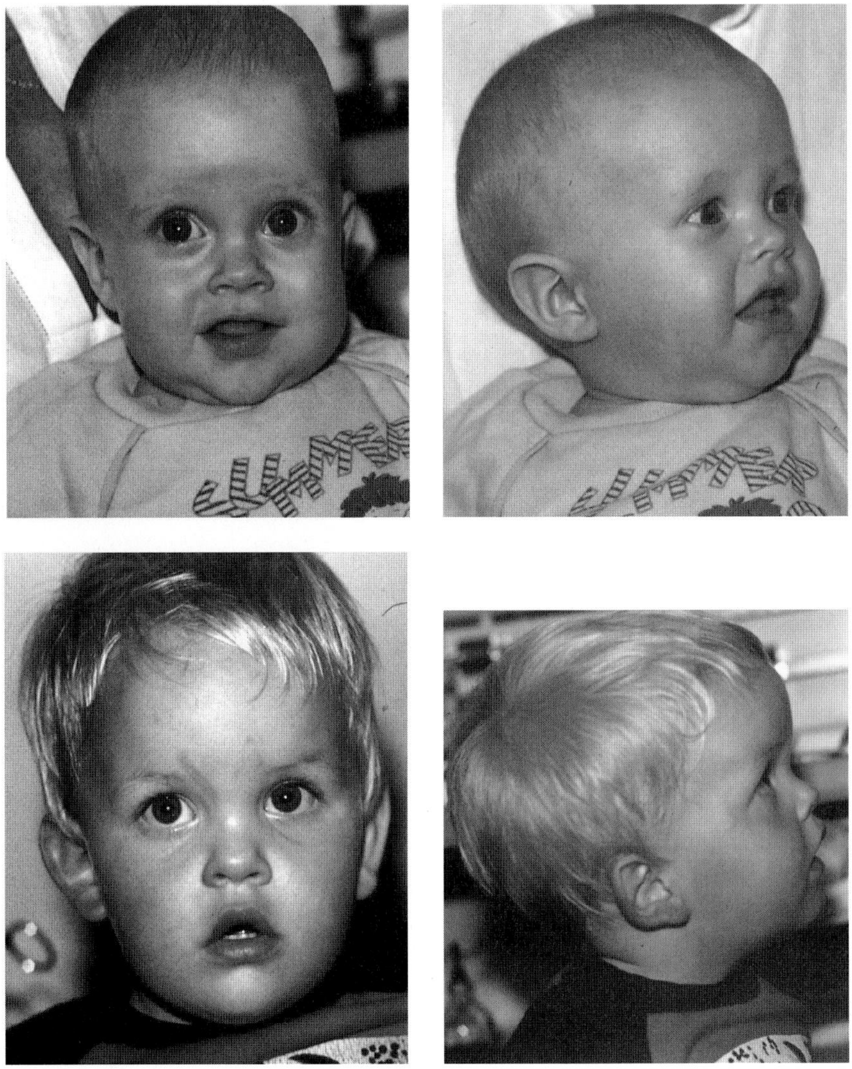

Stoll Syndrome. Brothers at ages 9 months (A), 33 months (B), showing macrocephaly, frontal bossing, hypertelorism, depressed nasal bridge, anteverted nostrils, and malar hypoplasia. Courtesy of Dr. Claude Stoll, University of Strasbourg, Strasbourg, France.

HETEROZYGOTE EXPRESSION. Two carrier females were reported to have the same facial appearance as affected males, but normal cognitive function.

IMAGING. Normal cranial ultrasonography and tomography.

COMMENT. The craniofacial phenotype, based on a single family, appears different from other XLMR syndromes.

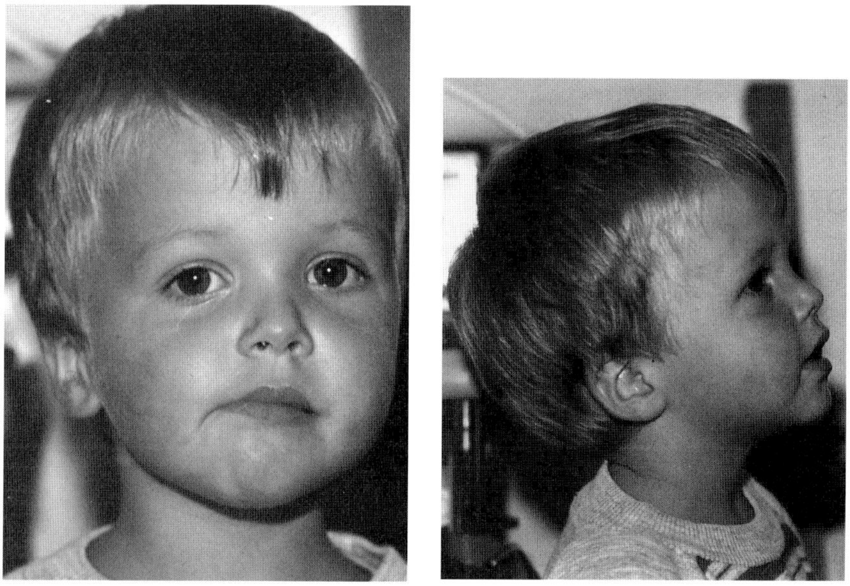

C

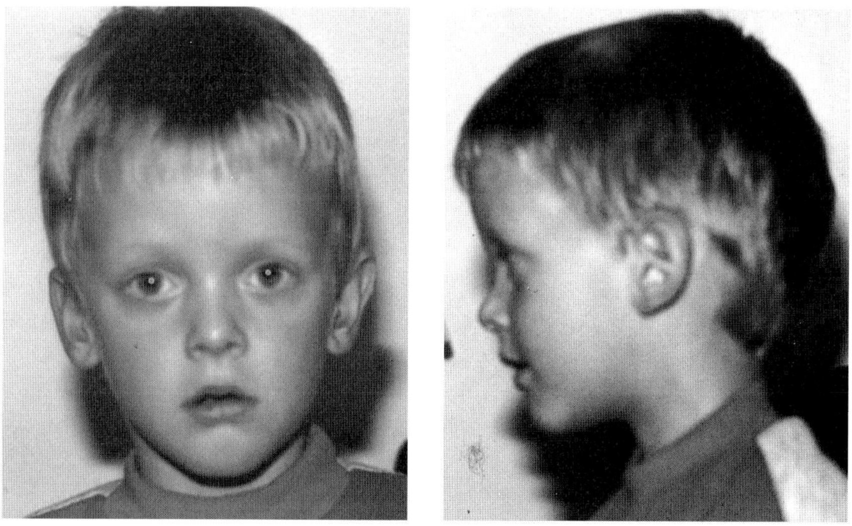

D

Stoll Syndrome. (continued) 4 years (C), and 6 years (D) showing macrocephaly, frontal bossing, hypertelorism, depressed nasal bridge, anteverted nostrils, and malar hypoplasia. Courtesy of Dr. Claude Stoll, University of Strasbourg, Strasbourg, France.

REFERENCE

Stoll C, Géraudel A, Chauvin A: New X-linked syndrome of mental retardation, short stature, and hypertelorism. Am J Med Genet 39:474, 1991.

Differential Matrix

Syndrome	Short Stature	Hyper-telorism	Hypotonia	Comments
Stoll	+	+	+	Forehead prominence, depressed nasal root, anteverted nares
Coffin-Lowry	+	+	+	Microcephaly, anteverted nares, tented upper lip, prominent lips, large mouth, large ears, soft hands with tapered digits, pectus carinatum
Proud	+	+	+	Hearing loss, vision loss, agenesis of corpus callosum, cryptorchidism, inguinal hernias, ataxia, spasticity, seizures
Vasquez	+	+	+	Microcephaly, gynecomastia, obesity, hypogonadism
XLMR-hypotonic facies (Carpenter-Waziri) (Holmes-Gang) (Juberg-Marsidi)	+	+	+	Microcephaly, small testes, telecanthus, small triangular nose, tented upper lip, open mouth, spacing of teeth, genital anomalies, musculoskeletal anomalies, hemoglobin H inclusions in erythrocytes
Aarskog	+	+	0	Downslanting palpebral fissures, ptosis, cupped ears, anteverted nares, brachydactyly, horizontal palmar crease, midfoot varus, joint laxity, shawl scrotum, cryptorchidism, inguinal hernias
Atkin-Flaitz	+	+	0	Macrocephaly, downslanting palpebral fissures, broad nasal tip, thick lower lip, brachydactyly, seizures
Cranioorodigital	+	+	0	Hearing impairment, prominent forehead, flat/ broad nasal bridge, downslanting palpebral fissures, flat midface, cleft palate, blunted flexed overlapping fingers, rockerbottom feet, hypoplastic fibulae, subluxed/dislocated joints
Otopalatodigital I	+	+	0	Conductive hearing impairment, prominent brow, broad nasal root, downslanting palpebral fissures, cleft palate, blunted distal phalanges, irregular curvature and spacing of digits, limitation of elbow movement
XLMR-psoriasis	0	+	+	Open mouth, large ears, seizures, psoriasis
Chudley-Lowry	+	0	+	Bitemporal narrowing, almond-shaped eyes, depressed nasal bridge, tented upper lip, open mouth, hypogonadism, obesity
Miles-Carpenter	+	0	+	Microcephaly, ptosis, small palpebral fissures, open mouth, pectus excavatum, scoliosis, long hands, camptodactyly, rockerbottom feet, arch fingerprints, spasticity, unsteady gait
Smith-Fineman-Myers	+	0	+	Microcephaly, ptosis, flat philtrum, scoliosis, midfoot varus, narrow feet, seizures
Wittwer	+	0	+	Microcephaly, microphthalmia, hearing loss, vision loss, genitourinary anomalies, seizures

Sutherland-Haan Syndrome

(Sutherland Syndrome, MRXS3, formerly MRX2, MIM 309470)

Definition. XLMR with short stature, microcephaly, small testes, and spastic diplegia. The gene maps to the region between MAOA (Xp11.3) and DXS1125 (Xq12), lod score 4.34.

Somatic Features. Short stature, microbrachycephaly, small testes, and spastic diplegia dominate the phenotype. Major malformations are exceptional, one male having imperforate anus and a second having anal stenosis. Facial manifestations include upslanted palpebral fissures, strabismus, maxillary hypoplasia, and in some cases large ears and mild prognathism. There is a tendency to lean body mass and pectus excavatum, scoliosis, stiffness of small joints, and pes cavus. Special senses appear normal except for one case of deafness possibly related to recurrent otitis and mastoiditis.

Growth and Development. Intrauterine growth appears mildly impaired with birth weights in the lower centiles. Postnatal growth is similarly slow with adult height and head circumference usually below −2 SD. The testicular volume measures in the lower centiles and is possibly related to delay in puberty and decreased body hair. There is mild to moderate delay of speech and motor milestones.

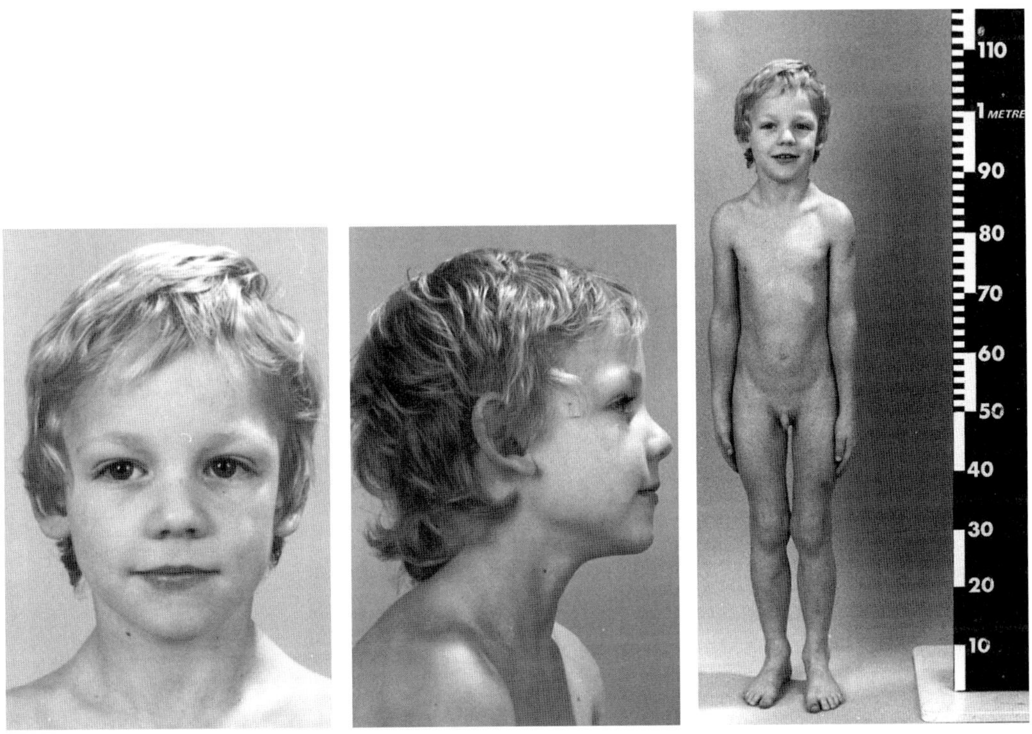

A

Sutherland-Haan Syndrome. Five-year-old male with microcephaly and normal facial appearance (A)

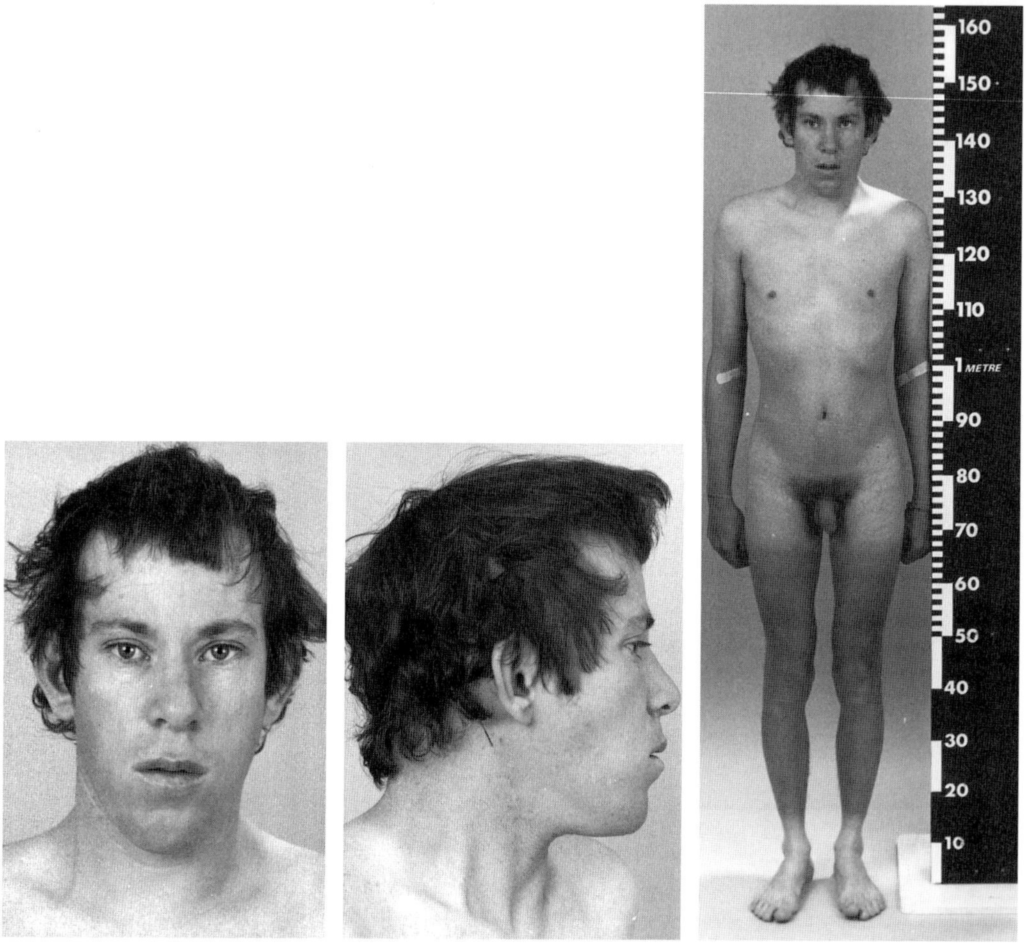

B

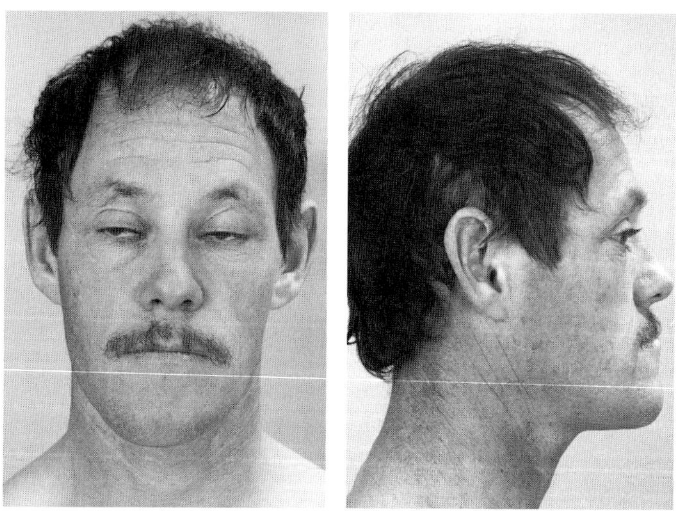

C

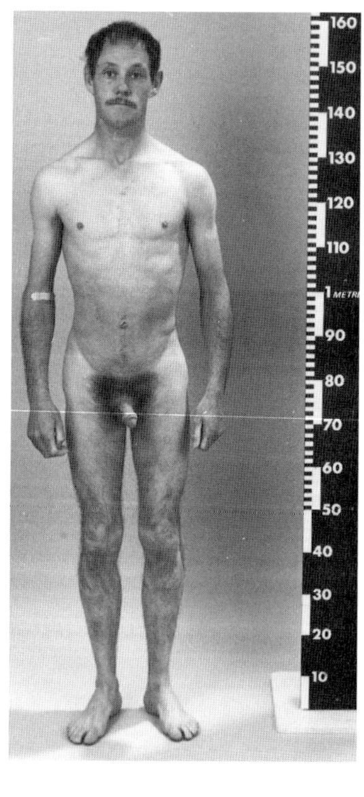

Sutherland-Haan Syndrome. (continued) 28-year-old with microbrachycephaly, short stature, asthenic body build, long face, and upslanting palpebral fissures (B); 34-year-old with microbrachycephaly, maxillary hypoplasia, and asthenic body build (C). Courtesy of Dr. Grant Sutherland, Women's and Children's Hospital, Adelaide, Australia.

COGNITIVE FUNCTION. Affected males exhibit a wide range of cognitive function from low normal to moderate impairment.

NEUROLOGICAL FINDINGS. Several males experienced poor feeding during infancy. Increased muscle tone and hyperreflexia of lower limbs may be noted by early childhood, is of mild to moderate severity, and does not appear progressive.

HETEROZYGOTE EXPRESSION. Carrier females show no cognitive or somatic abnormalities.

IMAGING. Prominent ventricles secondary to mild cerebral atrophy were found in one affected male on CT scan.

COMMENT. Only one family has been reported. Eight males were affected in three generations. The major features—short stature, microcephaly, and small testes—are shared with Renpenning syndrome. The two syndromes also share overlapping linkage limits in Xp11. Although the index family with Renpenning syndrome lacked the musculoskeletal features and spastic diplegia of Sutherland-Haan syndrome, allelism cannot be excluded.

REFERENCES

Gedeon A, Haan E, Mulley J: Gene localization for Sutherland-Haan syndrome (SHS:MIM 309470). Am J Med Genet 64:78, 1996.

Sutherland GR, Gedeon AK, Haan EA, et al.: Linkage studies with the gene for an X-linked syndrome of mental retardation, microcephaly and spastic diplegia. Am J Med Genet 30:493, 1988.

Differential Matrix

Syndrome	Micro-cephaly	Short Stature	Small Testes	Comments
Sutherland-Haan	+	+	+	Upslanting palpebral fissures, asthenic habitus, pectus excavatum, scoliosis, stiff joints, pes cavus, spasticity
XLMR-hypotonic facies (Carpenter-Waziri) (Holmes-Gang) (Juberg-Marsidi)	+	+	+	Telecanthus, small triangular nose, tented upper lip, open mouth, spacing of teeth, genital anomalies, musculoskeletal anomalies, hemoglobin H inclusions in erythrocytes
Chudley-Lowry	+	+	+	Bitemporal narrowing, almond-shaped eyes, depressed nasal bridge, tented upper lip, open mouth, hypogonadism, hypotonia, obesity
Renpenning	+	+	+	Upslanting palpebral fissures
X-linked hereditary bullous dystrophy	+	+	+	Upslanting palpebral fissures, protruding ears, digits short and tapered, cardiac defects, bullous dystrophy, early death from pulmonary infection
Miles-Carpenter	+	+	0	Ptosis, small palpebral fissures, open mouth, pectus excavatum, scoliosis, long hands, camptodactyly, rockerbottom feet, arch fingerprints, spasticity, unsteady gait
Pettigrew	+	0	+	Microcephaly or hydrocephaly, long face with macrostomia and prognathism, Dandy-Walker malformation, spasticity, seizures, contractures, choreoathetosis, iron deposits in basal ganglia

TELECANTHUS-HYPOSPADIAS SYNDROME

(Hypertelorism-Hypospadias Syndrome, Opitz BBB Syndrome, Opitz G syndrome, MIM 300000)

DEFINITION. XLMR with telecanthus, high broad nasal root, and hypospadias. An X chromosome locus on Xp22 is the site of one causative gene; a second locus is located in 22q11.

SOMATIC FEATURES. Structural anomalies of the midline dominate the somatic phenotype. Telecanthus, broad and high nasal root, dysplastic or posteriorly rotated ears, and cleft lip and palate are placed on an oval facial background with narrow forehead. Epicanthus, bifid uvula, high palate, micrognathia and clefts or other anomalies of the pharynx, larynx, and trachea may occur. The cranium may be marked by a metopic ridge, scaphocephaly, brachycephaly, oxycephaly, or asymmetry. Cardiac malformations, including septal defects, patent ductus ate-

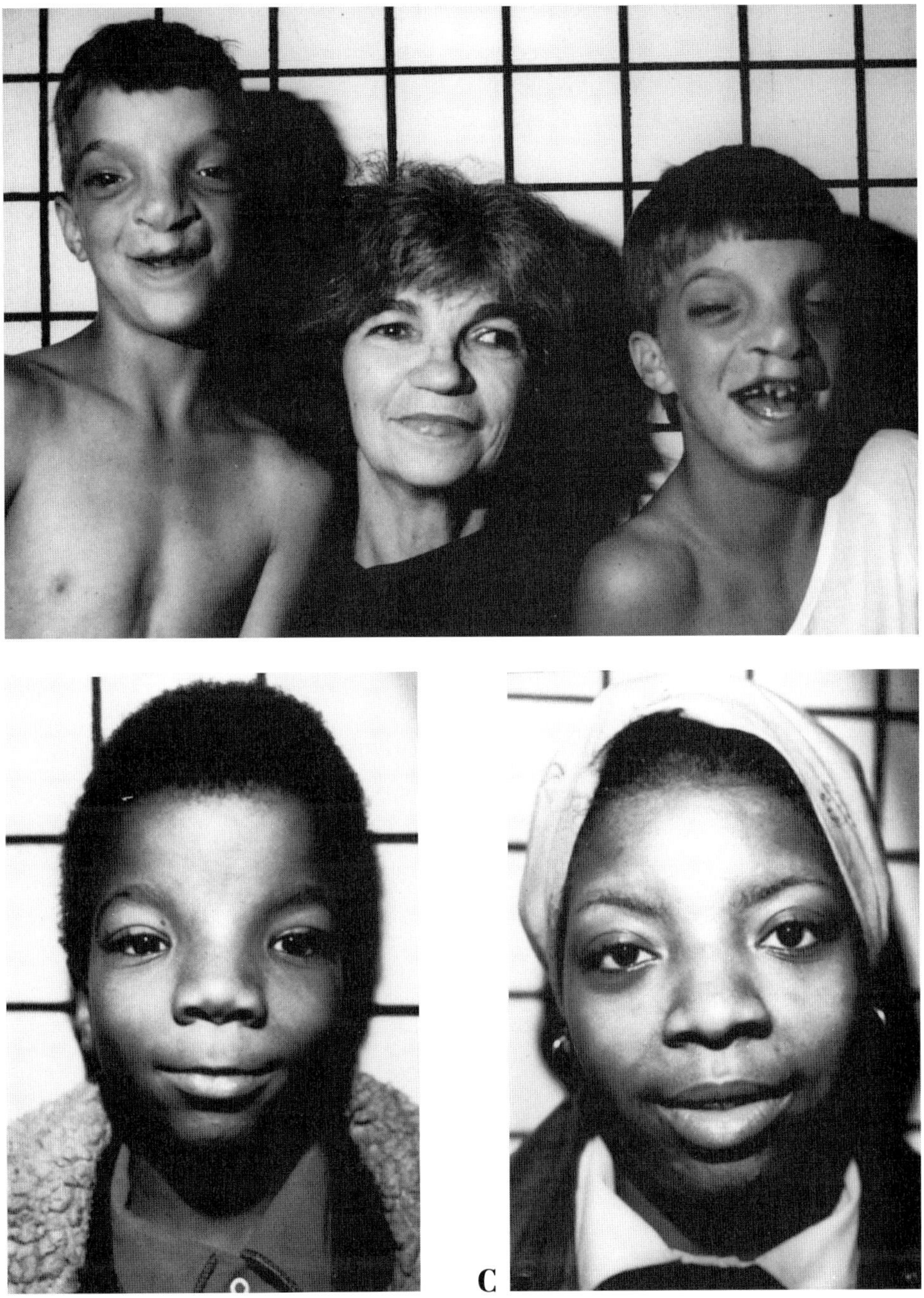

Telecanthus-Hypospadias Syndrome. Twin brothers at age 8 years showing telecanthus and bilateral cleft lip and palate, and their mother with telecanthus and broad nasal tip (A); 8-year-old male with telecanthus and high broad nasal bridge (B); mother of boy in B with telecanthus (C). Courtesy of Dr. Cathy Stevens, T.C. Thompson Children's Hospital, Chattanooga, TN.

riosus, coarctation of the aorta, and pulmonary valve incompetence occur in a minority. Hypospadias occurs in almost all males, but with variable meatal placement. Cryptorchidism, hypoplastic or cleft scrotum, inguinal hernias, and imperforate anus also occur. Stridor, dysphagia, gastroesophageal reflux, aspiration, and hoarse/weak cry may complicate the early course. Early death has occurred.

GROWTH AND DEVELOPMENT. About a third have microcephaly and short stature.

COGNITIVE FEATURES. Most males have developmental delay, poor school performance, or mild cognitive deficits as assessed by testing.

HETEROZYGOTE EXPRESSION. Carrier females typically have telecanthus but uncommonly have other facial features. Cognitive function is normal.

IMAGING. None.

COMMENT. Discovery of two gene loci, one autosomal (22q11.2) and one X chromosomal (Xp22), has helped to resolve the controversy regarding the genetic basis of the telecanthus-hypospadias syndrome.

REFERENCES

Christian JC, Bixler D, Blythe SC, et al.: Familial telecanthus with associated congenital anomalies. In: *The Clinical Delineation of Birth Defects. II. Malformation Syndromes.* D Bergsma, ed. The National Foundation-March of Dimes, New York, Birth Defects Orig Art Ser V(2):82, 1969.

May M, Huston S, Wilroy S, et al.: Linkage analysis in a family with Opitz GBBB syndrome refines the location of the gene to a 4 cM region. Am J Med Genet 68:244, 1997.

Opitz JM, Summitt RL, Smith DWG: The BBB syndrome. Familial telecanthus with associated congenital anomalies. In: *The Clinical Delineation of Birth Defects. II. Malformation Syndromes.* D Bergsma, ed. The National Foundation–March of Dimes, New York, Birth Defects Orig Art Ser V(2):86, 1969.

Robin NH, Feldman GJ, Aronson AL, et al.: Opitz syndrome is genetically heterogeneous, with one locus on Xp22, and a second locus on 22q11.2. Nat Genet 11:459, 1995.

Robin NH, Opitz JM, Meunke M: Opitz G/BBB syndrome: clinical comparisons of families linked to Xp22 and 22q , and a review of the literature. Am J Med Genet 62:305, 1996.

Stevens CA, Wilroy RS: The telecanthus-hypospadias syndrome. J Med Genet 25:536, 1988.

Differential Matrix

Syndrome	Tele-canthus	Cardiac Defects	Urogenital Anomalies	Comments
Telecanthus-hypospadias	+	+	+	High broad nasal root, dysplastic ears, cleft lip/palate, abnormal cranial contour or symmetry
XLMR-hypotonic facies (Carpenter-Waziri) (Holmes-Gang) (Juberg-Marsidi)	+	+	+	Microcephaly, short stature, small testes, small triangular nose, tented upper lip, open mouth, spacing of teeth, genital anomalies, musculoskeletal anomalies, hemoglobin H inclusions in erythrocytes
Golabi-Ito-Hall	+	+	0	Microcephaly, short stature, high nasal root, cupped ears, thoracic asymmetry, sacral dimple, dry/brittle/sparse hair, cutis marmorata, nail hypoplasia
MIDAS	+	+	0	Microphthalmia, ocular dysgenesis, corneal opacification, dermal aplasia, dysgenesis of corpus callosum, cardiomyopathy
Opitz FG	+	+	0	Macrocephaly, broad forehead, downslanted palpebral fissures, everted lower lip, dysgenesis of corpus callosum, imperforate anus, constipation, flat thumbs and great toes, hypotonia
Simpson-Golabi-Behmel	+	+	0	Somatic overgrowth, supernumerary nipples, polydactyly
Lenz microphthalmia	0	+	+	Microcephaly, microphthalmia, ocular dysgenesis, malformed ears, cleft lip/palate, thumb duplication or hypoplasia, narrow shoulders
X-linked hereditary bullous dystrophy	0	+	+	Microcephaly, short stature, upslanting palpebral fissures, protruding ears, short and tapered digits, bullous dystrophy, small testes, early death from pulmonary infection
Proud	+	0	+	Microcephaly, hearing loss, vision loss, agenesis of corpus callosum, cryptorchidism, inguinal hernias, ataxia, spasticity, seizures
XLMR-psoriasis	+	0	+	Hypertelorism, open mouth, large ears, hypotonia, seizures, psoriasis

URBAN SYNDROME

Assignment of XLMR syndrome status is tentative, being based on the clinical report of two brothers with short stature, small hands and feet with digital contractures, osteoporosis, obesity, and genital anomalies. Both had low birth weight

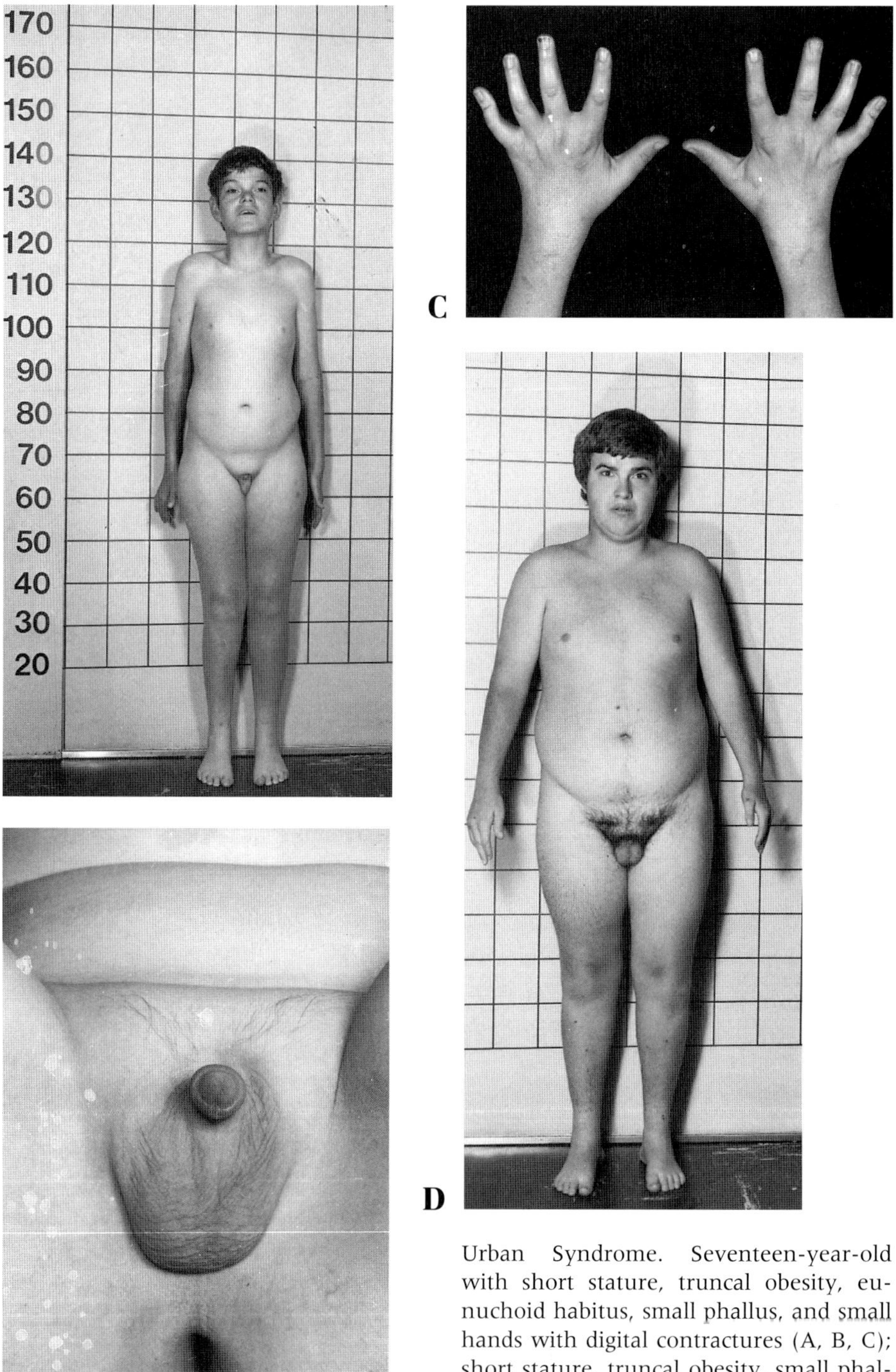

A B C D

Urban Syndrome. Seventeen-year-old with short stature, truncal obesity, eunuchoid habitus, small phallus, and small hands with digital contractures (A, B, C); short stature, truncal obesity, small phallus, and small hands with digital contractures in a 20-year-old (D–F). Courtesy of Dr. Walter Meyer, III, University of Texas Medical Branch at Galveston, Galveston.

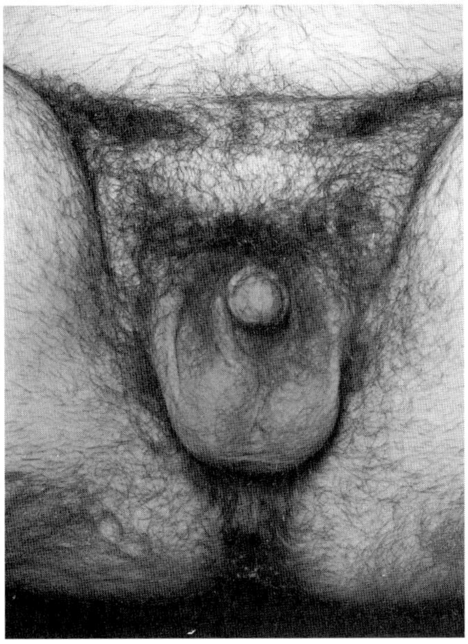

E

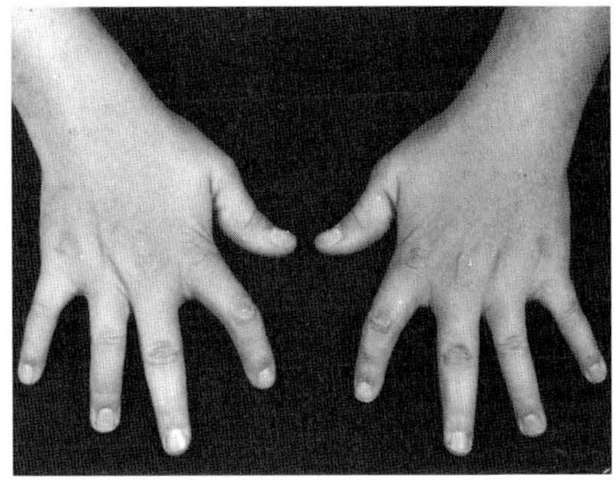

F

Urban Syndrome. (continued)

at term gestation. Craniofacial manifestations were upslanting palpebral fissures, lateral extension of the eyebrows, and tented upper lip. One brother had strabismus and small optic discs. Both had abnormalities of eye movement. Skeletal manifestations included wormian bones in the lambdoid sutures, small hands and feet with wasting of the intrinsic muscles and finger contractures, narrow iliac wings, osteoporosis, and fractures with inadequate provocation. The body acquired a eunuchoid shape and truncal obesity. At age 20 years, the older brother had moderate facial, axillary, and body hair, small penis, and large testes (4.5 × 5 cm). The younger brother had small penis, scant pubic hair, and undescended testes.

Speech and motor milestones were moderately delayed. IQ measurements were 67 and 71 during the teenage years. During childhood, both brothers had chronic constipation. They had low serum thyroxine and T_3 resin uptake.

The findings in these two males are suggestive of those in XLMR syndromes with obesity, hypotonia, hypogonadism (e.g., Börjeson-Forssman-Lehmann, Chudley-Lowry, Vasquez, and Wilson-Turner syndromes). Hypotonia was never noted in these brothers, however, and the oldest appears moderately masculinized and has normal gonadotropins.

REFERENCE

Urban MD, Rogers JG, Meyer WJ: Familial syndrome of mental retardation, short stature, contractures of the hands, and genital anomalies. J Pediatr 94:52, 1979.

VACTERL-Hydrocephalus Syndrome

(Hunter-MacMurray Syndrome, VACTERL-H Syndrome, MIM 314390)

Definition. XLMR with hydrocephaly and vertebral, tracheoesophageal, renal, and limb malformations. The gene has not been localized.

Somatic Features. A wide array of malformations affecting nearly all systems contributes to the seriousness and early lethality in this entity. Only the heart appears to be exempt. Hydrocephaly, the manifestation that distinguishes the syndrome from sporadic VACTERL association, is due to aqueductal stenosis. Microphthalmia, cleft palate, and apparently low-set ears may be the only other craniofacial features. Radial deficiency with club hands and absent thumbs are the typical limb anomalies. Genitalia may be hypoplastic or abnormally formed. Imperforate anus and a number of internal malformations—tracheoesophageal fissure, abnormal lung lobation, accessory spleens, intestinal atresia, and ectopic

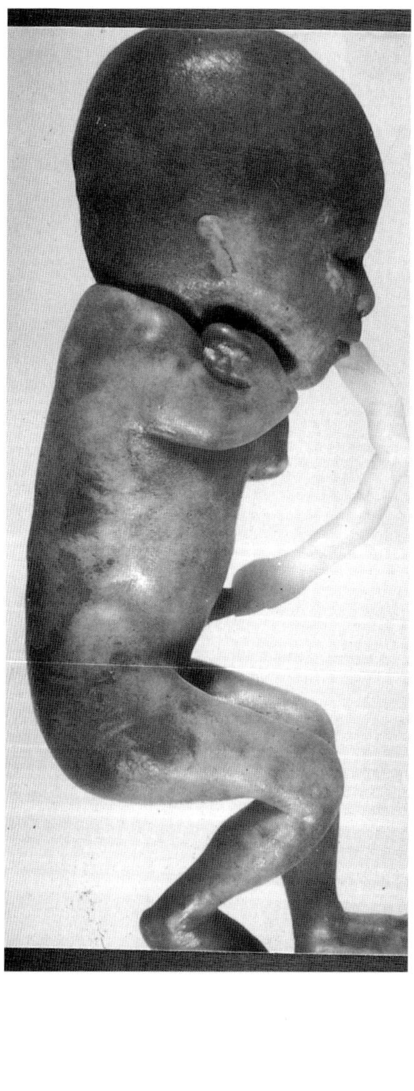

A

VACTERL-Hydrocephalus Syndrome. Newborn infant with hydrocephaly, small ears, and radial aplasia (A).

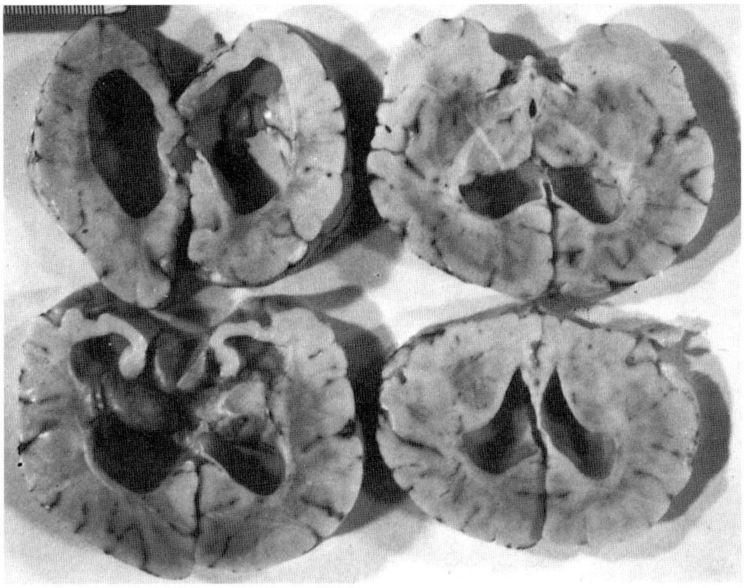

B

VACTERL-Hydrocephalus Syndrome. (continued) Hydrocephaly on cut brain sections (B). Courtesy of Dr. Ursula Froster, University of Leipzig, Leipzig, Germany.

or horseshoe kidney—complete the phenotype. Most infants die in the neonatal period.

GROWTH AND DEVELOPMENT. Intrauterine growth retardation and hydrocephaly combine to give the appearance of marked craniotruncal disproportion.

COGNITIVE FEATURES. Early lethality precludes definitive assessment of cognitive abilities but severe impairment is presumed based on the marked hydrocephaly and the developmental course of the few survivors.

HETEROZYGOTE EXPRESSION. None reported.

NEUROPATHOLOGY. Although hydrocephaly due to stenosis or other anomaly of the aqueduct of Sylvius is the usual postmortem finding, other structural defects of the brain have been reported.

IMAGING. Prenatal ultrasound has documented hydrocephaly and upper limb anomalies in most cases.

COMMENT. Only a minority of cases of concurrence of hydrocephaly and VACTERL anomalies can be accounted for by this X-linked syndrome. The larger number represent cases with autosomal recessive inheritance and sporadic cases in which causation is not identified.

REFERENCES

Evans JA, Stranc LC, Kaplan P, et al.: VACTERL with hydrocephalus: further delineation of the syndrome(s). Am J Med Genet 34:177, 1989.

Froster UG, Wallner SJ, Reusche E, et al.: VACTERL with hydrocephalus and branchial arch defects: prenatal, clinical, and autopsy findings in two brothers. Am J Med Genet 62:169, 1996.

Hunter AGW, MacMurray B: Malformations of the VATER association plus hydrocephalus in a male infant and his maternal uncle. Proc Greenwood Genet Cntr 6:146, 1987.
Lurie IW, Ferencz C: VACTERL-hydrocephaly, DK-phocomelia, and cerebro-cardio-radio-reno-rectal community. Am J Med Genet 70:144, 1997.
Vandenborne K, Beemer F, Fryns JP, et al.: VACTERL with hydrocephalus. A distinct entity with a variable spectrum of multiple congenital anomalies. Genet Couns 4:199, 1993.

Differential Matrix

Syndrome	Hydro-cephaly	Limb Anomalies	Early Lethality	Comments
VACTERL-hydrocephalus	+	+	+	Vertebral anomalies, radial limb defects, tracheal and esophageal anomalies, renal malformations, anal anomalies
X-linked hydrocephaly-MASA spectrum	+	+	+	Adducted thumbs, spastic paraplegia, dysgenesis of corpus callosum
Hydrocephly-cerebellar agenesis	+	0	+	Absent cerebellar hemispheres, hypotonia, seizures

VASQUEZ SYNDROME

DEFINITION. XLMR with short stature, microcephaly, hypotonia, obesity, hypogonadism, and gynecomastia. The gene has not been localized.

SOMATIC FEATURES. Craniofacial manifestations include microbrachycephaly, narrow bifrontal diameter, small eyes, and upslanting palpebral fissures. Cleft soft palate was present in one case. Truncal obesity and eunuchoid habitus with cubitus valgus and genu valgum become obvious with age. Hands and feet are normal size but the hands have ulnar deviation, and fifth finger clinodactyly and camptodactyly may be present. One patient had thoracolumbar kyphoscoliosis. The genitalia are underdeveloped and evidence of hypogonadism with gynecomastia, incomplete virilization, and high-pitched voice are obvious. Hypotonia, obvious prenatally by decreased fetal movement, persists into adult life.

GROWTH AND DEVELOPMENT. Only limited information is available on growth. Birth weight was reduced in one infant. Short stature appears consistent and head circumference has been small in all except one case.

NEUROLOGICAL FINDINGS. Hypotonia is the major neuromuscular abnormality. Seizures occurred in one case.

HETEROZYGOTE EXPRESSION. None.

IMAGING. Not available.

LABORATORY. The serum testosterone response to human chorionic gonadotropin stimulation was consistent with hypogonadotrophic hypogonadism. Testicular biopsy

→

Vasquez Syndrome. Thirty-month-old with short stature, rounded face, and obesity (A, B); 18-year-old with short stature, obesity, gynecomastia, eunuchoid habitus, cubitus valgum, and decreased virilization (C); 19-year-old with short stature, obesity, gynecomastia, eunuchoid habitus, decreased virilization, and genu valgum (D). Courtesy of Dr. Juan Sotos, Children's Hospital, Columbus, OH.

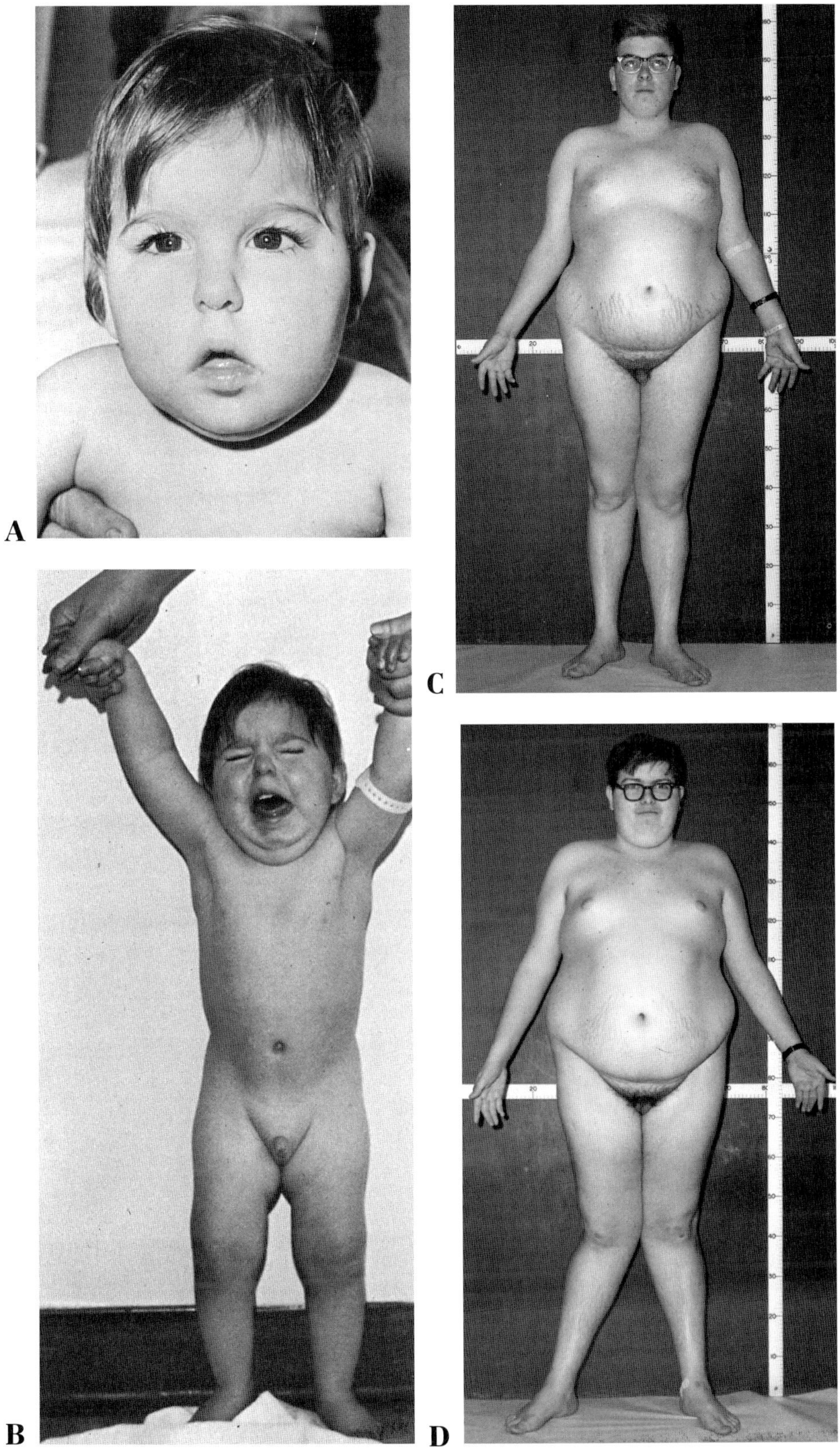
A
B
C
D

has shown abnormal lining of the seminiferous tubules, presence of mononuclear and inflammatory cells, and decreased Leydig cells, spermatogonia, and spermatids.
COMMENT. Hypotonia, hypogonadism, and obesity constitute a triad of clinical findings present in several XLMR syndromes. To date, only two separate linkage regions have been identified: the pericentromeric region (encompassing loci for XLMR–hypotonic facies, Wilson-Turner, and Chudley-Lowry syndromes) and Xq26-q27.2 (Börjeson-Forssman-Lehmann syndrome).

REFERENCE

Vasquez SB, Hurst DL, Sotos JF: X-linked hypogonadism, gynecomastia, mental retardation, short stature, and obesity—a new syndrome. J Pediatr 94:56, 1979.

Differential Matrix

Syndrome	Obesity	Hypotonia	Hypo-gonadism	Comments
Vasquez	+	+	+	Short stature, microcephaly, gynecomastia
Börjeson-Forssman-Lehmann	+	+	+	Short stature, microcephaly, coarse face, large ears, gynecomastia, narrow sloped shoulders, visual impairment, tapered digits
Chudley-Lowry	+	+	+	Short stature, bitemporal narrowing, almond-shaped eyes, depressed nasal bridge, tented upper lip, open mouth
MEHMO	+	+	+	Short stature, microcephaly, edematous hands and feet, equinovarus deformity, seizures, early childhood death
Wilson-Turner	+	+	+	Normal growth, small hands and feet, tapered digits, gynecomastia, emotional lability
Pettigrew	0	+	+	Dandy-Walker malformation, spasticity, seizures, microcephaly or hydrocephaly, long face with macrostomia and prognathism, small testes, contractures, choreoathetosis, iron deposits in basal ganglia
XLMR-hypotonic facies (Carpenter-Waziri) (Holmes-Gang) (Juberg-Marsidi)	0	+	+	Short stature, microcephaly, telecanthus, small triangular nose, tented upper lip, open mouth, spacing of teeth, genital anomalies, musculoskeletal anomalies, hemoglobin H inclusions in erythrocytes
Urban	+	0	+	Short stature, small hands and feet, digital contractures, osteoporosis
XLMR-panhypopituitarism	+	0	+	Short stature, small sella turcica, deficiency of pituitary, thyroid, adrenal, and gonadal hormones
Young-Hughes	+	0	+	Short stature, small palpebral fissures, cupped ears, ichthyosiform scaling

WAISMAN-LAXOVA SYNDROME

(Waisman Syndrome, XLMR-Parkinson, MIM 311510)

DEFINITION. XLMR with macrocephaly, stabismus, parkinsonian rigidity and tremors, and seizures. The gene is localized distal to DXS98 in Xq27.3, maximal lod score 5.19.

SOMATIC FEATURES. Although normal at birth, the head circumference increases thereafter and generally exceeds the 98th centile throughout childhood and adult life. Frontal prominence accompanies the macrocephaly. Otherwise, the craniofacial appearance is not distinctive, although high palate and crowded teeth occur in most and protruding ears in some. Multiple diffuse pigmented papules occurred on the trunk in several cases.

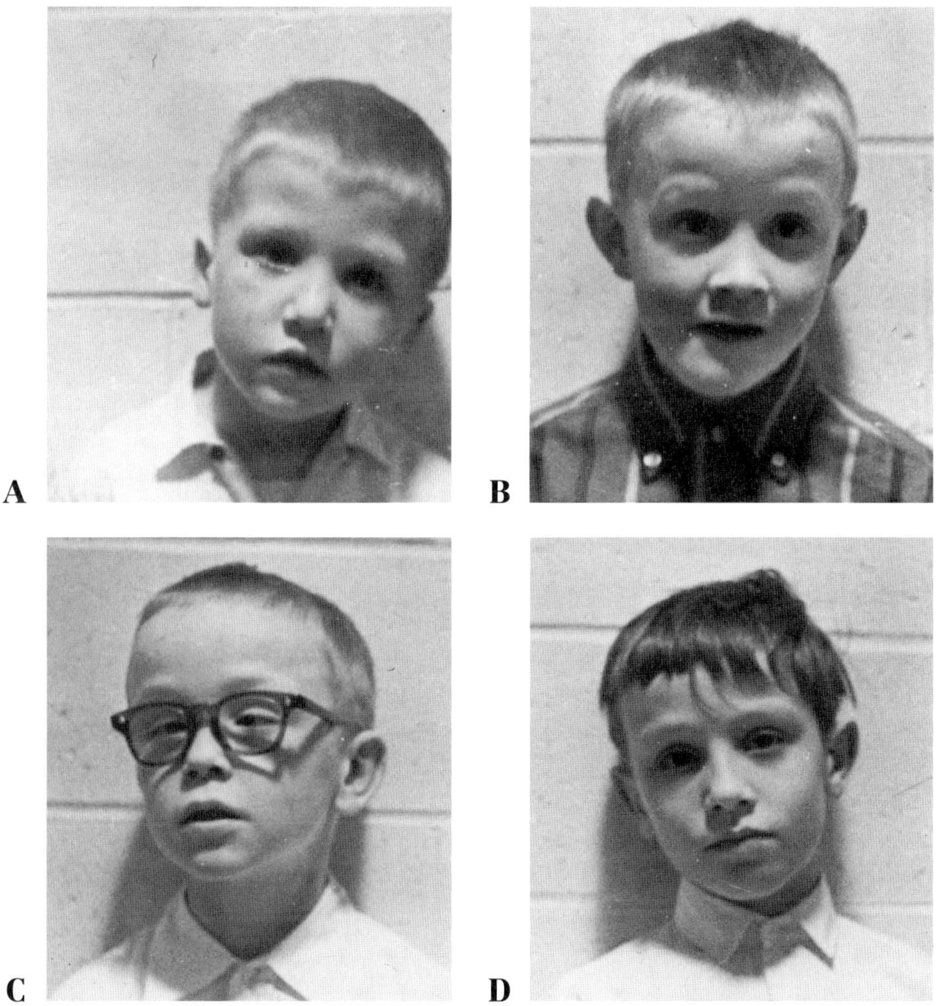

Waisman-Laxova Syndrome. Normal facial features in six affected males at ages 4, 6, 8, and 9.

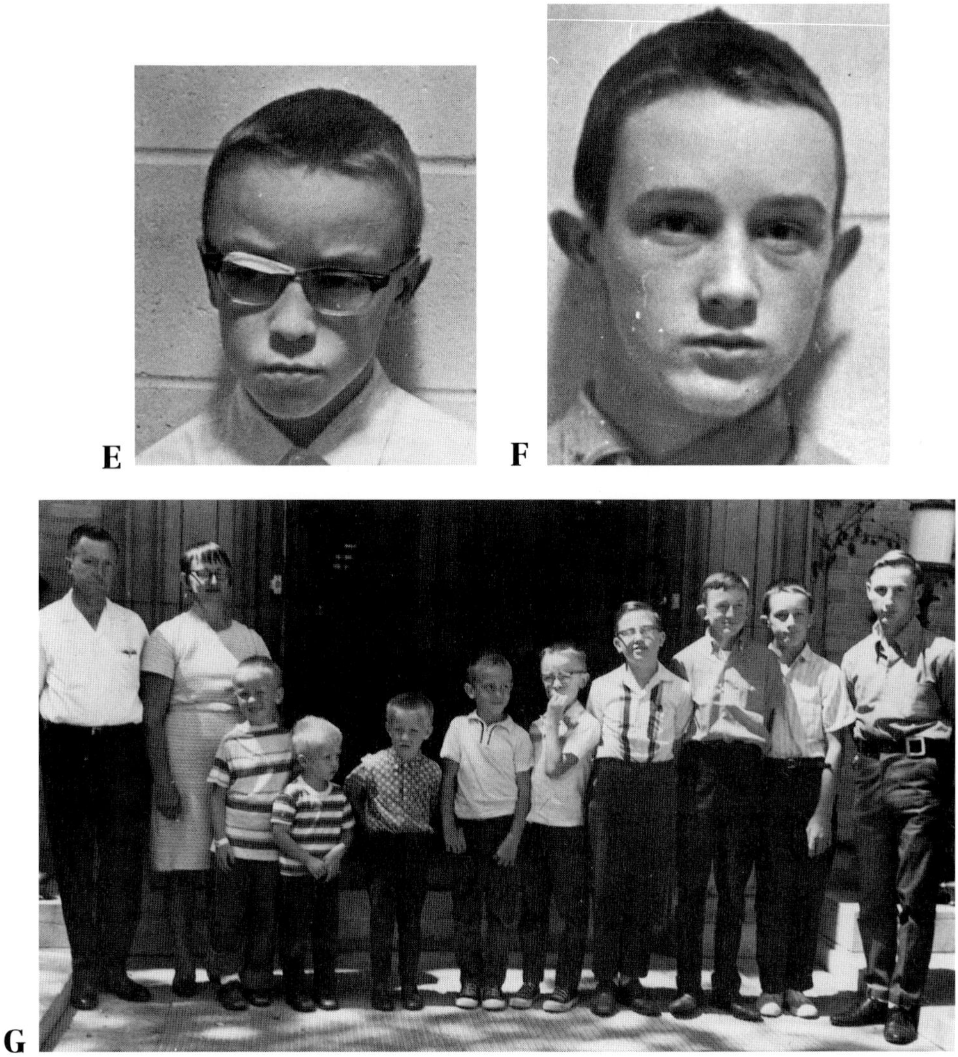

Waisman-Laxova Syndrome. (continued) Normal facial features in six affected males at ages 10 and 15 years (E–F); family group showing affected males; unaffected brothers are first, third, and fourth from right (G). Courtesy of Dr. Renata Laxova, University of Wisconsin–Madison, Madison, WI.

GROWTH AND DEVELOPMENT. Intrauterine growth is normal. Postnatal height and weight are also normal, but macrocephaly with frontal bossing becomes apparent by early childhood. All developmental milestones are moderately delayed. Walking and first words begin by about 2 years and use of sentences is delayed until after age 4–5 years.

COGNITIVE FEATURES. IQ measurements range from below 30 to 70.

NEUROLOGICAL FINDINGS. Neurological signs dominate the phenotype and have been documented as early as age 2 years. A general paucity of movement, tremors of the trunk and limbs, choreoathetoid movements, persistence of frontal lobe reflexes, cogwheel rigidity of the upper limbs, slow and shuffling gait, stooped posture, and hypokinetic dysarthria occur in most affected males. Seizures occur less often.

IMAGING. Pneumoencephalography and cranial CT show brain enlargement with normal ventricles and no calcifications.

COMMENT. In the absence of hydrocephaly, macrocephaly is an uncommon finding among the XLMR syndromes. Fragile X, mucopolysaccharidosis II, Atkin-Flaitz, Lujan, and Simpson-Golabi-Behmel syndromes may have macrocephaly without hydrocephaly. The phenotypes of these XLMR syndromes are sufficiently distinctive such that they should not be confused with Waisman-Laxova syndrome.

REFERENCES

Gregg RG, Metzenberg AB, Hogan K, et al.: Waisman syndrome, a human X-linked recessive basal ganglia disorder with mental retardation: localization to Xq27.3—qter. Genomics 9:701, 1991.

Laxova R, Brown ES, Hogan K, et al.: An X-linked recessive basal ganglia disorder with mental retardation. Am J Med Genet 21:681, 1985.

Differential Matrix

Syndrome	Spasticity	Choreo-athetosis	Tremors & Rigidity	Comments
Waisman-Laxova	+	+	+	-
Arena	+	+	+	Muscle hypoplasia, club foot, iron deposits in basal ganglia, ataxia, dystonia
Pettigrew	+	+	+	Dandy-Walker malformation, seizures, microcephaly or hydrocephaly, long face with macrostomia and prognathism, small testes, contractures, iron deposits in basal ganglia
Gustavson	+	0	+	Microcephaly, short stature, optic atrophy with blindness, large ears, deafness, joint contractures, rockerbottom feet, brain undergrowth, hydrocephaly, cerebellar hypoplasia, seizures
Lesch-Nyhan	+	+	+	Self-mutilation, hyperuricemia
Schimke	+	+	0	Microcephaly, sunken eyes, downslanting palpebral fissures, narrow nose, spacing of teeth, cupped ears, hypotonia, abducens palsy, hearing loss, vision loss, contractures
XLMR-hydrocephaly-basal ganglia calcifications	+	+	0	Hydrocephaly, calcifications of basal ganglia, muscle hypoplasia, sensory impairment
XLMR-spastic paraplegia-athetosis	+	+	+	Nystagmus, weakness, dysarthria, muscle wasting, contractures
Pelizaeus-Merzbacher	+	0	+	Optic atrophy, nystagmus, hypotonia, ataxia, dystonia, CNS dysmyelination
PPM-X	+	0	+	Macroorchidism, psychosis, parkinsonian features

WARKANY SYNDROME

(Intrauterine Growth Retardation–Microcephaly Mental Retardation Syndrome, MIM 308400)

The designation Warkany syndrome is based on a single family with six affected males in three generations. Limited details were provided on two brothers who

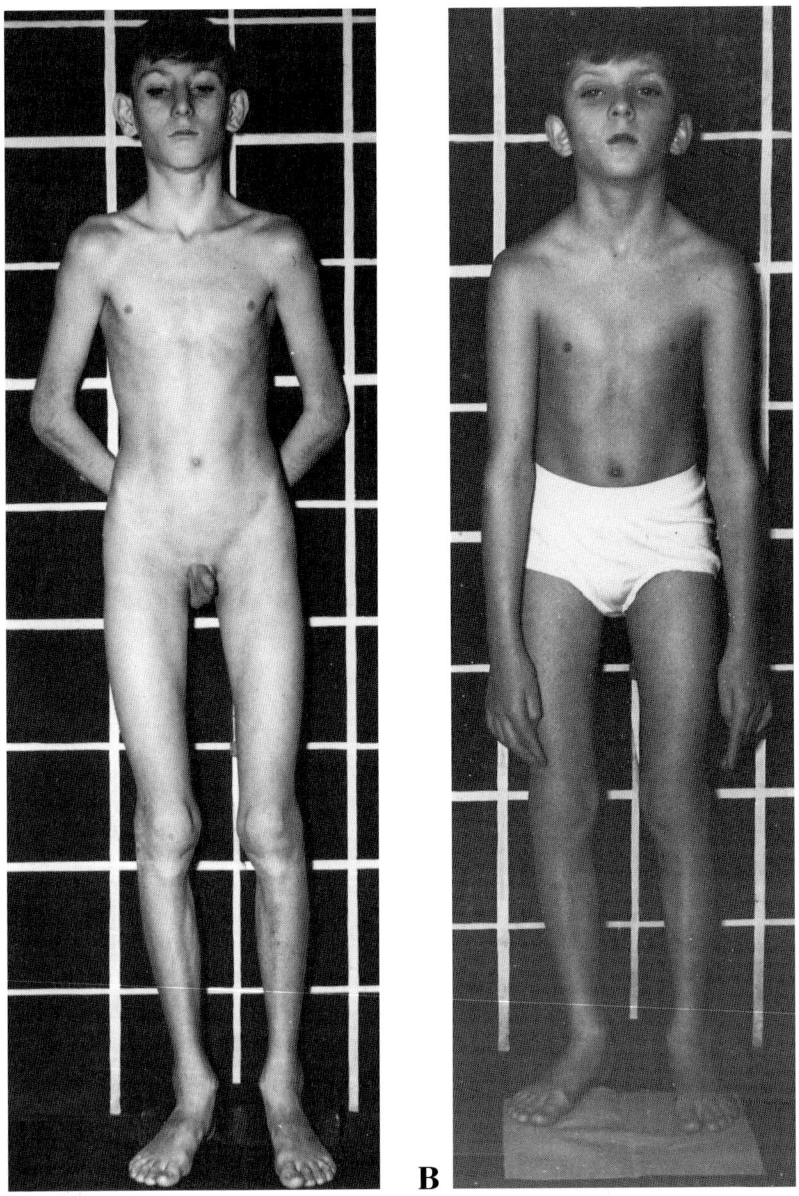

A B

Warkany Syndrome. Brothers at ages 12 years (A) and 14 years (B) showing microcephaly, cupped ears, general asthenic habitus, and short stature. Courtesy of Dr. Wladimir Wertelecki, University of South Alabama College of Medicine, Mobile.

had intrauterine growth retardation, short stature, and microcephaly. One brother had ptosis, cupped ears, thin neck, and flat chest. Developmental milestones were moderately delayed and IQ measurements were approximately 50. Carrier females had intrauterine growth retardation but normal postnatal growth and development.

REFERENCES

Warkany J, Monroe BB, Sutherland BS: Intrauterine growth retardation. Am J Dis Child 102:249, 1961.

Warkany J: Intrauterine growth retardation. In: Congenital Malformations. Notes and Comments. J Warkany, ed. Year Book Medical, Chicago, 1971, p.143.

WIEACKER-WOLFF SYNDROME

(XLMR–Muscle Atrophy–Contractures–Oculomotor Apraxia, MIM 314580)

DEFINITION. XLMR with foot contractures, distal muscle atrophy, dysarthria, and oculomotor apraxia. The gene has been localized to markers between PFC (Xp11.3-p11.23) and DXS339 (Xq11.2-q13), lod score 4.89.

SOMATIC FEATURES. Musculoskeletal findings date from birth, appear slowly progressive, and are most striking in the lower limbs. Usually described as clubbed at birth, the feet are contracted at all joints; calcaneovalgus position and rocker-bottom appearance are usual. The toes are crowded with flexion contractures. The legs taper distally, giving the appearance of muscle underdevelopment or wasting of the muscles, especially the peroneal muscles. The upper limbs are similarly involved but to a less severe degree. Evidence that neuropathic involvement is widespread includes generalized weakness, mild ptosis, sluggish reaction of the pupils to light and convergence, defective horizontal and vertical eye movement, strabismus, dysarthria, and kyphoscoliosis. Muscle biopsy shows muscle cell atrophy suggestive of a neuropathy. Sensation and nerve conduction appear normal.

GROWTH AND DEVELOPMENT. Details of growth are not available. Acquisition of motor skills and speech is moderately delayed.

COGNITIVE FEATURES. Older individuals appear more severely impaired than those younger, perhaps reflecting less exposure to educational opportunities in times past. Alternatively, there may be progressive loss of cognitive abilities.

NEUROLOGICAL FINDINGS. An underlying neuropathy best explains the generalized muscle weakness, distal muscle atrophy, and contractures.

HETEROZYGOTE EXPRESSION. None.

LABORATORY. Motor and sensory nerve conduction velocities, serum creatine kinase, and electroencephalography are normal. Muscle biopsy shows atrophic muscle cells dispersed in a neuropathogenic fashion.

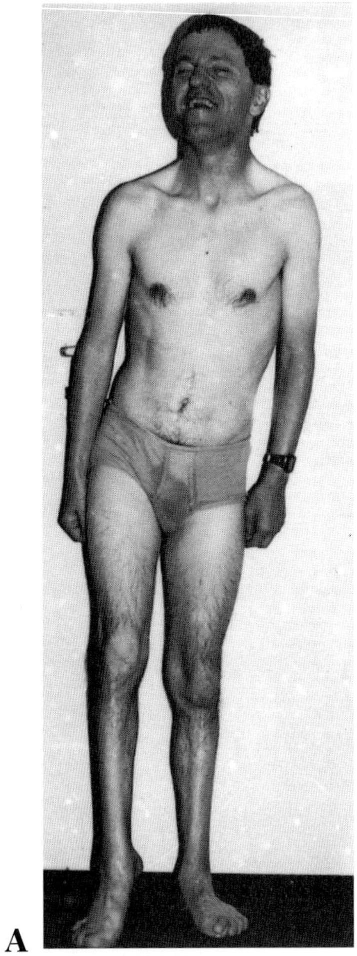

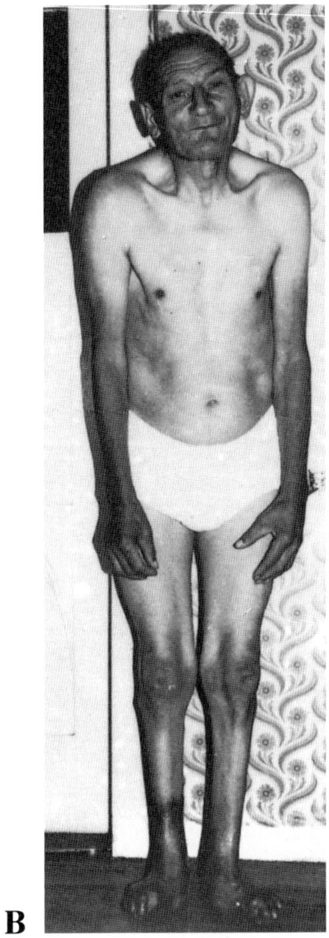

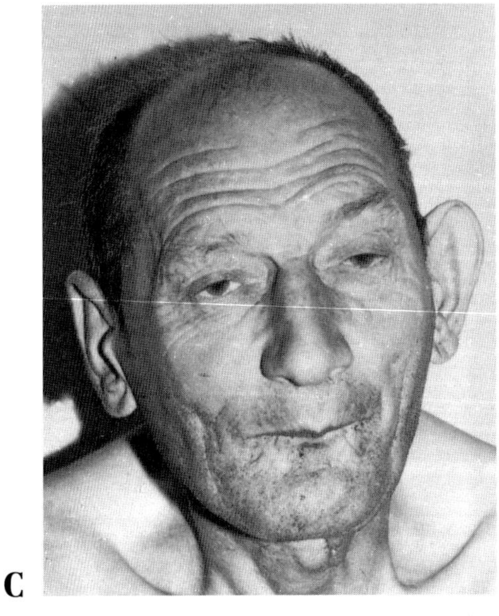

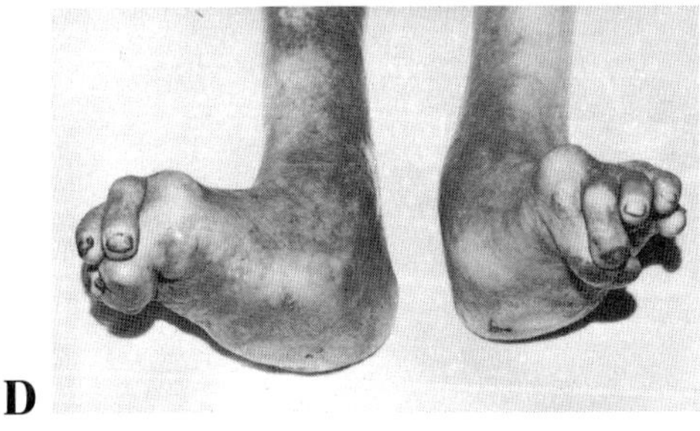

Wieacker-Wolff Syndrome. Scoliosis, muscle wasting of the distal limbs, and foot contractures in a 33-year-old (A) and his 63-year-old uncle (B–D). Courtesy of the *American Journal of Medical Genetics*, copyright © 1985, Alan R. Liss, Inc.

IMAGING. Normal.

COMMENT. Although underdevelopment of the skeletal musculature and weakness may be present in several XLMR syndromes, contractures at birth are described only in Wieacker-Wolff syndrome.

REFERENCE

Kloos DU, Jakubiczka S, Wienker T, et al.: Localization of the gene for Wieacker-Wolff syndrome in the pericentromeric region of the X chromosome. Hum Genet 100:426, 1997.

Wieacker P, Wolff G, Wienker TF, et al.: A new X-linked syndrome with muscle atrophy, congenital contractures, and oculomotor apraxia. Am J Med Genet 20:597, 1985.

Differential Matrix

Syndrome	Muscle Hypoplasia or Atrophy	Contractures	Ocular Palsies	Comments
Wieacker-Wolff	+	+	+	Weakness, distal muscle atrophy, dysarthria
Christianson	+	+	+	Short stature, microcephaly, general asthenia, seizures, ophthalmoplegia
Allan-Herndon-Dudley	+	+	0	Large ears with cupping or abnormal architecture, childhood hypotonia, dysarthria, athetosis, ataxia, spastic paraplegia
Apak ataxia-spastic diplegia	+	+	0	Short stature, clubfoot, ataxia, spastic paraplegia
Arena	+	+	0	Clubfoot, iron deposits in basal ganglia, ataxia, spastic paraplegia, rigidity, dystonia
Duchenne muscular dystrophy	+	+	0	Hypertrophy of calf muscle, elevated muscle enzymes, progressive weakness, loss of reflexes, muscle wasting
Goldblatt spastic paraplegia	+	+	0	Optic atrophy, exotropia, nystagmus, ataxia, spastic paraplegia, dysarthria
XLMR-spastic paraplegia-athetosis	+	+	0	Nystagmus, weakness, dysarthria, spastic paraplegia, muscle wasting
Schimke	0	+	+	Microcephaly, sunken eyes, downslanting palpebral fissures, narrow nose, spacing of teeth, cupped ears, hypotonia, abducens palsy, hearing loss, vision loss, spasticity, choreoathetosis

WILSON-TURNER SYNDROME

(Wilson Syndrome, MRXS6, MIM 309589)

DEFINITION. XLMR with obesity, gynecomastia, tapered digits, small feet, and emotional lability. The gene localizes between DXS426 (Xp11) and DXS990 (Xq21), lod score 6.1.

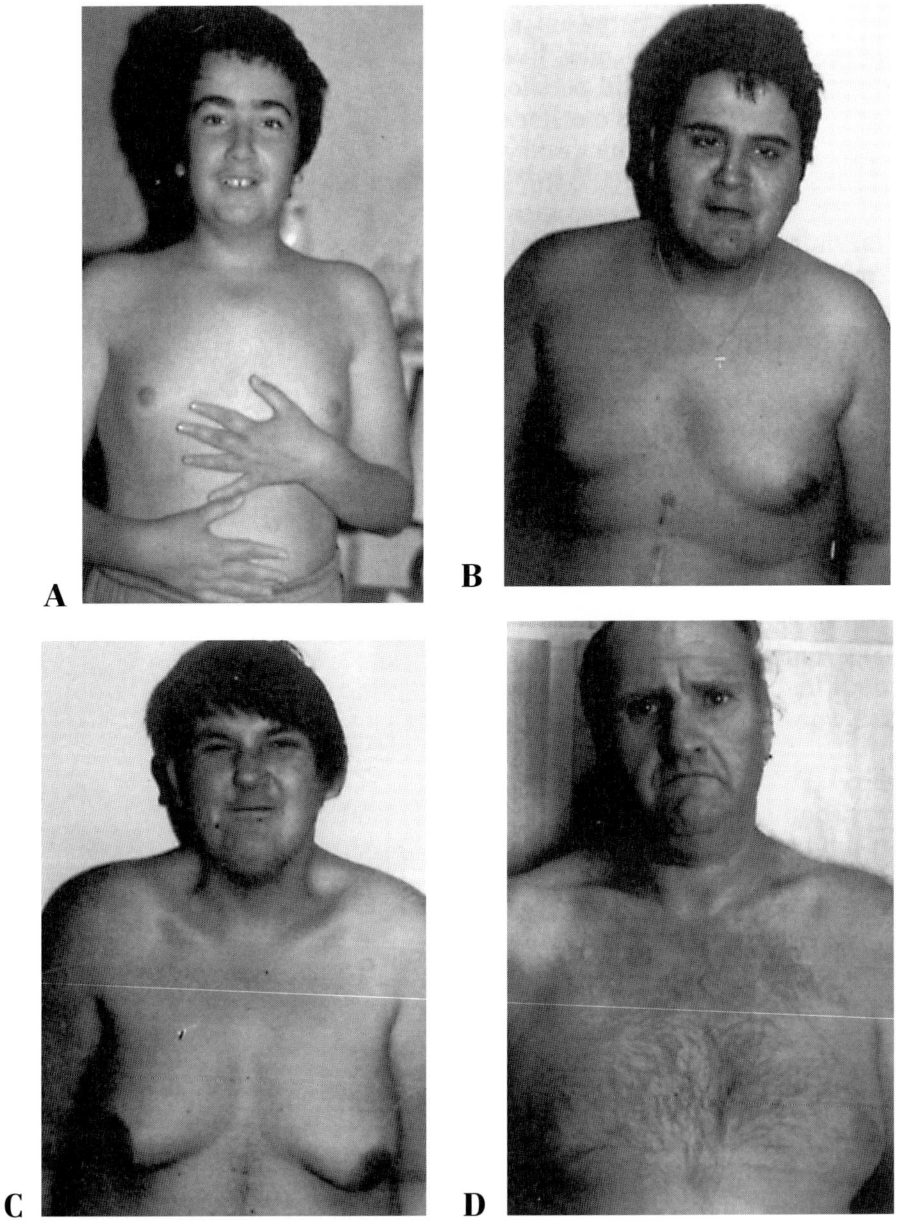

Wilson-Turner Syndrome. Heavy eyebrows, synophrys, gynecomastia, and obesity in affected males at ages 13 years (A), 19 years (B), 25 years (C), and 48 years (D). Courtesy of the *American Journal of Medical Genetics*, copyright © 1991, Wiley-Liss, Inc.

SOMATIC FEATURES. Patients lack distinctive facial features except for heavy eyebrows. They have normal stature and cranial growth. The hands tend to be small and tapering and the feet are small. Truncal obesity and gynecomastia or lipomastia become apparent at puberty. Genital development varies from normal to hypogenitalism with small penis and small or undescended testes. Body hair tends to be scant; pubic hair varies with genital development. Some males have pes planus, others pes cavus.

GROWTH AND DEVELOPMENT. Normal prenatal and postnatal growth is reported with most males becoming obese and developing gynecomastia at puberty. Developmental milestones are globally delayed with speech more severely impaired. Some males have little or no speech.

COGNITIVE FEATURES. Variable but usually mild to moderate impairment of cognitive function occurs.

BEHAVIORAL MANIFESTATIONS. In general, affected males are quiet with a cheerful temperament, although several have appeared easily upset, tearful, or aggressive.

NEUROLOGICAL FINDINGS. Poor muscle tone and excessive drooling during infancy have been noted in some cases, but not in others. Stuttering appears quite common.

HETEROZYGOTE EXPRESSION. None.

LABORATORY. A disturbance of hypothalmic-pituitary-gonadal axis has been suspected on the basis of decreased or low normal androgens with normal follicle-stimulating hormone (FSH) and luteinizing hormone (LH).

COMMENT. Wilson-Turner syndrome shares the phenotypic triad of hypotonia, hypogonadism, and obesity with another XLMR syndrome (Chudley-Lowry syndrome) which maps to the pericentromeric region.

REFERENCES

Gedeon A, Mulley J, Turner G: Gene localisation for Wilson-Turner syndrome (WTS:MIM 309585). Am J Med Genet 64:80, 1994.

Wilson M, Mulley J, Gedeon A, et al.: New X-linked syndrome of mental retardation, gynecomastia, and obesity is linked to DXS255. Am J Med Genet 40:406, 1991.

Differential Matrix

Syndrome	Obesity	Hypo-gonadism	Hypotonia	Comments
Wilson-Turner	+	+	+	Normal growth, small hands and feet, tapered digits, gynecomastia, emotional lability
Börjeson-Forssman-Lehmann	+	+	+	Short stature, microcephaly, coarse facies, large ears, gynecomastia, narrow sloped shoulders, visual impairment, tapered digits
Chudley-Lowry	+	+	+	Short stature, bitemporal narrowing, almond-shaped eyes, depressed nasal bridge, tented upper lip, open mouth
MEHMO	+	+	+	Short stature, microcephaly, edematous hands and feet, equinovarus deformity, seizures, early childhood death
Vasquez	+	+	+	Short stature, microcephaly, gynecomastia
Urban	+	+	0	Short stature, small hands and feet, digital contractures, osteoporosis
Young-Hughes	+	+	0	Short stature, small palpebral fissures, cupped ears, ichthyosiform scaling
XLMR-panhypopituitarism	+	+	0	Short stature, small sella turcica, deficiency of pituitary, thyroid, adrenal, and gonadal hormones
Pettigrew	0	+	+	Dandy-Walker malformation, spasticity, seizures, microcephaly or hydrocephaly, long face with macrostomia, small testes, contractures, choreoathetosis, iron deposits in basal ganglia
XLMR-hypotonic facies (Carpenter-Waziri) (Holmes-Gang) (Juberg-Marsidi)	0	+	+	Microcephaly, short stature, telecanthus, small triangular nose, tented upper lip, open mouth, spacing of teeth, genital anomalies, musculoskeletal anomalies, hemoglobin H inclusions in erythrocytes

WITTWER SYNDROME

DEFINITION. XLMR with growth failure, microcephaly with large fontanels, frontal prominence, hypertelorism, long philtrum, thin upper lip, cupped ears, blindness, hearing loss, and seizures. Concordance for markers in Xp22.3 suggests localization.

SOMATIC FEATURES. Recessed eyes, bringing the forehead and cheeks into prominence, give the face a distinctive appearance. Craniofacial appearance is further

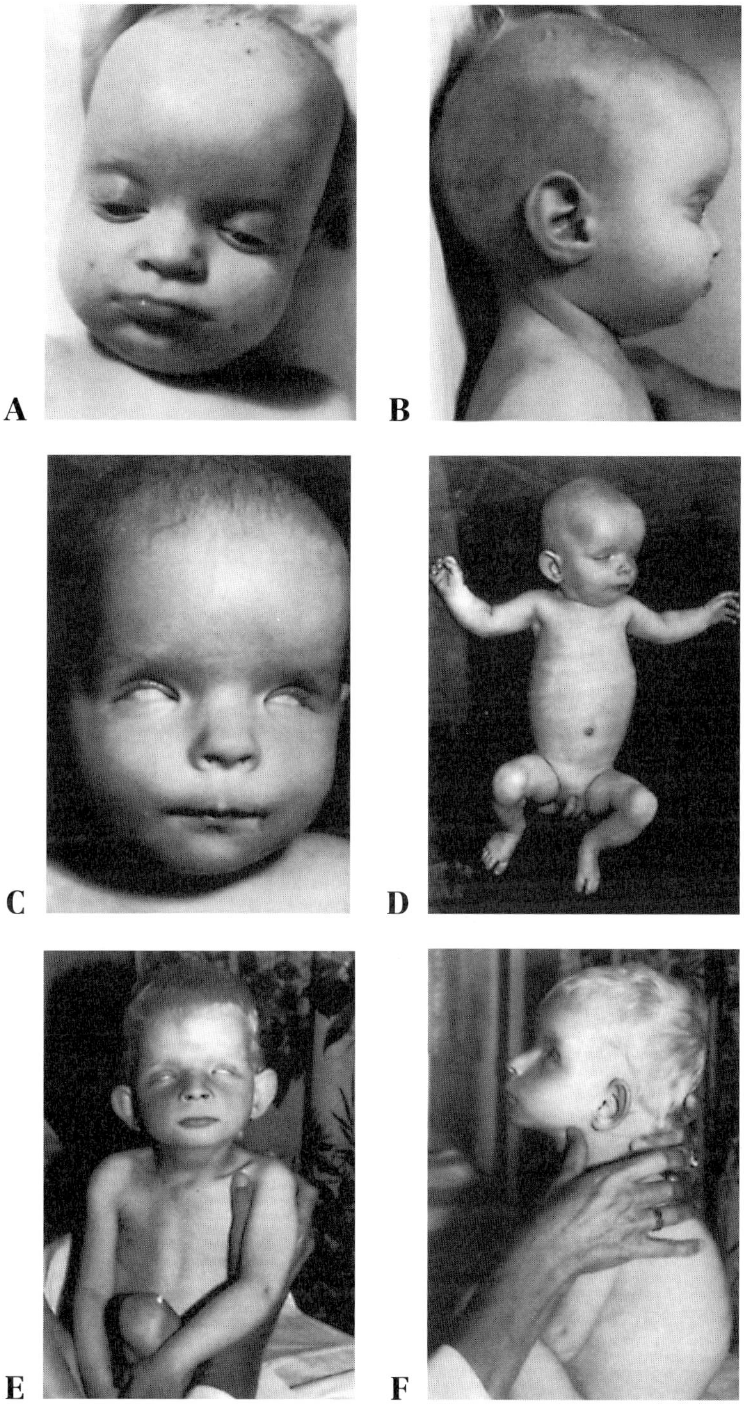

Wittwer Syndrome. Four-month-old male with prominent forehead, retracted midface, hypertelorism, downslanted palpebral fissures, and thin upper lip (A, B); prominent forehead, hypertelorism, epicanthal folds, downslanted palpebral fissures, retracted midface, long philtrum, thin upper lip, cupped ears, microphthalmia, and sclerocornea in a cousin at age 6 months (C, D); and 5 years (E, F). Courtesy of the American Journal of Medical Genetics, Copyright © 1995, Wiley-Liss, Inc.

characterized by large fontanels, downslanting palpebral fissures, hypertelorism, epicanthus, anteverted nares, long philtrum, thin upper lip, and cupped ears. One infant had microphthalmia and sclerocornea and another had optic atrophy. Minor skeletal anomalies may include finger 5 clinodactyly, single palmar creases, bell-shaped chest, clubfoot with camptodactyly, and delayed bone maturation. Cryptorchidism, epispadias, vesicoureteral reflux, and hydronephrosis have been described. Blindness dates from birth and hearing loss is evident early in childhood.

GROWTH AND DEVELOPMENT. Intrauterine growth is impaired and all postnatal growth parameters fall far below the normal centiles. All developmental milestones lag markedly behind. Speech and independent ambulation are never achieved.

COGNITIVE FEATURES. Severe impairment based on childhood developmental progress.

NEUROLOGICAL FINDINGS. Generalized seizures develop during infancy. Weakness and poor muscle tone persist throughout childhood.

HETEROZYGOTE EXPRESSION. Mild mental retardation was described in one mother.

NEUROPATHOLOGY. Postmortem examination of one infant showed cerebellar atrophy and hydrocephalus.

IMAGING. Cranial ultrasound and CT were normal in two infants. The CT suggested dysgenesis of the corpus callosum in another infant, but this was not confirmed at autopsy.

COMMENT. This entity is based on a description of three affected males, sons of sisters by three partners.

REFERENCE

Wittwer B, Kircheisen R, Leutelt J, et al.: New X-linked mental retardation syndrome with the gene mapped tentatively in Xp22.3. Am J Med Genet 64:42, 1996.

Differential Matrix

Syndrome	Blindness	Hearing Loss	Genitourinary Anomalies	Comments
Wittwer	+	+	+	Growth deficiency, microcephaly, microphthalmia, hypertelorism, hypotonia, seizures
Proud	+	+	+	Microcephaly, agenesis of corpus callosum, cryptorchidism, inguinal hernias, ataxia, spasticity, seizures
Arts	+	+	0	Growth deficiency, paucity of muscles, hypotonia, areflexia, ataxia, seizures, childhood death
Gustavson	+	+	0	Microcephaly, short stature, optic atrophy with blindness, large ears, joint contractures, rockerbottom feet, brain undergrowth, hydrocephaly, cerebellar hypoplasia, spasticity, seizures
Norrie	+	+	0	Ocular dysgenesis and degeneration, adult-onset hearing loss
Mohr-Tranebjaerg (Jensen)	+	+	0	Neurologic deterioration with childhood onset, dystonia, spasticity
Paine	+	+	0	Microcephaly, short stature, optic atrophy, spasticity, seizures
Schimke	+	+	0	Microcephaly, sunken eyes, downslanting palpebral fissures, narrow nose, spacing of teeth, cupped ears, hypotonia, abducens palsy, spasticity, choreoathetosis, contractures
X-linked ataxia-deafness-dementia	+	+	0	Optic atrophy, spastic paraplegia, ataxia, hypotonia, seizures, childhood death
Cerebrooculogenital	+	0	+	Short stature, microcephaly, hydrocephaly, agenesis of corpus callosum, microphthalmia, ptosis, hypospadias, cryptorchidism, clubfoot, spasticity
Goltz	+	0	+	Cataracts, ocular dysgenesis, linear areas of dermal aplasia, cutaneous adipose herniations, dystrophic nails, abnormal teeth and hair, vertebral anomalies, limb reduction defects
Lenz microphthalmia	+	0	+	Microcephaly, microphthalmia, ocular dysgenesis, malformed ears, cleft lip/palate, cardiac anomalies, thumb duplication or hypoplasia, narrow shoulders
Lowe	+	0	+	Short stature, cataracts, hypotonia, aminoaciduria, progressive renal disease

X-LINKED AGENESIS OF THE CORPUS CALLOSUM

(Menkes-Kaplan Syndrome, MIM 304100)

Maldevelopment of the corpus callosum may occur as an isolated and perhaps asymptomatic finding or may coexist with other anomalies. XLMR syndromes that may have dysgenesis of the corpus callosum include Aicardi, Bertini, Brooks, cerebrooculogenital, Kang, X-linked lissencephaly, Lujan, MIDAS, Optiz FG, oral-facial-digital I, Proud, pyruvate dehydrogenase deficiency, and X-linked hydrocephaly–MASA syndromes. Although a number of families with apparently X-linked partial or complete agenesis of the corpus callosum have been reported, it is not clear that they do not represent one of these syndromes.

Boyd et al. and others have noted that dysgenesis of the corpus callosum may be a frequent finding in some families with X-linked hydrocephaly–MASA spectrum. The families reported by Menkes et al. and Kaplan may, in fact, be examples of this spectrum. Menkes et al. reported five cases with agenesis of the corpus callosum who experienced severe developmental impairment and seizures beginning in the neonatal period. Kaplan reported a 2-year-old boy with developmental retardation, small head size, enlarged ventricles, hypoplasia of the inferior vermis and cerebellum, right ptosis, adducted thumbs, upper limb weakness, and Hirschsprung disease. The child's maternal uncle had mental retardation, microcephaly, and agenesis of the corpus callosum.

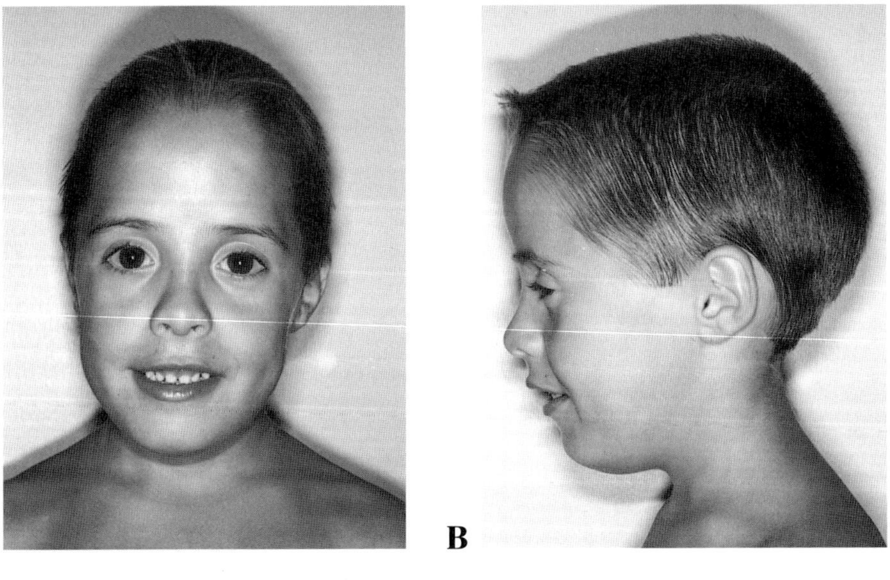

A B

X-Linked Agenesis of the Corpus Callosum. Seven-year-old male with total agenesis of the corpus callosum (A–B).

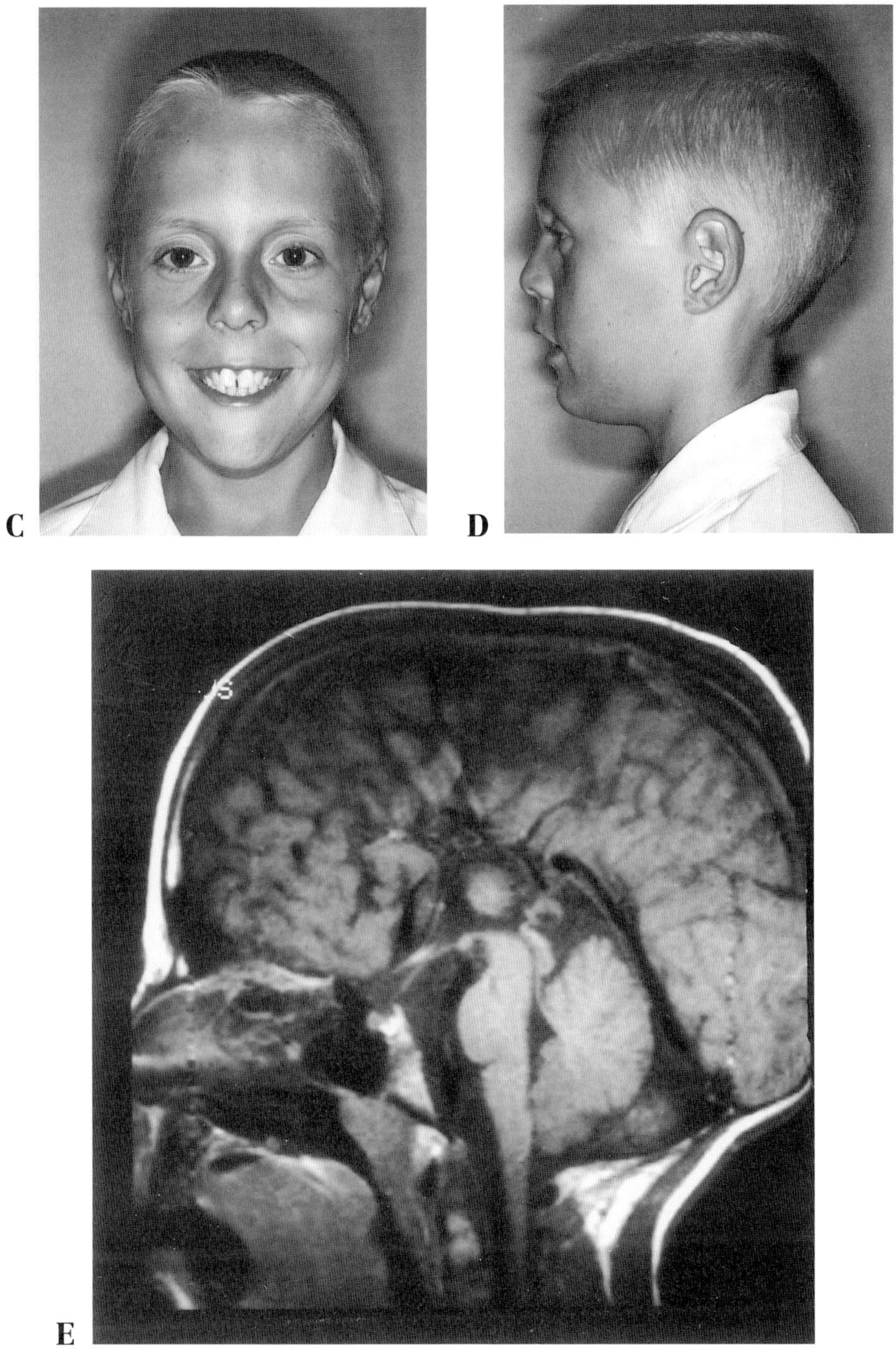

X-Linked Agenesis of the Corpus Callosum. (continued) Brother of patient in A and B at age 9 years with total agenesis of the corpus callosum (C, D); sagittal MRI scan of patient shown in C and D showing absence of the corpus callosum (E).

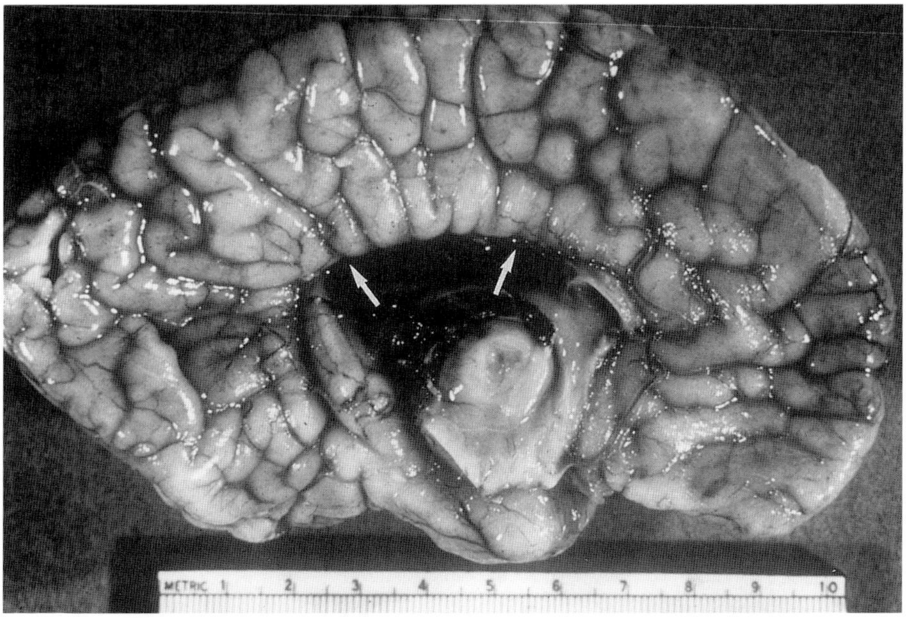

F

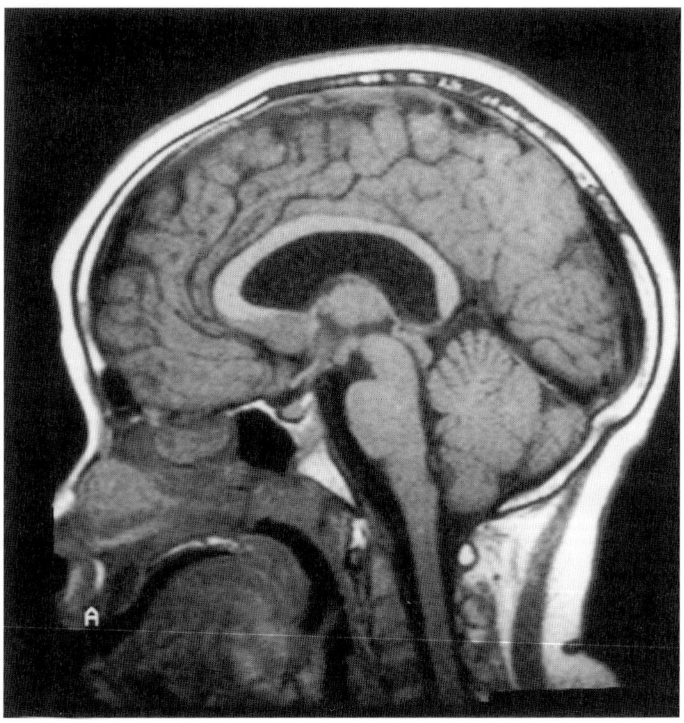

G

X-Linked Agenesis of the Corpus Callosum. (continued) Sagittal brain section showing absence of the corpus callosum [arrows] (F); sagittal MRI scan of a child with macrocephaly and normal-appearing corpus callosum (G). Illustrations A–E courtesy of Dr. E.M. Honey, University of Pretoria, Republic of South Africa.

REFERENCES

Boyd E, Schwartz CE, Schroer RJ, et al.: Agenesis of the corpus callosum associated with MASA syndrome. Clin Dysmorphol 2:332, 1993.

Kaplan P: X linked recessive inheritance of agenesis of the corpus callosum. J Med Genet 20:122, 1983.

Menkes JH, Philippart M, Clark DB: Hereditary partial agenesis of corpus callosum. Arch Neurol 11:198, 1964.

Serville F, Lyonnet S, Pelet A, et al.: X-linked hydrocephalus: clinical heterogeneity at a single gene locus. Eur J Pediatr 51:515, 1992.

X-Linked Ataxia-Deafness-Dementia

(XLMR-Ataxia-Deafness, Schmidley Syndrome, MIM 301790)

Definition. XLMR with optic atrophy, deafness, hypotonia, progressive ataxia, and seizures. The condition has not been mapped.

Somatic Features. No distinctive somatic features have been described. Optic atrophy is demonstrable during the first year. Neurological signs appear in early infancy and progress steadily to demise in midchildhood.

Growth and Development. Developmental milestones lag from the outset. Affected boys fail to walk independently and have little or no speech. Growth parameters have not been described.

Neurological Findings. Recurrent episodes of choking, dysphagia, or vomiting with lethargy, weakness, and incoordination lasting several days punctuate a course of poor developmental progress and neurological deterioration. Deafness, optic atrophy, and esotropia are noted by 1 year. Paralysis of ocular move-

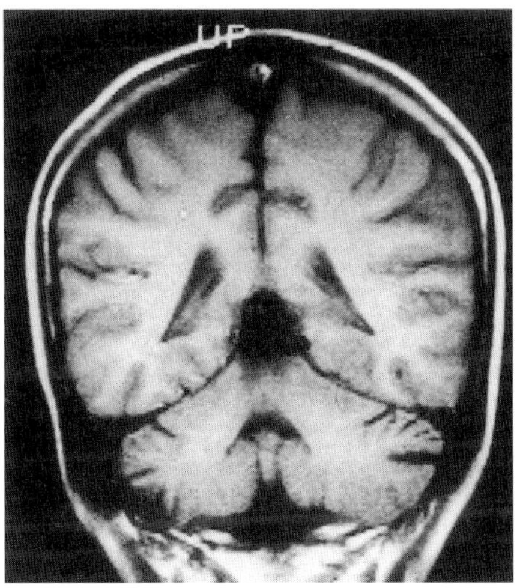

X-Linked Ataxia-Deafness-Dementia. Magnetic resonance image showing prominent cerebellar folia and enlarged fourth ventricle. Courtesy of Dr. Morris Levinsohn, Beachwood, Ohio.

ments may occur late in the course. Neuromuscular findings include ataxia of head, trunk and limbs, dysmetria, tremors, head titubation, depressed deep tendon reflexes, and hypotonia. Seizures develop after a few years and death from pneumonia occurs by age 2 years. Spasticity may be a late manifestation.

HETEROZYGOTE EXPRESSION. One mother had two episodes in adult life with ataxia and confusion. Brain imaging showed cerebellar atrophy and enlargement of the fourth ventricle.

NEUROPATHOLOGY. Postmortem examination has shown neuronal loss and gliosis in the brain stem and cerebellum. The dentate nucleus and inferior olive are invariably involved. Diffuse gliosis was present in the cerebellum with loss of myelinated fibers in the white matter and loss of Purkinje and granule cells in the cortex.

COMMENT. Although the recurrence of vomiting, lethargy, and incoordination suggests a metabolic disturbance, none has been found. A similar condition but without deafness and recurrent episodes of vomiting, lethargy, and incoordination has been reported by Malamud and Cohen.

REFERENCES

Malamud N, Cohen P: Unusual form of cerebellar ataxia with X-linked inheritance. Neurology 8:261, 1958.

Schmidley JW, Morris W, Levinsohn MW, et al.: Infantile X-linked ataxia and deafness: a new clinicopathologic entity. Neurology 37:1344, 1987.

Differential Matrix

Syndrome	Ataxia	Hearing Loss	Vision Loss	Comments
X-linked ataxia-deafness-dementia	+	+	+	Optic atrophy, spastic paraplegia, hypotonia, childhood death
Arts	+	+	+	Growth deficiency, paucity of muscles, hypotonia, areflexia, seizures, childhood death
Gustavson	+	+	+	Microcephaly, short stature, optic atrophy with blindness, large ears, joint contractures, rockerbottom feet, brain undergrowth, hydrocephaly, cerebellar hypoplasia, spasticity, seizures
Mohr-Tranebjaerg (Jensen)	+	+	+	Neurologic deterioration with childhood onset, dystonia, spasticity
Proud	+	+	+	Microcephaly, agenesis of corpus callosum, cryptorchidism, inguinal hernias, spasticity, seizures
Adrenoleukodystrophy	0	+	+	Adrenal insufficiency, diffuse skin pigmentation, spastic paraplegia, progressive neurologic deterioration and dementia, elevated long chain fatty acids in plasma
Paine	0	+	+	Microcephaly, short stature, optic atrophy, spasticity, seizures
Schimke	0	+	+	Microcephaly, sunken eyes, downslanting palpebral fissures, narrow nose, spacing of teeth, cupped ears, hypotonia, abducens palsy, spasticity, choreoathetosis, contractures
Wittwer	0	+	+	Growth deficiency, microcephaly, microphthalmia, hypertelorism, genitourinary anomalies, hypotonia, seizures
Goldblatt spastic paraplegia	+	0	+	Optic atrophy, exotropia, nystagmus, spastic paraplegia, dysarthria, muscle hypoplasia, contractures
Pelizaeus-Merzbacher	+	0	+	Optic atrophy, nystagmus, hypotonia, spasticity, dystonia, CNS dysmyelination

X-LINKED ATAXIA-DEMENTIA

(XLMR-Ataxia, MIM 301840)

DEFINITION. X-linked progressive ataxia, pyramidal signs, and adult-onset dementia. Close linkage has not been found but most of Xp and distal Xq (Xq26-qter) have been excluded.

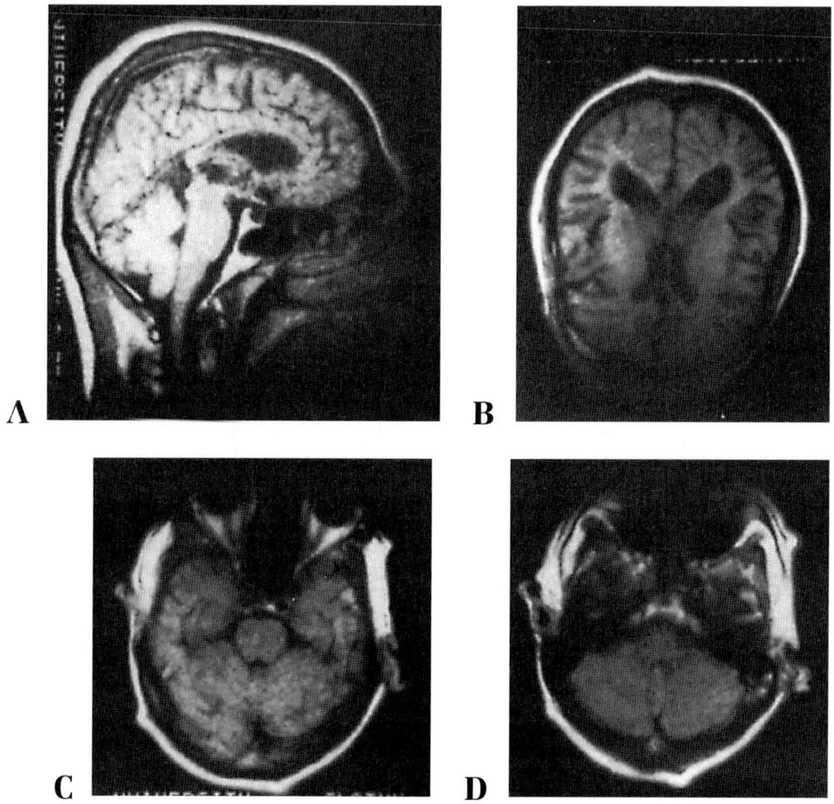

X-Linked Ataxia-Dementia. Midsagittal (A) and axial (B–D) magnetic resonance images of brain of 55-year-old man showing generalized cortical atrophy, but normal pons and cerebellum. Courtesy of Dr. Martin Farlow, Indiana University School of Medicine, Indianapolis, Indiana.

SOMATIC FEATURES. Affected males have no distinctive facial features or growth aberrations. Motor and language milestones are moderately delayed and clumsiness and tremors mark childhood. Incoordination of gait and intention tremor are demonstrable but mild during childhood. Ataxia and pyramidal tract signs progressively intensify during adult life and may lead to near-total incapacitation in the fourth or fifth decades. Muscle weakness and extrapyramidal signs do not occur. Cognitive impairment is not apparent during childhood although some affected persons have not completed secondary schooling. Dementia begins in early adulthood, heralded by forgetfulness, confusion, disorientation, and loss of cognitive skills. Mood swings with emotional lability accompany the dementia.

GROWTH AND DEVELOPMENT. No abnormalities of growth are reported. Motor and language milestones are delayed with walking and first words between ages 2 and 3 years.

COGNITIVE FEATURES. Impairment during childhood has not been documented. Cognitive deterioration begins as early as the fourth decade and progresses.

Neurological Findings. Progressive neurological changes dominate the clinical picture: The clumsiness of childhood evolves by early adult life into frank incoordination, unsteady gait, intention tremors, increased tone and deep tendon reflexes, and Babinski signs. Lower limbs are affected to a greater degree.

Imaging. CT and MRI show cortical atrophy but no specific abnormality of cerebellum, olivary nuclei, or white matter.

Comment. The findings in X-linked ataxia-dementia have also been reported as cerebello-olivary degeneration. Patients with similar neurologic course but without dementia have been reported by Spira et al. and Shokier. A more severe deterioration was noted in a family with mental retardation, ataxia, tremors, dysarthria, extrapyramidal signs, and death in childhood, reported by Malamud and Cohen. Adult-onset dementia, ataxia, and pyramidal signs occur in Mohr-Tranebjaerg syndrome but the optic atrophy, blindness, and mutation in the XLMR-dystonia-deafness protein (DDP) gene have not been found in the ataxia-dementia syndrome. Adrenoleukodystrophy may be excluded by normal long-chain fatty acids and the absence of leukodystrophy on brain imaging.

REFERENCES

Carter RH, Sukavanjana C: Familial cerebello-olivary degeneration with late development of rigidity and dementia. Neurology 6:876, 1956.

Farlow MR, DeMyer W, Dlouhy SR, et al.: X-linked recessive inheritance of ataxia and adult-onset dementia: clinical features and preliminary linkage analysis. Neurology 37:602, 1987.

Malamud N, Cohen P: Unusual form of cerebellar ataxia with sex-linked inheritance. Neurology 8:261, 1958.

Shokeir MHK: X-linked cerebellar ataxia. Clin Genet 1:225, 1970.

Spira PJ, McLeod JG, Evans WA: A spinocerebellar degeneration with X-linked inheritance. Brain 102:27, 1979.

Tranebjaerg L, Lou H, Andreesen J: New X-linked syndrome with apraxia, ataxia, and mental deficiency: clinical, cytogenetic and neuropsychological studies in two Danish families. Am J Med Genet 43:498, 1992.

Differential Matrix

Syndrome	Ataxia	Spasticity	Tremors or Rigidity	Comments
X-linked ataxia-dementia	+	+	+	Adult-onset dementia
Arena	+	+	+	Muscle hypoplasia, clubfoot, iron deposits in basal ganglia, dystonia
Pelizaeus-Merzbacher	+	+	+	Optic atrophy, nystagmus, hypotonia, dystonia, CNS dysmyelination
Pettigrew	+	+	+	Dandy-Walker malformation, seizures, microcephaly or hydrocephaly, long face with macrostomia, small testes, contractures, choreoathetosis, iron deposits in basal ganglia
Adrenoleukodystrophy	+	+	0	Adrenal insufficiency, diffuse skin pigmentation, progressive neurologic deterioration and dementia, elevated long chain fatty acids in plasma
Allan-Herndon-Dudley	+	+	0	Large ears with cupping or abnormal architecture, muscle hypoplasia, childhood hypotonia, contractures, dysarthria, athetosis
Apak ataxia-spastic diplegia	+	+	0	Short stature, clubfoot, muscle hypoplasia
Goldblatt spastic paraplegia	+	+	0	Optic atrophy, exotropia, nystagmus, dysarthria, muscle hypoplasia, contractures
Mohr-Tranebjaerg (Jensen)	+	+	0	Hearing loss, vision loss, neurologic deterioration with childhood onset, dystonia
X-linked hydrocephaly-MASA spectrum	+	+	0	Hydrocephaly, adducted thumbs, dysgenesis of corpus callosum
XLMR-ataxia-deafness-dementia	+	+	0	Optic atrophy, vision loss, hearing loss, hypotonia, seizures, childhood death
Lesch-Nyhan	0	+	+	Choreoathetosis, self-mutilation, hyperuricemia
PPM-X	0	+	+	Macroorchidism, psychosis, parkinsonian features
Waisman-Laxova	0	+	+	-
XLMR-spastic paraplegia-athetosis	0	+	+	Nystagmus, weakness, dysarthria, muscle wasting, contractures
XLMR-ataxia-apraxia	+	0	+	Prominent forehead, large ears, uncoordinated movements, hypotonia, seizures

X-LINKED BRANCHIAL ARCH SYNDROME

(Toriello Branchial Arch Syndrome, MIM 301950)

DEFINITION. XLMR with microcephaly, branchial arch defects, hearing loss, and cryptorchidism.
SOMATIC FEATURES. Microcephaly, hypertelorism, sparseness of lateral eyebrows, epicanthus, ptosis, downslanting palpebral fissures, flat malar area, high broad nasal bridge, anteverted nares, cupped and/or low-set ears, preauricular pits, high palate, long upper lip, flat philtrum, and micrognathia give a distinctive appearance. Facial and limb asymmetry, broad neck, and cryptorchidism may occur. The ear canals may be stenotic and mixed hearing loss is typical.
GROWTH AND DEVELOPMENT. Head circumference is small and stature tends to be in the lower percentiles.
COGNITIVE FEATURES. No formal testing available but cognitive function is considered mildly delayed.
NEUROLOGICAL FINDINGS. Normal.
HETEROZYGOTE EXPRESSION. None.
COMMENT. The phenotype is based on a single family with three affected males. On the basis of pedigree structure, microcephaly, and cryptorchidism, they appear to differ from other branchial arch syndromes (Treacher Collins, otofaciocervical, branchioskeletogenital, branchiootorenal, and oculoauriculovertebral syndromes).

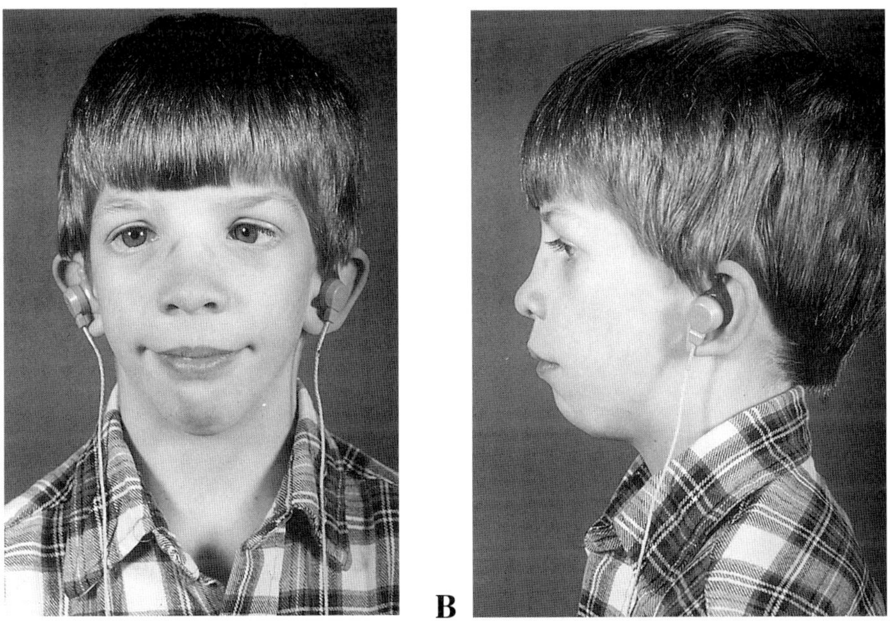

A B

X-Linked Branchial Arch Syndrome. Microcephaly, triangular face, sparse lateral eyebrows, downslanting palpebral fissures, broad nasal bridge, malar hypoplasia, micrognathia, and cupped ears in a 10-year-old boy (A–C).

C 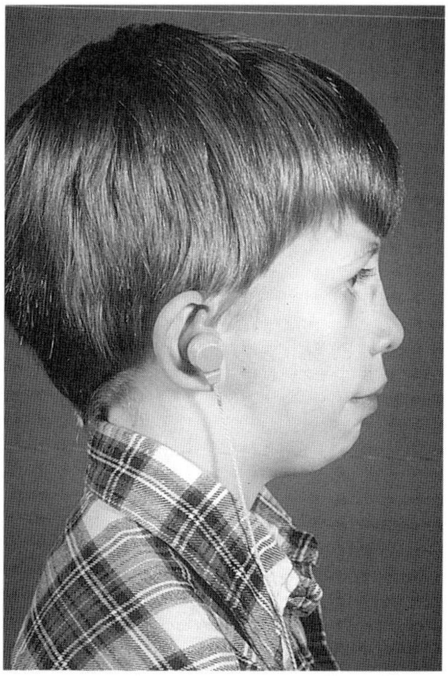

D 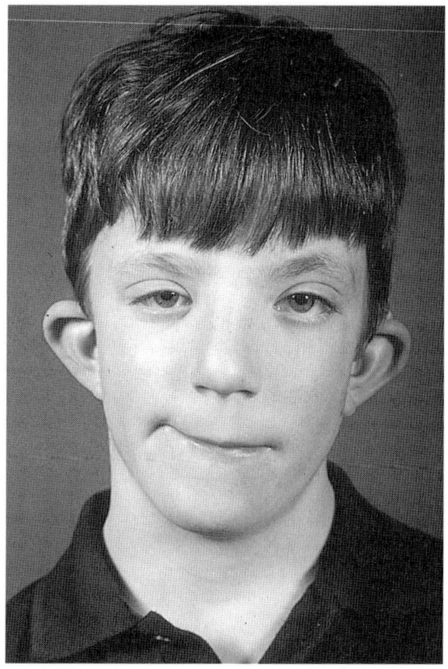

E 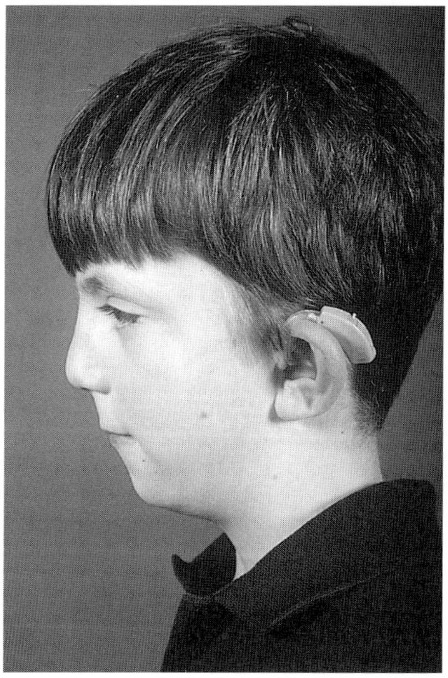

F 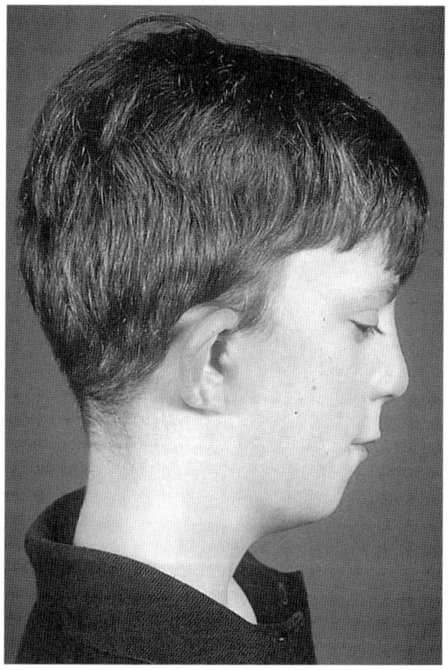

X-Linked Branchial Arch Syndrome. (continued) Microcephaly, triangular face, sparse lateral eyebrows, downslanting palpebral fissures, broad nasal bridge, malar hypoplasia, micrognathia, and cupped ears in a 10-year-old boy (A–C); microcephaly, facial asymmetry, ptosis, high and broad nasal bridge, cupped ears, smooth philtrum with thin upper lip, epicanthus, sparse lateral eyebrows and micrognathia in a 10-year-old cousin (D–F). Courtesy of Dr. James Higgins, Spectrum Health, Grand Rapids, Michigan.

REFERENCE

Toriello HV, Higgins JV, Abrahamson J, et al.: X-linked syndrome of branchial arch and other defects. Am J Med Genet 21:137, 1985.

Differential Matrix

Syndrome	Micro-cephaly	Malformed Ears	Hearing Loss	Comments
X-linked branchial arch	+	+	+	Branchial arch defects, micrognathia, facial and limb asymmetry
Coffin-Lowry	+	+	+	Short stature, bitemporal narrowing, almond-shaped eyes, depressed nasal bridge, tented upper lip, open mouth, hypogonadism, hypotonia, obesity
Gustavson	+	+	+	Short stature, optic atrophy with blindness, large ears, joint contractures, rockerbottom feet, brain undergrowth, hydrocephaly, cerebellar hypoplasia, spasticity, seizures
Lenz microphthalmia	+	+	+	Microphthalmia, ocular dysgenesis, cleft lip/palate, cardiac and genitourinary anomalies, thumb duplication or hypoplasia, narrow shoulders
Proud	+	+	+	Vision loss, agenesis of corpus callosum, cryptorchidism, inguinal hernias, ataxia, spasticity, seizures
Schimke	+	+	+	Sunken eyes, downslanting palpebral fissures, narrow nose, spacing of teeth, hypotonia, abducens palsy, vision loss, spasticity, choreoathetosis, contractures
XLMR-hypotonic facies (Carpenter-Waziri) (Holmes-Gang) (Juberg-Marsidi)	+	+	+	Short stature, small testes, telecanthus, small triangular nose, tented upper lip, open mouth, spacing of teeth, genital anomalies, musculoskeletal anomalies, hemoglobin H inclusions in erythrocytes
Paine	+	0	+	Short stature, optic atrophy, vision loss, spasticity, seizures
Pettigrew	+	0	+	Dandy-Walker malformation, spasticity, seizures, microcephaly or hydrocephaly, long face with macrostomia, small testes, contractures, choreoathetosis, iron deposits in basal ganglia
Wittwer	+	0	+	Growth deficiency, microphthalmia, vision loss, hypertelorism, genitourinary anomalies, hypotonia, seizures

X-Linked Hereditary Bullous Dystrophy

(Macular-Type Bullous Dystrophy, MIM 302000)

Definition. XLMR with short stature, microcephaly, alopecia, macular bullous dystrophy, tapered fingers, and hypogenitalism. The gene maps distal to DXS998 in Xq27.3.

Somatic Features. Microcephaly, scalp alopecia, upslanting palpebral fissures, and protruding ears give the face its characteristic appearance. The corneas may be cloudy. Alopecia begins before birth or during the first year of life. Bullous lesions usually make their appearance during the first year as well. The lesions consist of macules or papules on sun-exposed surfaces, particularly the face and dorsal surface of the hands and lips. Some lesions are vesicular and leave hypopigmented or hyperpigmented areas upon resolution. Cutaneous cancer has been noted in at least one case. Cataracts may develop in adult life. The teeth are normal and nail dystrophy has been noted in only one case. The fingers are short and tapered and may show acrocyanosis. The testes may be small or undescended. Incompletely characterized heart defects appear to be common. One case had pulmonary valve stenosis and a right-sided conduction defect. Death in childhood or early adult life from pulmonary infections is not unusual.

Growth and Development. Markedly slow growth is evident at birth and catch-up growth does not occur. All growth parameters are affected.

Cognitive Features. Most cases appear to have mental retardation, although the severity has not been reported.

Heterozygote Expression. None.

Imaging. Except for its small size, brain structure is normal.

Comment. Although a defect in the immune system has been suspected as an underlying factor in the respiratory infections that lead to death in childhood or early adult life, no such defect has been demonstrated.

REFERENCES

Lungarotti MS, Martello C, Barboni G, et al.: X-linked mental retardation, microcephaly, and growth delay associated with hereditary bullous dystrophy macular type: report of a second family. Am J Med Genet 51:598, 1994.

Mendes da Costa S, Van der Valk JW: Typus maculatus der bullosen hereditären dystrophie. Arch Derm Syph 91:1, 1908.

Wijker M, Ligtenberg JL, Schoute F, et al.: The gene for hereditary bullous dystrophy, X-linked macular type, maps to the Xq27.3-qter region. Am J Hum Genet 56:1096, 1995.

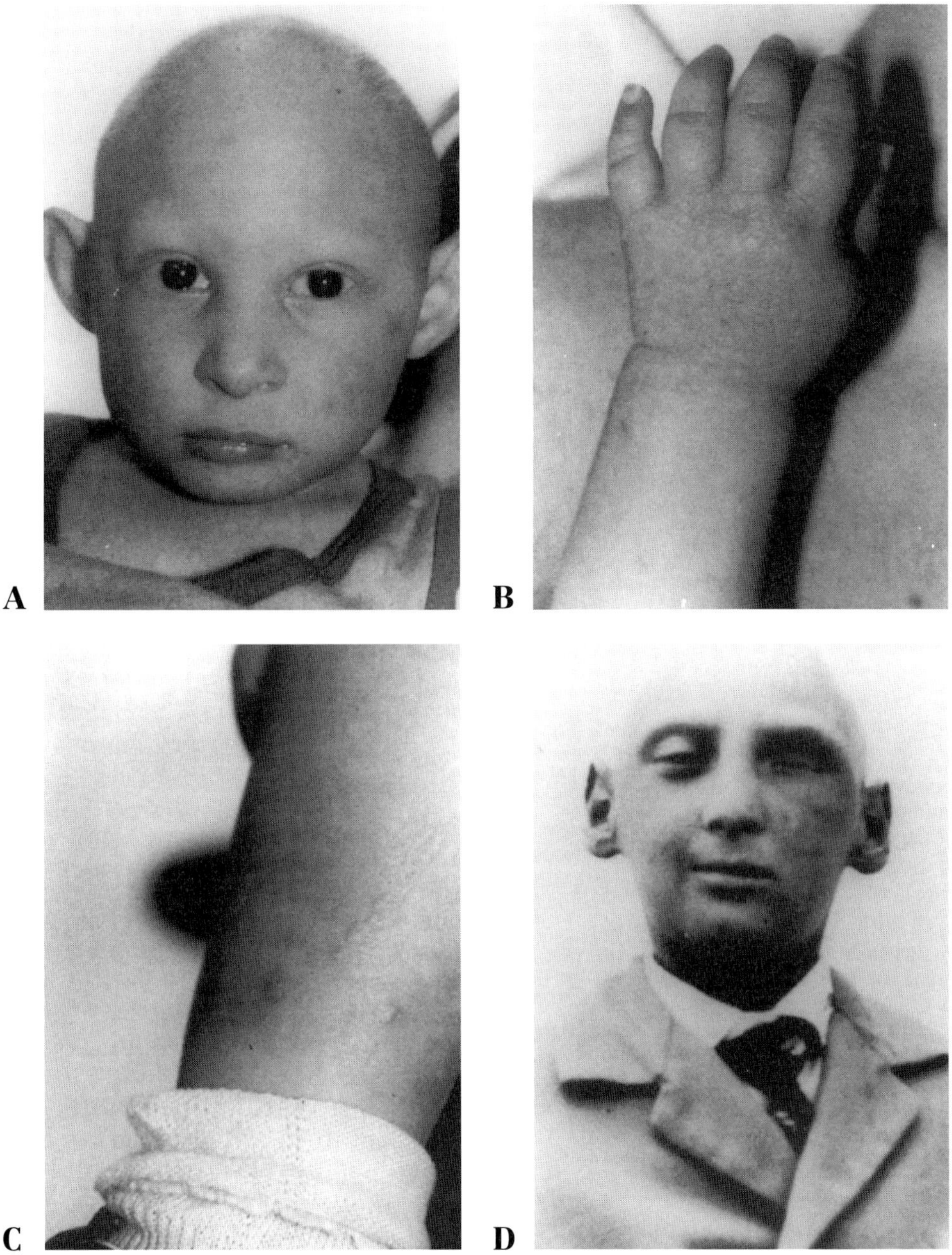

X-Linked Hereditary Bullous Dystrophy. Microcephaly, alopecia, protruding ears, upslanting palpebral fissures, tapered fingers and macular, papular, and vesicular lesions on the forearm and legs (A–C); microcephaly and alopecia in a maternal uncle (D). Courtesy of Dr. Serena Lungarotti, University of Perugia, Perugia, Italy.

Differential Matrix

Syndrome	Micro-cephaly	Cutaneous Lesions	Cardiac Defects	Comments
X-linked hereditary bullous dystrophy	+	+	+	Short stature, upslanting palpebral fissures, protruding ears, digits short and tapered, bullous dystrophy, small testes, early death from pulmonary infection
Golabi-Ito-Hall	+	+	+	Short stature, telecanthus, high nasal root, cupped ears, cardiac malformation, thoracic asymmetry, sacral dimple, dry/brittle/sparse hair, cutis marmorata, nail hypoplasia
Cantu	+	+	0	Short stature, alopecia, hyperpigmented lesions, follicular keratosis, cortical atrophy, seizures, pancytopenia
Goltz	+	+	0	Cataracts, ocular dysgenesis, linear areas of dermal aplasia, cutaneous adipose herniations, dystrophic nails, abnormal teeth and hair, vertebral anomalies, limb reduction defects, genitourinary anomalies
Fitzsimmons	0	+	+	Pes cavus, hyperkeratosis of palms and soles, dystrophic nails, spastic paraplegia
MIDAS	0	+	+	Microphthalmia, ocular dysgenesis, corneal opacification, dermal aplasia, dysgenesis of corpus callosum, cardio-myopathy

X-LINKED HYDROCEPHALY–MASA SPECTRUM

(Complicated Spastic Paraplegia, Spastic Paraplegia 1, XLMR–Clasp Thumb, Mental Retardation–Aplasia–Shuffling Gait–Adducted Thumbs Syndrome, X-Linked Hydrocephalus–Stenosis of Aqueduct of Sylvius, L1 Syndrome, MIM 303350, 312900, 307000)

DEFINITION. XLMR with hydrocephalus, adducted thumbs, and spastic paraplegia. The causative gene, L1 cell adhesion molecule, is located in distal Xq28.

SOMATIC FEATURES. Severe hydrocephalus leads to intrauterine or neonatal death in many cases. Dilation of the cerebral ventricles, present in about half of

→

X-Linked Hydrocephaly–MASA Syndrome. Infant showing massive hydrocephaly and clasp thumb (A); massive hydrocephaly on sagittal magnetic resonance imaging (B); clasp thumb in newborn infant (C); adult with microcephaly and flexed positioning of thumbs (D–F). Figures B and C courtesy of Dr. Connie Schrander-Stumpel, Clinical Genetics Center, Maastricht, Netherlands.

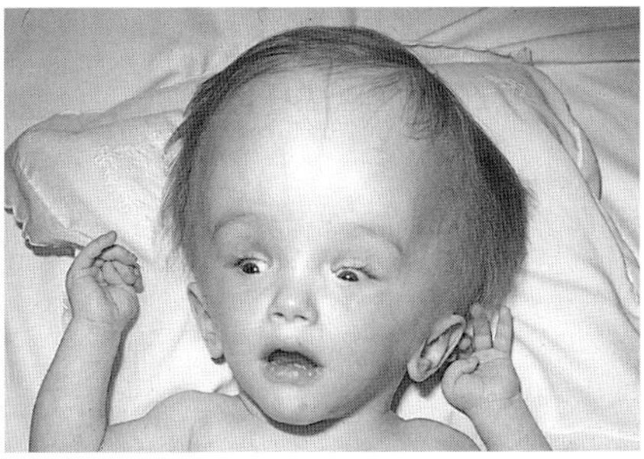
A

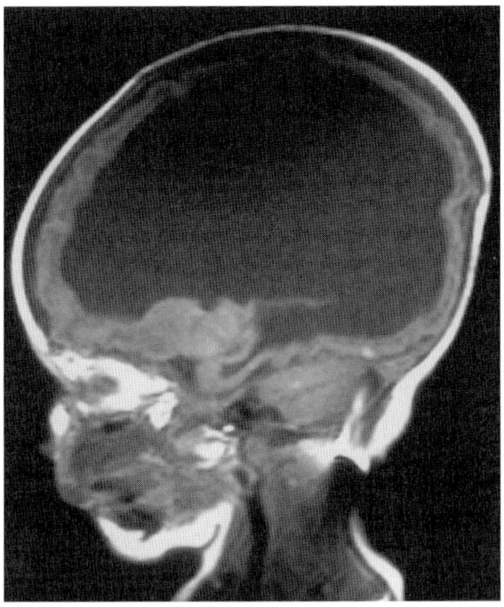
B

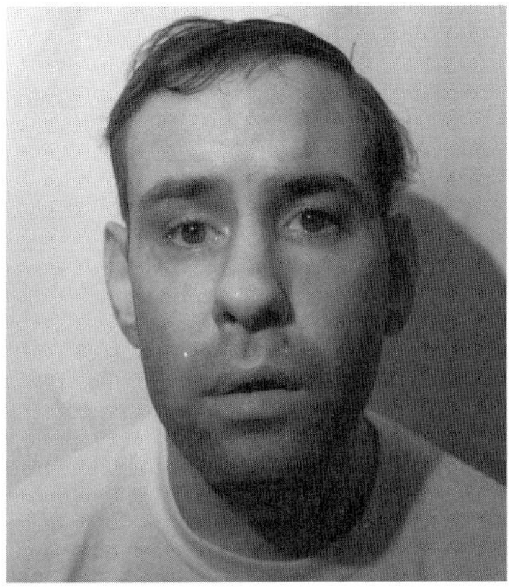
D

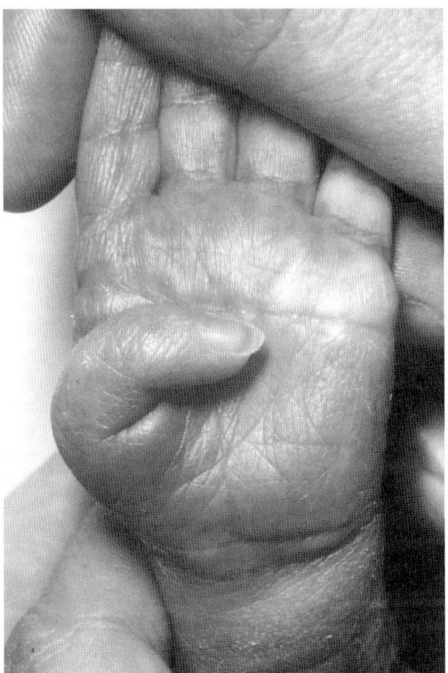
C

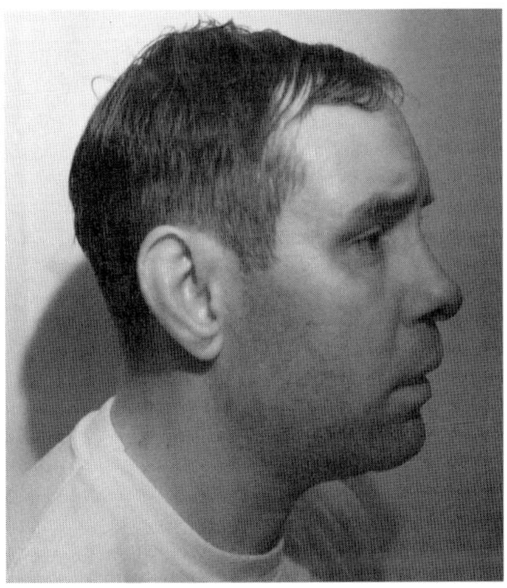
E

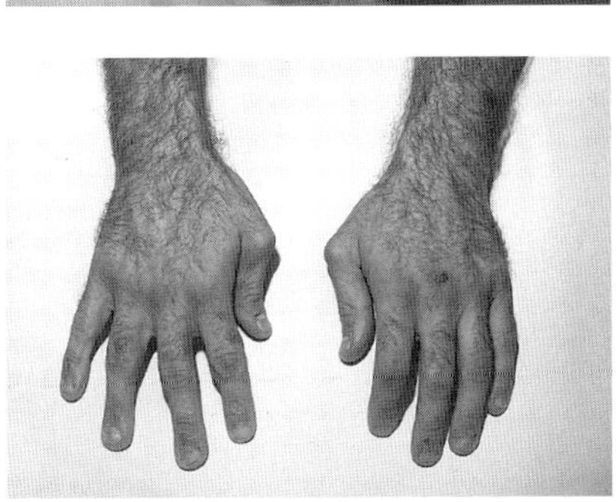
F

survivors, underlies the variable macrocephaly. Dygenesis of the corpus callosum has been noted in a third of cases. Although a wide range of craniofacial features other than the large head size have been described, none has proven to be consistently present. Clasp thumb, secondary to deficiency of the extensor pollicis muscle or abductor pollicis muscle, or hypoplasia of the thumb with underdevelopment of the thenar eminence is found in most cases.

GROWTH AND DEVELOPMENT. In most cases, statural growth is normal but may measure in the lower centiles. Hip and knee flexion may falsely lower the height measurement. Macrocephaly of variable degree occurs and is dependent at least in part on dilation of the cerebral ventricles. Motor and speech milestones are mildly to moderately delayed. Slow motor development is most notable in males with hypotonia.

COGNITIVE FEATURES. Impairment of cognitive function is quite variable; some patients function in the lower range of normal while others have profound mental retardation. There appears to be a correlation between the severity of cognitive impairment and degree of hydrocephaly.

NEUROLOGICAL FINDINGS. Although motor and speech development is delayed from the outset, neurological changes are delayed in some patients until later in childhood or the teen years. Hypotonia in early childhood is associated with slow motor development. Spasticity, manifest by hyperactive deep tendon reflexes, Babinski signs, shuffling gait, and less so by increased muscle tone, usually begins in school age. The severity of mental retardation tends to correlate with the degree of hydrocephaly and the level of spasticity.

HETEROZYGOTE EXPRESSION. Carrier females usually show no evidence of hydrocephaly, thumb anomalies, gait disturbance, spasticity, or cognitive impairment. Skewed X-inactivation has been suggested as the explanation for expression (cognitive function lower than noncarrier sisters, hydrocephalus, adducted thumbs) in a few carrier females.

COMMENT. Linkage analysis and mutational analysis of the L1CAM gene has permitted the inclusion of four entities previously considered separate—X-linked hydrocephalus, MASA syndrome, XLMR–clasp thumb syndrome, and complicated spastic paraplegia 1—into a single spectrum. Preliminary evidence suggests that the phenotype can be correlated with the type of mutation affecting the L1CAM gene. Mutations that result in truncated L1CAM protein give rise to a severe phenotype. This probably results from the loss of the extracellular domain responsible for cell–cell and cell–matrix interactions. Mutations affecting the cytoplasmic domain at the carboxyl end are not as severe since only the cytoplasmic signal pathway is affected. Lastly, missense mutations in the extracellular domains produce a variety of phenotypes. The length of infant survival is associated with the location of missense mutations; those in key residues of either the immunoglobulin (Ig) or fibronectin (FN) domains result in survival of less than 1 year.

REFERENCES

Bianchine JW, Lewis RC Jr: The MASA syndrome: a new heritable mental retardation syndrome. Clin Genet 5:298, 1974.

Bickers DA, Adams RD: Hereditary stenosis of the aqueduct of Sylvius as a cause of congenital hydrocephalus. Brain 72:246, 1949.
Boyd E, Schwartz CE, Schroer RJ, et al.: Agenesis of the corpus callosum associated with MASA syndrome. Clin Dysmorphol 2:332, 1993.
Jouet M, Rosenthal A, MacFarlane J, et al.: A missense mutation confirms the L1 defect in X-linked hydrocephalus. Nat Genet 4:331, 1993.
Schrander-Stumpel C, Höweler C, Jones M, et al.: The spectrum of X-linked hydrocephalus (HSAS), MASA syndrome, and complicated spastic paraplegia (SPG1): clinical review with six additional families. Am J Med Genet 56:1, 1995.
Vits L, Van Camp G, Coucke P, et al.: MASA syndrome is due to mutations in the neural cell adhesion gene L1CAM. Nat Genet 7:408, 1994.

Differential Matrix

Syndrome	Hydro-cephaly	Agenesis of Corpus Callosum	Spasticity	Comments
X-linked hydrocephaly-MASA spectrum	+	+	+	Adducted thumbs
Brooks	+	+	+	Microcephaly, short stature, deep-set eyes, blepharophimosis, cupped ears, bulbous nose, small mouth, thin upper lip, pectus excavatum, flexion contractures
Kang	+	+	+	Microcephaly, frontal prominence, telecanthus, small nose, short hands, seizures, downslanted mouth, brachydactyly
Proud	+	+	+	Microcephaly, hearing loss, vision loss, cryptorchidism, inguinal hernias, ataxia, seizures
Pyruvate dehydrogenase deficiency	0	+	+	Lactic acidosis, microcephaly, hypotonia, ataxia, dysarthria, CNS anomalies
Gustavson	+	0	+	Microcephaly, short stature, optic atrophy with blindness, large ears, deafness, joint contractures, rockerbottom feet, brain undergrowth, cerebellar hypoplasia, seizures
Pettigrew	+	0	+	Dandy-Walker malformation, seizures, microcephaly or hydrocephaly, long face with macrostomia and prognathism, small testes, contractures, choreoathetosis, iron deposits in basal ganglia
VACTERL-hydrocephalus	+	0	+	Vertebral anomalies, radial limb defects, tracheal and esophageal anomalies, renal malformations, anal anomalies
XLMR-hydrocephaly-basal ganglia calcifications	+	0	+	Calcifications of basal ganglia, muscle hypoplasia, sensory impairment

X-LINKED LISSENCEPHALY

(X-Linked Lissencephaly–Agenesis of Corpus Callosum, Subcortical Band Heterotopia, MIM 300067)

DEFINITION. XLMR with microcephaly, defect in neuronal migration, hypoplastic genitalia, hypotonia, spasticity, and seizures. The gene, doublecortin (DCX), is located in Xq22.3.

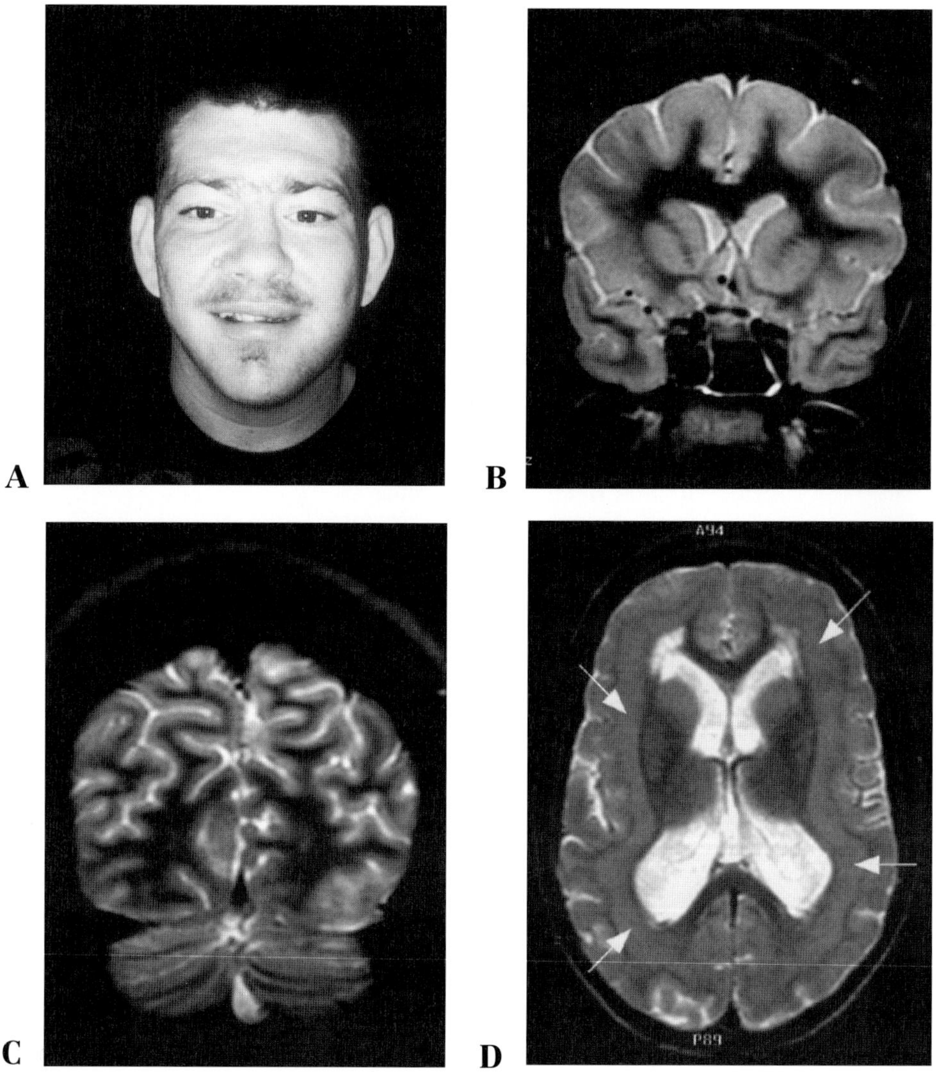

X-Linked Lissencephaly. Microcephaly, upslanted palpebral fissures, and otherwise normal facies in a 32-year-old male (A); coronal section of frontal cortex as seen with MRI showing pachygyria (B); coronal section from posterior parietal cortex showing normal gyral pattern (C); axial section from carrier female showing subcortical band heterotopia [arrows] (D). Illustration D courtesy of Dr. Joseph Gleeson, Beth Israel Deaconess Medical Center, Boston.

SOMATIC FEATURES. The craniofacial features are not distinctive and major malformations outside the central nervous system do not occur. Cranial size is small and the brain has variable evidence of defective neuronal migration. In males, this is usually evident as frontal pachygyria, and in females as subcortical band heterotopia. Less commonly, males have agyria, polymicrogyria, and dysgenesis of the corpus callosum. The genitalia are underdeveloped.

GROWTH AND DEVELOPMENT. Males have very limited development and have failure of growth including microcephaly.

NEUROLOGICAL FINDINGS. Beginning soon after birth, males develop seizures of a variety of types—tonic, tonic-clonic, myoclonic, and infantile spasms. Hypotonia, spasticity, or both (truncal hypotonia with hypertonia and hyperreflexia of the limbs) occur.

NATURAL HISTORY. Seizures begin soon after birth and are poorly controlled by anticonvulsants. There is little psychomotor progress, limited environmental interaction, and poor growth. Death occurs the first year of life, usually in the first months.

HETEROZYGOTE EXPRESSION. Females often have mild to moderate mental retardation, but some have normal intelligence and others severe mental retardation. In childhood, there may be psychomotor delay, behavioral problems, and hyperactivity. Seizures usually begin in childhood, but may not begin until young adulthood, and are of various types—tonic, tonic-clonic, atonic, atypical absence, partial complex, infantile spasms, Lennox-Gastaut.

NEUROPATHOLOGY. Neuronal migration defect with agygria and pachygyria in males and subcortical band heterotopia in females.

IMAGING. In males, pachygyria (particularly frontal), agygria (posterior), agenesis of corpus callosum, dilated ventricles, and cerebellar vermis hypoplasia occur. In females, there is a layer of gray matter heterotopia between the cortex and ventricles, separated from the cortex by white matter. The thickness of this heterotopic band correlates with the severity of the cognitive impairment and of the seizures.

REFERENCES

Berry-Kravis E, Israel J: X-linked pachygyria and agenesis of the corpus callosum: evidence for X chromosome lissencephaly locus. Ann Neurol 36:229, 1994.

des Portes V, Pinard JM, Smadja D, et al.: Dominant X linked subcortical laminar heterotopia and lissencephaly syndrome (XSCLH/LIS): evidence for the occurrence of mutation in males and mapping of a potential locus in Xq22. J Med Genet 34:177, 1997.

des Portes V, Pinard JM, Billuart P, et al.: A novel CNS gene required for neuronal migration and involved in X-linked subcortical laminar heterotopia and lissencephaly syndrome. Cell 92:51, 1998.

Dobyns WB, Andermann E, Andermann F, et al.: X-linked malformations of neuronal migration. Neurology 47:321, 1996.

Gleeson JG, Allen KM, Fox JW, et al.: *Doublecortin,* a brain specific gene mutated in human X-linked lissencephaly and double cortex syndrome, encodes a putative signaling protein. Cell 92:63, 1998.

Sossey-Alaoui K, Hartung AJ, Guerrini R, et al.: Human *doublecortin (DCX)* and the homologous gene in mouse encode a putative Ca^{2+}-dependent signaling protein which is mutated in human X-linked neuronal migration defects. Hum Mol Genet 7:1327, 1998.

Srivastava AK, Ross ME, Allen KM, et al.: X-linked lissencephaly and SBH (XLIS): mapping of a novel neuronal migration gene. Am J Hum Genet 59 (Suppl):A55, 1996.

Differential Matrix

Syndrome	Lissencephaly or Cerebral Heterotopia	Dysgenesis of Corpus Callosum	Seizures	Comments
X-linked lissencephaly	+	+	+	Defect in neuronal migration resulting in frontal pachygyria in males and subcortical band heterotopia in carrier females, hypotonia, spasticity, genital hypoplasia
Aicardi	+	+	+	Ocular dysgenesis, lacunar retinopathy, costovertebral anomalies
Bertini	0	+	+	Macular degeneration, hypotonia, ataxia, childhood death, hypoplasia of cerebellar vermis and corpus callosum, developmental delays and regression, postnatal growth impairment
Brooks	0	+	+	Microcephaly, short stature, deep-set eyes, blepharophimosis, cupped ears, bulbous nose, small mouth, thin upper lip, pectus excavatum, flexion contractures
Kang	0	+	+	Microcephaly, frontal prominence, telecanthus, small nose, short hands, downslanted mouth, brachydactyly
Opitz FG	0	+	+	Macrocephaly, broad forehead, downslanted palpebral fissures, everted lower lip, cardiac defects, imperforate anus, constipation, broad flat thumbs and great toes, hypotonia
Proud	0	+	+	Microcephaly, hearing loss, vision loss, cryptorchidism, inguinal hernias, ataxia, spasticity
Pyruvate deyhydrogenase deficiency	0	+	+	Lactic acidosis, microcephaly, hypotonia, ataxia, dysarthria, CNS anomalies

X-LINKED OPTIC ATROPHY

(Went syndrome, Optic Atrophy–2, MIM 311050)

DEFINITION. XLMR with optic atrophy, ataxia, tremors, absent ankle deep tendon reflexes, and emotional lability. The gene has not been mapped.

SOMATIC FEATURES. Major malformations or craniofacial manifestations do not occur. Ocular and neurologic findings predominate. Bilateral optic atrophy begins early, perhaps being present at birth, and is slowly progressive. The optic discs appear pale and commonly are cupped. Retinal vessels may have abnormal origin and course. Peripheral visual fields are normal, but central scotomas or enlarged physiological blind spots have been demonstrated. Color vision may be defective as a secondary phenomenon. Neurologic dysfunction presents in the form of gait disturbance, ataxia, tremors, dysdiadochokinesis, hyperactive deep tendon reflexes at the knees but absent ankle reflexes, and Babinski signs. The Achilles tendons may be short. Clubfoot or kyphosis may occur.

GROWTH AND DEVELOPMENT. Details of growth have not been reported.

COGNITIVE FEATURES. Early schooling difficulties have been noted, in part related to visual impairment. Adults show mild cognitive impairment.

BEHAVIORAL MANIFESTATIONS. Emotional lability has been described in some cases.

NEUROLOGICAL FINDINGS. Neurological abnormalities, primarily involuntary movements, pathological reflexes, gait disturbances, dysdiadochokinesis, and dysarthria vary in severity and time of onset. Typically, the deep tendon reflexes at the knees are hyperactive and at the ankles depressed or absent.

HETEROZYGOTE EXPRESSION. Carrier females have normal ocular and neurological findings.

COMMENT. The phenotype is based on a single family with eight affected males in three generations. It is possible that this entity stems from a contiguous gene deletion syndrome rather than a single gene mutation.

REFERENCES

Völker-Dieben HJ, Van Lith GHM, Went LN, et al.: A family with sex-linked optic atrophy (ophthalmological and neurological aspects). Doc Ophthalmol 37:307, 1974.

Went LN, De Vries-De Mol EC, Völker-Dieben HJ: A family with apparently sex-linked optic atrophy. J Med Genet 12:94, 1975.

Differential Matrix

Syndrome	Vision Loss	Tremors	Abnormal Deep Tendon Reflexes	Comments
X-linked optic atrophy	+	+	+	Optic atrophy, ataxia, dysarthria, gait disturbance, emotional lability
X-linked ataxia-deafness-demetia	+	+	+	Optic atrophy, hearing loss, spastic paraplegia, ataxia, hypotonia, seizures, childhood death
Arts	+	0	+	Growth deficiency, paucity of muscles, hypotonia, areflexia, ataxia, deafness, seizures, childhood death
Gustavson	+	0	+	Microcephaly, short stature, large ears, deafness, joint contractures, rockerbottom feet, brain undergrowth, hydrocephaly, cerebellar hypoplasia, spasticity, seizures
Mohr-Tranebjaerg (Jensen)	+	0	+	Hearing loss, neurologic deterioration with childhood onset, dystonia, spasticity
Paine	+	0	+	Microcephaly, short stature, optic atrophy, hearing loss, spasticity, seizures
Proud	+	0	+	Microcephaly, hearing loss, agenesis of corpus callosum, cryptorchidism, inguinal hernias, ataxia, spasticity, seizures
Schimke	+	0	+	Microcephaly, sunken eyes, downslanting palpebral fissures, narrow nose, spacing of teeth, cupped ears, hypotonia, abducens palsy, hearing loss, spasticity, choreoathetosis, contractures

X-LINKED SPASTIC PARAPLEGIA, TYPE 7

(X-Linked Spastic Paraplegia)

DEFINITION. XLMR with nystagmus, reduced vision, absent speech and ambulation, bowel and bladder dysfunction, and spastic quadriplegia. The gene is located between AR (Xq11.2-q12) and DXS458 (Xq23), lod score 2.91.

SOMATIC FEATURES. Malformations or distinctive craniofacial features have not been described.

GROWTH AND DEVELOPMENT. Head circumference is normal; details of statural growth are not available. Language and motor milestones are severely delayed from infancy with failure of speech and independent ambulation.

COGNITIVE FEATURES. Severe impairment.

NEUROLOGICAL FINDINGS. Nystagmus is present for a time but disappears before adolescence. Spasticity, evident during the second 6 months of life, appears first in the lower limbs and progresses to affect all limbs.

A 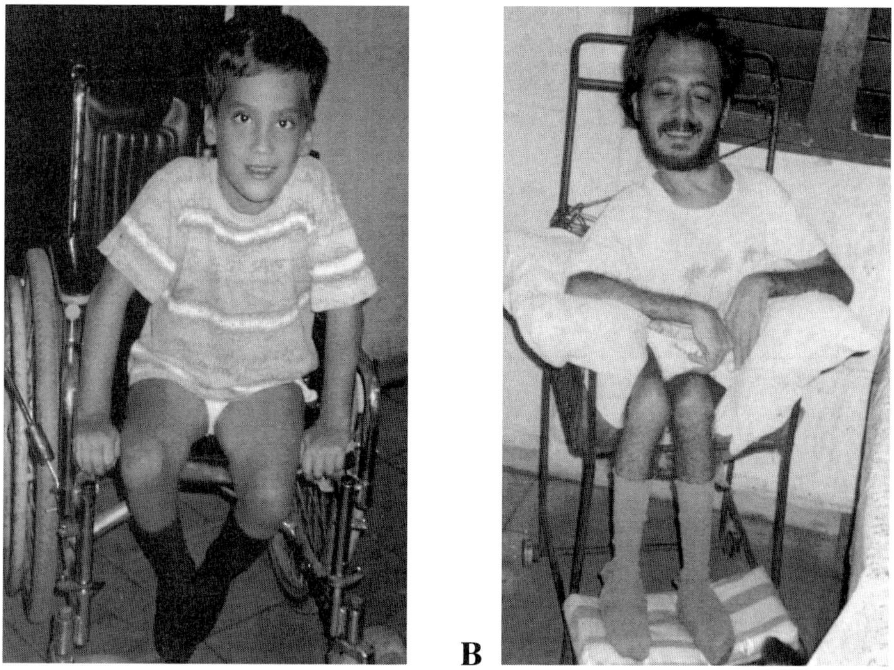 B

X-Linked Spastic Paraplegia, Type 7. Affected males in childhood and adult life showing progressive muscle wasting and spasticity. Courtesy of Dr. Ulrich Müller, Universität Giessen, Giessen, Germany.

HETEROZYGOTE EXPRESSION. None.

IMAGING. Not available.

COMMENT. Spastic paraplegia type 7 is the most recently described X-linked type. The proteolipid protein gene responsible for the Pelizaeus-Merzbacher type of spastic paraplegia (SPG2) is located within the mapping limits. Extensive search for a mutation in the PLP gene has been negative.

REFERENCES

Saugier-Veber P, Munnich A, Bonneau D, et al.: X-linked spastic paraplegia and Pelizaeus-Merzbacher disease are allelic disorders at the proteolipid protein locus. Nat Genet 6:257, 1994.

Steinmüller R, Lantigua-Cruz A, Garcia-Garcia R, et al.: Evidence of a third locus in X-linked recessive spastic paraplegia. Hum Genet 100:287, 1997.

Differential Matrix

Syndrome	Spasticity	Impaired Vision	Absent Ambulation	Comments
X-linked spastic paraplegia, type 7	+	+	+	Nystagmus, absent speech, bowel and bladder dysfunction
Cerebrooculogenital	+	+	+	Short stature, microcephaly, hydrocephaly, agenesis of corpus callosum, microphthalmia, ptosis, hypospadias, cryptorchidism, clubfoot
Goldblatt spastic paraplegia	+	+	+	Optic atrophy, exotropia, nystagmus, ataxia, dysarthria, muscle hypoplasia, contractures
Gustavson	+	+	+	Microcephaly, short stature, optic atrophy with blindness, large ears, deafness, joint contractures, rockerbottom feet, brain undergrowth, hydrocephaly, cerebellar hypoplasia, seizures
Paine	+	+	+	Microcephaly, short stature, optic atrophy, hearing loss, seizures
X-linked ataxia-deafness-dementia	+	+	+	Optic atrophy, ataxia, hypotonia, seizures, childhood death
XLMR-blindness-seizures-spasticity	+	+	+	Poor growth, postnatal microcephaly, clubfoot, seizures, contractures, scoliosis, hypomyelination
Pelizaeus-Merzbacher	+	+	0	Optic atrophy, nystagmus, hypotonia, ataxia, dystonia, CNS dysmyelination
Apak ataxia-spastic diplegia	+	0	+	Short stature, club foot, muscle hypoplasia, ataxia
Arena	+	0	+	Muscle hypoplasia, clubfoot, iron deposits in basal ganglia, ataxia, rigidity, dystonia

X-Linked Mental Retardation-Arch Fingerprints-Hypotonia Syndrome

Definition. XLMR with distinctive facies, poor muscle tone, tapered fingers, arch fingerprints, genu valgum, and absent deep tendon reflexes. The syndrome maps to Xq13.

Somatic Features. The face appears large in relation to the cranium and has a squarish configuration. Subcutaneous tissues of the upper eyelids, helices of the ears, alae nasi, and columella are thickened. The upper lip is arched, especially during childhood, and permanent teeth appeared small in two affected males.

Overall decreased muscle tone is reflected in persistent drooling, cupped ears, arched upper lip, genu valgum, absent reflexes, and perhaps in the tapered fingers and thickened soft tissues of the eyelids, ears, and nose. Presumably de-

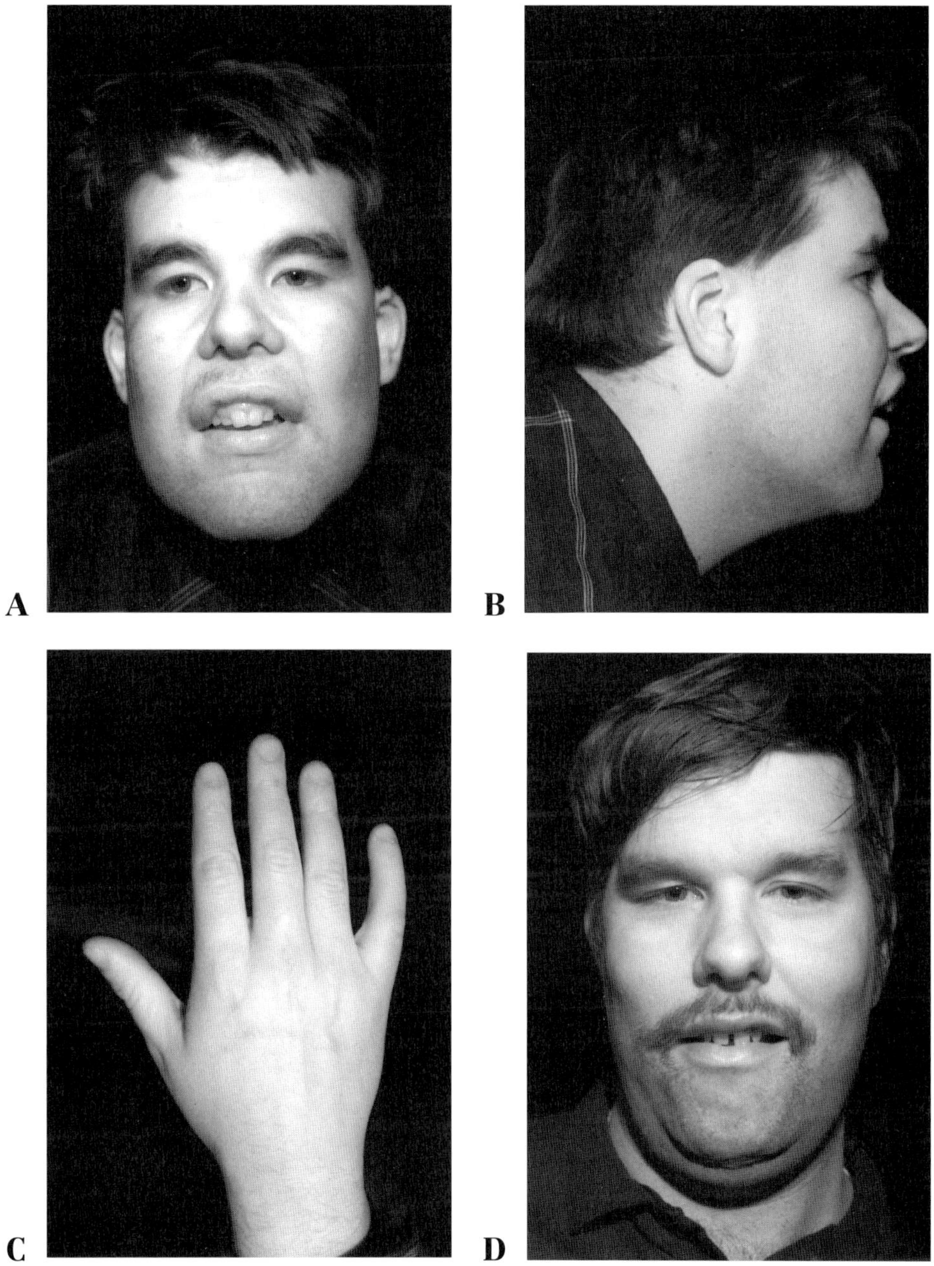

XLMR–Arch Fingerprints–Hypotonia. Large squarish face, heavy eyelids, thickened helices, thickened alae nasi, broad philtrum with tented upper lip, and tapered fingers in a 28-year-old male (A–C); similar features in 32-year-old brother (D).

E F

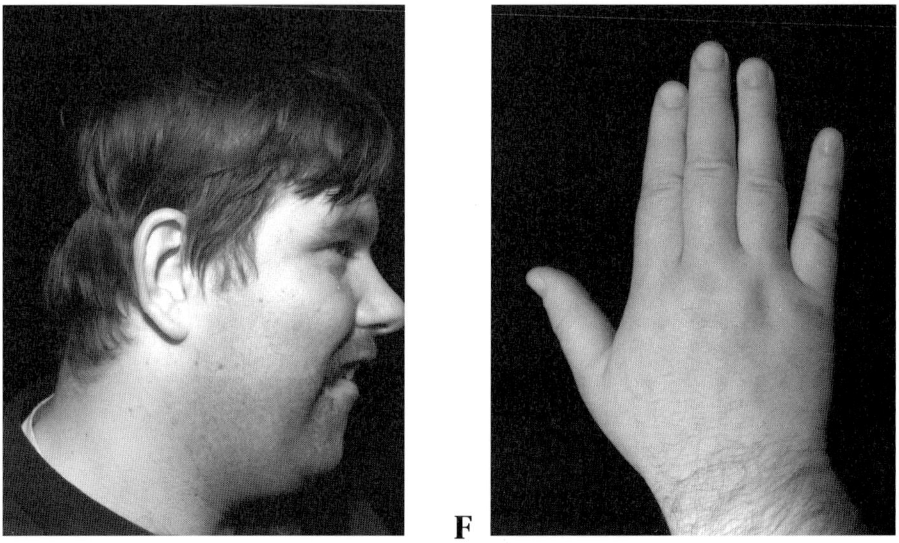

XLMR–Arch Fingerprints–Hypotonia. (continued) Large squarish face, heavy eyelids, thickened helices, thickened alae nasi, broad philtrum with tented upper lip and tapered fingers in 32-year-old brother (D–F) of male shown in A–C.

creased muscle tone contributes, in part, to the delay in motor milestones. The cause for decreased muscle tone and absent deep tendon reflexes has not been identified.

An excessive number of fingerprint arches and low loops were found in the three living males. The average ridge count was 28 in two affected males and 154 in five unaffected brothers. There was associated tapering of the digits and small distal phalanges. None of the five unaffected brothers or two obligate carrier females has excessive arches or low total ridge counts.

GROWTH AND DEVELOPMENT. Intrauterine and postnatal growth are comparable in affected and unaffected males except that affected males are heavier. Sexual maturation occurs at the appropriate time.

COGNITIVE FEATURES. Motor and language development is moderately delayed with adult IQs measuring between 40 and 50.

NEUROLOGICAL FINDINGS. Deep tendon reflexes are absent.

NEUROPATHOLOGY. None.

IMAGING. None.

COMMENT. This syndrome has certain similarities (hypotonia, open mouth with arched upper lip, tapered digits) with XLMR–hypotonic facies (α-thalassaemia mental retardation: ATR-X) syndrome, but differs in many other manifestations (severity of mental retardation, absent speech, seizures, lack of bowel or bladder control, constipation, telecanthus or hypertelorism, small, triangular nose, spacing of teeth, small and simple ears, genital anomalies, short stature, brachydactyly) of that entity. Dermatoglyphics have not been reported in XLMR–hypotonic facies syndrome. Both syndromes map to Xq13. One patient lacked hemoglobin H inclusions that have been found in XLMR–hypotonic facies syndrome.

Excessive fingerprint arches have been found in several chromosomal and single-gene disorders. Coffin-Lowry, Miles-Carpenter, and Chudley syndromes are distinctive XLMR syndromes in which excessive arches have been reported. Coffin-Lowry syndrome has distinctive facial and skeletal features, heterozygote manifestations, and gene localization to Xp22. Miles-Carpenter syndrome maps close to the entity reported here but may be distinguished by microcephaly, facial asymmetry, rockerbottom feet, contractures, and spastic paraplegia. There are a number of similarities between the syndrome reported here and the condition reported by Chudley et al. That condition, characterized by moderate–severe mental retardation, has bitemporal narrowing, almond-shaped eyes, small nose, open mouth with arched upper lip, short stature, low fingerprint ridge count, obesity, hypogonadism, genu valgum, and brachydactyly. It has not been mapped.

REFERENCES

Stevenson RE, Häne B, Arena JF, et al.: Arch fingerprints, hypotonia, and areflexia associated with X linked mental retardation. J Med Genet 34:465, 1997.

Differential Matrix

Syndrome	Hypotonic Facies	Tapered Digits	Excessive Fingerprint Arches	Comments
XLMR-arch fingerprints-hypotonia	+	+	+	Genu valgum, areflexia, hypotonia
Coffin-Lowry	+	+	+	Short stature, microcephaly, hypertelorism, anteverted nares, tented upper lip, prominent lips and large mouth, large ears, soft hands, pectus carinatum
Chudley-Lowry	+	+	+	Short stature, bitemporal narrowing, almond-shaped eyes, depressed nasal bridge, tented upper lip, open mouth, hypogonadism, obesity
XLMR-hypotonic facies (Carpenter-Waziri) (Holmes-Gang) (Juberg-Marsidi)	+	+	0	Short stature, microcephaly, telecanthus, small triangular nose, tented upper lip, open mouth, spacing of teeth, genital anomalies, musculoskeletal anomalies, hemoglobin H inclusions in erythrocytes
Wilson-Turner	+	+	0	Normal growth, small hands and feet, obesity, hypogonadism, gynecomastia, emotional lability

XLMR-ATAXIA-APRAXIA

(Tranebjaerg Syndrome II)

DEFINITION. XLMR with ataxia and dyspraxia with variable cognitive function.

SOMATIC FEATURES. Major malformations do not occur and craniofacial manifestations are incompletely described. Prominent high forehead, cupped ears, and thin upper lip are evident in the published photographs. Although the head circumference is said to be increased, the measurements provided are near the 50th centile. Clubfoot was noted in two boys.

GROWTH AND DEVELOPMENT. Prenatal and postnatal growth was normal. Developmental milestones were mildly delayed.

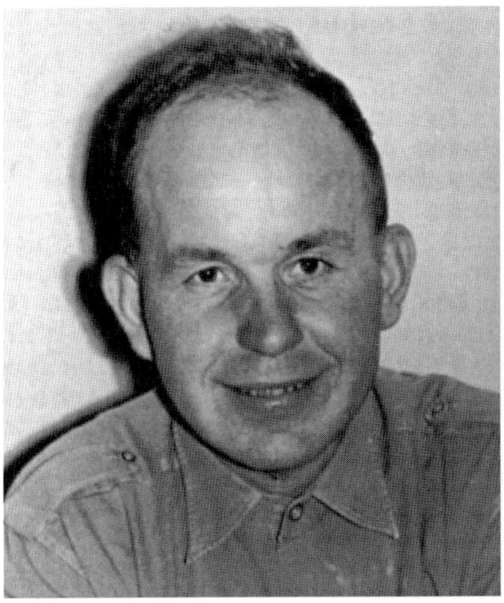
A

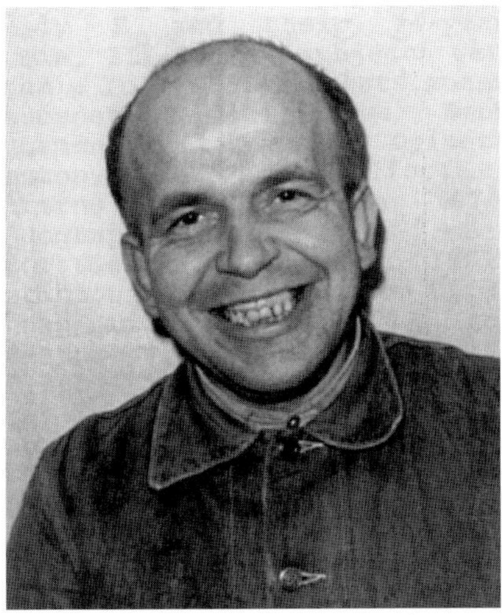
B

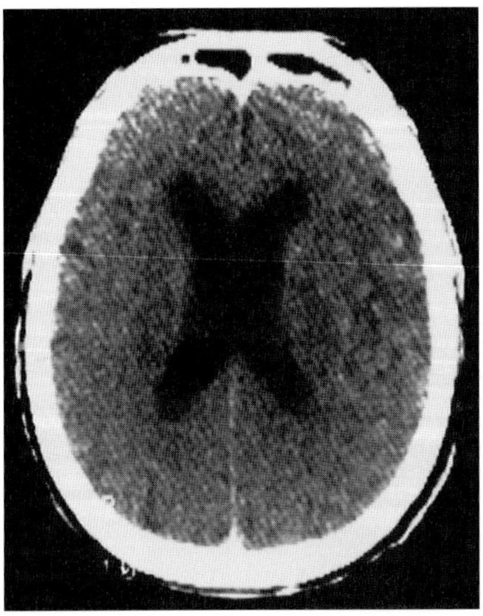
C

XLMR-Ataxia-Apraxia. Brothers at ages 31 and 33 years showing prominent forehead and large ears (A, B); enlarged lateral ventricles on cranial tomography of older brother (C). Courtesy of Dr. Lisbeth Tranebjaerg, University Hospital, Tromsø, Norway.

COGNITIVE FEATURES. Verbal and performance assessments show considerable discordance, with verbal function measuring below average, but within the normal range. In one family, performance measures were in the mildly impaired range; in the second family, measures were in the low-normal range.
NEUROLOGICAL FINDINGS. Nonprogressive ataxia and dyspraxia manifest as inability to copy simple geometric figures; incoordination of limbs and of ocular and tongue movements are noted from early childhood. Hypotonia, tremors, and seizures also occur.
HETEROZYGOTE EXPRESSION. One carrier female had mild constructional dyspraxia and dysgraphia but normal intellectual function.
IMAGING. Brain atrophy was described in two individuals.
COMMENT. Two families, one with six affected males and the other with three affected males, were reported by Tranebjaerg et al.

REFERENCE

Tranebjaerg L, Lou H, Andresen J: New X-linked syndrome with apraxia, ataxia, and mental deficiency: clinical, cytogenetic and neuropsychological studies in two Danish families. Am J Med Genet 43:498, 1992.

Differential Matrix

Syndrome	Ataxia	Hypotonia	Tremors	Comments
XLMR-ataxia-apraxia	+	+	+	Prominent forehead, large ears, uncoordinated movements, seizures
Pelizaeus-Merzbacher	+	+	+	Optic atrophy, nystagmus, spasticity, dystonia, CNS dysmyelination
XLMR-ataxia-deafness-dementia	+	+	+	Optic atrophy, vision loss, hearing loss, spastic paraplegia, seizures, childhood death
Allan-Herndon-Dudley	+	+	0	Large ears with cupping or abnormal architecture, muscle hypoplasia, childhood hypotonia, contractures, dysarthria, athetosis, spastic paraplegia
Pettigrew	+	+	0	Dandy-Walker malformation, spasticity, seizures, microcephaly or hydrocephaly, long face with macrostomia, small testes, contractures, choreoathetosis, iron deposits in basal ganglia
Oral-facial-digital I	0	+	+	Sparse scalp hair, dystopia canthorum, flat midface, hypoplastic alae nasi, hypertrophic and aberrant oral frenuli, intraoral clefts and pseudoclefts, lingual hamartomas, brachydactyly, syndactyly, clinodactyly, structural brain anomalies, polycystic kidneys
X-linked ataxia-dementia	+	0	+	Spastic paraplegia, adult-onset dementia

XLMR-BLINDNESS-SEIZURES-SPASTICITY

(Hamel Syndrome)

DEFINITION. XLMR with postnatal-onset microcephaly and poor growth, clubfoot, progressive loss of vision, spasticity, seizures, digital contractures, hypomyelination, and early childhood death. The gene is localized between DXS337 (Xp11.3) and PGK (Xq12), lod score 3.30.

SOMATIC FEATURES. Major malformations and distinctive craniofacial changes do not occur. Apart from calcaneovalgus foot deformation, appearance at birth is normal. Neurological deterioration begins within a few months and is manifest as loss of vision, waning of interest in the environment, failure to achieve motor and language milestones, seizures, and spasticity. Global growth failure results in microcephaly and short stature. Pale optic discs, strabismus, and digital contractures are noted and unexplained febrile episodes occur. Death occurs within a few years.

GROWTH AND DEVELOPMENT. Intrauterine growth appears normal but slowing of all growth parameters occurs in infancy. Little developmental progress is made during infancy and the early childhood years.

COGNITIVE FEATURES. Severe impairment.

NEUROLOGICAL FINDINGS. The first neurological sign appears at about age 3 months with progressive loss of vision, spasticity, and seizures. Hearing appears normal. Clubfoot is present at birth and scoliosis and digital contractures develop secondary to the spasticity.

HETEROZYGOTE EXPRESSION. None.

NEUROPATHOLOGY. Brain examination has been possible in two cases. The brains were small and showed mild hypomyelination of the cerebrum and cerebellum.

IMAGING. Not available.

COMMENT. Although a number of XLMR syndromes are localized to the pericentromeric region, XLMR-blindness-seizures-spasticity is the only severe neurodegenerative disorder thus far linked to the region.

REFERENCE

Hamel BC, Wesseling P, Renier WO, et al.: A new X linked neurodegenerative syndrome with mental retardation, blindness, convulsions, spasticity, mild hypomyelination, and early death maps to the pericentromeric region. J Med Genet 36:140, 1999.

Differential Matrix

Syndrome	Optic Atrophy or Blindness	Spastic Paraplegia	Seizures	Comments
XLMR-blindness-seizures-spasticity	+	+	+	Poor growth, postnatal microcephaly, clubfoot, contractures, scoliosis, hypomyelination
Cerebrooculogenital	+	+	+	Short stature, microcephaly, hydrocephaly, agenesis of corpus callosum, microphthalmia, ptosis, hypospadias, cryptorchidism, clubfoot
Gustavson	+	+	+	Microcephaly, short stature, large ears, deafness, joint contractures, rockerbottom feet, brain undergrowth, hydrocephaly, cerebellar hypoplasia
Paine	+	+	+	Microcephaly, short stature, hearing loss
Pelizaeus-Merzbacher	+	+	+	Nystagmus, hypotonia, ataxia, dystonia, CNS dysmyelination
Proud	+	+	+	Microcephaly, hearing loss, agenesis of corpus callosum, cryptorchidism, inguinal hernias, ataxia
Schimke	+	+	+	Microcephaly, sunken eyes, downslanting palpebral fissures, narrow nose, spacing of teeth, cupped ears, hypotonia, abducens palsy, hearing loss, choreoathetosis, contractures
X-Linked ataxia-deafness-dementia	+	+	+	Hearing loss, ataxia, hypotonia, childhood death
Adrenoleukodystrophy	+	+	0	Adrenal insufficiency, diffuse skin pigmentation, progressive neurologic deterioration and dementia, elevated long chain fatty acids in plasma
Goldblatt spastic paraplegia	+	+	0	Exotropia, nystagmus, ataxia, dysarthria, muscle hypoplasia, contractures
Mohr-Tranebjaerg (Jensen)	+	+	0	Hearing loss, neurologic deterioration with childhood onset, dystonia
X-linked spastic paraplegia, type 7	+	+	0	Nystagmus, reduced vision, absent speech and ambulation, bowel and bladder dysfunction
Wittwer	+	0	+	Growth deficiency, microcephaly, microphthalmia, hearing loss, hypertelorism, genitourinary anomalies, hypotonia

XLMR-CLEFT LIP/CLEFT PALATE

(XLMR-Facial Clefting, Breslau-Siderius Syndrome)

DEFINITION. XLMR with cleft lip and cleft palate, long face, broad nose, and large hands. The gene is located between DXS337 (Xp11.3) and DXS990 (Xq21.3), lod score 2.78.

A 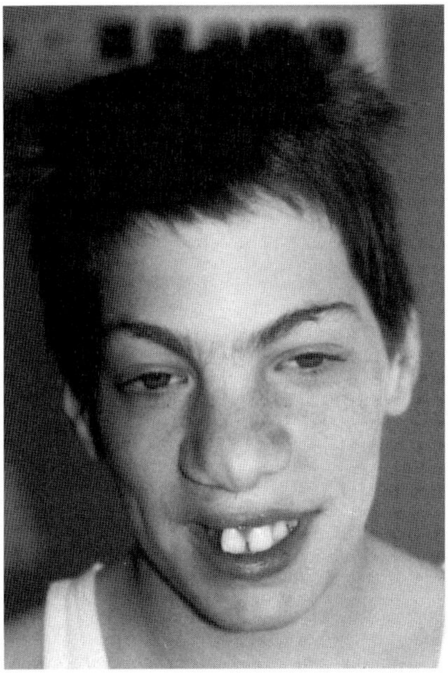

B 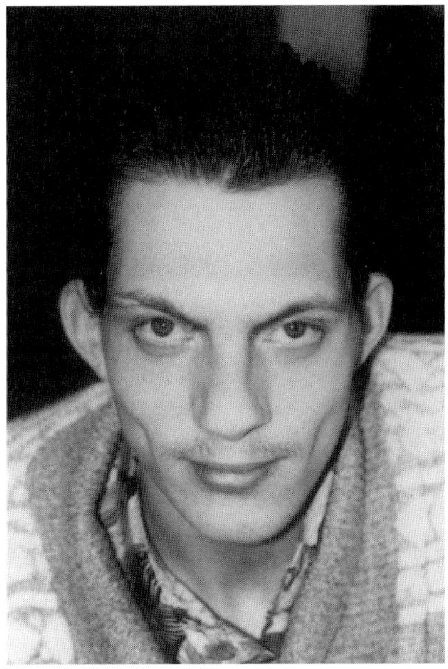

C 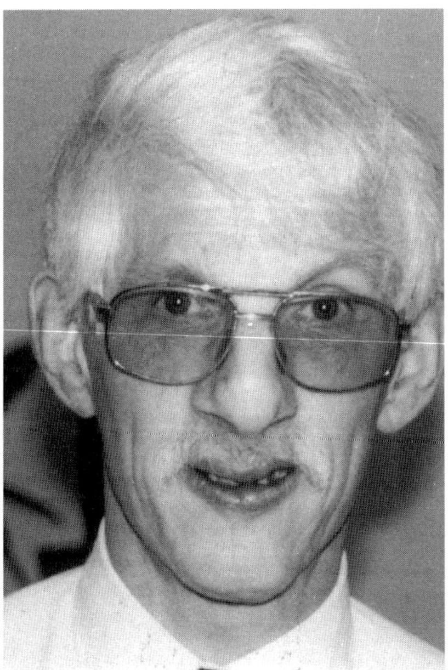

XLMR–Cleft Lip/Cleft Palate. Teenager and adults with long face, broad nasal root and nasal tip (A, B, C). Teenager (A) has synophrys and repaired cleft lip and cleft palate. Adult (C) has repaired cleft lip and palate. Courtesy of Dr. Ben Hamel, University Hospital, Nijmegen, The Netherlands.

Somatic Features. The phenotype is based on observations in three cases. Craniofacial manifestations include normal head circumference, long face, fullness of the nasal root, broad nasal tip, cleft lip, and cleft palate. Cupping of the ears was present in two cases, synophrys and low posterior hairline in one case, thoracic scoliosis and postaxial polydactyly in one case. The testes were retractile in two cases and in one of these cases they were small. Total hand length was near or above the 97th centile.

Growth and Development. Intrauterine and postnatal growth were normal. Although details are not available, developmental delay was noted from early childhood.

Cognitive Features. Mild to borderline impairment.

Behavioral Manifestations. Behavior in two cases is described as unpredictable with aggressive outbursts and uncontrollable with short attention span.

Neurological Findings. None.

Heterozygote Expression. None.

Imaging. Normal.

Comment. A number of X-linked mental retardation syndromes (Aarskog, Aicardi, Cranioorodigital, Lenz, Oral-facial-digital I, Simpson-Golabi-Behmel, and Telecanthus-hypospadias syndromes) may have cleft lip and cleft palate, at least occasionally. Cleft palate alone has been reported in XLMR-hypotonic facies, Otopalatodigital, Snyder-Robinson, and Vasquez syndromes. Isolated median cleft lip occurs in Pallister W syndrome. Of these, only Aarskog and XLMR-hypotonic facies syndromes map to the same region as XLMR–Cleft Lip/Cleft Palate. These three conditions may be easily distinguished on clinical grounds.

REFERENCE

Siderius LE, Hamel BCJ, van Bokhoven H, et al.: X-linked mental retardation associated with cleft lip/cleft palate maps to Xp11.3-q21.3. Am J Med Genet 85:216, 1999.

Differential Matrix

Syndrome	Orofacial Clefting	Hyper-telorism or Broad Nose	Large Hands	Comments
XLMR-cleft lip/ cleft palate	+	+	+	Long face, broad nasal tip, long hands
Aarskog	+	+	0	Short stature, downslanting palpebral fissures, ptosis, cupped ears, anteverted nares, brachydactyly, horizontal palmar crease, midfoot varus, joint laxity, shawl scrotum, cryptorchidism, inguinal hernias
Cranioorodigital	+	+	0	Undergrowth, hearing impairment, prominent forehead, downslanting palpebral fissures, flat midface, cleft palate, blunted flexed overlapping fingers, rockerbottom feet, hypoplastic fibulae, subluxed/dislocated joints
Oral-facial-digital I	+	+	0	Sparse scalp hair, dystopia canthorum, flat midface, hypoplastic alae nasi, hypertrophic and aberrant oral frenuli, lingual hamartomas, brachydactyly, syndactyly, clinodactyly, structural brain anomalies, polycystic kidneys
Otopalatodigital I	+	+	0	Short stature, conductive hearing impairment, prominent brow, apparent ocular hypertelorism, downslanting palpebral fissures, blunted distal phalanges, irregular curvature and spacing of digits, limitation of elbow movement
Simpson-Golabi-Behmel	+	+	0	Somatic overgrowth, supernumerary nipples, polydactyly
Telecanthus-hypospadias	+	+	0	Dysplastic ears, abnormal cranial contour or symmetry

XLMR-EPILEPSY

(Epilepsy–Mental Retardation in Females, formerly MIM 121250)

DEFINITION. XLMR with epilepsy limited to females. The gene is located in Xq22 between loci DXS1220 and DXS6804, lod score 4.15.

SOMATIC FEATURES. Malformations or distinctive craniofacial features do not appear to be a component of this syndrome. Individual cases have had cataracts, microcephaly, syndactyly, or strabismus, perhaps unrelated findings. Neurological manifestations begin during infancy (age 4–18 months) with the onset of generalized or partial seizures. Seizures increase in frequency for a period of time but decrease by age 2–3 years. Coincident with the seizures is developmental regression. Ultimately, the deterioration results in marked cognitive impairment in some individuals but less severe impairment in others. The more severely impaired show stereotyped movements, handwringing, hand flapping and loss of some fine motor skills.

GROWTH AND DEVELOPMENT. Details of intrauterine and postnatal growth have not been reported. Only one girl has had microcephaly. Developmental milestones appear normal until the onset of seizures.

COGNITIVE FEATURES. A range of impairment exists from profound to mild.

NEUROLOGICAL FINDINGS. Generalized, partial, and minor seizures have been described, usually with onset in infancy. During or following a period of developmental and cognitive regression, patients may develop hyperflexia and stereotypic repetitive activities such as handwringing or hand flapping.

HETEROZYGOTE EXPRESSION. Only carrier females have seizures and mental regression. Hemizygous males manifest no seizures or symptoms.

COMMENT. A single family with affected females in four generations has been reported by several observers. Males who carry the gene do not experience seizures or developmental regression and appear normally fertile. This sparing of males in an apparently X-linked dominant disorder is unique.

REFERENCES

Fabisiak K, Erickson R: A familial form of convulsive disorder with or without mental retardation limited to females: extension of a pedigree limits possible genetic mechanisms. Clin Genet 38:353, 1990.

Juberg RC, Hellman CD: A new familial form of convulsive disorder and mental retardation limited to females. J Pediatr 79:726, 1971.

Page DC: Save the Males! Nat Genet 17:3, 1997.

Ryan SG, Chance PF, Zou C-H, et al.: Epilepsy and mental retardation limited to females: an X-linked dominant disorder with male sparing. Nat Genet 17:92, 1997.

Differential Matrix

Syndrome	Developmental regression	Repetitive Stereotypic Hand Movements	Seizures	Comments
XLMR-epilepsy	+	+	+	-
Rett	+	+	+	Acquired microcephaly, truncal ataxia, autistic features
Pyruvate dehydrogenase deficiency	+	0	+	Lactic acidosis, microcephaly, hypotonia, ataxia, dysarthria, brain anomalies
Ornithine transcarbamylase deficiency	+	0	+	Chronic or intermittent hyperammonemia, microcephaly, protein-induced vomiting and lethargy, ataxia

XLMR–HYDROCEPHALY–BASAL GANGLIA CALCIFICATIONS

(Fried Syndrome)

DEFINITION. XLMR with hydrocephaly, calcification of the basal ganglia, and spastic diplegia. The gene has been localized between KAL and DXS989 in Xp22.
SOMATIC FEATURES. Except for macrocephaly, which is found only among those with hydrocephaly, the craniofacial manifestations are not distinctive. The ears may be prominent with outfolding of the upper portion. In adult life, the face may appear elongated with some coarsening. From early childhood, the muscles appear hypoplastic or atrophic. The small muscles of the hands are especially affected. Kyphoscoliosis, genu valgum, and pes planus are also evident.
GROWTH AND DEVELOPMENT. On the basis of limited information, intrauterine growth appears to be normal. Adult stature is variable with some measurements below the third centile. Head circumference is normal except in the presence of hydrocephaly. Developmental milestones lag from birth in most cases.
COGNITIVE FEATURES. Severe impairment.
NEUROLOGICAL FINDINGS. Although the onset of spasticity has not been well documented, increased muscle tone, weakness, hyperactive deep tendon reflexes, and clonus are apparent by early adult life. Sensory loss and impairment of coordination have also been documented.
HETEROZYGOTE EXPRESSION. None.
IMAGING. Cranial tomography shows enlarged ventricles and calcification of the basal ganglia.

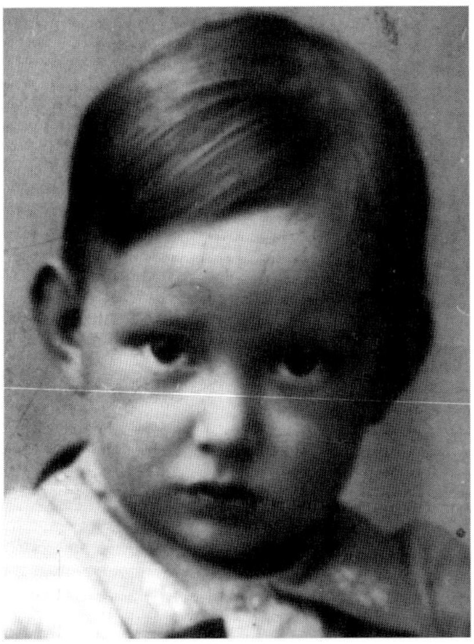

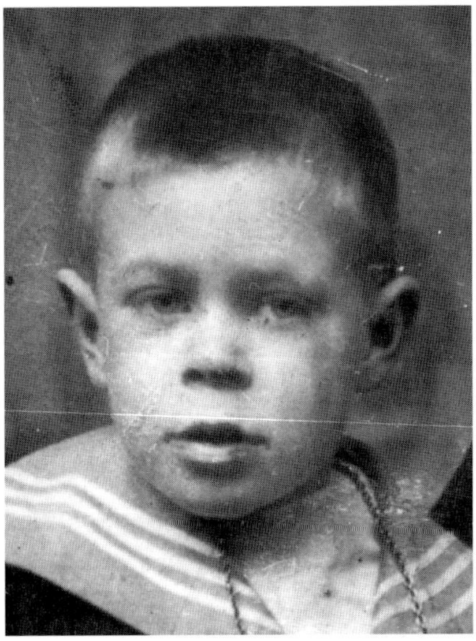

XLMR–Hydrocephaly–Basal Ganglia Calcifications. Facial appearance in six affected boys showing no consistent distinctive manifestations other than cupping of the ears. Courtesy of Dr. Kalman Fried, ASAF Harofe Hospital, Zerifin, Israel.

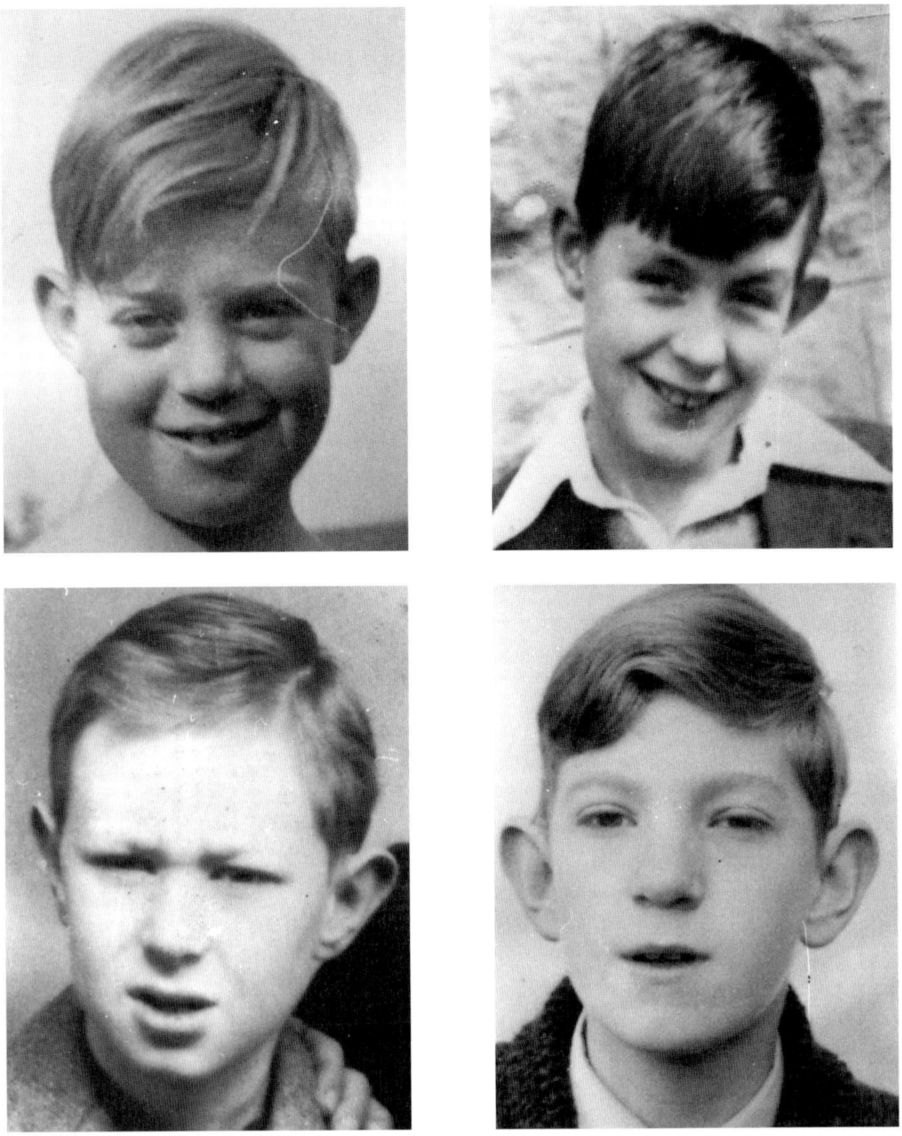

XLMR–Hydrocephaly–Basal Ganglia Calcifications. (continued)

COMMENT. Prior to localization of the gene in Xq22, this entity was considered to be the same as the MASA syndrome. There are thus at least two XLMR syndromes with hydrocephaly and spastic paraplegia as predominant manifestations.

REFERENCES

Fried K: X-linked mental retardation and/or hydrocephalus. J Med Genet 10:17, 1973.

Strain L, Wright AF, Bonthron DT: Fried syndrome is a distinct X linked mental retardation syndrome mapping to Xp22. J Med Genet 34:535, 1977.

Differential Matrix

Syndrome	Muscle Hypoplasia	Iron Deposits or Calcification of Basal Ganglia	Spastic Paraplegia	Comments
XLMR-hydrocephaly-basal ganglia calcifications	+	+	+	Hydrocephaly, sensory impairment
Arena	+	+	+	Clubfoot, ataxia, rigidity, dystonia
Gustavson	+	+	+	Microcephaly, short stature, optic atrophy with blindness, large ears, deafness, joint contractures, rockerbottom feet, brain undergrowth, hydrocephaly, cerebellar hypoplasia, seizures
Schimke	0	+	+	Microcephaly, sunken eyes, downslanting palpebral fissures, narrow nose, spacing of teeth, cupped ears, hypotonia, abducens palsy, hearing loss, vision loss, choreoathetosis, contractures

XLMR-Hypogammaglobulinemia

(Chudley Hypogammaglobulinemia Syndrome, XLMR-Hypogamma-globulinemia-Ataxia-Seizures)

Definition. XLMR with prominent glabella, synophrys, prognathism, single palmar creases, hirsutism, progressive weakness and gait disturbance, seizures, and hypogammaglobulinemia. The gene maps between DXS1170 (Xq21.33) and DXS8067 (Xq23), lod score 2.23.

Somatic Features. Major malformations do not occur. The craniofacies are characterized by normal head size, hypertelorism, prominent glabella, synophrys, and prognathism. Single palmar creases and generalized hirsutism may also be present. Small cerebellar size was present in one case. Another case had a bifid uvula, diastasis rectus, an undescended testis, mild scoliosis, and macrocephaly, the latter finding evident in his father as a coincidental trait.

Growth and Development. Intrauterine and postnatal growth appears normal. Developmental milestones lag from infancy, with speech delayed to a greater degree than motor skills.

Cognitive Features. Moderate impairment.

Neurological Findings. Generalized tonic–clonic seizures date from childhood or early adolescence. Two older males had progressive weakness and ataxia with gait disturbance in their forties, findings not present in a younger cousin at age 22 years. Tight heel cords and brisk deep tendon reflexes were demonstrated in one of the older males and abnormal peripheral nerve conduction in the other.

Heterozygote Expression. None.

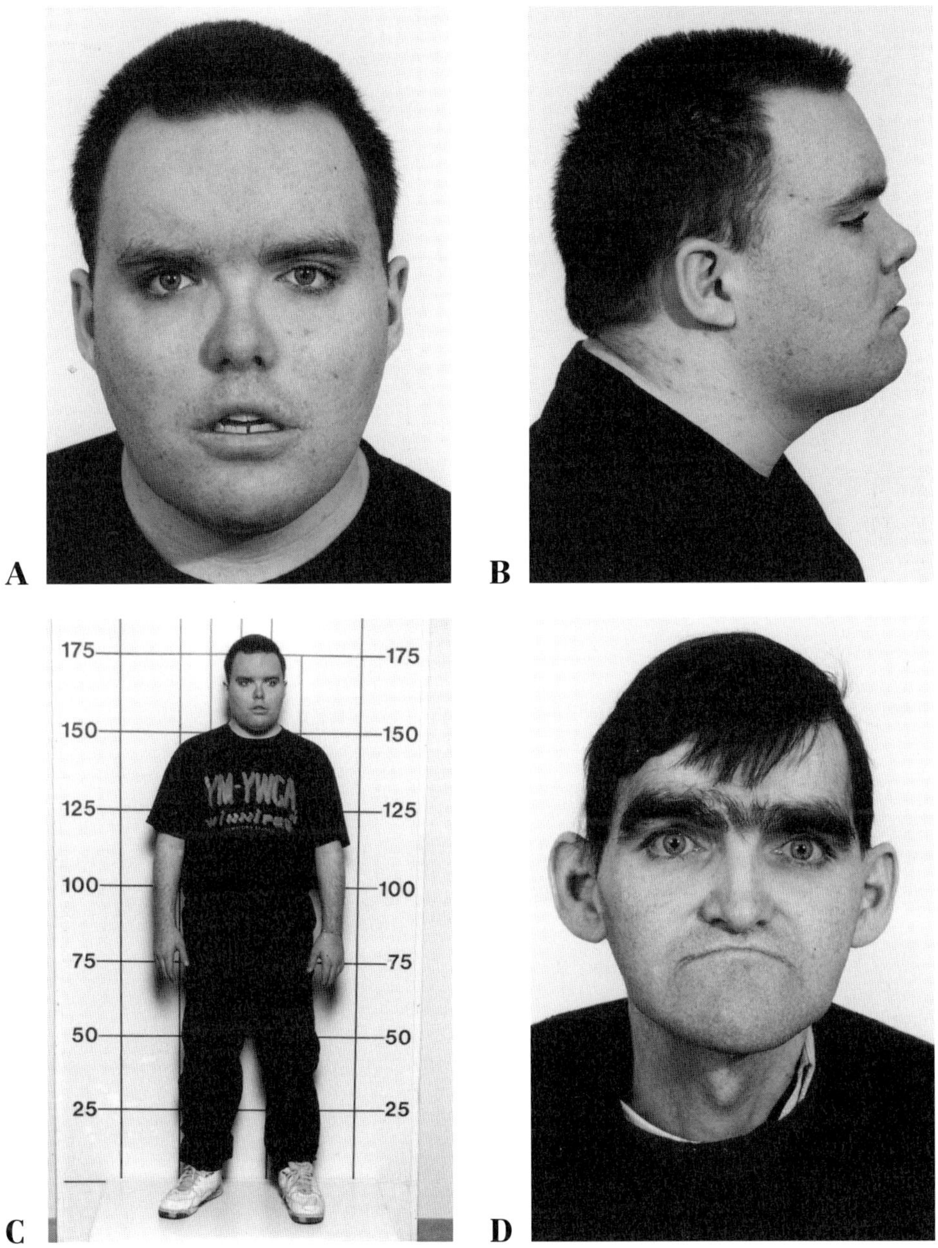

XLMR-Hypogammaglobulinemia. Hypertelorism, mild synophrys, underbite, and prognathism at age 22 years (A–C); heavy eyebrows, synophrys, hypertelorism, short philtrum, and prognathism in a 43-year-old maternal uncle (D–F). Courtesy of Dr. Albert Chudley, Children's Hospital, Winnipeg, Manitoba, Canada.

E 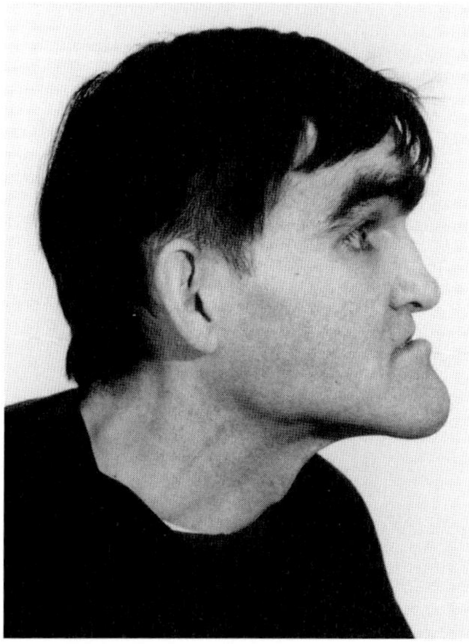

F 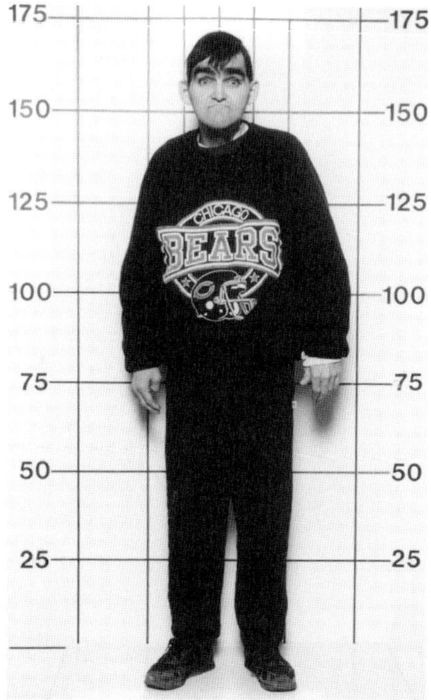

XLMR-Hypogammaglobulinemia. (continued)

IMAGING. Cranial tomography showed cerebellar atrophy in one case and normal anatomy in another. The latter was the youngest of the three cases reported and had not yet developed progressive weakness and ataxia.

LABORATORY. Hypogammaglobulinemia with low IgG and absent secretory IgA was present in two of the three cases reported. The third case had low normal IgM, IgG, and IgA.

COMMENT. The gene for Bruton-type X-linked agammaglobulinemia (Btk) is located within the mapping limits of Chudley hypogammaglobulinemia syndrome. Since Bruton agammaglobulinemia is not associated with mental retardation, ataxia, and seizures, the possibility of a contiguous gene deletion syndrome was considered by Chudley et al. A search for a deletion involving the 5′ and 3′ untranslated regions of the Btk gene was negative.

REFERENCE

Chudley AE, Tackels DC, Lubs HA, et al.: X-linked mental retardation syndrome with seizures, hypogammaglobulinemia, and progressive gait disturbance is regionally mapped between Xq21.33 and Xq23. Am J Med Genet 85:255, 1999.

Differential Matrix

Syndrome	Ataxia	Seizures	Hypogamma-globulinema	Comments
XLMR-hypogamma-globulinemia	+	+	+	Prominent glabella, synophrys, prognathism, hirsutism, weakness, gait disturbance
Arts	+	+	0	Growth deficiency, paucity of muscles, hypotonia, areflexia, deafness, vision loss, childhood death
Gustavson	+	+	0	Microcephaly, short stature, optic atrophy with blindness, large ears, deafness, joint contractures, rockerbottom feet, brain undergrowth, hydrocephaly, cerebellar hypoplasia, spasticity
Pelizaeus-Merzbacher	+	+	0	Optic atrophy, nystagmus, hypotonia, spasticity, dystonia, CNS dysmyelination
Proud	+	+	0	Microcephaly, hearing loss, vision loss, agenesis of corpus callosum, cryptorchidism, inguinal hernias, spasticity
X-linked ataxia-deafness-dementia	+	+	0	Optic atrophy, vision loss, hearing loss, spastic paraplegia, hypotonia, childhood death

XLMR-HYPOSPADIAS

Goldblatt et al. reported three brothers with normal stature, microcephaly, trigonocephaly, synophrys, midface hypoplasia, beaked nose, posteriorly rotated ears with folded helicies and arched palate. Hypotonia and joint hypermobility were present. There was fifth finger clinodactyly and nail "breaking." Two of the brothers had glandular hypospadias and the third had a hooded prepuce. Mild to moderate developmental impairment was present. Other cases have not been reported. Craniofacial features are different from the telecanthus-hypospadias syndrome (Opitz BBB, C syndrome), which maps to Xp22.

REFERENCE

Goldblatt J, Wallis C, Viljoen D (1987) A new hypospadias—mental retardation syndrome in three brothers. Am J Dis Child 141:1168–1169.

A B C

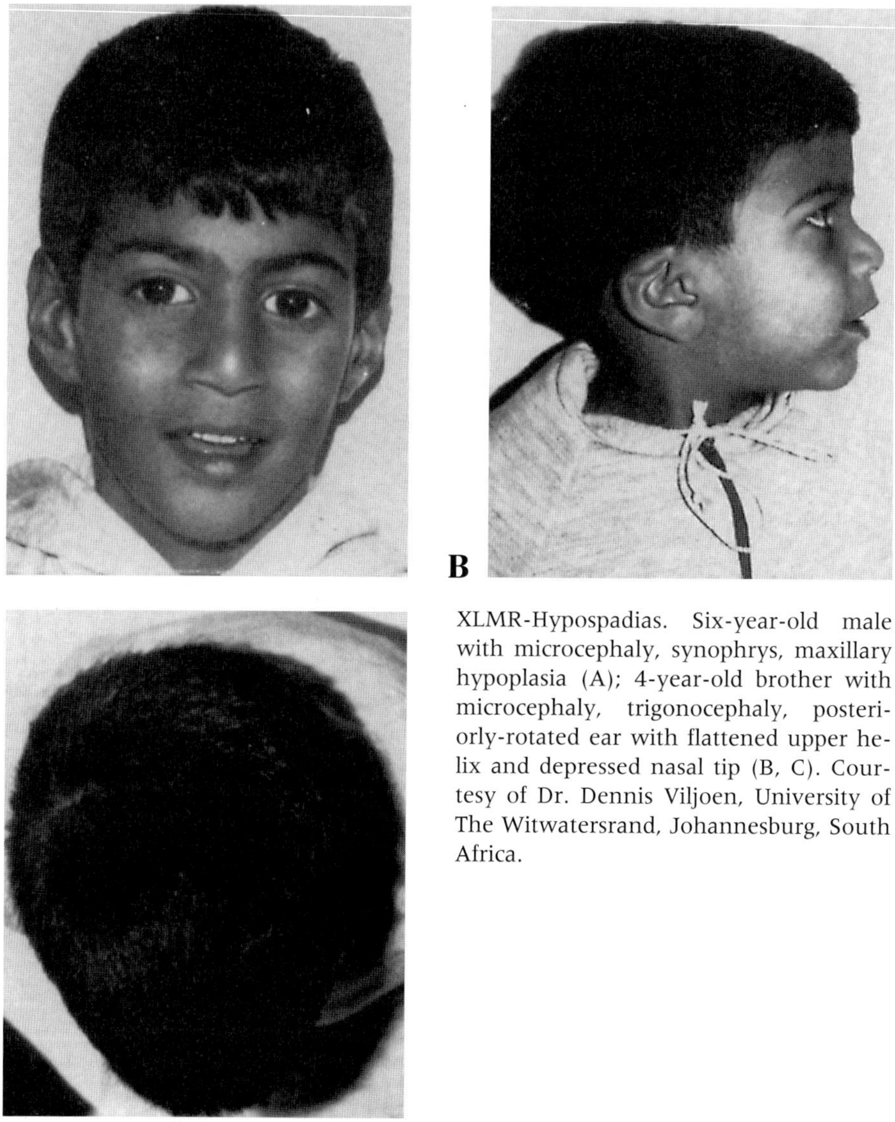

XLMR-Hypospadias. Six-year-old male with microcephaly, synophrys, maxillary hypoplasia (A); 4-year-old brother with microcephaly, trigonocephaly, posteriorly-rotated ear with flattened upper helix and depressed nasal tip (B, C). Courtesy of Dr. Dennis Viljoen, University of The Witwatersrand, Johannesburg, South Africa.

XLMR–HYPOTONIA–RECURRENT INFECTIONS

(Lubs-Arena Syndrome)

DEFINITION. XLMR with hypotonic facies, hypertelorism, downslanting palpebral fissures, gastroesophageal reflux, recurrent respiratory infections, and seizures. The gene is localized distal to DXS8103 in Xq28, lod score 3.42.

SOMATIC FEATURES. Major malformations do not occur. Hypotonic facies with hypertelorism, downslanting palpebral fissures, posteriorly rotated or abnormally sculpted ears, short nose with a flat nasal bridge, and large open mouth are the major somatic findings. Cardiomegaly was present at postmortem examination

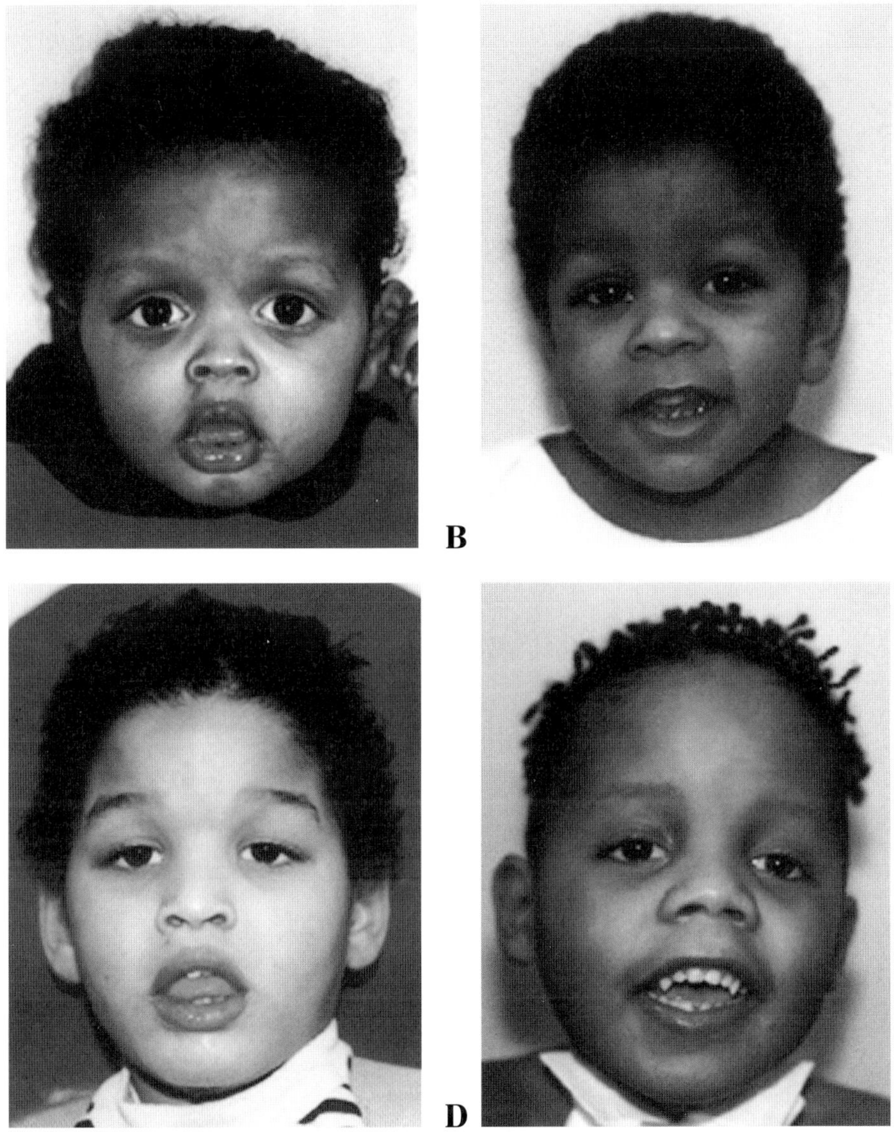

A B C D

XLMR–Hypotonia–Recurrent Infections. Affected males at ages 2, 3, 5, and 7 years (A–D) showing hypertelorism, downslanted palpebral fissures, short nose with anteverted nostrils, and tenting of the upper lip. Courtesy of Drs. Herbert Lubs and Fernando Arena, University of Miami School of Medicine, Miami, Florida.

in two cases. Cerebral atrophy is the only abnormality present on cranial imaging. Swallowing problems and gastroesophageal reflux appear due to cerebral dysfunction rather than structural anomalies of the gastrointestinal tract. Similarly, recurrent pulmonary infections appear to be due to aspiration rather than a defect in the immune system. A relentless deterioration of nervous system function leads to death by age 10 years.

GROWTH AND DEVELOPMENT. Although birth weight is impaired, the velocity of all growth parameters appears normal postnatally. Developmental milestones are delayed from infancy and developmental regression begins prior to age 5 years.
COGNITIVE FEATURES. Severe impairment.
NEUROLOGICAL FINDINGS. Hypotonia exists from infancy and rapid neurological deterioration manifest by loss of motor and language skills, seizures, loss of vision and hearing, spasticity, and decreased responsiveness usually begins before age 5 years. The neurological deterioration is further complicated with swallowing difficulty, gastroesophageal reflux, and recurrent respiratory infections.
HETEROZYGOTE EXPRESSION. Carrier females may have mild cognitive impairment but do not experience neurologic abnormalities or recurrent infections. Language function is affected to the greatest degree and emotional lability is evident.
NEUROPATHOLOGY. Three postmortem examinations have yielded inconsistent findings. No gross or microscopic changes other than ischemia and vascular congestion were present in two cases, both of whom died at 8 years. Normal cerebral cortex, small hippocampi, loss of Purkinje cells, and evidence of meningitis, encephalitis, and anoxia were present in a third patient, who died at age 5 years.
IMAGING. Cerebral atrophy.
LABORATORY. Immunoglobulins, acyl carnitine profile, and lysosomal enzymes are normal. In one case, skeletal muscle obtained at postmortem showed variability in size of muscle fibers with centralization of nuclei. In two other cases, there was cardiomegaly with biventricular hypertrophy.
COMMENT. Barth syndrome, which maps to Xq28 and is due to mutations in the G4.5 gene, has cardiomyopathy and childhood death but lacks the mental retardation and nervous system deterioration seen in XLMR–hypotonia–recurrent infections. Pai et al. have reported another syndrome with hypertelorism, seizures, recurrent infections, and childhood death which maps to the same region. The clinical manifestations were sufficiently inconsistent, however, to prompt the authors to consider the phenotype nonsyndromic.

REFERENCES

Lubs H, Abidi F, Blaymore J, et al.: An XLMR syndrome characterized by multiple respiratory infections, hypertelorism, severe CNS deterioration and early death localizes to distal Xq28. Am J Med Genet, in press, 1999.

Pai GS, Häne B, Joseph M, et al.: A new X-linked recessive syndrome of mental retardation and mild dysmorphism maps to Xq28. Am J Med Genet 34:529, 1997.

Differential Matrix

Syndrome	Hypotonic Facies	Develop-mental Regression	Seizures	Comments
XLMR-hypotonia-recurrent infections	+	+	+	Hypertelorism, downslanting palpebral fissures, gastroesophageal reflux, recurrent infections, childhood death
Rett	0	+	+	Acquired microcephaly, truncal ataxia, repetitive hand movements, autistic features
XLMR-epilepsy	0	+	+	Repetitive stereotypic hand movements
Proud	+	0	+	Microcephaly, hearing loss, vision loss, agenesis of corpus callosum, cryptorchidism, inguinal hernias, ataxia, spasticity
Smith-Fineman-Myers	+	0	+	Microcephaly, ptosis, flat philtrum, scoliosis, midfoot varus, narrow feet, hypotonia
XLMR-psoriasis	+	0	+	Hypertelorism, open mouth, large ears, hypotonia, psoriasis

XLMR–Hypotonic Facies Syndrome

(α-Thalassemia Mental Retardation, Cerebrofaciogenital Syndrome, ATR-X, MIM 301040)

Definition. XLMR with short stature, microcephaly, hypotonic facies with hypertelorism, small nose, open mouth and prominent lips, brachydactyly, genital anomalies, hypotonia, and, in some cases, hemoglobin H inclusions in erythrocytes. The gene, X-linked nuclear protein (XNP), is located in Xq13.3.

Somatic Features. Most somatic manifestations can be noted from birth and in part may appear more distinctive in early childhood than later in life. Microcephaly is the rule and is often present at birth. Facial characteristics include telecanthus or hypertelorism, epicanthus, flat nasal bridge, maxillary hypoplasia, small triangular nose, anteverted nares, open mouth with prominent lips, and wide spacing of the incisors. There is a tendency toward coarsening of the facial features with age. Many minor anomalies of the skeleton may be noted: brachydactyly, tapering fingers, clinodactyly, digital contractures, overlapping digits, pes planus, varus and valgus foot deformations, kyphosis, scoliosis, pectus carinatum, and dimples over the lower spine. Ambiguous genitalia occur uncommonly but most cases have some genital anomaly including hypospadias, cryptorchidism, or genital hypoplasia. Major malformations are rare but cleft palate and cardiac septal defects have been described.

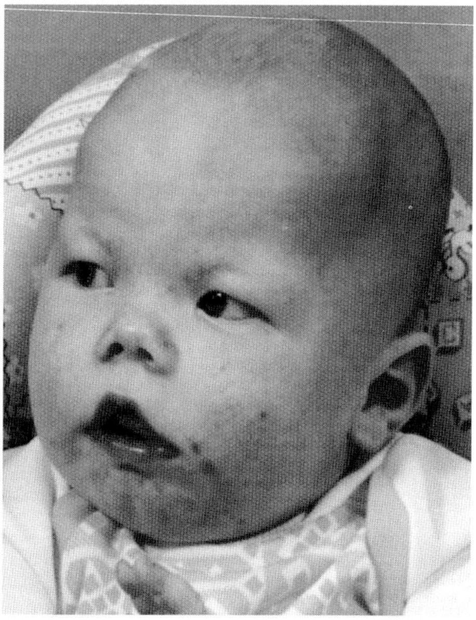

A

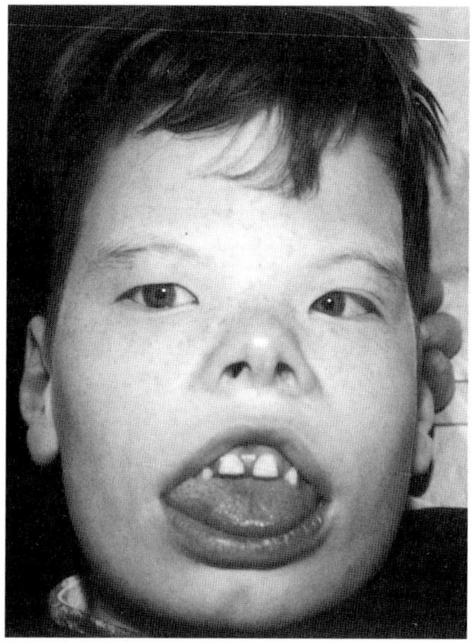

B

XLMR–Hypotonic Facies. Microcephaly, hypertelorism, telecanthus, depressed nasal bridge, short triangular nose, anteverted nostrils, full lips, and tented upper lip at age 6 months (A) and 21 years (B).

GROWTH AND DEVELOPMENT. Most patients will ultimately have short stature. In some cases it is apparent from birth and in others it appears to begin or to become more pronounced at puberty. Puberty is often delayed. Development is globally and profoundly delayed. Walking is delayed until late childhood and other motor skills come late as well. Speech is absent or severely limited.

BEHAVIORAL MANIFESTATIONS. Generally described as affectionate but some suggestion of outbursts of laughter or crying.

NEUROLOGICAL FINDINGS. Hypotonia dominates the neuromuscular phenotype and undoubtedly contributes to the somatic appearance as well.

HETEROZYGOTE EXPRESSION. Although hypertelorism and maxillary hypoplasia have been noted, there is little evidence for expression in carrier females. Carriers may in some cases be identified by rare HgbH inclusions in erythrocytes. The usual absence of manifestations in carriers serves as an important means of clinical differentiation from Coffin-Lowry syndrome. Carriers typically have marked skewing of X chromosome inactivation with preferential inactivation of the chromosome carrying the XNP mutation.

NATURAL HISTORY. These patients are obviously and profoundly affected from birth. In addition to the slow developmental progress, infancy is compromised by poor feeding, vomiting and esophageal reflux, recurrent respiratory and urinary infections, apneic or cyanotic spells, and constipation. Most do not develop meaningful speech and motor skills are markedly impaired.

LABORATORY. A mild microcytic anemia may be present. Inclusions in erythrocytes stained with brilliant cresyl blue for hemoglobin H (β_4 tetramers) or hemoglobin electrophoresis offer convenient methods for screening for XLMR–Hypotonic Facies syndrome. However, many cases do not have significant levels of HgbH to be detected by electrophoresis and erythrocyte inclusions may be rare, necessitating repeated screening. Other cases may lack hemoglobin abnormalities altogether. Diagnostic confirmation depends on mutational analysis of the responsible gene.

COMMENT. Although the first cases of XLMR–hypotonic facies syndrome were ascertained because of mild hematologic abnormalities, subsequent cases were identified because of somatic manifestations. Three other named XLMR syndromes (Juberg-Marsidi, Carpenter-Waziri, and Holmes-Gang syndromes) have been shown to have mutations of XNP. Of the named XLMR syndromes, no less than 10% are candidates for allelism with XLMR–hypotonic facies syndrome based on phenotypic findings. These include XLMR–arch fingerprints–hypotonia, Brooks, Chudley-Lowry, Miles-Carpenter, Proud, Smith-Fineman-Myers, Vasquez, Young-Hughes, and XLMR-psoriasis syndromes.

Coffin-Lowry syndrome may be easily confused with the XLMR–hypotonic facies syndrome, especially in early childhood. The frequent presence of carrier manifestations, large fleshy hands and fingers, skeletal abnormalities, and absence of genital anomalies in Coffin-Lowry syndrome serve as distinguishing features. Mutational analysis, XNP in XLMR–hypotonic facies syndrome, and Rsk-2 in Coffin-Lowry can confirm the correct diagnosis in most cases.

REFERENCES

Donnai D, Clayton-Smith J, Gibbons RJ, et al.: The non-deletion α-thalassemia/mental retardation syndrome. Further support for X linkage. J Med Genet 28:742, 1991.

Gibbons RJ, Suthers GK, Wilkie AOM, et al.: X-linked α-thalassemia/mental retardation (ATR-X) syndrome: localization to Xq12-q21.31 by X inactivation and linkage analysis. Am J Hum Genet 51:1136, 1992.

Gibbons RJ, Brueton L, Buckle VJ, et al.: Clinical and hematologic aspects of the X-linked α-thalassemia/mental retardation syndrome (ATR-X). Am J Med Genet 55:288, 1995.

Gibbons RJ, Picketts DJ, Villard L, et al.: Mutations in a putative global transcriptional regulator cause X-linked mental retardation with α-thalassemia (ATR-X syndrome). Cell 80:837, 1995.

Villard L, Gecz J, Mattei JF, et al.: XNP mutation in a large family with Juberg-Marsidi syndrome. Nat Genet 12:359, 1996.

Wilkie AOM, Gibbons RJ, Higgs DR, et al.: X-linked α-thalassaemia/mental retardation: spectrum of clinical features in three related males. J Med Genet 28:738, 1991.

Differential Matrix

Syndrome	Micro-cephaly	Hypotonic facies	Urogenital anomalies	Comments
XLMR-hypotonic facies (Carpenter-Waziri) (Holmes-Gang) (Juberg-Marsidi)	+	+	+	Short stature, telecanthus, small triangular nose, tented upper lip, open mouth, spacing of teeth, genital anomalies, musculoskeletal anomalies, hemoglobin H inclusions in erythrocytes
Proud	+	+	+	Hearing loss, vision loss, agenesis of corpus callosum, cryptorchidism, inguinal hernias, ataxia, spasticity, seizures
Smith-Fineman-Myers	+	+	+	Ptosis, flat philtrum, scoliosis, midfoot varus, narrow feet, seizures, hypotonia
Coffin-Lowry	+	+	0	Short stature, hypertelorism, anteverted nares, tented upper lip, prominent lips and large mouth, large ears, soft hands with tapered digits, pectus carinatum
Miles-Carpenter	+	+	0	Short stature, ptosis, small palpebral fissures, open mouth, pectus excavatum, scoliosis, long hands, camptodactyly, rockerbottom feet, arch fingerprints, spasticity, unsteady gait
Chudley-Lowry	0	+	+	Short stature, bitemporal narrowing, almond-shaped eyes, depressed nasal bridge, tented upper lip, open mouth, hypogonadism, hypotonia, obesity
XLMR-psoriasis	0	+	+	Hypertelorism, strabismus, large ears, macrostomia, psoriasis, seizures
Vasquez	+	0	+	Short stature, gynecomastia, obesity, hypotonia, hypogonadism
XLMR-hypospadias	+	0	+	Trigonocephaly, synophrys, beaked nose, dysplastic ears, joint hyperextensibility, hypotonia

XLMR–Ichthyosis–Hypogonadism

(Rud Syndrome, MIM 308200)

Definition. XLMR with ichthyosis, hypogonadism, anosmia, and seizures. This combination of manifestations probably results from deletions of variable magnitude in Xp22.3 rather than from mutations in a single gene. The entry is included for historical reasons.

Somatic Features. Craniofacial features appear normal although alopecia including absent eyebrows and eyelashes has been reported. Ichthyosis is present from birth or very soon thereafter. It may begin as a general erythema and progress to thick scales which darken with age. The trunk and extensor surfaces are most extensively affected; the palms, soles and flexion creases are spared. Most patients have underdevelopment of the genitalia and hypogonadism. The penis is small and testes small or undescended. Uncommonly, hypospadias is present. Sexual hair does not develop and gynecomastia occurs in a minority. Generalized or psychomotor seizures occur in most patients, with usual onset at the end of the first decade. Nystagmus and anosmia have been noted in some cases.

GROWTH AND DEVELOPMENT. Short stature occurs in most cases.

COGNITIVE FEATURES. Variable impairment has been described with IQs ranging from low normal range to severe impairment.

NEUROLOGICAL FINDINGS. Seizures occur in most cases. Nystagmus, strabismus, and anosmia are less consistently present.

HETEROZYGOTE EXPRESSION. Carriers have normal cognitive function and no somatic manifestations.

LABORATORY. Deletions of Xp22 may result in reduced levels of steroid sulfatase, testosterone, and gonadotropins. Normal steroid sulfatase and hypergonadotrophic hypogonadism are likely caused by genocopies.

COMMENT. Traupe has pointed out that the two patients, a male and an unrelated female, described by Rud had dissimilar disorders and neither had mental retardation. The diagnosis, Rud syndrome, to describe ichthyosis, hypogonadism, mental retardation, and seizures, is thus inappropriate. Further, it appears probable that this constellation of findings cannot be attributed to a single gene mutation but rather to a contiguous gene deletion. The clinical heterogeneity is based in large measure on the extent of the deletion. Ichthyosis is associated with deletion of the steroid sulfatase (aryl sulfatase C) gene, hypogonadotrophic hypogonadism and anosmia with deletion of the Kallman syndrome gene, and, presumably, mental retardation and seizures with a different gene in the neighborhood.

REFERENCES

Münke M, Kruse K, Goos M, et al.: Genetic heterogeneity of the ichthyosis, hypogonadism, mental retardation, and epilepsy syndrome. Eur J Pediatr 141:8, 1983.

Perrin JCS, Idemoto JY, Sotos JF, et al.: X-linked syndrome of congenital ichthyosis, hypogonadism, mental retardation and anosmia. Birth Defects Orig Art Ser XII(5):267, 1976.

Rud E: Et Tilfaelde af Infantilisme med Tetani, Epilepsi, Polyneuritis, Ichthyosis og Anaemi of Pernicios Type. Hospitalstidende 70:525, 1927.

Rud E: Et Tilfaelde af Hypogenitalisme (Eunuchoidismus feminus) med partiel Gigantisme og Ichthyosis. Hospitalstidende 72:426, 1929.

Traupe H: The Ichthyoses. A Guide to Clinical Diagnosis, Genetic Counseling, and Therapy. Springer-Verlag, Berlin, 1989.

XLMR–INFANTILE SPASMS

(West Syndrome, MIM 308350)

DEFINITION. XLMR with infantile spasms and hypsarrhythmia. The gene has been localized between DXS274 (Xp21.3) and the adrenal hypoplasia locus (Xp22.1), lod score 3.97.

SOMATIC FEATURES. Malformations or distinctive craniofacial manifestations do not occur.

GROWTH AND DEVELOPMENT. Intrauterine and postnatal growth are normal. Developmental milestones slow after the onset of infantile spasms, usually within the first 6 months of life.

COGNITIVE FEATURES. Severe impairment.

NEUROLOGICAL FINDINGS. Prior to the onset of seizures, affected males appear normal and experience normal growth and development. Seizures, usually in the form of infantile spasms, begin between 2 and 8 months. Typically, infantile spasms follow a brief period of atonia and consist of clusters of flexion and extension movements of the limbs, neck, and trunk. Early childhood death is not uncommon.

HETEROZYGOTE EXPRESSION. None.

LABORATORY. Metabolic studies are normal. A hypsarrhythmia pattern—multifocal spikes and high-voltage slow waves throughout the cortex—is usually found on electroencephalography.

IMAGING. Cranial imaging is usually normal except for mild dilation of the cerebral ventricles.

COMMENT. A period of normal infantile development followed by stagnation of developmental progress and loss of skills is seen in few XLMR syndromes. This phenomenon appears related to the seizures in XLMR–infantile spasms and in XLMR-epilepsy. In other cases, the regression appears secondary to episodic or persistent metabolic abnormalities.

REFERENCES

Claes S, Devriendt K, Lagae L, et al.: The X-linked infantile spasms syndrome (MIM 308350) maps to Xp11.4-Xpter in two pedigrees. Ann Neurol 42:360, 1997.

Feinberg AP, Leahy WR: Infantile spasms: case report of sex-linked inheritance. Dev Med Child Neurol 19:524, 1977.

Rugtveit J: X-linked mental retardation and infantile spasms in two brothers. Dev Med Child Neurol 28:544, 1986.

Differential Matrix

Syndrome	Developmental Regression	Seizures	EEG Hypsarrhythmia Pattern	Comments
XLMR-infantile spasms	+	+	+	Early childhood death
Bertini	+	+	0	Macular degeneration, hypotonia, ataxia, childhood death, hypoplasia of cerebellar vermis and corpus callosum, postnatal growth impairment
Menkes	+	+	0	Growth deficiency, sparse kinky hair, hypothermia, pallor, limited movement, hypertonicity, metaphyseal widening and spurs, arterial tortuosity, childhood death
Ornithine transcarbamylase deficiency	+	+	0	Chronic or intermittent hyperammonemia, microcephaly, protein-induced vomiting and lethargy, ataxia
Pelizaeus-Merzbacher	+	+	0	Optic atrophy, nystagmus, hypotonia, spasticity, ataxia, dystonia, CNS dysmyelination
Pyruvate dehydrogenase deficiency	+	+	0	Lactic acidosis, microcephaly, hypotonia, ataxia, dysarthria, CNS anomalies
Rett	+	+	0	Acquired microcephaly, truncal ataxia, repetitive hand movements, autistic features
XLMR-epilepsy	+	+	0	Repetitive stereotypic hand movements

XLMR–Isolated Growth Hormone Deficiency

Definition. XLMR with short stature, gynecomastia, isolated growth hormone deficiency, and infantile behavior. The gene is located between DXS424 (Xq24) and FRAXA (Xq27.3), lod score 3.26.

Somatic Features. Short stature is obvious from childhood and gynecomastia occurs after puberty.

Growth and Development. Intrauterine growth may be normal but height lags from birth. Ultimate height reaches 135–139 cm. Bone age lags significantly behind and statural growth may continue into the midtwenties. The age of puberty has not been documented but genitalia appear normal in adults although secondary sexual characteristics may be incompletely virilized.

Neurological Findings. None.

Heterozygote Expression. None.

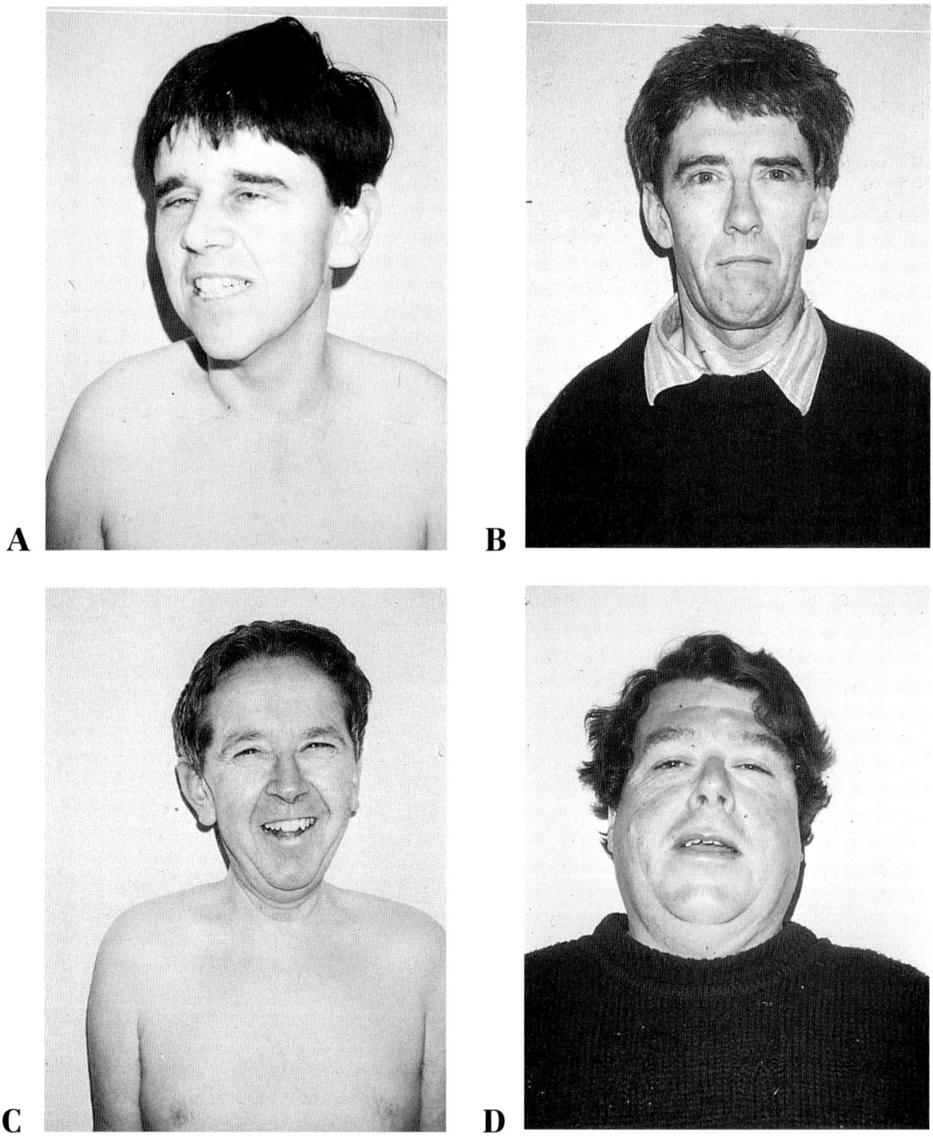

XLMR–Isolated Growth Hormone Deficiency. Narrow palpebral fissures but otherwise variable facial appearance in brothers at ages 39, 45, and 50 years (A–C) and a maternal cousin at age 45 years (D). Courtesy of Dr. Ben Hamel, University Hospital, Nijmegen, The Netherlands.

Behavioral Manifestations. Several adults are described as having infantile behavior.

Imaging. Radiographs show a small sella turcica.

Laboratory. Isolated growth hormone deficiency with normal thyroid, adrenal, and gonadal hormones.

Comment. XLMR–isolated growth hormone deficiency maps within the mapping limits of XLMR–panhypopituitarism, suggesting that the two entities may be allelic.

REFERENCE

Hamel BCJ, Smits APT, Otten BJ, et al.: Familial X-linked mental retardation and isolated growth hormone deficiency. Am J Med Genet 64:35, 1996.

Differential Matrix

Syndrome	Short Stature	Gyneco-mastia	Growth Hormone Deficiency	Comments
XLMR-isolated growth hormone deficiency	+	+	+	-
Börjeson-Forssman-Lehmann	+	+	0	Obesity, hypotonia, hypogonadism, microcephaly, coarse facies, large ears, narrow sloped shoulders, visual impairment, tapered digits
Chudley-Lowry	+	+	0	Bitemporal narrowing, almond-shaped eyes, depressed nasal bridge, tented upper lip, open mouth, hypogonadism, hypotonia, obesity
Vasquez	+	+	0	Microcephaly, obesity, hypotonia, hypogonadism
XLMR-panhypopituitarism	+	0	+	Hypogenitalism, small sella turcica, deficiency of pituitary, thyroid, adrenal, and gonadal hormones

XLMR-MACROCEPHALY

DEFINITION. XLMR with macrocephaly in affected males and carrier females. The gene is localized in the pericentromeric region between DXS1068 (Xp11.23) and DXS1125 (Xq12), lod score 3.30.

SOMATIC FEATURES. Macrocephaly occurs in males and carrier females, but not in nonaffected siblings. Apart from macrocephaly, downslanting palpebral fissures, obesity, and elbow limitation, the phenotype is not notable. Testicular volume is normal. Tapered fingers with short terminal phalanges and nails were present in one case.

GROWTH AND DEVELOPMENT. Details of childhood growth are not available. Although all developmental milestones are delayed, speech lags to a greater degree than motor skills.

COGNITIVE FEATURES. Mild to moderate impairment.

NEUROLOGICAL FINDINGS. None.

HETEROZYGOTE EXPRESSION. Carrier females have macrocephaly, obesity, and mild mental retardation. Seizures have occurred in one carrier.

IMAGING. Cranial tomography in one male was normal at age 1 year.

COMMENT. Macrocephaly of all causes occurs twice as frequently among individuals with mental retardation as in the general population. Commonly, the

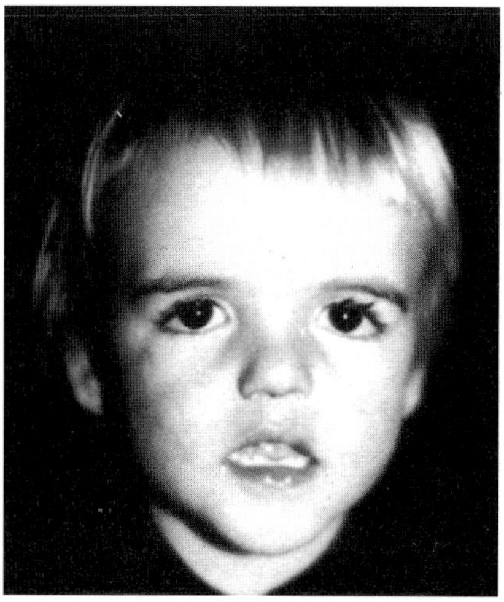
A

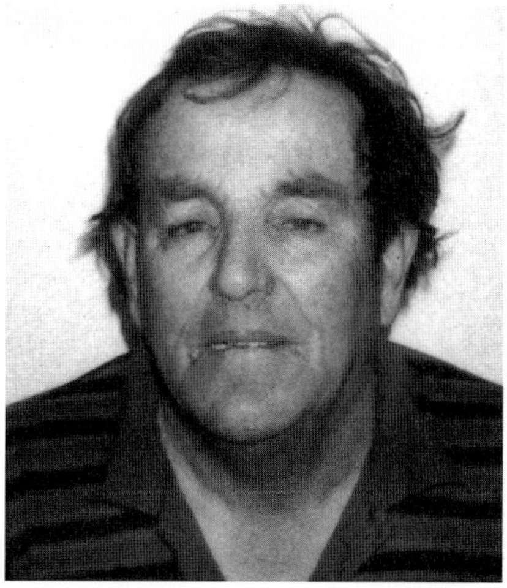
B

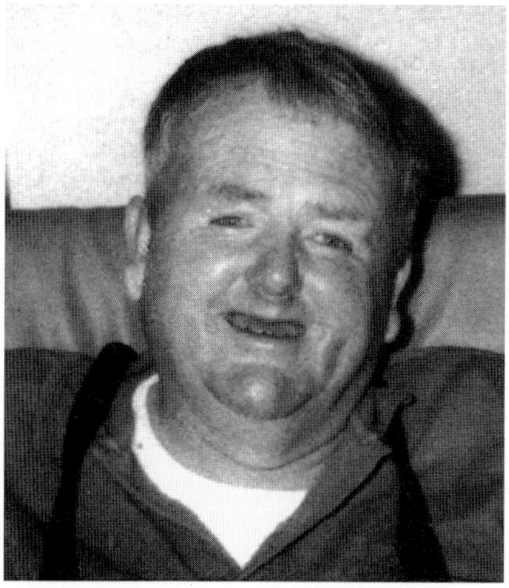
C

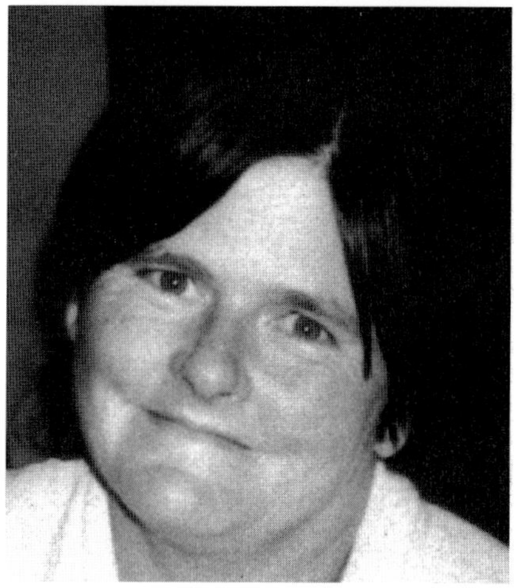
D

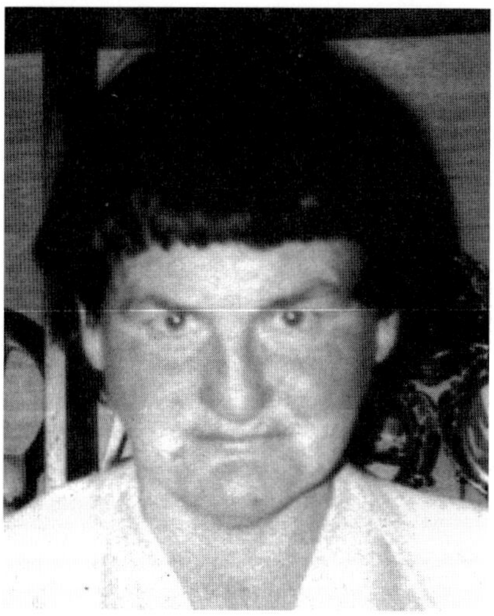
E

XLMR-Macrocephaly. Macrocephaly and downslanting palpebral fissures in a boy age 2 years (A); macrocephaly and downslanting palpebral fissures and prominence of the tip of the chin in adult cousins (B, C); macrocephaly and prominence of the tip of the chin in adult carrier females (D, E). Courtesy of Dr. Gillian Turner, Prince of Wales Children's Hospital, Randwick, New South Wales, Australia.

macrocephaly is due to hydrocephaly. Macrocephaly due to a large brain without hydrocephaly occurs in a number of XLMR syndromes, including Atkin-Flaitz, Clark-Baraitser, fragile X, mucopolysaccharidosis IIA, PPM-X, Waisman-Laxova, XLMR-macrocephaly, and XLMR-macrocephaly-macroorchidism syndromes.

REFERENCE

Turner G, Gedeon A, Mulley J: X-linked mental retardation with heterozygous expression and macrocephaly: pericentromeric gene localization. Am J Med Genet 51:575, 1994.

Differential Matrix

Syndrome	Macro-cephaly	Obesity	Carrier Female Manifestations	Comments
XLMR-macrocephaly	+	+	+	Downslanting palpebral fissures, elbow limitation
Atkin-Flaitz	+	+	+	Short stature, hypertelorism, downslanting palpebral fissures, broad nasal tip, thick lower lip, brachydactyly, seizures
Clark-Baraitser	+	+	+	Large stature, dental abnormalities, broad nasal tip, thick lower lip, macroorchidism
Fragile X	+	0	+	Normal or excessive growth, prominent forehead, long face, midface hypoplasia, large ears, prominent mandible, macroorchidism
Lujan	+	0	+	Marfanoid habitus, asthenic build, long face, prominent forehead, high palate, micrognathia, long digits, pectus excavatum, joint hyperextensibility, seizures, hyperactivity
PPM-X	+	0	+	Macroorchidism, spastic paraplegia, psychosis, parkinsonian features
Waisman-Laxova	+	0	+	Spasticity
XLMR-macrocephaly-macroorchidism	+	0	+	Elongated face, prominent mandible, macroorchidism, clumsiness, repetitive movements

XLMR–MACROCEPHALY–MACROORCHIDISM

(XLMR–Macroorchidism, MIM 309530)

DEFINITION. XLMR with normal stature, variable macrocephaly and macroorchidism, and normal FMR1 analysis. Although multiple causes may produce this phenotype, one gene has been located between DXS991 (Xp11) and DXS1002 (Xq21), lod score 2.96.

SOMATIC FEATURES. Macrocephaly contributes to the triangular facial shape and downslanting palpebral fissures. Prominence of the mandible has been noted in some cases. Macroorchidism becomes obvious after puberty.

GROWTH AND DEVELOPMENT. Details of childhood growth and development are not available. In adulthood, stature is normal and head circumference large. Speech appears impaired to a greater degree than motor skills.

A 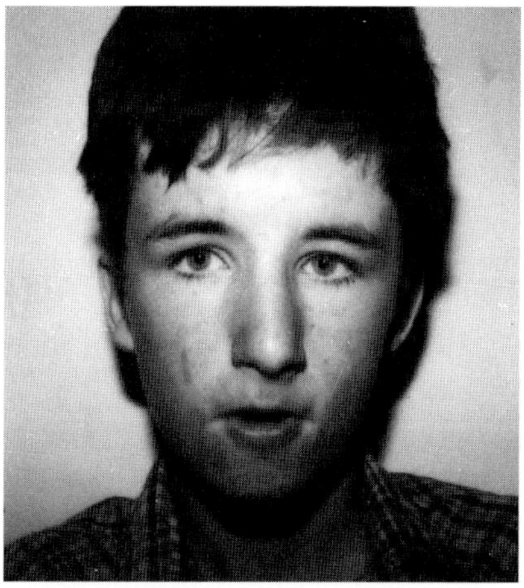

B 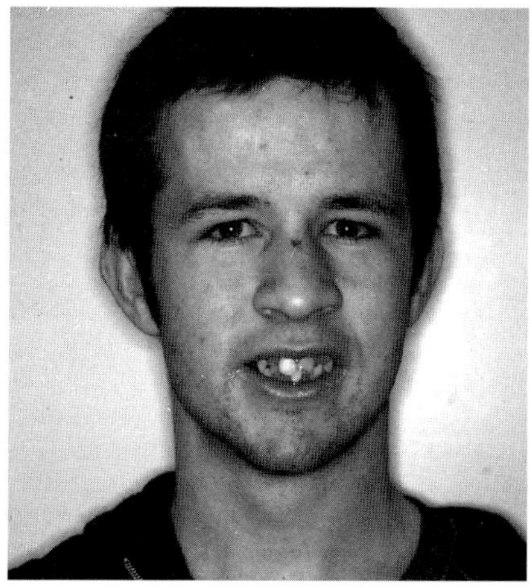

C 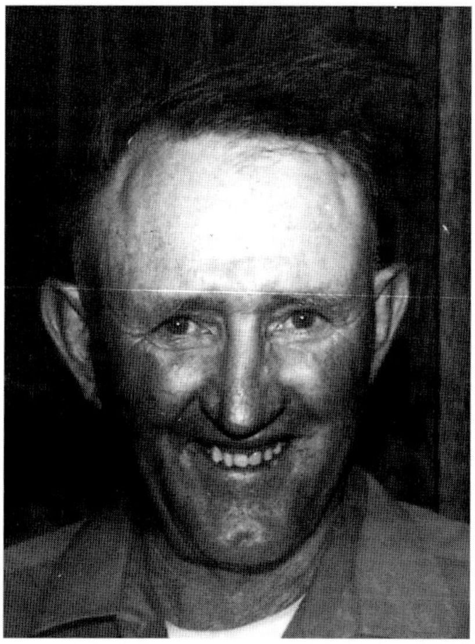

XLMR-Macrocephaly-Macroorchidism. Brothers at ages 17 and 22 years showing macrocephaly and downslanting palpebral fissures (A, B); maternal uncle at age 56 years with macrocephaly and prominence of the mandible (C). Courtesy of Dr. John Johnson, Shodair Hospital, Helena, Montana.

COGNITIVE FEATURES. Moderate impairment is usual with IQ measurements between 35 and 50.

HETEROZYGOTE EXPRESSION. Mild cognitive impairment may occur in carrier females.

COMMENT. Once the phenotype of the fragile X syndrome was delineated, individuals with similar phenotypes but negative fragile X testing were identified. Prominent among these individuals were those with mental retardation and macroorchidism with or without macrocephaly or other craniofacial manifestations of the fragile X syndrome. Proops et al., Tariverdian et al., and Johnson et al. have reported affected brothers or families that appear to follow a pattern of X-linked transmission. Proops described three adult brothers who were small with relatively large heads, square facial shape, prominent ears, high arched palate, stubby hands and feet, macroorchidism, limited language, and pleasant quiet demeanors. Three nephews also had mental retardation and short stature but showed a less consistent phenotype. Carrier females appeared to have mild mental retardation. This family, designated MRX2, shows linkage to DXS989 in Xp22 (Hu et al., 1994).

Tariverdian et al. reported two half brothers with elongated face, dense eyebrows, long nose, prominent jaw, and macroorchidism. Growth was normal. Severe mental retardation, aggressive behaviors, clumsy "unskilled movement" and gait, repetitive hand movements, dysarthria, and echolalia were present. The mother had a prominent chin and mild mental impairment. Cranial tomography in the younger brother showed slight enlargement of the third ventricle, a subarachnoid cyst in the left temporal region, and an area of density in the pons.

Johnson et al. studied a family with 10 males with moderate mental retardation, macrocephaly, and macroorchidism. However, not all affected males had macrocephaly and macroorchidism, while some of the nonretarded brothers did. Several carrier females had mild mental retardation. The responsible gene was mapped to the pericentromeric region between Xp11 and Xq12.

Fryns et al. (1986) and Chiurazzi et al. (1994) have reported similar sporadic or familial cases.

REFERENCES

Chiurazzi P, de Graaff E, Ng J, et al.: No apparent involvement of the FMR1 gene in five patients with phenotypic manifestations of the fragile X syndrome. Am J Med Genet 51:309, 1994.

Fryns JP, Dereymaeker A, Hoefnagels M, et al.: Partial fragile(X) phenotype with megalotestes in fragile(X)-negative patients with acquired lesions of the central nervous system. Am J Med Genet 23:213, 1986.

Hu L-J, Blumenfeld-Heyberger S, Hanauer A, et al.: Non-specific X-linked mental retardation: linkage analysis in MRX2 and MRX4 families revisited. Am J Med Genet 51:569, 1994.

Johnson JP, Nelson R, Schwartz CE: A family with mental retardation, variable macrocephaly and macroorchidism, and linkage to Xq12-q21. J Med Genet 35:1026, 1998.

Proops R, Mayer M, Jacobs PA: A study of mental retardation in children in the Island of Hawaii. Clin Genet 23:81, 1983.

Tariverdian G, Froster-Iskenius U, Deuschl G, et al.: Mental retardation, acromegalic face, and megalotestes in two half-brothers: a specific form of X-linked mental retardation without fra(X) (q)? Am J Med Genet 38:208, 1991.

Differential Matrix

Syndrome	Macro-cephaly	Macro-orchidism	Carrier Female Manifestations	Comments
XLMR-macrocephaly-macroorchidism	+	+	+	Elongated face, prominent mandible, clumsiness, repetitive movements
XLMR-macrocephaly	+	+	+	Downslanting palpebral fissures, obesity, elbow limitation
Atkin-Flaitz	+	+	+	Short stature, hypertelorism, downslanting palpebral fissures, broad nasal tip, thick lower lip, brachydactyly, seizures
Clark-Baraitser	+	+	+	Large stature, obesity, dental abnormalities, broad nasal tip, thick lower lip
Fragile X	+	+	+	Normal or excessive growth, prominent forehead, long face, midface hypoplasia, large ears, prominent mandible
Lujan	+	+	+	Marfanoid habitus, asthenic build, long face, prominent forehead, high palate, micrognathia, long digits, pectus excavatum, joint hyperextensibility, seizures, hyperactivity
PPM-X	0	+	+	Spastic paraplegia, psychosis, parkinsonian features
Waisman-Laxova	+	0	+	Spasticity

XLMR–PANHYPOPITUITARISM

(MIM 312000)

DEFINITION. XLMR with short stature and hypogenitalism associated with panhypopituitarism. The gene has been mapped between DXS425 (Xq25) and DXS102 (Xq26.3), lod score 4.12.

SOMATIC FEATURES. Major malformations or craniofacial abnormalities do not occur. The sella turcica is small. Short stature becomes apparent in infancy and, untreated, persists into adult life. Hypogenitalism may be obvious before puberty and thereafter is associated with variable degrees of hypogonadism, including decreased sexual hair and truncal obesity. Some affected males have died during

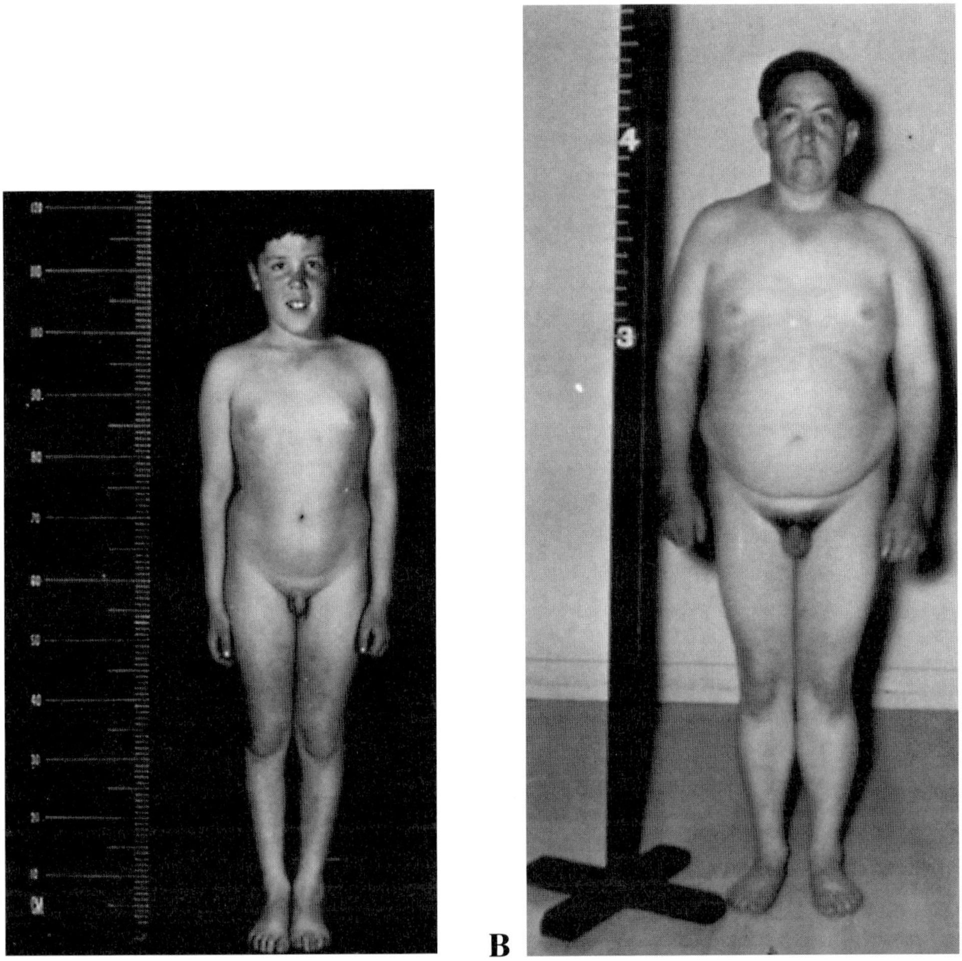

A B

XLMR-Panhypopituitarism. Eleven-year-old male with short stature (A); 30-year-old uncle with short stature, obesity, and diminished virilization as manifestation of panhypopituitarism (B). Reprinted from *Birth Defects: Original Article Series* VII(6), 1971, Courtesy of the March of Dimes National Foundation.

the newborn period with hypoplasia of the adrenal glands documented at autopsy.

GROWTH AND DEVELOPMENT. Intrauterine growth is usually normal, but slowing of bone growth occurs during the first year. Puberty is delayed and virilization is incomplete. Language skills lag behind motor skills.

COGNITIVE FEATURES. Lower cognitive function than in nonaffected siblings can be expected, but with mental retardation of mild degree present in a minority.

HETEROZYGOTE EXPRESSION. None.

LABORATORY. Growth hormone deficiency consistently occurs. Other endocrine abnormalities are more variable, but may include low levels of other pituitary hormones, thyroxine, cortisol, and sex hormones.

COMMENT. The location of XLMR–panhypopituitarism overlaps the mapping limits of XLMR–isolated growth hormone deficiency, suggesting the possibility that these two XLMR syndromes are allelic. Secondary hypothyroidism may contribute, at least in part, to the mental retardation in XLMR–panyhypopituitarism.

REFERENCES

Phelan PD, Connelly J, Martin FIR, et al.: X-linked recessive hypopituitarism. Birth Defects Orig Art Ser VII(6):24, 1971.

Lagerström-Fermér M, Sundvall M, Johnsen E, et al.: X-linked recessive panhypopituitarism associated with a regional duplication in Xq25-q26. Am J Hum Genet 60:910, 1997.

Differential Matrix

Syndrome	Short Stature	Hypo-genitalism	Obesity	Comments
XLMR-panhypopituitarism	+	+	+	Small sella turcica, deficiency of pituitary, thyroid, adrenal, and gonadal hormones
Börjeson-Forssman-Lehmann	+	+	+	Hypotonia, microcephaly, coarse facies, large ears, gynecomastia, narrow sloped shoulders, visual impairment, tapered digits
Chudley-Lowry	+	+	+	Bitemporal narrowing, almond-shaped eyes, depressed nasal bridge, tented upper lip, open mouth, hypotonia
Urban	+	+	+	Small hands and feet, digital contractures, osteoporosis
Young-Hughes	+	+	+	Small palpebral fissures, cupped ears, ichthyosiform scaling
Vasquez	+	+	+	Microcephaly, gynecomastia, hypotonia
Cerebrooculogenital	+	+	0	Microcephaly, hydrocephaly, agenesis of corpus callosum, microphthalmia, ptosis, hypospadias, cryptorchidism, clubfoot, spasticity
Sutherland-Haan	+	+	0	Microcephaly, upslanting palpebral fissures, asthenic habitus, pectus excavatum, scoliosis, stiff joints, pes cavus, spasticity
X-linked hereditary bullous dystrophy	+	+	0	Microcephaly, upslanting palpebral fissures, protruding ears, short and tapered digits, cardiac defects, bullous dystrophy, early death from pulmonary infection
XLMR-hypotonic facies (Carpenter-Waziri) (Holmes-Gang) (Juberg-Marsidi)	+	+	0	Microcephaly, telecanthus, small triangular nose, tented upper lip, open mouth, spacing of teeth, genital anomalies, musculoskeletal anomalies, hemoglobin H inclusions in erythrocytes
Wilson-Turner	0	+	+	Normal growth, small hands and feet, tapered digits, gynecomastia, hypotonia, emotional lability

XLMR-PSORIASIS

(Tranebjaerg Syndrome I, MIM 309480)

DEFINITION. XLMR with hypertelorism, large ears, macrostomia with arched upper lip, prominent lips, hypotonia, childhood-onset psoriasis, and seizures. The gene has not been mapped.

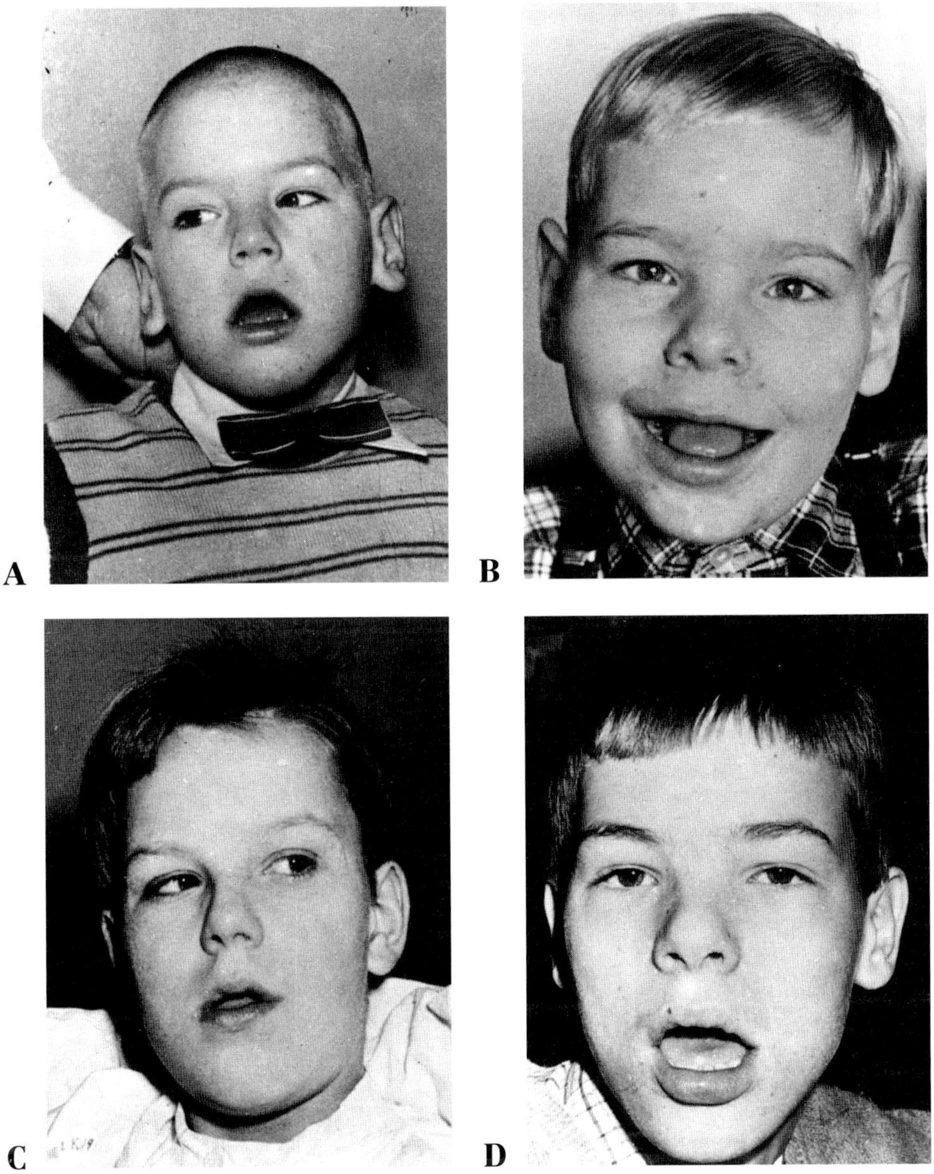

XLMR-Psoriasis. Short nose, tented upper lip, prominent ears, and everted lower lip in four affected members of the same family at ages 6, 8, 10, and 14 years. Courtesy of Dr. Lisbeth Tranebjaerg, University Hospital, Tromsø, Tromsø, Norway, and The American Journal of Medical Genetics, © 1988, Wiley-Liss, Inc.

SOMATIC FEATURES. Patients have hypotonic facies with hypertelorism, large open mouth and prominent lips, thickening of the alae nasi, and large ears. The nares may be anteverted and the palate high. Skeletal features include horizontal palmar creases, proximally placed thumbs, hyperextensible joints, and clinodactyly 5. Cryptorchidism may occur. Psoriasis occurs during childhood, affecting the scalp, trunk, elbows, knees, palms, soles, genital area and popliteal fossas. The cutaneous changes begin as nonspecific and generalized erythroderma or dry scaling skin and progress to typical localized psoriatic plaques.

GROWTH AND DEVELOPMENT. Intrauterine and postnatal growth progresses at a normal rate. Marked delay of developmental milestones is evident from infancy.

COGNITIVE FEATURES. Severe impairment.

NEUROLOGICAL FINDINGS. Seizures with onset in early childhood are described.

HETEROZYGOTE EXPRESSION. None.

LABORATORY. Skin biopsy shows changes of psoriasis. Normal steroid sulfatase activity has been demonstrated in fibroblasts.

COMMENT. Except for the normal cranial circumference, the craniofacial manifestations resemble those of XLMR-hypotonic facies syndrome (α-thalassemia mental retardation). Psoriasis has been described in no other XLMR syndrome.

REFERENCE

Tranebjaerg L, Svejgaard A, Lykkesfeldt G: X-linked mental retardation associated with psoriasis: a new syndrome? Am J Med Genet 30:263, 1988.

Differential Matrix

Syndrome	Hypotonic Facies	Hypo-genitalism	Ectodermal Changes	Comments
XLMR-psoriasis	+	+	+	Hypertelorism, open mouth, large ears, hypotonia, seizures, psoriasis
Wittwer	+	+	0	Growth deficiency, microcephaly, microphthalmia, hearing loss, vision loss, hypertelorism, genitourinary anomalies, hypotonia, seizures
XLMR-hypotonic facies (Carpenter-Waziri) (Holmes-Gang) (Juberg-Marsidi)	+	+	0	Microcephaly, short stature, telecanthus, small triangular nose, tented upper lip, open mouth, spacing of teeth, musculoskeletal anomalies, hemoglobin H inclusions in erythrocytes
X-linked hereditary bullous dystrophy	0	+	+	Microcephaly, short stature, upslanting palpebral fissures, protruding ears, short and tapered digits, cardiac defects, bullous dystrophy, early death from pulmonary infection

XLMR–Retinitis Pigmentosa

(XLMR–Microcephaly–Retinitis Pigmentosa Syndrome)

Definition. XLMR with microcephaly and retinitis pigmentosa. The gene has not been localized, although preliminary evidence suggests a location between Xp21 and Xq21.

Somatic Features. Microcephaly, possibly of postnatal onset, occurs as the only consistent nonocular manifestation. Myopia, pigmentary retinopathy, narrowing of the retinal arterioles, choroidal degeneration, and pallid optic discs may be noted in the first 2 years of life. Nystagmus may be present from infancy. Constricted visual fields, night blindness, and poor vision result from the retinitis pigmentosa. Cataracts may develop in adulthood.

Growth and Development. Growth impairment appears to be a variable component of this syndrome. Low birth weight has been recorded in one case and adult short stature in another.

Cognitive Features. Mild impairment.

Neurological Findings. Seizures have occurred in one case. Although poor vision may be apparent from infancy or early childhood, blindness may be delayed until late childhood or early adult life. Nystagmus has occurred in infancy in one case and in later childhood in another.

Heterozygote Expression. Cognitive function is normal. In early adult life, carriers may develop myopia, constricted visual fields, choroidal degeneration, and night blindness.

Laboratory. Electroretinogram and visual evoked responses are abnormal.

Comment. Two X-linked genes for retinitis pigmentosa have been mapped, RP2 at Xp11.3 and RP3 at Xp21.1. The possibility that XLMR–microcephaly–retinitis pigmentosa is caused by a deletion of contiguous genes cannot be excluded at present.

REFERENCE

Aldred MA, Dry KL, Knight-Jones EB, et al.: Genetic analysis of a kindred with X-linked mental handicap and retinitis pigmentosa. Am J Hum Genet 55:916, 1994.

Schwahn U, Lenzner S, Dong J, et al.: Positional cloning of the gene for X-linked retinitis pigmentosa 2. Nat Genet 19:327, 1998.

Differential Matrix

Syndrome	Microcephaly	Vision Loss	Nystagmus	Comments
XLMR-retinitis pigmentosa	+	+	+	Bone-spicule-type retinitis pigmentosa
Cerebrooculogenital	+	+	+	Short stature, hydrocephaly, agenesis of corpus callosum, microphthalmia, ptosis, hypospadias, cryptorchidism, clubfoot, spasticity
Paine	+	+	+	Short stature, optic atrophy, hearing loss, spasticity, seizures
Proud	+	+	+	Hearing loss, agenesis of corpus callosum, cryptorchidism, inguinal hernias, ataxia, spasticity, seizures
Gustavson	+	+	0	Short stature, large ears, deafness, joint contractures, rockerbottom feet, brain undergrowth, hydrocephaly, cerebellar hypoplasia, spasticity, seizures
Lenz microphthalmia	+	+	0	Microphthalmia, ocular dysgenesis, malformed ears, cleft lip/palate, cardiac and genitourinary anomalies, thumb duplication or hypoplasia, narrow shoulders
Schimke	+	+	0	Sunken eyes, downslanting palpebral fissures, narrow nose, spacing of teeth, cupped ears, hypotonia, abducens palsy, hearing loss, spasticity, choreoathetosis, contractures
Wittwer	+	+	0	Growth deficiency, microphthalmia, hearing loss, hypertelorism, genitourinary anomalies, hypotonia, seizures
Goldblatt spastic paraplegia	0	+	+	Optic atrophy, exotropia, ataxia, spastic paraplegia, dysarthria, muscle hypoplasia, contractures
Lowe	0	+	+	Short stature, cataracts, hypotonia, aminoaciduria, progressive renal failure

XLMR–SPASTIC PARAPLEGIA–ATHETOSIS

(Baar-Gabriel syndrome, MIM 312890)

DEFINITION. XLMR with spastic paraplegia, weakness, dysarthria, and nystagmus. A gene locus has not been mapped.

SOMATIC FEATURES. No distinctive facial features or major malformations occur. Facial muscles show very little movement. Positional abnormalities of the limbs may be present at birth. Wasting, contractures, and kyphoscoliosis accompany the neurologic abnormalities.

GROWTH AND DEVELOPMENT. Prenatal growth is normal or nearly so. Speech may appear at the normal time but is slurred. Weakness, wasting, and contractures prevent normal ambulation.

COGNITIVE FEATURES. Considerable variability of cognitive function, both intrafamilial and interfamilial, has been observed. Severe impairment, however, is the rule.

NEUROLOGICAL FINDINGS. Neurologic signs dominate the clinical picture from early in childhood. Spastic tetraparesis with greater involvement of the lower limbs is typical. Muscle tone and deep tendon reflexes are increased and Babinski signs present. Secondary muscle wasting, weakness, and kyphoscoliosis may occur. Cerebellar signs include nystagmus, unsteadiness, and dysmetria of the upper limbs. Athetoid movements of the upper limbs occur as well. Speech is dysarthric, gag reflex is exaggerated, and tongue movements spastic. Even among infants whose limbs appear spared at birth, nystagmus or unsteadiness of gaze indicates involvement.

HETEROZYGOTE EXPRESSION. None.

IMAGING. Not available.

COMMENT. The X-linked spastic paraplegias with mental retardation are a large and heterogeneous group. Two major types–Complicated spastic paraplegia 1 and Complicated spastic paraplegia 2—have been mapped and the genes — L1 cell adhesion molecule (L1CAM) and proteolipid protein (PLP)—have been cloned. SPG1 is allelic to X-linked hydrocephaly–MASA spectrum and SPG2 to Pelizaeus-Merzbacher syndrome. XLMR–spastic paraplegia–athetosis may, in fact, be allelic to one of these syndromes. Numerous additional spastic paraplegia loci have been mapped and include Allan-Herndon-Dudley, Apak, Arena, Lesch-Nyhan, Mohr-Tranebjaerg, and Pettigrew syndromes. X-linked spastic paraplegias without mental retardation may represent separate or allelic disorders (e.g., the family reported by Johnston and McKusick and updated by Thurmon et al. and Zatz et al. is due to a mutation in PLP).

REFERENCES

Baar HS, Gabriel AM: Sex-linked spastic paraplegia. Am J Ment Defic 71:13 1966.

Bundy S, Griffiths MT: Recurrence risks in families of children with symmetrical spasticity. Dev Med Child Neurol 19:179, 1977.

Haldane JBS: The partial sex-linkage of recessive spastic paraplegia. J Genet 41:141, 1941.

Johnston AW, McKusick VA: A sex-linked recessive form of spastic paraplegia. Am J Hum Genet 14:83, 1962.

Paskind HA, Stone TT: Familial spastic paralysis. Arch Neuro Psychia 30:481, 1933.

Thurman TF, Walker BA, Scott CI, et al.: Two kindreds with a sex-linked recessive form of spastic paraplegia. Birth Defects Orig Art Ser VII(1):219, 1971.

Zatz M, Penha-Serrano C, Otto PA: X-linked recessive type of pure spastic paraplegia in a large pedigree: absence of detectable linkage with Xq. J Med Genet 13:217, 1976.

Differential Matrix

Syndrome	Spasticity	Cerebellar Signs	Seizures	Comments
XLMR-spastic paraplegia-athetosis	+	+	+	Nystagmus, weakness, dysarthria, spastic paraplegia, muscle wasting, contractures
Goldblatt spastic paraplegia	+	+	+	Optic atrophy, exotropia, nystagmus, ataxia, spastic paraplegia, dysarthria, muscle hypoplasia, contractures
Paine	+	+	+	Microcephaly, short stature, optic atrophy, vision and hearing loss
Pelizaeus-Merzbacher	+	+	+	Optic atrophy, nystagmus, hypotonia, ataxia, dystonia, CNS dysmyelination
Pettigrew	+	+	+	Dandy-Walker malformation, microcephaly or hydrocephaly, long face with macrostomia and prognathism, small testes, contractures, choreoathetosis, iron deposits in basal ganglia
Proud	+	+	+	Microcephaly, hearing loss, vision loss, agenesis of corpus callosum, cryptorchidism, inguinal hernias, ataxia
X-linked-ataxia-deafness-dementia	+	+	+	Optic atrophy, vision loss, hearing loss, ataxia, hypotonia, childhood death
Adrenoleukodystrophy	+	+	0	Adrenal insufficiency, diffuse skin pigmentation, progressive neurologic deterioration and dementia, elevated very long chain fatty acids in plasma
Allan-Herndon-Dudley	+	+	0	Large ears with cupping or abnormal architecture, muscle hypoplasia, childhood hypotonia, contractures, dysarthria, athetosis, ataxia
Apak ataxia-spastic diplegia	+	+	0	Short stature, clubfoot, muscle hypoplasia, ataxia
Arena	+	+	0	Muscle hypoplasia, clubfoot, iron deposits in basal ganglia, ataxia, rigidity, dystonia
Cerebrooculogenital	+	+	0	Short stature, microcephaly, hydrocephaly, agenesis of corpus callosum, microphthalmia, ptosis, hypospadias, cryptorchidism, clubfoot
Lesch-Nyhan	+	+	0	Choreoathetosis, self-mutilation, hyperuricemia
Mohr-Tranebjaerg (Jensen)	+	+	0	Hearing loss, vision loss, neurologic deterioration with childhood onset, dystonia

Schimke	+	+	0	Microcephaly, sunken eyes, downslanting palpebral fissures, narrow nose, spacing of teeth, cupped ears, hypotonia, choreoathetosis, contractures
X-linked hydrocephaly-MASA spectrum	+	+	0	Hydrocephaly, adducted thumbs, spastic paraplegia, dysgenesis of corpus callosum
Bertini	0	+	+	Macular degeneration, hypotonia, ataxia, childhood death, hypoplasia of cerebellar vermis and corpus callosum, developmental delays and regression, postnatal growth impairment
Christianson	0	+	+	Short stature, microcephaly, general asthenia, contractures, ophthalmoplegia
Gustavson	+	0	+	Microcephaly, short stature, optic atrophy with blindness, large ears, deafness, joint contractures, rockerbottom feet, brain undergrowth, hydrocephaly, cerebellar hypoplasia

XLMR–Thyroid Aplasia–Cutis Verticis Gyrata

(Åkesson Syndrome, MIM304200)

Åkesson reported a single case with short stature, cutis gyrata over the vertex of the scalp, signs of myxedema, diastasis rectus, ulnar deviation of the hands, and severe mental retardation with aphasia. The head circumference was normal. Autopsy showed thyroid aplasia and no gross brain abnormalities. Four other males in two generations were mentally retarded by history but it is not known whether they had cretinism or cutis gyrata of the scalp.

REFERENCE

Åkesson HO: Cutis verticis gyrata thyroaplasia and mental deficiency. Acta Genet Med Gem 14:200, 1965.

XLMR with Thyroxine-Binding Globulin Deficiency

(TBG Deficiency–Mental Retardation)

Definition. XLMR with thyroxine-binding globulin deficiency.

Somatic Features. No consistent somatic manifestations have been reported among males with TBG deficiency and mental retardation. Individual cases have had short stature, muscular build, hypertelorism, high palate, seizures, conductive hearing loss, and ataxic gait.

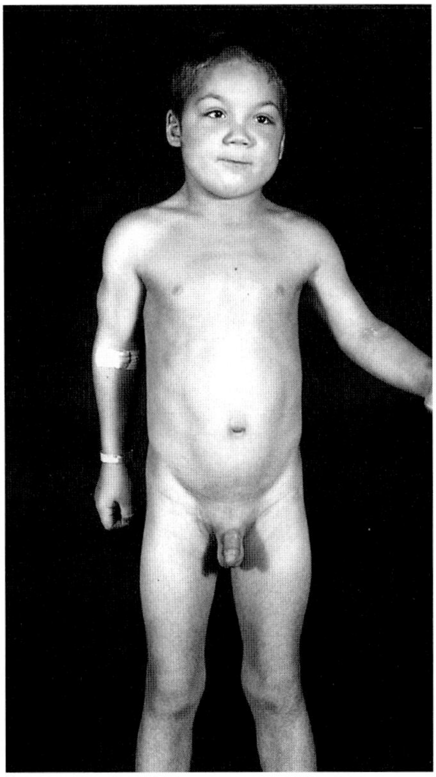

XLMR With Thyroxine-Binding Globulin Deficiency. Short stature, hypertelorism and muscular build in a 7-year-old male with thyroid-binding globulin deficiency. Courtesy of Dr. Theodore AvRuskin, Brookdale Hospital Medical Center, Brooklyn, New York.

GROWTH AND DEVELOPMENT. If prenatal growth impairment occurs, it is mild. In some cases, postnatal stature has been normal; in others, significantly shortened. Developmental milestones lag from the outset with speech delay being more severe than motor delay.

COGNITIVE FEATURES. Moderate impairment.

HETEROZYGOTE EXPRESSION. Carrier females may have low thyroxine-binding capacity but have normal growth and cognitive function.

LABORATORY. Growth hormone, adrenal steroids, and glucose metabolism are normal. Serum thyroxine is low and thyroxine-binding globulin is low or absent. Delayed bone age may be found in patients with short stature.

COMMENT. Thyroxine-binding globulin is the major serum-binding protein for triiodothyronine (T_3) and thyroxine (T_4). When absent or deficient, serum total T_3 and T_4 may be low, whereas free T_3 and T_4 may be elevated. Patients with TBG deficiency are generally euthyroid and do not have mental or neurologic impairments. For this reason, it might be suspected that XLMR associated with TBG deficiency is due to a contiguous gene deletion rather than to a mutation of the TBG gene. The TBG gene has been mapped to Xq22.2.

REFERENCE

AvRuskin TW, Braverman LE, Crigler JF: Thyroxine-binding globulin deficiency and associated neurological deficit. Pediatrics 50:638, 1972.

YOUNG-HUGHES SYNDROME

DEFINITION. XLMR with short stature, obesity, hypergonadotrophic hypogonadism, chronic dermatitis, strabismus, and seizures. The gene has not been localized.

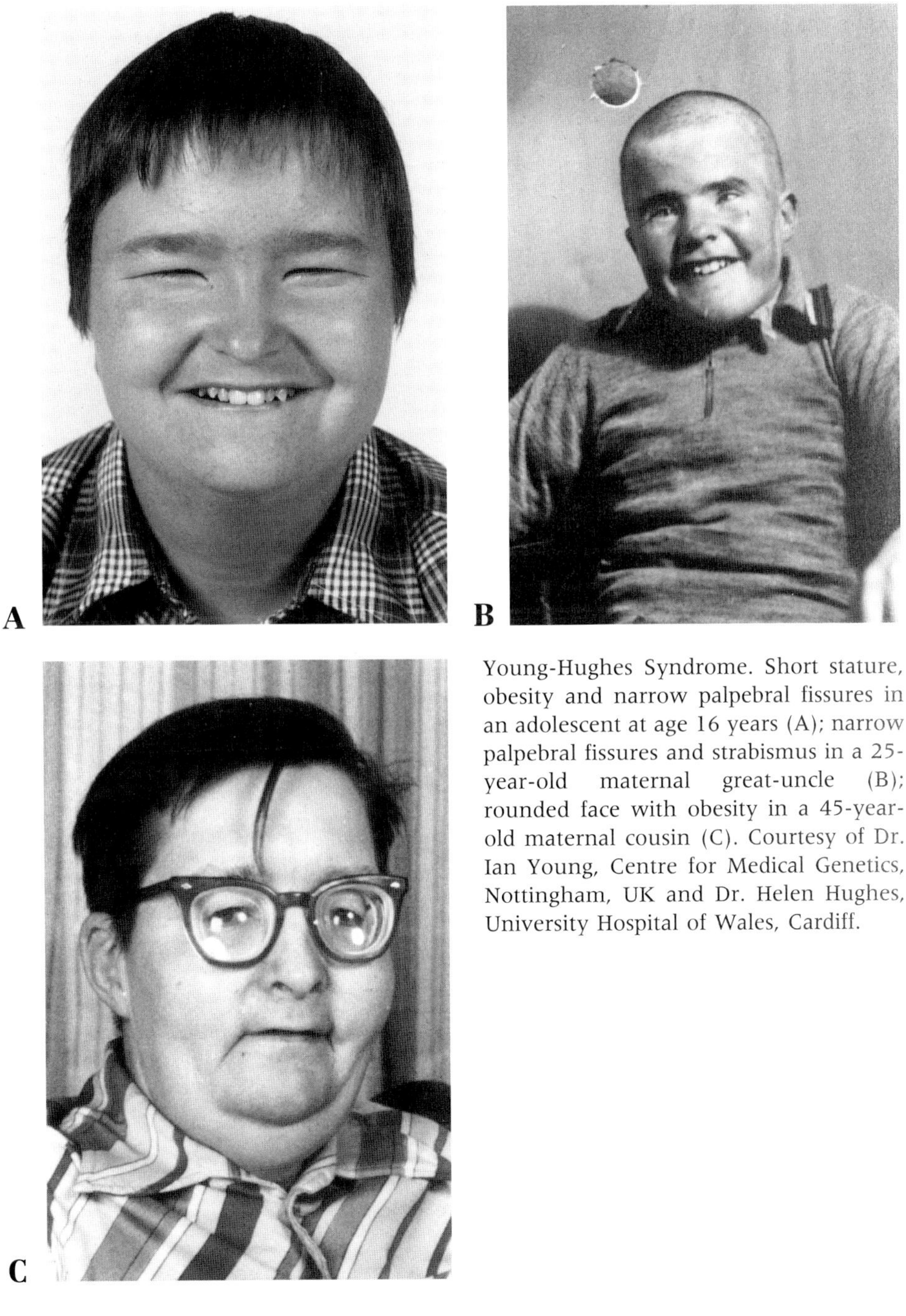

Young-Hughes Syndrome. Short stature, obesity and narrow palpebral fissures in an adolescent at age 16 years (A); narrow palpebral fissures and strabismus in a 25-year-old maternal great-uncle (B); rounded face with obesity in a 45-year-old maternal cousin (C). Courtesy of Dr. Ian Young, Centre for Medical Genetics, Nottingham, UK and Dr. Helen Hughes, University Hospital of Wales, Cardiff.

Somatic Features. The facies show short palpebral fissures, strabismus, and low-set and cupped ears. Optic nerve hypoplasia, nystagmus, and myopia may be present. Short stature, obesity, underdevelopment of the genitalia, and scant sexual hair dominate the phenotype. The skin is chronically and variably affected with dryness, atopia, ichthyosiform scaling, and excoriation. Generalized seizures appear common. The voice is high pitched.

Growth and Development. Low birth weight is followed by short stature and obesity during childhood and beyond. Developmental milestones are globally delayed. Speech development appears more delayed than motor development.

Cognitive Features. Severe cognitive impairment with IQ measurements below 30.

Behavioral Manifestations. All affected males have been good-natured, gentle, and affectionate.

Neurological Findings. No neurologic manifestations except seizures have been noted.

Heterozygote Expression. Carrier females have normal intelligence and normal stature and exhibit none of the somatic features seen in affected males.

Laboratory. Low testosterone, elevated gonadotropins, and normal steroid sulfatase.

Comment. Short stature and obesity commonly accompany XLMR syndromes with hypogonadism. The type of hypogonadism, severity of cognitive impairment, and association with other somatic or neurologic manifestations are useful in discriminating these syndromes. In no case has the underlying gene been identified, although several of the hypogonadism–short stature–obesity syndromes have been regionally mapped.

REFERENCE

Young ID, Hughes HE: Sex-linked mental retardation, short stature, obesity and hypogonadism: report of a family. J Ment Defic Res 26:153, 1982.

Differential Matrix

Syndrome	Short Stature	Obesity	Hypo-genitalism	Comments
Young-Hughes	+	+	+	Small palpebral fissures, cupped ears, ichthyosiform scaling
Börjeson-Forssman-Lehmann	+	+	+	Hypotonia, hypogonadism, microcephaly, coarse facies, large ears, gynecomastia, narrow sloped shoulders, visual impairment, tapered digits
Chudley-Lowry	+	+	+	Bitemporal narrowing, almond-shaped eyes, depressed nasal bridge, tented upper lip, open mouth, hypogonadism, hypotonia
MEHMO	+	+	+	Hypotonia, microcephaly, edematous hands and feet, equinovarus deformity, seizures, early childhood death
Urban	+	+	+	Small hands and feet, digital contractures, osteoporosis
Vasquez	+	+	+	Microcephaly, gynecomastia, hypotonia
Wilson-Turner	0	+	+	Normal growth, small hands and feet, tapered digits, gynecomastia, hypotonia, emotional lability
Cerebrooculogenital	+	0	+	Microcephaly, hydrocephaly, agenesis of corpus callosum, microphthalmia, ptosis, hypospadias, cryptorchidism, clubfoot, spasticity
Renpenning	+	0	+	Microcephaly, upslanting palpebral fissures
Sutherland-Haan	+	0	+	Microcephaly, upslanting palpebral fissures, asthenic habitus, pectus excavatum, scoliosis, stiff joints, pes cavus, spasticity
X-linked hereditary bullous dystrophy	+	0	+	Microcephaly, upslanting palpebral fissures, protruding ears, short and tapered digits, cardiac defects, bullous dystrophy, early death from pulmonary infection
XLMR-hypotonic facies (Carpenter-Waziri) (Holmes-Gang) (Juberg-Marsidi)	+	0	+	Microcephaly, telecanthus, small triangular nose, tented upper lip, open mouth, spacing of teeth, genital anomalies, musculoskeletal anomalies, hemoglobin H inclusions in erythrocytes

Index